Nutritional Neuroscience

Nutritional Neuroscience

Editor: Henry Christian

AMERICAN
MEDICAL PUBLISHERS
www.americanmedicalpublishers.com

AMERICAN
MEDICAL PUBLISHERS
www.americanmedicalpublishers.com

Cataloging-in-Publication Data

Nutritional neuroscience / edited by Henry Christian.
p. cm.
Includes bibliographical references and index.
ISBN 979-8-88740-345-8
1. Nervous system--Diseases--Nutritional aspects. 2. Nervous system--Diseases--Diet therapy.
3. Brain--Diseases--Nutritional aspects. 4. Diet in disease. 5. Neurosciences. 6. Nutrition. I. Christian, Henry.
RC386.2 .N88 2023
616.8--dc23

American Medical Publishers,
41 Flatbush Avenue,
1st Floor, New York,
NY 11217, USA

ISBN 979-8-88740-345-8 (Hardback)

Contents

Preface

I am honored to present to you this unique book which encompasses the most up-to-date data in the field. I was extremely pleased to get this opportunity of editing the work of experts from across the globe. I have also written papers in this field and researched the various aspects revolving around the progress of the discipline. I have tried to unify my knowledge along with that of stalwarts from every corner of the world, to produce a text which not only benefits the readers but also facilitates the growth of the field.

Nutritional neuroscience is an area of study which focuses on the impact which diverse constituents of diet have on neurochemistry, cognition, behavior and neurobiology. A few of such diet components are minerals, protein and vitamins. Minerals such as iron, zinc, copper and manganese can impact the development of the brain based on their deficiency or excess. The deficiency and overload of iron has the potential to disrupt the central nervous system function. Deficiency of zinc can lead to various disorders such as anorexia, depression and memory impairment while its excess can hinder the absorption of copper. The imbalance of vitamins in a person's body can also lead to degenerative and developmental diseases. This book is a compilation of research papers that discuss the most vital concepts and developments in the field of nutritional neuroscience. It consists of contributions made by international experts. This book will help the readers in keeping pace with the rapid changes in this field.

Finally, I would like to thank all the contributing authors for their valuable time and contributions. This book would not have been possible without their efforts. I would also like to thank my friends and family for their constant support.

Editor

1

Kinetic Modeling of pH-Dependent Oxidation of Dopamine by Iron and its Relevance to Parkinson's Disease

Yingying Sun [1], A. Ninh Pham [1], Dominic J. Hare [2,3] and T. David Waite [1]*

[1] Water Research Centre, School of Civil and Environmental Engineering, The University of New South Wales, Sydney, NSW, Australia, [2] Atomic Pathology Laboratory, Melbourne Dementia Research Centre at the Florey Institute of Neuroscience and Mental Health and The University of Melbourne, Parkville, VIC, Australia, [3] Department of Clinical Pathology, The University of Melbourne, Parkville, VIC, Australia

***Correspondence:**
T. David Waite
d.waite@unsw.edu.au

Parkinson's disease is the second most common neurodegenerative disease. While age is the most significant risk factor, the exact cause of this disease and the most effective approaches to mitigation remain unclear. It has long been proposed that dopamine may play a role in the pathology of Parkinson's disease in view of its ability to generate both protein-modifying quinones such as aminochrome and reactive oxygen species, especially in the presence of pathological iron accumulation in the primary site of neuron loss. Given the clinically measured acidosis of *post-mortem* Parkinson's disease brain tissue, the interaction between dopamine and iron was investigated over a pH range of 7.4 to 6.5 with emphasis on the accumulation of toxic quinones and generation of reactive oxygen species. Our results show that the presence of iron accelerates the formation of aminochrome with ferrous iron (Fe[II]) being more efficient in this regard than ferric iron (Fe[III]). Our results further suggest that a reduced aminochrome rearrangement rate coupled with an enhanced turnover rate of Fe[II] as a result of brain tissue acidosis could result in aminochrome accumulation within cells. Additionally, under these conditions, the enhanced redox cycling of iron in the presence of dopamine aggravates oxidative stress as a result of the production of damaging reactive species, including hydroxyl radicals.

Keywords: pH, iron, dopamine, aminochrome, oxidative stress, Parkinson's disease

INTRODUCTION

Parkinson's disease is the second most common neurodegenerative disorder after Alzheimer's disease (Guttmacher et al., 2003). Even though the exact cause of Parkinson's disease is still unknown, two main pathological indicators are observed in the *post-mortem* brain; namely (i) loss of dopamine-producing neurons in the substantia nigra pars compacta (SNc; Kordower et al., 2013) and (ii) the widespread deposition of amyloid-like Lewy bodies rich in α-synuclein both in the SNc and other brain regions where overt neurodegeneration is not observed (Surmeier et al., 2017).

Accumulation of iron (Fe) in the SNc is an additional pathological feature common to all forms of Parkinson's disease (Ayton and Lei, 2014) that appears to precede the onset of clinical symptoms (Berg et al., 2015). Unlike synucleinopathy, brain Fe accumulation beyond that observed in normal aging is an early-stage event (He et al., 2015) restricted to the degenerating nigrostriatal pathway in Parkinson's disease (Wang et al., 2016) with this association supporting a potential causative role of Fe in neuron loss. In healthy neurons, Fe uptake is primarily *via* transferrin receptor mediated endocytosis, which releases labile Fe into the cytosol for immediate distribution to various organelles and Fe-storage and regulatory proteins. In dopaminergic neurons a small amount of Fe is bound to neuromelanin, a biopolymer formed during the oxidation of dopamine (DA). The labile iron pool is thought to be transient and consists primarily of both ferrous (Fe[II]) and ferric (Fe[III]) species bound to low molecular weight ligands such as citrate and ATP (Double et al., 2002; Hare et al., 2013). While characterization of the labile Fe pool in a living system, particularly human tissue, remains an analytical challenge (New et al., 2018), it has been argued that an increase in reactive Fe in the labile iron pool may contribute to generation of reactive oxygen species (ROS) in Parkinson's disease at levels above those that can normally be attenuated by endogenous antioxidant mechanisms (Ward et al., 2014). Biochemically, Fe-mediated generation of ROS is primarily *via* traditional Fenton/Haber-Weiss chemistry (Equations 1, 2) where cytosolic iron cycles between Fe[II] and Fe[III] to produce a range of harmful oxidants, including superoxide ($O_2^{\bullet-}$), hydrogen peroxide (H_2O_2) and hydroxyl radicals ($^{\bullet}OH$; Graham et al., 1978; Halliwell and Gutteridge, 1984; Segura-Aguilar et al., 2014; Sun et al., 2016):

$$\text{Fe[III]} + O_2^{\bullet-} \rightarrow \text{Fe[II]} + O_2 \quad (1)$$

$$\text{Fe[II]} + H_2O_2 \rightarrow \text{Fe[III]} + {}^{\bullet}OH + OH^- \quad (2)$$

The Fenton/Haber-Weiss reaction is not, however, unique to dopaminergic neurons and normal Fe accumulation with age occurs in other neuroanatomical regions (Acosta-Cabronero et al., 2016) without causing generalized cell loss. Numerous antioxidant mechanisms, including superoxide dismutase 1 (SOD1), reduced glutathione (GSH) and glutathione peroxidase, and vitamin E-mediated scavenging of $O_2^{\bullet-}$, H_2O_2 and $^{\bullet}OH$, attenuate potential ROS-induced neurotoxicity from gradual increase in Fe levels, suggesting that dysfunction of attenuating mechanisms is involved in Fe-mediated dopaminergic cell death in Parkinson's disease (Zecca et al., 2004).

An emerging theory, supported by initial observations of Fe dysregulation dating back nearly 100 years (Lhermitte et al., 1924), suggests that abnormal interactions between Fe and DA represent a biochemical mechanism unique to the microchemical environment of vulnerable neurons (Hare et al., 2014). Healthy dopaminergic neurons have particularly high endogenous oxidative load, owing to their extensive and complex axonal network, large soma and high metabolic output (Blesa et al., 2015). Further, cytosolic DA present in the mid-μM range in these neurons (Mosharov et al., 2009) gives rise to a pathway of Fe-mediated ROS generation independent of Fenton/Haber-Weiss chemistry (Hare and Double, 2016). Dopamine-derived quinones, such the DA *o*-quinone (DAQ) and aminochrome (DAC) can also be produced *via* the Fe-driven generation of the transient precursor DA semiquinone ($DA^{\bullet-}$) intermediary (Hare and Double, 2016; Sun et al., 2018b). It is unclear if endogenous antioxidant enzymes are capable of attenuating damage from DA-quinone production, though one proposed mechanism involves polymerization as the dark pigment, neuromelanin (Zhang et al., 2012).

As a major neurotoxic metabolite of DA, DAC has been used as a preclinical model compound to examine neurotoxicity in view of its apparent ability to cause indiscriminate neuronal damage, including mitochondrial dysfunction (Herrera et al., 2016; Segura-Aguilar and Huenchuguala, 2018), likely *via* lipid peroxidation and disruption of membrane integrity. It has been proposed that DAC can induce aggregation of α-synuclein and eventual Lewy body deposition through formation of a DAC-synuclein adduct (Berman and Hastings, 1999; Conway et al., 2001; Bianco et al., 2002; Norris et al., 2005), and α-synuclein mRNA has a predicted iron-response element in the 5′-untranslated region similar to the Fe-storage protein ferritin (Friedlich et al., 2007), suggesting this hallmark protein of Parkinson's disease also plays a role in Fe-mediated toxicity within vulnerable neurons. Previous studies also reported that the presence of DA quinones may also aggravate oxidative stress as a result of the inactivation in the electron transport chain of mitochondrial complexes I and III and the subsequent leakage of electrons from the respiratory chain (Stokes et al., 1999; Adam-Vizi, 2005; Lin and Beal, 2006; Gautier et al., 2008).

Much of our understanding of Fe-mediated DA oxidation has come from *ex vivo* studies where the chemical environment remains relatively constant, or *in vivo* investigations using cell culture or simple animal models of parkinsonism (Jiang et al., 2013; Panicker et al., 2015; Sampson et al., 2016). While useful and of most relevance, *in vivo* experiments generally provide insight into the overall consequence of the whole process with limited insights regarding the exact pathway, or pathways, of DA transformation. As such, it is unlikely that location of the most toxic intermediates or their relative concentrations will be determined in such studies with resultant restrictions in identifying the most efficacious therapeutic strategies targeting toxic DA metabolites. While previous work has firmly established that aberrant reactions between Fe and DA give rise to increased levels of free radicals and oxidative stress markers (Hermida-Ameijeiras et al., 2004; Jiang et al., 2013), comparatively little attention has been paid to the quantitative study of the DA intermediates that are directly implicated in causing neuronal dysfunction. Mitochondrial complex I inhibition by DA quinones and subsequent mitochondrial dysfunction has been identified as a possible molecular basis of neurodegeneration in Parkinson's disease (Schapira, 1994) and resulting intraneuronal acidosis is likely to decrease cytoplasmic pH (Balut et al., 2008) and influence the kinetics of Fe-mediated DA oxidation *in vivo*. Further, while the frequently observed decrease in pH of *post-mortem* brain tissue in the numerous tissue biobanks may result from *ex vivo* handling (Hare et al., 2012), physiological effects of

Abbreviations: 6-OHDA, 6-hydroxydopamine; AFO, amorphous iron oxide; DA, dopamine (1-amino-2-(3,4-dihydroxyphenyl)ethane); $DA^{\bullet-}$, semiquinone radical; DAC, dopaminochrome; DAL, leukoaminochrome; DAQ, dopamine-*o*-quinone; DHI, 5,6-dihydroxyindole; ECF, extracellular fluid; Fe[II], inorganic ferrous ion; Fe[III], inorganic ferric ion; $Fe^{[III]}DA$, *mono*-complex; $Fe^{[III]}DA_2$, *bis*-complex; $Fe^{[III]}DA_3$, *tris*-complex; $Fe[III]_T$, total inorganic Fe[III]; H_2O_2, hydrogen peroxide; LMCT, ligand to metal charge transfer; MQ, Milli-Q water; $O_2^{\bullet-}$, superoxide; $^{\bullet}OH$, hydroxyl radical; ROS, reactive oxygen species; SNc, substantia nigra pars compacta; TOR, turnover rate.

cardiorespiratory failure, cerebrovascular accident and end-stage neurodegenerative diseases generally result in lower brain tissue pH ranging from 7.0 to ~ 6.0 (Hardy et al., 1985; Yates et al., 1990; Harrison et al., 1995; Monoranu et al., 2009; Genoud et al., 2017). Mitochondrial dysfunction, which is a cardinal feature of neurodegenerative disease (Lin and Beal, 2006), also decreases tissue pH *via* leakage of protons into the cytosol (Brand and Nicholls, 2011). Thus, a reduction in brain tissue pH as a result of disease progression may have a substantial role in accelerating the progression of Fe-mediated DA oxidation in Parkinson's disease.

To demonstrate the relevance of interplay between Fe and DA to Parkinson's disease under acidified conditions mimicking predicted effects of disease-specific *pre-mortem* and non-specific *post-mortem* changes, we examined interactions between DA and Fe *in vitro* at a range of pH values–from pH 7.4, the typical pH of extracellular fluid (ECF) to pH 6.5, which is the reported average pH value of human Parkinson's disease tissue from the Sydney Brain Bank (Genoud et al., 2017) (though the specific location within the brain from which these samples were drawn was not reported). In the majority of previous studies, biochemical assays were undertaken at pH 7.4 as opposed to intraneuronal values that are typically around 6.96 to 7.05. This is a major limitation given that the transformation and fate of a range of biochemical compounds such as DA is strongly dependent upon pH. As Fe-mediated DA oxidation is an aerobic process, we also examined the effects of dissolved O_2 concentration within aqueous systems with respect to both the kinetics of Fe[II] oxidation and the production of reactive DA intermediates. In order to facilitate accurate and precise determination of reactive and unstable quinone intermediates, these investigations of the influence of pH and oxygen concentration on Fe-mediated DA oxidation have been performed *ex vivo*. These fundamental studies are critical for understanding Fe-DA reaction kinetics and set the stage for future studies where the techniques described are applied to the study of both the formation of neurotoxic DA metabolites in the Parkinson's disease brain and to the new therapies designed to prevent abnormal reactions of Fe within dopaminergic neurons that account for the changing pH of a degenerating dopaminergic neuron.

MATERIALS AND METHODS

Chemical and Reagents

All analytical grade chemicals were purchased from Sigma-Aldrich (Castle Hill, Australia) or as otherwise stated. All solutions were prepared using 18 MΩ·cm ultrapure Milli-Q water (MQ; Merck-Millipore, Bayswater, Australia). All glassware was acid washed in 5% HCl (v/v) for at least 1 week, then thoroughly rinsed in MQ before use. Stock solutions were stored in amber glass bottles at 4°C prior to use. To mimic the intracellular environment and focus on the effect of pH on iron catalyzed oxidation of DA, all experiments were performed in a light-free environment at a controlled temperature of 22 ± 0.6°C. This temperature, rather than a physiological temperature of 37°C was selected to allow direct comparison with previous work at pH 7.4. Investigation of the effect of temperature on the processes of interest in this work would be worthwhile though it should be

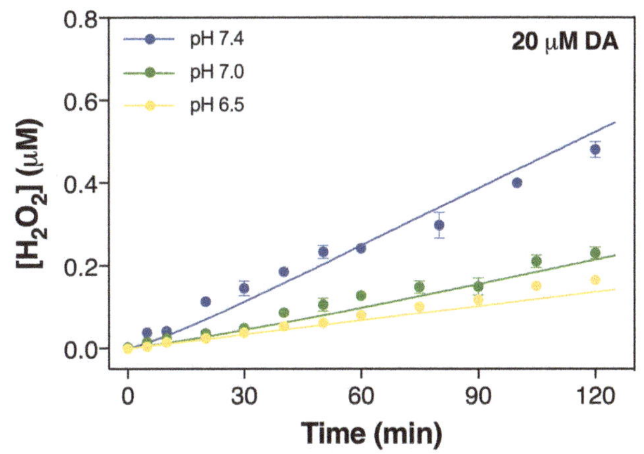

FIGURE 1 | Formation of H_2O_2 *via* the oxidation of 20 μM DA in the absence of added iron at pH 6.5, pH 7.0, and pH 7.4 in 0.1 M NaCl solution. Error bars are standard errors from triplicate measurements and solid lines represent the model fit.

recognized that thermodynamic and kinetic data for many of the key reactions underpinning these processes has been obtained by other investigators in the temperature range 20–25°C. Details of the preparation of stock and working solutions can be found in **Supplementary Materials.**

Preparation of Buffer Solutions

In general, despite often being considered "chemically inert" (Yu et al., 1997; Thiel et al., 1998), buffers such as 3-(N-morpholino)propanesulfonic acid (MOPS), 2-(N-morpholino)ethanesulfonic acid (MES) and 4-(2-hydroxyethyl)piperazine-1-ethanesulfonic acid (HEPES) may still exert an influence on the spectroscopic measurement and/or formation of different target substances. As such, to eliminate any buffer induced experimental artifacts, studies were undertaken in 0.1 M NaCl, 2 mM $NaHCO_3$ solutions containing 10 mM of MOPS, MES or HEPES by taking into consideration their pH control range and the influence they may exert on the measurement. Specifically, MOPS was used for the measurement of the generation of $Fe^{[III]}DA_2$, DAC and H_2O_2 over pH 6.5–7.4 (**Figures 1–4** and **Supplementary Figure 5**) as it does not exhibit spectrum broadening effects. For the measurement of Fe[II], MES was used at pH 6.5, while HEPES was used at both pH 7.0 and 7.4 (**Figure 4** and **Supplementary Figure 7**) as a result of the pH control range of these buffers and the negligible buffer facilitated reduction of Fe[III] in the presence of ferrozine (FZ; 4-[3-pyridin-2-yl-5-(4-sulfophenyl)-1,2,4-triazin-6-yl]benzenesulfonate) at pHs below 7.0.

Control of Dissolved O_2 Content in Buffer Solutions

For experiments using variable O_2 concentrations (0, 2.5, and 5% dissolved O_2), buffer solutions prepared above were sparged with special gas mixtures (297 ± 6 ppm CO_2 with or without 5% O_2, in Ar; BOC Gases, Preston, Australia) for at least 1 h before the addition of DA and Fe (see Control of Dissolved O_2 Content in

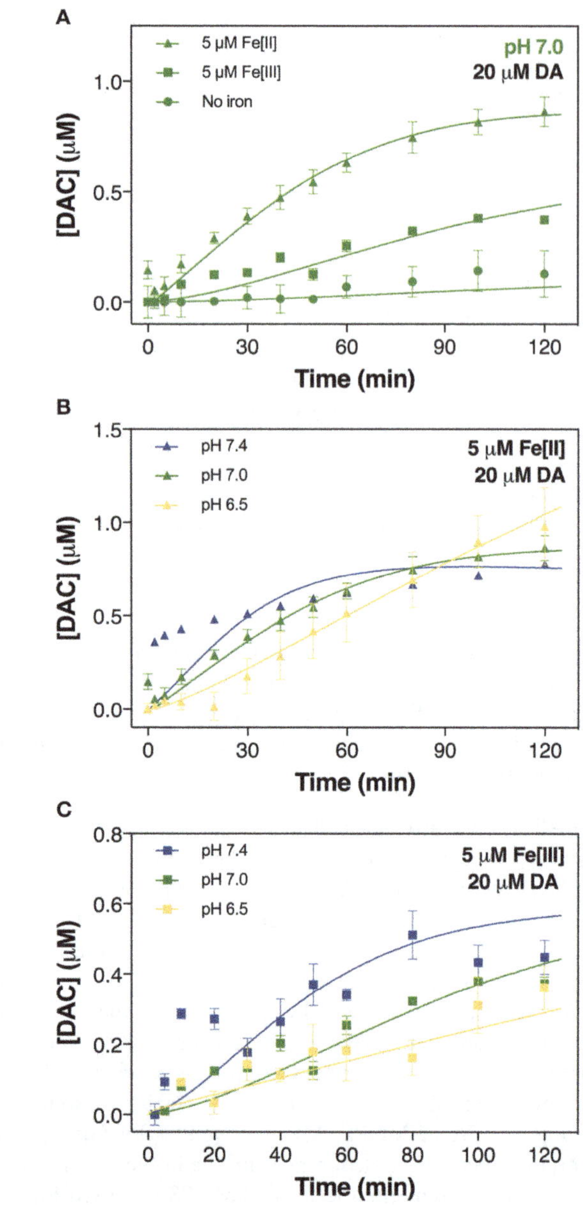

FIGURE 2 | Formation of DAC in air-saturated (21% O_2) 0.1 M NaCl solutions containing 20 μM DA and 5 μM iron (both Fe[III] and Fe[II]) at pH 7.0 **(A)**, in solutions containing 20 μM DA and 5 μM Fe[II] **(B)** and 5 μM Fe[III] **(C)** at pH 6.5, pH 7.0, and pH 7.4. Error bars are standard errors from triplicate measurements and solid lines represent the model fit.

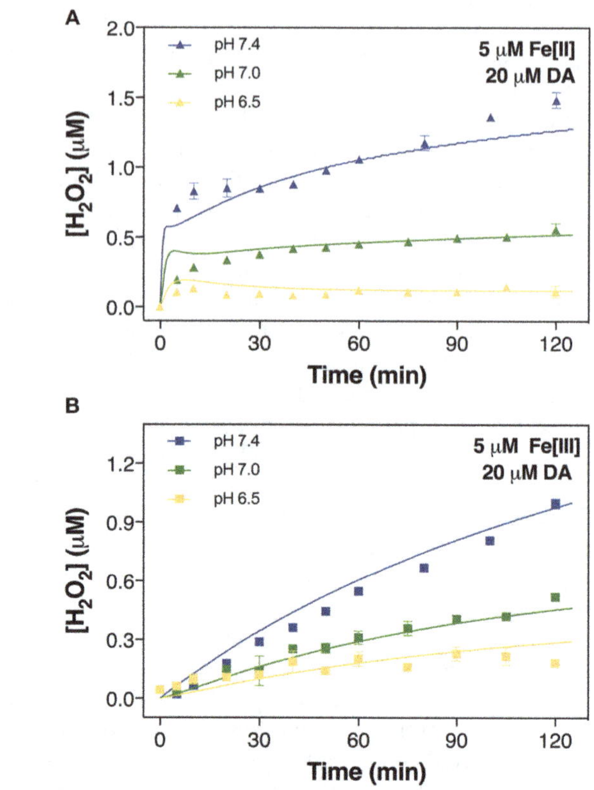

FIGURE 3 | Formation of H_2O_2 in air-saturated (21% O_2) 0.1 M NaCl solutions containing 20 μM DA and 5 μM Fe[II] **(A)** and 5 μM Fe[III] **(B)** at pH 6.5, pH 7.0, and pH 7.4. Error bars are standard errors from triplicate measurements and solid lines represent the model fit.

Buffer Solutions). Constant O_2 concentration was maintained by continuous sparging with the gas mixture over the course of the entire experiment.

Analytical Methods

pH Measurements

All pH measurements were made using a Hanna Instruments HI9025 pH meter (Keysborough, Australia) with a glass electrode and Ag-AgCl reference electrode. The pH meter and electrode were calibrated prior to each experiment using NIST-traceable buffer solutions (pH 4.01, 7.01, and 10.01).

Ferrous Iron Quantification

Quantitative measurements of Fe[II] were made using the modified FZ method as the reduction of DA bound iron occurs in the presence of FZ at low pH (Garg et al., 2013). The UV absorbance of $Fe^{III}FZ_3$ (both from inorganically and organically bound Fe[II]) was monitored at 562 nm with baseline correction at 690 nm. The concentration of total Fe[II] was then calculated per the following (Garg et al., 2013):

$$[\mathrm{Fe[II]}] = \frac{\left(A_{562} - \epsilon_{\mathrm{Fe[III]}} \times [\mathrm{Fe}]_T \times l\right)}{\left(\varepsilon_{\mathrm{Fe[II]}} - \varepsilon_{\mathrm{Fe[III]}}\right) \times l} \qquad (3)$$

where A_{562} is the recorded absorbance at 562 nm, $\varepsilon_{\mathrm{Fe[II]}}$ and $\varepsilon_{\mathrm{Fe[III]}}$ are the molar absorption coefficients of the $Fe^{III}FZ$ complex at 562 nm arising from the presence of Fe[II] and Fe[III], respectively. $[\mathrm{Fe}]_T$ is the total iron concentration, and l is the path length (10 cm).

Iron-Dopamine Complex Measurements

The concentration of $Fe^{III}DA_2$ was determined spectrophotometrically by measuring the absorbance at

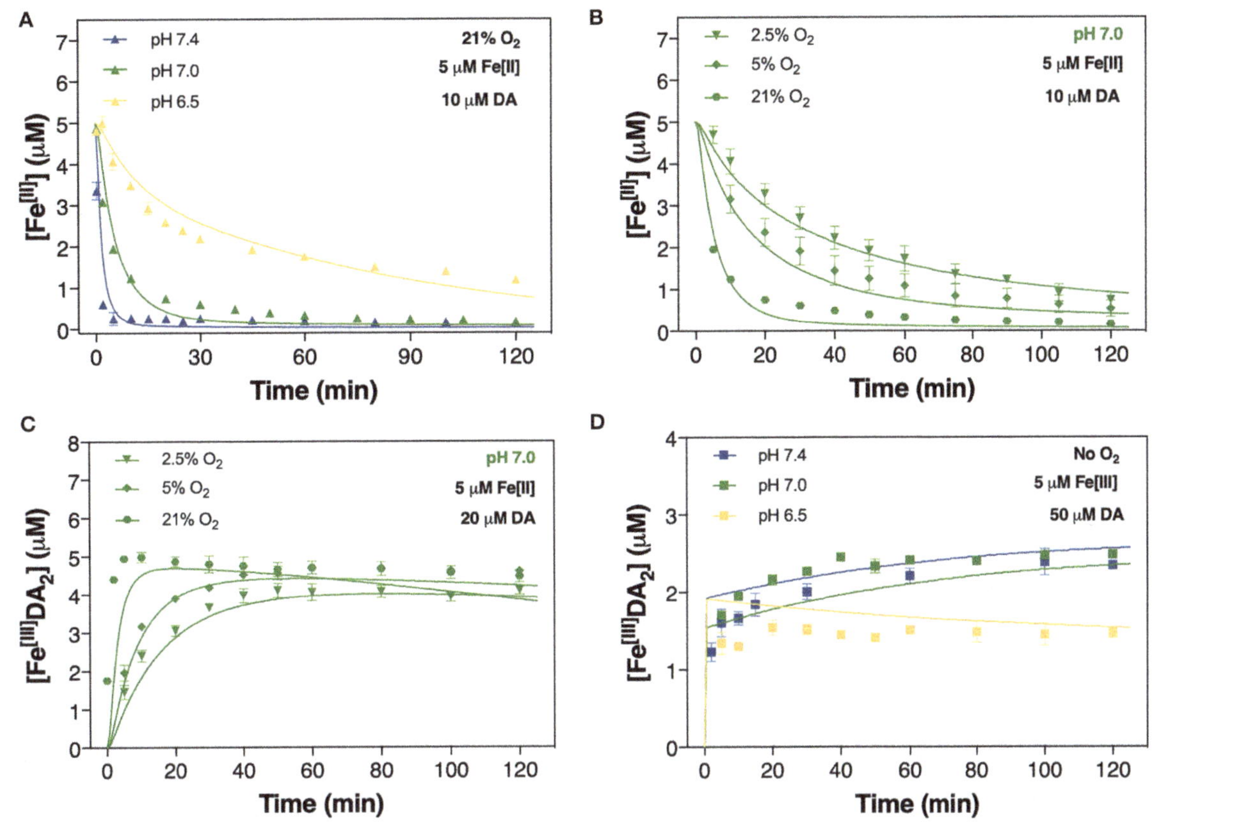

FIGURE 4 | Oxidation of 5 μM Fe[II] at pH 6.5, pH 7.0, and pH 7.4 in air-saturated (21% O_2) 0.1 M NaCl solutions containing 10 μM DA **(A)**; oxidation of 5 μM Fe[II] at pH 7.0 in the presence of 2.5, 5, and 21% O_2 **(B)**; and the formation of $Fe^{III}DA_2$ **(C)** in 0.1 M NaCl solutions in the same O_2 conditions. Formation of $Fe^{III}DA_2$ in 0.1 M deoxygenated NaCl solutions containing 5 μM Fe[III] and 50 μM DA at pH 6.5, pH 7.0, and pH 7.4 **(D)**. Error bars are standard errors from triplicate measurements and solid lines represent the model fit. The experimental data at pH 7.4 was taken from Sun et al. (2016).

580 nm with baseline correction at 850 nm. Calibration curves for quantification of the concentration of $Fe^{[III]}DA_2$ were constructed from measurements performed under anoxic conditions (Sun et al., 2016). Given the low concentrations and weak absorptivity of the *mono*-complex, the effect of this species on the measurement was considered negligible. It should be noted, however, that the $Fe^{[III]}DA$ complex is a precursor to the formation of the highly neurotoxic 6-OHDA quinone (Hare and Double, 2016). The molar absorptivity of $Fe^{[III]}DA_2$ was determined to be 3,121 M^{-1} cm^{-1} which was within 7% of the previously published value (Sever and Wilker, 2004). As a result of the slightly acidic pH and DA concentration used in this study, the extent of formation of the *tris*-complex should be negligible (Kowalchyk et al., 1995; Sun et al., 2018a). Even though the spectrum of DAC can overlap with that of the $Fe^{[III]}DA_2$ complex at 580 nm, the influence of DAC was not considered given the low concentration present (nominally <1 μM) under all conditions investigated herein (Pezzella et al., 1997) and the small molar absorptivity of DAC at 580 nm (ε_{580} = 439 $M^{-1}cm^{-1}$).

Hydrogen Peroxide Measurements

The H_2O_2 formed from Fe-mediated DA oxidation was quantified using the modified DPD method (Bader et al., 1988; Voelker and Sulzberger, 1996; Sun et al., 2016). Briefly, 1 mM DTPA was added to quench H_2O_2 generation at each time point in each assay (Sun et al., 2016). To eliminate interference from subsequent H_2O_2 generation and/or consumption as a result of the presence of high Fe[II] concentrations, 500 μM BPY was added prior to DTPA addition (Voelker and Sulzberger, 1996).

Quantitative data were interpolated by linear regression analysis of absorbance at 551 nm by increasing concentrations of H_2O_2 in 0.1 M NaCl with 60 μM DPD and 500 U/L HRP added, including a standard blank. No apparent interferences arising from the presence of moderate Fe[III] (5 μM) and DA (30 μM) were identified (**Supplementary Figure 1**). In order to enhance the accuracy of the measurements and remove potential interference arising from DA residuals on H_2O_2 absorbance measurements, the corresponding amount of DA, which was exactly the same as that used in a specific experiment set, was added to develop calibration curves for the experiments containing high concentrations of Fe[II].

Aminochrome Quantification

The concentration of DAC was determined by measuring absorbance at 475 nm with baseline correction at 850 nm (**Supplementary Figure 2**; Herlinger et al., 1995; Pham and Waite, 2014). The molar absorptivity derived from the calibration curves indicated that the precursor DAQ was unlikely to exert any influence on the measurement of DAC while most phenolic organics, including DA (**Supplementary Figure 3**) and 5,6-dyhydroxyindole (DHI), only absorb at around 280 nm (Il'ichev and Simon, 2003). As such, the influence arising from the rearrangement products of DAC should be minimal at 475 nm. Absorbance at a particular wavelength is the sum of the absorbances contributed from different species, thus spectral overlap may cause false-positive measurements. Given the coexistence of $Fe^{[III]}DA_2$ and DAC in solutions containing iron and DA, the concentration of each species was determined by solving the linear equations as described previously (Sun et al., 2018b); i.e.,

$$A_{475} = \left(\varepsilon_{475}^{Fe^{[III]}DA_2} C_{Fe^{[III]}DA_2} l\right) + \left(\varepsilon_{475}^{DAC} C_{DAC} l\right) \quad (4)$$

where A is the total absorbance at 475 nm, ε_i^j is the molar absorptivity of species j at wavelength i, C_j is the concentration of species j and l is the pathlength (10 cm). The concentration of $Fe^{[III]}DA_2$ was initially quantified based on the absorbance at 580 nm as DAC absorbed negligibly at this wavelength.

Calibration curves of DAC were developed by adding different concentrations of the freshly prepared DAC working solution into the air-saturated MOPS buffer solutions at pH 7.0 (Sun et al., 2018a). The molar absorptivity of DAC calculated in this study ($\varepsilon_{475\ nm} = 3{,}245\ M^{-1}cm^{-1}$) is similar to that reported by Segura-Aguilar and Lind (1989) ($\varepsilon_{475} = 3{,}085\ M^{-1}cm^{-1}$) and Pham and Waite (2014) ($\varepsilon_{475} = 3{,}281\ M^{-1}cm^{-1}$).

Speciation and Kinetic Modeling

The pH-dependent distributions of DA, Fe[III] and Fe[II] species were determined using the program Visual Minteq (Gustafsson, 2005). Details of the distributions are shown in **Supplementary Figure 4** with stability constants used in this study provided in **Supplementary Table 1**.

The kinetic model developed to describe the experimental data at pH 6.5, 7.0, and 7.4 was implemented using the software Kintek Explorer (Johnson et al., 2009). Specifically, the kinetic model is a set of reactions describing the key processes involved in the interplay between Fe and DA. To apply the model for the quantification of the time-dependent transformation of reactants, intermediates and products, the rate constant for each key process was either adopted from previous work or fitted in this study. The "goodness of fit" was judged by the ability of the reaction set used (and the associated set of coupled differential equations representing the rate expressions for each reaction) to describe the time-dependent transformation of a range of substances. If the model provided a poor description of the data, it indicated either a flaw in the reaction set or rate constant(s) used. In addition to the data collected in the current work, portions of the experimental data collected at pH 7.4 described by Sun et al. (2016) were used to complement this dataset and fully elucidate the effect of pH on DA oxidation. Given the critical role of dissociation of DA bound Fe at lower pH and the improved constraints provided by analysis of DAC, slight amendments were applied to the kinetic model previously developed for pH 7.4 (Sun et al., 2016).

RESULTS

Development and Rationale of Experimental Model

Given the relatively complicated model developed in this study, several intermediates were measured in order to better constrain the rate constants used herein. Briefly, (i) generation of DAC and H_2O_2 (shown in **Figures 1–3**) are used to constrain the rate constants for transformation of DA both in the absence and presence of iron including those for the oxidation of DA and leukoaminochrome (DAL) and cyclization of DAQ; (ii) decay of Fe[II] and formation of Fe-DA complexes in the presence of O_2 (shown in **Figures 4A–C**) are used to constrain the rate constant for the DA-induced transformation of Fe; and (iii) formation of Fe[III]-DA complexes (shown in **Figure 4D** and **Supplementary Figure 5**) in the absence of O_2 is used to constrain the rate constants for *mono*-complex formation, DA-induced reductive dissolution of ferrihydrite (amorphous ferric oxyhydroxide; or AFO) as well as the dynamic equilibrium between the *mono*- and *bis*-complexes. Details of the various reactions hypothesized to play a role are presented in **Tables 1–3**. Sensitivity analysis was used to determine the relative importance of the proposed reactions. Specifically, the greater the variation of the relative residuals that occurred with the change in magnitude of the rate constant, the more influential the reaction is. The lowest point or the "shift point" shown in the sensitivity analysis represents the optimal rate constant for the overall model applied. To simplify the applied model, rate constants were maintained consistent with those deduced in our previous study (Sun et al., 2016) with the exception of those with significant sensitivity to change of pH.

The sensitivity of the model to changes in individual rate constant values, defined as the relative residual, r, was determined using the program Kintecus (Ianni, 2003) combined with a Visual Basic for Applications (VBA) program. Note that the relative residual is defined as:

$$r = \frac{1}{n}\sum_{i=1}^{n} \frac{|MP_i - ED_i|}{ED_i} \quad (5)$$

where MP_i is the model prediction, ED_i is the experimental data at the same condition and time interval and n represents the total number of measured data points.

As shown in **Supplementary Figures 6A,B**, significant influence of DAQ cyclization and DAC decay on the transformation of DA was observed at the two pH values investigated here (the results of previous studies at pH 7.4 are provided by Sun et al., 2016). The most sensitive point of the relative residual r increases in line with pH. This is in agreement with the proposed rate constants (**Tables 1–3**) in the main text as deprotonation is generally the prerequisite for DAQ cyclization and DAC decay. In contrast, a relatively insensitive relative residual r is observed below the deduced upper rate constant ($k_5 = 5.3 \times 10^6$) for the redox exchange between DAQ and DAL (Land et al., 2003; Sun et al., 2016), especially at pH 7.0 (**Supplementary Figure 6C**). As such, the rate constant of the

TABLE 1 | Modeled reactions and rate constants for the autoxidation of DA at pH 6.5, 7.0, and 7.4.

No.	reactions	Rate constants ($M^{-1}s^{-1}$ or s^{-1})			References
		pH 6.5	**pH 7.0**	**pH 7.4**	
1	$DA + O_2 \xrightarrow{k_1} O_2^{\bullet-} + DA^{\bullet-}$	$k_1 = 3.94 \times 10^{-3}$	$k_1 = 4.22 \times 10^{-3}$	$k_1 = 8.24 \times 10^{-3a}$	This study
2	$DA^{\bullet-} + O_2 \underset{k_{-2}}{\overset{k_2}{\rightleftharpoons}} O_2^{\bullet-} + DAQ$		$k_2 = 2.95 \times 10^3$		1
			$k_{-2} = 1.0 \times 10^9$		1
3	$DA^{\bullet-} + DA^{\bullet-} \xrightarrow{k_3} DA + DAQ$		$k_3 = 2.35 \times 10^8$		2
4	$DAQ \xrightarrow{k_4} DAL$	$k_4 = 1.23 \times 10^{-2}$	$k_4 = 1.0$	$k_4 = 4.45^a$	This study
5	$DAL + DAQ \xrightarrow{k_5} DA + DAC$		$k_5 = 5.30 \times 10^6$		3
6	$DAL + O_2 \xrightarrow{k_6} DAC + H_2O_2$	$k_6 = 1.17$	$k_6 = 1.31$	$k_6 = 5.12^a$	This study
7	$O_2^{\bullet-} + O_2^{\bullet-} \xrightarrow{k_7} H_2O_2 + O_2$	$k_7 = 1.90 \times 10^6$	$k_7 = 6.0 \times 10^5$	$k_7 = 1.90 \times 10^5$	4
8	$DA^{\bullet-} + O_2^{\bullet-} \xrightarrow{k_8} DAQ + H_2O_2$		$k_8 = 8.27 \times 10^{9b}$		5
9	$DAC \underset{\text{Iron}}{\xrightarrow{k_9}}$ Decay products[c]	$k_9 = 1.2 \times 10^{-6}$	$k_9 = 8 \times 10^{-5}$	$k_9 = 4 \times 10^{-4}$	This study

[a]Value modified from that used in Sun et al. (2016). [b]Rate constant taken from Sun et al. (2016). [c]The rate constant proposed for reaction 9 incorporates the influence of Fe. DA, dopamine; $DA^{\bullet-}$, semiquinone radical; DAQ, dopamine-o-quinone; DAC, aminochrome; DAL, leukoaminochrome; and $O_2^{\bullet-}$, superoxide. Refs: (1) Pham and Waite (2014); (2) Borovansky et al. (2006); (3) Land et al. (2003); (4) Zafiriou (1990) and (5) Sun et al. (2016).

TABLE 2 | Modeled reactions and rate constants for Fe[III]-catalyzed oxidation of DA at pH 6.5,7.0 and 7.4.

No.	reactions	Rate constants ($M^{-1}s^{-1}$ or s^{-1})			References
		pH 6.5	**pH 7.0**	**pH 7.4**	
10	$Fe[III] + Fe[III] \xrightarrow{k_{10}} AFO + nH^+$	$k_{10} = 1.0 \times 10^6$	$k_{10} = 3.4 \times 10^6$	$k_{10} = 5.0 \times 10^6$	6
11	$>Fe[III]_n + DA \xrightarrow{k_{11}} >Fe[III]_{n-1} + Fe^{[III]}DA$	$k_{11} = 0.599$	$k_{11} = 2.3$	$k_{11} = 2.34^b$	This study
12	$>Fe[III]_n + DA \xrightarrow{k_{12}} >Fe[III]_{n-1} + Fe[II] + DA^{\bullet-}$	$k_{12} = 0.008$	$k_{12} = 0.3$	$k_{12} = 0.6^b$	This study
13	$Fe[III] + DA \underset{k_{-13}}{\overset{k_{13}}{\rightleftharpoons}} Fe^{[III]}DA$	$k_{13} = 8.7 \times 10^4$	$k_{13} = 2.09 \times 10^5$	$k_{13} = 4.15 \times 10^{5a}$	This study
		$k_{-13} = 1.45$	$k_{-13} = 0.969$	$k_{-13} = 0.463$	This study
14	$Fe^{[III]}DA + DA \underset{k_{-14}}{\overset{k_{14}}{\rightleftharpoons}} Fe^{[III]}DA_2$		$k_{14} = 4.50 \times 10^5$		7
		$k_{-14} = 3.37 \times 10^{-4}$	$k_{-14} = 2.86 \times 10^{-4}$	$k_{-14} = 2.59 \times 10^{-4}$	This study
15	$Fe^{[III]}DA + O_2^{\bullet-} \xrightarrow{k_{15}} Fe^{[II]}DA + O_2$		$k_{15} = 1.50 \times 10^8$		8
16	$Fe^{[III]}DA \xrightarrow{k_{16}} Fe[II] + DA^{\bullet-}$		$k_{16} = 0.23$		9
17	$Fe^{[III]}DA_2 \xrightarrow{k_{17}} Fe[II] + DA + DA^{\bullet-}$		$k_{17} = 7.26 \times 10^{-5b}$		5
18	$Fe[III] + O_2^{\bullet-} \xrightarrow{k_{18}} Fe[II] + O_2$		$k_{18} = 1.50 \times 10^8$		10
19	$>Fe[III]_n + O_2^{\bullet-} \xrightarrow{k_{19}} >Fe[III]_{n-1} + Fe[II] + O_2$	$k_{19} = 4.84 \times 10^4$	$k_{19} = 3.70 \times 10^5$	$k_{19} = 3.70 \times 10^{5b}$	This study
20	$Fe[III] + DA^{\bullet-} \xrightarrow{k_{20}} Fe[II] + DAQ$		$k_{20} = 9.12 \times 10^9$		This study

[a]Modified value of the model developed at pH 7.4 in Sun et al. (2016). [b]Rate constant taken from Sun et al. (2016). DA, dopamine; $DA^{\bullet-}$, dopamine semiquinone radical; DAQ, dopamine-o-quinone; $O_2^{\bullet-}$, superoxide; Fe[III], inorganic ferric ion; $Fe[III]_t$, total inorganic Fe[III]; AFO, ferrihydrite; and Fe[II], inorganic ferrous ion. Refs: (6) Pham et al. (2006); (7) Blesa and Matijevi (1989); (8) Rose and Waite (2003); (9) El-Avaan et al. (1997) and (10) Rush and Bielski (1985).

redox exchange reaction at both pH 6.5 and 7.0 was consistent with these previously reported findings.

As shown in **Supplementary Figure 6D**, the DA-induced dissolution of AFO is an important process as the relative residual *r* is very sensitive to the change in the magnitude of the rate constant. A slight increase in the shift point with increase in pH is observed with this result in accord with the proposed rate constants applied. However, compared with that of DA-induced dissolution of AFO, the reductive dissolution after the adsorption of DA onto the surface of AFO (Reaction 12, **Table 2**) is relatively insensitive at both pH values used (**Supplementary Figure 6E**), indicating that reductive dissolution is not as important as DA-induced dissolution of AFO at each pH value investigated herein. As shown in **Supplementary Figures 6F,G**, the formation of both $Fe^{[III]}DA$ (Reaction 13, **Table 2**) and $Fe^{[II]}DA$ (Reaction 24, **Table 3**) are key reactions in this study as can be seen from the relative sensitivities of the relative residuals for these reactions. The rate constant for the formation of the *bis*-complex from $Fe^{[III]}DA$ with another DA molecule (Reaction 14, **Table 2**) is assumed to be similar to the rate

TABLE 3 | Modeled reactions and rate constants for Fe[II]-catalyzed oxidation of DA at pH 6.5, 7.0 and 7.4.

	No. reactions	Rate constants ($M^{-1}s^{-1}$ or s^{-1})			References
		pH 6.5	pH 7.0	pH 7.4	
21	$Fe[II] + O_2 \xrightarrow{k_{21}} Fe[III] + O_2^{\bullet-}$	$k_{21} = 0.0209$	$k_{21} = 0.0959$	$k_{21} = 0.77^b$	This study
22	$Fe[II] + O_2^{\bullet-} \xrightarrow{k_{22}} Fe[III] + H_2O_2$		$k_{22} = 1.0 \times 10^7$		10
23	$Fe[II] + H_2O_2 \xrightarrow{k_{23}} Fe[III] + {}^\bullet OH + OH^-$	$k_{23} = 1.72 \times 10^3$	$k_{23} = 4.79 \times 10^3$	$k_{23} = 1.33 \times 10^4$	11
24	$Fe[II] + DA \underset{k_{-24}}{\overset{k_{24}}{\rightleftharpoons}} Fe^{[II]}DA$	$k_{24} = 7.0 \times 10^2$	$k_{24} = 7.2 \times 10^2$	$k_{24} = 7.5 \times 10^{2b}$	This study
		$k_{-24} = 1.02 \times 10^{-2}$	$k_{-24} = 9.2 \times 10^{-3}$	$k_{-24} = 1.6 \times 10^{-3}$	This study
25	$Fe^{[II]}DA + O_2 \xrightarrow{k_{25}} Fe^{[III]}DA + O_2^{\bullet-}$	$k_{25} = 3.32$	$k_{25} = 19$	$k_{25} = 145^b$	This study
26	$Fe^{[II]}DA + H_2O_2 \xrightarrow{k_{26}} Fe^{[III]}DA + {}^\bullet OH + OH^-$	$k_{26} = 1.72 \times 10^3$	$k_{26} = 4.79 \times 10^3$	$k_{26} = 1.33 \times 10^4$	11
27	$Fe^{[II]}DA + O_2^{\bullet-} \xrightarrow{k_{27}} Fe^{[III]}DA + H_2O_2$		$k_{27} = 1.0 \times 10^7$		8
28	$Fe^{[II]}DA + DA^{\bullet-} \xrightarrow{k_{28}} Fe^{[III]}DA + DA$		$k_{28} = 1.92 \times 10^{5b}$		5
29	$Fe[II] + DA^{\bullet-} \xrightarrow{k_{29}} Fe^{[III]}DA + DA$		$k_{29} = 1.92 \times 10^{5b}$		5

[a]Modified value of the model developed at pH 7.4 in Sun et al. (2016). [b]rate constant taken from Sun et al. (2016). DA, dopamine; $DA^{\bullet-}$, dopamine semiquinone radical; $O_2^{\bullet-}$, superoxide; Fe[III], inorganic ferric ion; Fe[II], inorganic ferrous ion; H_2O_2, hydrogen peroxide; and ${}^\bullet OH$, hydroxyl radical. Refs: (11) González-Davila et al. (2005).

constant for water-loss from $Fe(OH)(H_2O)_5^{2+}$ of 4.50×10^5 $M^{-1}s^{-1}$ (Blesa and Matijevi, 1989) in view of the fact that the replacement of a coordinated H_2O by the additional DA molecule is generally faster than the formation of the *mono*-complex (Ludwig et al., 1995). The results of sensitivity analysis shown in **Supplementary Figure 6H** indicate that this assigned value should be reasonable for the sensitivity of relative residual *r*. Similar to the formation of the Fe-DA complexes, dissociation of these complexes is also of great significance given the considerable sensitivity of the rate constants over several orders of magnitude (**Supplementary Figures 6I–K**). In contrast to increase in the optimal value on decrease in pH (**Supplementary Figure 6I**), the increase in the dissociation rate constant shown in **Supplementary Figure 6J** is much less significant. This supports the supposition that dissociation is generally important at low pH with the *bis*-complex much more stable in view of the iron sequestration. As shown in **Supplementary Figure 6L**, relative insensitivity of the relative residual *r* is evident for the deduced rate constant (3.7×10^5 $M^{-1}s^{-1}$) for the reaction between superoxide and AFO (Reaction 19, **Table 2**). As such, in order to simplify the model, the rate constant of this reaction at high pH is considered to be the same as that proposed previously (Sun et al., 2016). However, a value for this rate constant of one order of magnitude lower is deduced from model fitting in this study at pH 6.5 with this lower value possibly a result of the increased proportion of $HO_2^\bullet$ at this lower pH and the subsequent reduced electrostatic attraction between superoxide and the AFO surface.

Theoretically, change in pH would typically result in variation of the Fe[II] oxidation rate in the presence of oxidants such as $DA^{\bullet-}$. However, as shown in **Supplementary Figure 6M**, considerable insensitivity of the relative residual is observed around the value proposed at physiological pH. As such, a consistent rate constant was used. Reduction of Fe[III] by $DA^{\bullet-}$ is important at pH 6.5 given the significant decrease in relative residuals on variation of the rate constant (from 1 to 10^{10} $M^{-1}s^{-1}$; shown in **Supplementary Figure 6N**). Therefore, the reaction between Fe[III] and $DA^{\bullet-}$ is considered in the proposed reaction scheme. The reduction of DA bound Fe[III] by $DA^{\bullet-}$ is not as significant as the reduction of Fe[III] in view of its lower reduction potential. As such, reduction of organically complexed Fe[III] by $DA^{\bullet-}$ is not considered in the reaction scheme.

Dopamine-Derived Free Radical Production Is pH Dependent

To assess how pH influences the generation of toxic DA metabolites, the autoxidation of DA over a range of pH was initially investigated with attention given to the accumulation of H_2O_2 and DAC. As shown in **Figure 1**, spontaneous oxidation of DA is highly pH-dependent with 20 μM DA producing H_2O_2 at rates of 0.08, 0.12, and 0.24 μM h^{-1} at pH 6.5, 7.0, and 7.4, respectively. On the other hand, <0.1 μM of DAC was produced at pH 7.0 in the absence of Fe (**Figure 2A**).

The oxidation of DA by O_2:

$$DA + O_2 \rightarrow DA^{\bullet-} + O_2^{\bullet-} \tag{6}$$

is often considered to be a critical step in the production of H_2O_2 and DAC. Firstly, $DA^{\bullet-}$ can disproportionate to form DAQ which subsequently cyclizes to DAL. DAC and H_2O_2 can then be produced either through the redox exchange between DAQ and DAL (Equation 7) or as a result of the direct oxidation of DAL (Equation 8), $O_2^{\bullet-}$ disproportionation (Equation 9) and/or the $O_2^{\bullet-}$-mediated transformation of radicals such as $DA^{\bullet-}$ (Equation 10; Hawley et al., 1967; Graham, 1978; Sun et al., 2016).

$$DAQ + DAL \rightarrow DA + DAC \tag{7}$$

$$DAL + O_2 \rightarrow DAC + H_2O_2 \tag{8}$$

$$O_2^{\bullet-} + O_2^{\bullet-} \rightarrow H_2O_2 + O_2 \tag{9}$$

$$O_2^{\bullet-} + DA^{\bullet-} \rightarrow DAQ + H_2O_2 \tag{10}$$

Among the various reactions shown above, the direct oxidation of DA by O_2 to $DA^{\bullet-}$ and $O_2^{\bullet-}$ (Equation 6) is expected to be rate limiting in view of the spin restriction inherent between DA and O_2 and, accordingly, exhibits a small rate constant (**Table 1**). With this in mind, any factors that influence this rate-limiting step (such as the presence of Fe[II] and Fe[III]; see Section Iron Accelerates Dopamine Oxidation) will alter the rate of formation of products arising from the oxidation of DA.

In general, the apparent oxidation rate of DA is determined by the contribution of different DA species. The pH-dependent formation of H_2O_2 shown in **Figure 1** is attributed, at least partially, to the increase in the proportion of deprotonated DA ions on increase in pH; i.e.,

$$k_{app} = \alpha_{H_2DA}k_{H_2DA+O_2} + \alpha_{HDA}k_{HDA^-+O_2} + \alpha_{DA^{2-}}k_{DA^{2-}+O_2} \quad (11)$$

where k_{app} is the apparent oxidation rate constant, α_i is the fraction of total DA species present as species i and k_i is the intrinsic oxidation rate constant of species i. Previous work has suggested that the abstraction of a hydrogen atom from the *mono*-deprotonated form of DA is the rate limiting step in the oxidation of DA (Herlinger et al., 1995). As such, it is not unexpected that an increase in the proportion of deprotonated DA on increase in pH would give rise to the enhanced generation of both $DA^{\bullet-}$ and $O_2^{\bullet-}$ *via* Equation 6, eventually resulting in the subsequent increase in the concentration of H_2O_2. Compared with the significantly enhanced production of H_2O_2 in the presence of iron (shown in section Iron Accelerates Dopamine Oxidation), while continuously formed, the toxicity induced by the autoxidation of DA is unlikely to be significant given the presence of *in vivo* oxidant removal enzymes, such as superoxide dismutase 1 (SOD1) and the glutathione peroxidases (GPx), though there is evidence that both enzymes are dysfunctional in Parkinson's disease (Cardoso et al., 2017; Trist et al., 2017, 2018). Additionally, the presence of DA-derived quinones is expected to be negligible (as shown in **Figure 2A**).

Iron Accelerates Dopamine Oxidation

In order to quantify the rate of generation of ROS and reactive quinones arising from the interaction between Fe and DA over pHs ranging from those of the physiological neuronal cytosol to those that have experienced disease-related and *post-mortem* acidosis, the accumulation of DAC and the concentrations of the key Fenton reagents–Fe[II] and H_2O_2-were subsequently investigated.

In contrast to the negligible production of DAC in the absence of Fe, a substantially higher concentration was generated in the presence of 5 μM iron at pH 7.0. In general, our results show that Fe[II] was more effective in catalyzing DAC production than was Fe[III] (**Figure 2A**). The initial rate of formation of DAC in the presence of both Fe[II] and Fe[III] increased significantly at pH 7.0 and 7.4 (**Figures 2B,C**). By contrast, the concentration of DAC plateaued in the latter stages of the 120 min assessment period at pH 7.4, more so in the presence of Fe[II].

Accordingly, labile Fe also accelerated the production of H_2O_2, again with Fe[II] being generally more efficient than Fe[III], particularly during the initial ~10 min following addition of reagents (**Figure 3A**). While H_2O_2 was continuously produced at pH 7.0 and 7.4 in the presence of both Fe species, at pH 6.5 only Fe[III] showed an increase in H_2O_2 production though the concentration present at t = 120 min was only ~10% of that produced at pH 7.4 (**Figure 3B**). For Fe[II], H_2O_2 concentration remained stable after a subtle increase from t = 0–10 min.

Accompanying the rapid generation of both DAC and H_2O_2 was a significant decrease in the concentration of Fe[II]. The apparent oxidation rate of Fe[II] significantly increased in the presence of DA. In the absence of DA, the concentration of Fe[II] halved over 2 h at pH 7.0 (**Supplementary Figure 7A**) while Fe[II] levels were near-totally depleted within 30 min in the presence of 10 μM DA at the same pH (**Figure 4A**).

According to the rate law:

$$-\frac{d\,[\mathrm{Fe[II]}]}{dt} = k[\mathrm{Fe[II]}][O_2] \quad (12)$$

the oxidation of Fe[II] depends on the concentration of dissolved O_2 present. As the O_2 concentration in brain tissue is typically in the range of 10–60 μM (Koppenol and Butler, 1985; Ndubuizu and Lamanna, 2007), which corresponds to <5% O_2 saturation in aqueous solutions, the effect of O_2 (at 2.5 and 5% saturation) on the transformation of Fe[II] in the presence of DA was examined at pH 7.0. As expected, both the rate and extent of Fe[II] oxidation decreased with lower O_2 concentration, with only a 10% decrease in Fe[II] concentration at pH 7.0 in 5% O_2 at t = 2 h compared with a 40% decrease at 21% O_2 saturation (**Supplementary Figure 7B**). Oxidation of Fe[II] followed an exponential decay on addition of 10 μM DA at pH 7.0 with initial Fe[II] exhausted after ~70 min in 21% O_2 and 80–90% loss at 2 h for physiologically-relevant O_2 concentrations (**Figure 4B**). Accordingly, the initial formation of $Fe^{III}DA_2$ was strongly dependent on O_2 concentration with markedly lower rates observed at 2.5 and 5% O_2 (**Figure 4C**).

Dopamine Induces Iron Mobilization

As predicted by thermodynamic and kinetic data, the majority of Fe[III] should be present in an insoluble phase, even in the presence of 20 μM DA. As such, the continuous generation of both DAC and H_2O_2 in the presence of Fe[III] shown in **Figures 2C, 3B** suggests that DA is capable of inducing the slow release of reactive soluble Fe species. Indeed, dissolution of precipitated Fe by DA may pose a potential risk in view of its contribution to the labile iron pool (Dixon and Stockwell, 2014) and subsequent DA oxidation. Thus, to understand the extent of DA-induced mobilization of Fe[III], the temporal change in concentration of $Fe^{[III]}DA_2$ was measured over the pH range of 6.5 to 7.4. To eliminate potential confounding effects of O_2-mediated transformation of both Fe and reducing radicals, $Fe^{[III]}DA_2$ formation was investigated under anoxic conditions. As shown in **Figure 4D**, $Fe^{[III]}DA_2$ formation increased gradually at pH 7.0 and 7.4 in the presence of high initial DA concentration (50 μM) though not at pH 6.5. At this pH 6.5, $Fe^{[III]}DA_2$ formation was ~60% of that produced at circumneutral pH; a trend conserved at a lower DA concentration (20 μM; **Supplementary Figure 5**).

Compared with pH 6.5, the increase in the overall concentration of $Fe^{III}DA_2$ at pH 7.0 and 7.4 can most likely be attributed to: (i) the reduced rate of LMCT resulting from the increased proportion of $Fe^{III}DA_2$ present, and (ii) more efficient formation of transient >Fe[III]-DA surface complexes that precede thermal detachment of DA-bound Fe (Equation 13) and/or DA-induced reductive dissolution (Equation 14):

$$>Fe[III]_n + DA \rightarrow\ >Fe[III]_{n-1} + Fe^{[III]}DA \quad (13)$$

$$>Fe[III]_n + DA \rightarrow\ >Fe[III]_{n-1} + Fe[II] + DA^{\bullet-} \quad (14)$$

Ex vivo Modeling Predicts Potential Toxicity of Iron-Mediated Dopamine Oxidation

The kinetic model developed in this study was used to infer potential long-term effects of the combined mechanisms of DA oxidation in the presence of Fe. Particular emphasis was given to the effect of system conditions on Fe turnover rate (TOR; used as a measure of Fe-specific catalysis) and associated hydroxyl radical and DAC production, encompassing changing DA and H_2O_2 concentrations and steady-state dissolved O_2. In this study, given the overall goodness of the model fit to the experimental data (**Figures 1–5**, **Supplementary Figures 5**, **7**), the TOR was determined from the oxidation rate of Fe[II] as predicted by the model under particular conditions (e.g., pH, total concentration of Fe, the concentration ratio of Fe to DA and O_2 content).

Dopamine Concentration Mediates Iron Redox Cycling

In general, cycling rate of Fe was highest during the initial phase of each experiment and was amplified by increasing concentration of DA (**Figure 5A**) and higher pH (**Supplementary Figure 9**). After the initial dynamic cycling period, the TOR steadily decreased and appeared to reach equilibrium after ~30 min. Both acidic pH (pH 6.5) and DA concentration dictated higher Fe TOR at the near-midpoint of the reaction time (t = 50 min); the presence of 30 μM DA induced a 10-fold increase in turnover rate compared to DA-absent conditions at pH 6.5 whereas at pH 7.0 and 7.4 the increase in TOR represented only 2 and 1.3-fold change, respectively (**Figure 5B**). From this, we conclude that the effect of DA on Fe TOR is much more substantial in acidic conditions with this likely contributing to the abeyance of H_2O_2 generation (shown in **Figure 3A**) and predicted increase in $^{\bullet}OH$ production as a result of both Fenton chemistry (Equations 1, 2) and Fe[II]-mediated DA oxidation (Reactions 23 and 26, **Table 3**).

Kinetic Modeling of Sustained Parkinsonian Oxidative Stress

As a result of the attenuation by endogenous antioxidants, including SOD1, GPx, and endogenous ascorbate ions (Harrison and May, 2009), *in vivo* steady-state concentrations of H_2O_2 stemming from normal mitochondrial respiration in the brain are estimated to be maintained at around 5 nM (Adam-Vizi, 2005). However, concomitant hypoxia thought to occur in the Parkinson's disease brain (Adams and Odunze, 1991) may result in both the accumulation of lactate as a result of the anaerobic conditions, which, in turn, may contribute to the decrease in pH, as well as a release of DA from chemically-isolated vesicles (Phebus et al., 1986).

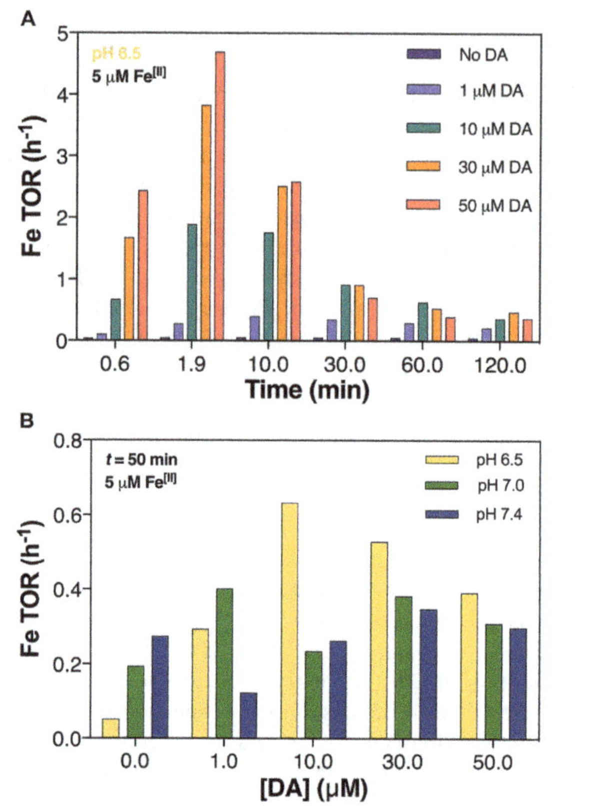

FIGURE 5 | Predicted turnover rate (TOR) of 5 μM Fe[II] in air-saturated (21% O_2) solutions with increasing DA concentrations at pH 7.0 **(A)** and at pH 6.5, pH 7.0, and pH 7.4 after 50 min **(B)**.

To predict the rate of $^{\bullet}OH$ generation in a chemical environment more reflective of continued replenishment of pro-oxidants in a DA neuron, the kinetic model was applied where pseudo-equilibrium was reached in the presence of a range of fixed H_2O_2 and DA concentrations. While it must be emphasized that this model is illustrative, as it is specific to only DA-derived oxidative stress, it represents an important advance in understanding the biochemical mechanism by which gradual neuronal Fe accumulation with age can become pathological in cells with both high metabolic output and an abundance of a pro-oxidant catecholamine in DA.

As shown in **Figure 6A**, at a fixed concentration of 50 μM DA, increased $^{\bullet}OH$ production rate was observed with increasing H_2O_2 concentration and decreasing O_2 concentrations over a 10–60 μM range typical of that within the brain (Ndubuizu and Lamanna, 2007). The increased production of hydroxyl radicals as H_2O_2 becomes more concentrated can be attributed to the relatively slow oxygenation rates at these conditions and the potential for active peroxidation of any Fe[II] present. In contrast, the effect of DA concentration on $^{\bullet}OH$ production as predicted by the model was more complex (**Figure 6B**; **Supplementary Figure 10**) as DA can both sequester

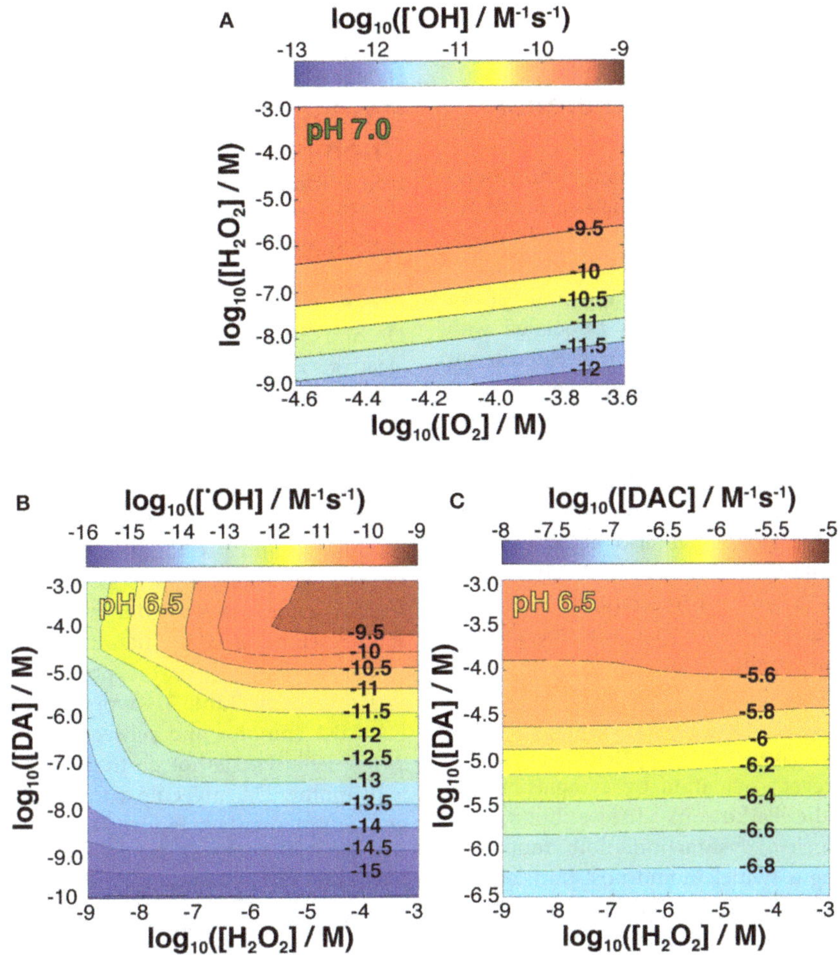

FIGURE 6 | Kinetic modeling of •OH production variability in the presence of 5 μM Fe[II] as a function of both fixed concentrations of O_2 and H_2O_2 and steady-state 50 μM DA at pH 7.0 **(A)**; and •OH **(B)** and DAC **(C)** production as a function of both fixed concentrations of H_2O_2 and DA at pH 6.5.

Fe[II] and Fe[III] in a variety of coordination complexes and mobilize Fe[III] from ferric oxide precipitates *via* DA induced dissolution. As a whole, DA concentrations under 0.1 μM produce minimal amounts of •OH regardless of the steady-state H_2O_2 concentration with this effect principally a result of there being insufficient labile Fe present to promote oxidation. In contrast, as DA concentrations exceed 10 μM, production of •OH is accelerated, provided the steady-state H_2O_2 concentration is in excess of ~100 nM, indicating that the leakage of DA at the later stage may aggravate the Fe and DA induced oxidative stress.

Again, the effect of increasing pH that promotes $Fe^{III}DA_2$ complex formation partially attenuates •OH production (**Supplementary Figure 10**), whereas $Fe^{III}DA$ production favored at pH 6.5 results in an increase in •OH generation rate (**Figure 6B**; **Supplementary Table 2**) compared to the behavior observed at both higher pH values and equivalent DA and H_2O_2 concentrations in an Fe-free environment.

Dopamine concentration had the largest effect on DAC production for all pH values investigated (**Figure 6C**; **Supplementary Figure 11**) with the highest rate of quinone formation observed at pH 6.5. On the other hand, while the model indicated H_2O_2 concentration had minimal influence on the rate of DAC formation at pH 6.5, low concentrations of H_2O_2 at pH 7.0 and pH 7.4 favor the accumulation of DAC, particularly at the lower range of DA concentrations used. Highlighting the versatility of Fe redox activity and why it is tightly regulated under normal physiological conditions, these results suggest that the oxidative load in a dopaminergic neuron arising from Fe-mediated •OH production at basal H_2O_2 levels are somewhat mitigated by the concomitant oxidation of Fe[II], effectively sequestering Fe in the ferric state, which is less active with respect to neurotoxic DAC production.

DISCUSSION

The value of this study is in the detailed kinetic and thermodynamic profiling of DA oxidation, which provides direct chemical evidence to support the involvement of this unique source of oxidative stress in a potentially pathogenic mechanism of dopaminergic neurotoxicity.

Iron, Dopamine, and Selective Neuronal Loss in Parkinson's Disease

Iron accumulates in multiple regions of the aging human brain (Acosta-Cabronero et al., 2016), and is most marked in the Fe-rich deep gray matter within the basal ganglia (Li et al., 2014). The degree of accumulation in Parkinson's disease patients is markedly higher in the SNc and putamen (Wang et al., 2016), where dopaminergic neurons project, and is associated with disease severity (Wallis et al., 2008), suggesting elevated levels of Fe are intrinsically linked to the biochemical mechanism underlying neuron loss (Hare et al., 2015). The disease-specific hyperaccumulation of Fe throughout the nigrostriatal pathway (He et al., 2015) indicates a particular vulnerability of dopaminergic neurons, and a lack of apparent pathology in non-Parkinson's-affected regions that also accumulate Fe during normal aging (Acosta-Cabronero et al., 2016) support the hypothesis that DA oxidation and free radical generation, occurring either independently of, or concurrent to, classical Fenton chemistry is a major source of oxidative stress in Parkinson's disease.

This characteristic feature may explain how two essential neurochemicals, which are normally segregated by vesicular confinement of DA to prevent oxidation by cytoplasmic Fe, are able to interact in the Parkinson's disease brain, and how they relate to α-synuclein dysfunction. Both mutations to the *SNCA* gene encoding α-synuclein and post-translational oxidative damage to the protein (Lotharius and Brundin, 2002b), the latter being an effect of elevated levels of Fe and Fenton-type ROS production, can lead to permeabilized vesicles that effectively "leak" DA into the pro-oxidant environment of the cytoplasm (Lotharius and Brundin, 2002a). This initial $^{\bullet}OH$-driven oxidative damage may trigger a cascade of free radical production that accelerates the rate of α-synuclein modifications, impaired vesicular transport, and DA oxidation, in turn, aggravating cell loss by triggering DAC-induced neurotoxicity.

Central to the view that elevated Fe facilitates DA breakdown is the notion of a labile Fe pool. The propensity of unbound cytoplasmic Fe[II] to react with by-products (such as H_2O_2) of mitochondrial respiration necessitates tight metabolic regulation of neuronal Fe levels involving various regulatory proteins (Moos et al., 2007), a number of which have been recognized as being dysfunctional in Parkinson's disease (Hare et al., 2013). Whether a labile Fe pool exists in actuality is the subject of much debate and both rapid oxidation of Fe[II] in the O_2-rich environment and obvious difficulties in directly speciating Fe within a living human neuron represent two analytical challenges that preclude obtaining conclusive evidence that Fe dyshomeostasis actively promotes increased oxidative stress in Parkinson's disease. Regardless, as nigral Fe accumulation is now recognized as an indisputable pathological feature of Parkinson's disease (Ayton and Lei, 2014; Wang et al., 2016), understanding the mechanism of how Fe promotes oxidative stress in dopaminergic neurons is critical as Fe chelation therapies enter clinical trials (Devos et al., 2014; Martin-Bastida et al., 2017; Moreau et al., 2018; Sun et al., 2018c).

Iron-Induced Dopamine Radical Production Is Independent of Fenton Chemistry

Iron-mediated DA oxidation differs from Fenton/Haber-Weiss chemistry in that, in addition to redox cycling of Fe[II]/Fe[III], both species are capable of forming intermediary complexes immediately preceding free radical production. For instance, both Fe[II] and Fe[III] are capable of *d* orbital "bridging" between DA and O_2, and inducing the subsequent accelerated transfer of electrons and generation of $DA^{\bullet -}$ and $O_2^{\bullet -}$ free radicals (Miller et al., 1990). The reactions and associated rate constants involved in Fe[II]/Fe[III] redox cycling and DA oxidation are listed in **Tables 2, 3.**

The particularly strong ability of Fe[II] to generate DAC and H_2O_2 evident in **Figures 2, 3** may result from the relative insolubility and precipitation of Fe[III] as AFO over the pH range investigated. This is an important factor to consider, as ferritin sequesters Fe within a protein nanocage in a chemical state resembling AFO (Jian et al., 2016). However, the ready oxidation of Fe[II] in the presence of DA (Reaction 24 and Reaction 25 in **Table 3**) favors the conversion of Fe[II] to the $Fe^{[III]}DA$ complex and subsequent $O_2^{\bullet -}$ generation (Sun et al., 2016). $Fe^{[III]}DA$ is not particularly stable and may either react with another DA molecule to form $Fe^{III}DA_2$ (shown in **Figure 4C** and **Supplementary Figure 7C**), reversibly react with $O_2^{\bullet -}$ to reform $Fe^{[III]}DA$ and O_2 or undergo ligand-to-metal charge transfer (LMCT) with release of Fe[II] and $DA^{\bullet -}$ as follows:

$$Fe^{[III]}DA \rightarrow Fe[II] + DA^{\bullet -} \quad (15)$$

Compared to the relatively inactive iron oxyhydroxide precipitates, the more soluble DA-bound Fe[III] oxidation product formed from ferrous DA complexes should enhance the production of both DAC and H_2O_2 by accelerating generation of both $DA^{\bullet -}$ and $O_2^{\bullet -}$ radicals.

Distinguishing iron-mediated dopamine oxidation from Fenton-generated ROS is important, as the free radicals produced do not have the multiple redundant detoxification pathways that exist for H_2O_2. While quinones are a relatively minor component of dopamine metabolism, which ordinarily favors providing a precursor for adrenaline biosynthesis or excretion from the central nervous system as homovanillic acid, it is unclear precisely how these highly-reactive species are neutralized. Several endogenous enzymes have been shown to interact with dopamine *o*-quinones, including SOD1, glutathione transferase (by way of glutathione conjugation) and macrophage migration inhibitory factor (Solano et al., 1999; Haque et al., 2003), though quinone detoxification would be considered a secondary function. In the absence of metal catalysis, polymerization of quinones to neuromelanin is a remarkably slow process with a normal aged brain containing only around 5 mg g^{-1} (Aime et al., 2000). Without an efficient mechanism of quinone removal, these products have greater neurotoxic potential. This is especially the case in human dopaminergic neurons, in light of recent data indicating that dopaminergic neurons derived from fibroblasts of sporadic and familial Parkinson's disease patients contain higher concentrations of DA and oxidation products than similarly-prepared murine cell cultures (Burbulla et al., 2017).

Relevance of Iron and pH to Disease Progression

The rapid formation of both DAC and H_2O_2 may be attributed to the pH-dependent oxidation of DA-bound Fe[II] shown in **Figure 4A**. Variation in pH reflecting transition from a physiologically normal microchemical environment to Parkin-associated mitochondrial dysfunction (Pickrell and Youle, 2015) and *post-mortem* acidosis (Donaldson and Lamont, 2013) had a marked effect on DAC and H_2O_2 production concomitant to pH-dependent oxidation of Fe[II]. The catechol moiety of DA is capable of forming a strong complex with Fe[III] (Avdeef et al., 1978; Sever and Wilker, 2004):

$$\mathrm{Fe[III]} + \mathrm{DA} \rightarrow \mathrm{Fe^{[III]}DA} \quad (16)$$

with the *mono*-complex ($Fe^{[III]}DA$) dominant at acidic pH and the *bis* $Fe^{[III]}DA_2$ complex favored at circumneutral pH (**Supplemental Figure 4**). At pH 6.5, the ratio of $[Fe^{[III]}DA_2]/[Fe^{[III]}DA]$ is $\sim$5 in conditions reflective of otherwise physiologically normal concentrations of Fe and DA. Once formed, radical generation would also occur, increasing potential protein and lipid peroxidation events with the rate of LMCT for $Fe^{[III]}DA$ (0.23 s^{-1}) substantially higher than that for $Fe^{[III]}DA_2$ (7.26×10^{-5} s^{-1}; El-Avaan et al., 1997; Sun et al., 2016). From the rate law

$$\frac{d\,[\mathrm{Fe[II]}]}{dt} = \frac{d\,[\mathrm{DA}^{\bullet -}]}{dt} = k[\mathrm{Fe^{[III]}DA}] \quad (17)$$

continuous generation of DAC at pH 6.5, especially in the presence of Fe[II], was unsurprising. The slightly higher concentrations of DAC formed in the presence of Fe[III], particularly during the initial half of the total reaction time assessed (**Figure 2C**), may be attributed to the more efficient Fe mobilization induced by DA at higher pH.

In contrast to the slower yet continuous generation of H_2O_2 at pH 7.0 and 7.4 (**Figure 3A**), the non-linear formation of DAC at these pHs (**Figure 2B**) suggests that DAC levels are maintained at a steady-state under physiological conditions through rearrangement of DAC and the subsequent formation of indoles or even possibly neuromelanin (**Supplementary Figure 8**). It is reasonable to deduce that the rearrangement of DAC coupled with the ensuing polymerization on increase in pH plays an important role in the removal of DAC.

It should be noted that the presence of metals, such as Fe and calcium (as Ca^{2+}) can also promote this process (Sun et al., 2018a). The model developed adequately describes the generation of reactive oxygen species and accumulation of DAC but comprehensive description of the specific role of Fe in DAC decomposition will require an expanded model. Regardless, the accumulation of protein-modifying DAC is likely to be enhanced at low pHs as a result of the presence of high concentrations of the active Fe[II] catalyst seen in both parkinsonian animal models (Hare et al., 2014; Billings et al., 2016) and the human Parkinson's disease brain (Dexter et al., 1991).

The cessation of H_2O_2 accumulation observed at pH 6.5 (**Figure 3A**) may be related to the high concentration of Fe[II] present in the solution. Under these conditions, the H_2O_2 initially generated as a result of DA-enhanced oxidation of Fe[II] is subsequently consumed *via* peroxidation of the remaining Fe[II]. Apart from the obvious pH-dependent oxidation process, attenuation of Fe[II] oxidation at pH 6.5 (**Figure 4A**), especially during the later stages of the reaction, suggests that Fe[II] may be regenerated under these conditions with the regeneration of Fe[II] related to formation of DA intermediates such as $DA^{\bullet -}$. Given the continuous generation of DAC (**Figure 2B**), the high concentrations of Fe[II] observed may, in turn, result from $DA^{\bullet -}$-induced reduction of ferric iron. Thermodynamically, the low reduction potential of the $DAQ/DA^{\bullet -}$ couple indicates that reduction of aqueous Fe[III] is feasible (Pham and Waite, 2014). Indeed, the rapid reduction of Fe[III] by 6-hydroxydopamine (6-OHDA) semiquinones has been proposed (Jameson and Linert, 2001) with 6-OHDA itself a neurotoxic breakdown product of DA that is facilitated by Fe (Hare and Double, 2016). However, as pH increases, it is expected that the majority of the Fe present would be efficiently converted into AFO and, with a low reduction potential at pH 7.0 (Watt et al., 1985), $DA^{\bullet -}$ is unable to mobilize Fe from AFO. It is of note that neuronal ferritin iron is stored in an AFO-like ferrihydrite core (Hagen et al., 2017) which is prone to mobilization under acidic conditions (La et al., 2017).

Considerations for Analysis of Dopamine Metabolites in *Post-mortem* Tissue

When viewed within the context of existing literature, the results described here present something of a conundrum for those wishing to quantify DAC and related DA oxidation products in human SNc tissue. While acidosis occurring in degenerating neurons may contribute to the progression of Parkinson's disease by increasing the rate of oxidant generation and accumulation of DAC, *post-mortem* decreases in tissue pH, stemming from sample handling, exposure to the environment after removal at autopsy, and even *post-mortem* interval may present inaccurate assessment of DA oxidation.

Considering mitochondrial dysfunction is common to most neurodegenerative diseases (Lin and Beal, 2006), it is not surprising that data supplied from tissue housed in the Sydney Brain Bank, where 72% of cases with a neurodegenerative disease, including pathologically-diagnosed Parkinson's disease, exhibited tissue pH as low as 5.86 (Genoud et al., 2017). Tissue pH that deviates from normal physiology, regardless of whether the cause is endogenous or artifact, will undoubtedly alter the speciation of DA and Fe, and rate of formation, reactivity and fate of toxic DA intermediates (El-Avaan et al., 1997; Pham et al., 2006; Sun et al., 2015, 2016, 2018a). Accordingly, to avoid any misinterpretation of DA metabolites, quantitative assessment of DA metabolism in *post-mortem* tissue should account for multiple confounding factors that influence tissue pH.

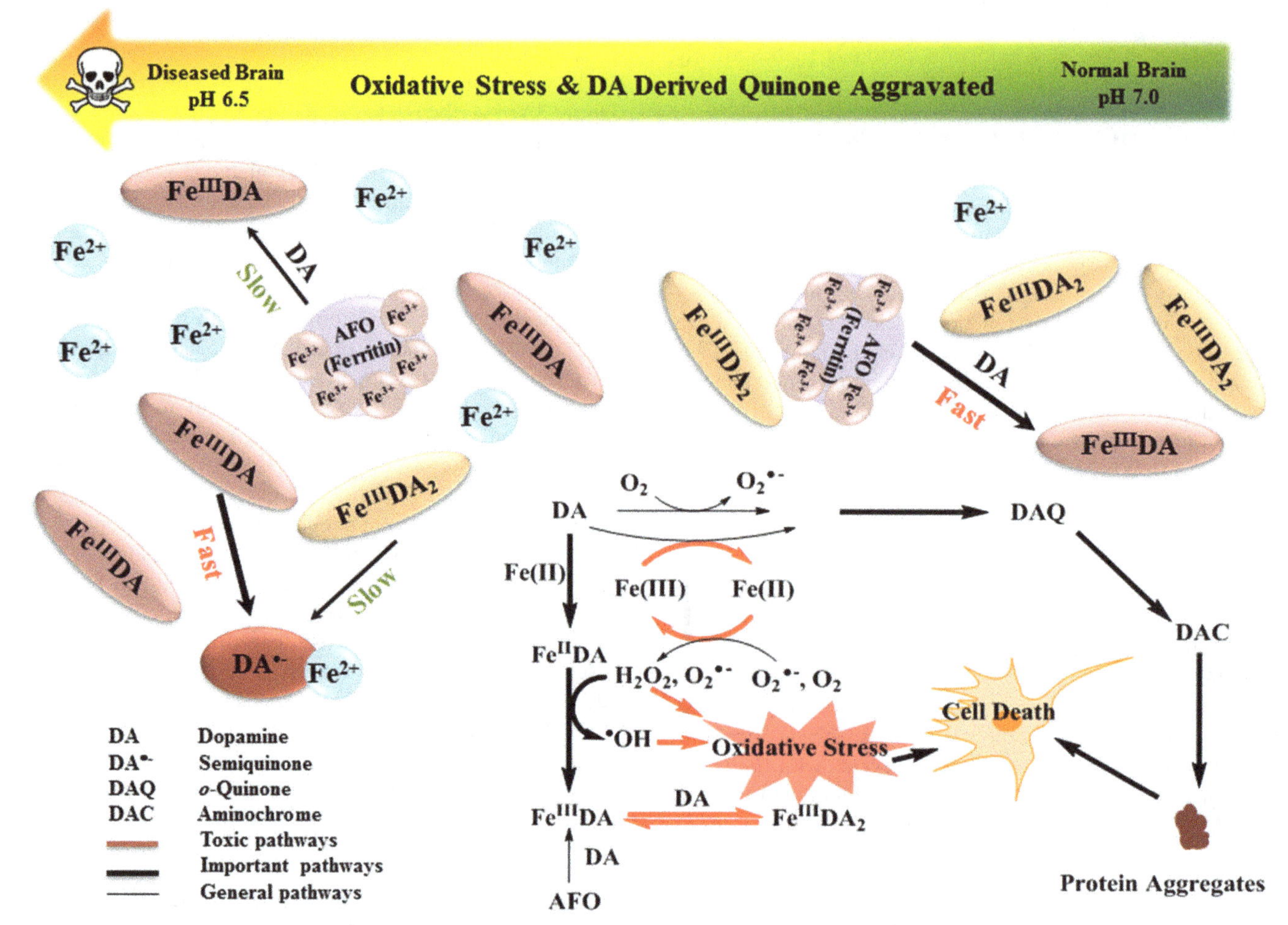

FIGURE 7 | Schematic showing the relative importance of the various reactions involved in the interplay between DA and Fe. Expected changes in key metabolites on decrease in pH are also shown.

CONCLUSIONS

The results of this study indicate that the formation of DA bound Fe[II] and Fe[III] complexes as well as the cyclization and rearrangement of DA-derived quinones are the most important pathways of DA metabolism, with each process heavily dependent on pH. A schematic showing the relative importance of these processes together with expected changes in key metabolites on decrease in pH is presented in **Figure 7**. The presence of Fe can accelerate the oxidation of DA and the accumulation of deleterious protein-modifying DAC with Fe[II] being more efficient in this regard than Fe[III]. Although DAC was slowly formed at pH 6.5, the decrease in the rearrangement rate of this species in acidic conditions resulted in long-term accumulation of DAC. As a result of both the rapid reduction of the unbound-Fe[III] by $DA^{\bullet -}$ and the enhanced LMCT that occurs with the change in the speciation of DA-bound Fe, a substantially higher concentration of Fe[II] was generated at pH 6.5 compared to that at pH 7.0 and 7.4. Even though the presence of both Fe[III] and Fe[II] resulted in increased accumulation of H_2O_2, the enhanced Fe[II] regeneration coupled with the slow rate of oxygenation of Fe[II] at pH 6.5 gave rise to substantially greater potential for the peroxidation of Fe[II] with concomitant enhanced generation of $^{\bullet}OH$. Model predictions indicate that, in the presence of the same concentrations of DA and H_2O_2, acidosis in the Parkinson's disease brain results in an increase in DAC accumulation and DA-mediated production of hydroxyl radicals, with these potential toxicants likely to further aggravate the progression of Parkinson's disease and severity of symptoms arising from DA denervation.

The model developed in this study places emphasis on the purely chemical interactions between Fe and DA and is of particular value in facilitating prediction of the long-term consequences of these interactions by incorporating a range of conditions resulting from the complicated *in vivo* homeostasis of dopaminergic neurons such as continuous DA leakage into the cytosol and increased steady-state concentrations of H_2O_2 as a result of the dysfunctional of antioxidant enzymes. It is also important to view these data within the broader biochemical context of Parkinson's disease neuropathology as a result of the limitations of current techniques. Regardless, the data presented here shows that pH, Fe and H_2O_2 concentrations are intrinsically linked in the rate of formation of neurotoxic DA metabolites.

AUTHOR CONTRIBUTIONS

All the authors were involved in the experiments design. YS conducted the experiments and prepared the manuscript. AP, DH, and TW revised the manuscript. All authors reviewed the results and approved the final version of the manuscript.

ACKNOWLEDGMENTS

The authors would like to acknowledge the Sydney Brain Bank for advice regarding the pH measurements of *post-mortem* brain tissue from patients with neurodegenerative disease. The Sydney Brain Bank is supported by The University of New South Wales and Neuroscience Research Australia. We also gratefully acknowledge the China Scholarship Council and the University of New South Wales for scholarship support to YYS; and the National Health and Medical Research Council's Career Development Fellowship (Industry) support to DJH (GNT1122981). Supplementary data associated with this article can be found in the online version.

REFERENCES

Acosta-Cabronero, J., Betts, M. J., Cardenas-Blanco, A., Yang, S., and Nestor, P. J. (2016). *In vivo* MRI mapping of brain iron deposition across the adult lifespan. *J. Neurosci.* 36, 364–374. doi: 10.1523/JNEUROSCI.1907-15.2016

Adams, J. D., and Odunze, I. N. (1991). Oxygen free radicals and Parkinson's disease. *Free Radic. Biol. Med.* 10, 161–169. doi: 10.1016/0891-5849(91)90009-R

Adam-Vizi, V. (2005). Production of reactive oxygen species in brain mitochondria: contribution by electron transport chain and non-electron transport chain sources. *Antioxid. Redox Signal.* 7, 1140–1149. doi: 10.1089/ars.2005.7.1140

Aime, S., Bergamasco, B., Casu, M., Digilio, G., Fasano, M., Giraudo, S., et al. (2000). Isolation and 13C-NMR characterization of an insoluble proteinaceous fraction from substantia nigra of patients with parkinson's disease. *Mov. Disord.* 15, 977–981. doi: 10.1002/1531-8257(200009)15:5<977::AID-MDS1032>3.0.CO;2-Q

Avdeef, A., Sofen, S. R., Bregante, T. L., and Raymond, K. N. (1978). Coordination chemistry of microbial iron transport compounds. 9. stability constants for catechol models of enterobactin. *J. Am. Chem. Soc.* 100, 5362–5370. doi: 10.1021/ja00485a018

Ayton, S., and Lei, P. (2014). Nigral iron elevation is an invariable feature of Parkinson's disease and is a sufficient cause of neurodegeneration. *Biomed. Res. Int.* 2014, 1–9. doi: 10.1155/2014/581256

Bader, H., Sturzenegger, V., and Hoigne, J. (1988). Photometric method for the determination of low concentrations of hydrogen peroxide by the peroxidase catalyzed oxidation of N, N-diethyl-*p*-phenylenediamine (DPD). *Water Res.* 22, 1109–1115. doi: 10.1016/0043-1354(88)90005-X

Balut, C., Vandeven, M., Despa, S., Lambrichts, I., Ameloot, M., Steels, P., et al. (2008). Measurement of cytosolic and mitochondrial pH in living cells during reversible metabolic inhibition. *Kidney Int.* 73, 226–232. doi: 10.1038/sj.ki.5002632

Berg, D., Postuma, R. B., Adler, C. H., Bloem, B. R., Chan, P., Dubois, B., et al. (2015). MDS research criteria for prodromal Parkinson's disease. *Mov. Disord.* 30, 1600–1611. doi: 10.1002/mds.26431

Berman, S. B., and Hastings, T. G. (1999). Dopamine oxidation alters mitochondrial respiration and induces permeability transition in brain mitochondria. *J. Neurochem.* 73, 1127–1137. doi: 10.1046/j.1471-4159.1999.0731127.x

Bianco, C. L., Ridet, J., Schneider, B., Deglon, N., and Aebischer, P. (2002). α-Synucleinopathy and selective dopaminergic neuron loss in a rat lentiviral-based model of Parkinson's disease. *Proc. Natl. Acad. Sci. U.S.A.* 99, 10813–10818. doi: 10.1073/pnas.152339799

Billings, J. L., Hare, D. J., Nurjono, M., Volitakis, I., Cherny, R. A., Bush, A. I., et al. (2016). Effects of neonatal iron feeding and chronic clioquinol administration on the Parkinsonian human A53T transgenic mouse. *ACS Chem. Neurosci.* 7, 360–366. doi: 10.1021/acschemneuro.5b00305

Blesa, J., Trigo-Damas, I., Quiroga-Varela, A., and Jackson-Lewis, V. R. (2015). Oxidative stress and Parkinson's disease. *Front. Neuroanat.* 9:91. doi: 10.3389/fnana.2015.00091

Blesa, M. A., and Matijevi,ć, E. (1989). Phase transformations of iron oxides, oxohydroxides, and hydrous oxides in aqueous media. *Adv. Colloid Interface Sci.* 29, 173–221. doi: 10.1016/0001-8686(89)80009-0

Borovansky, J., Edge, R., Land, E. J., Navaratnam, S., Pavel, S., Ramsden, C. A., et al. (2006). Mechanistic studies of melanogenesis: the influence of *N*-substitution on dopamine quinone cyclization. *Pigment Cell Res.* 19, 170–178. doi: 10.1111/j.1600-0749.2006.00295.x

Brand, M. D., and Nicholls, D. G. (2011). Assessing mitochondrial dysfunction in cells. *Biochem. J.* 435, 297–312. doi: 10.1042/BJ20110162

Burbulla, L. F., Song, P., Mazzulli, J. R., Zampese, E., Wong, Y. C., Jeon, S., et al. (2017). Dopamine oxidation mediates mitochondrial and lysosomal dysfunction in Parkinson's disease. *Science* 357, 1255–1261. doi: 10.1126/science.aam9080

Cardoso, B., Hare, D., Bush, A., and Roberts, B. (2017). Glutathione peroxidase 4: a new player in neurodegeneration? *Mol. Psychiatry* 22, 328–335. doi: 10.1038/mp.2016.196

Conway, K. A., Rochet, J.-C., Bieganski, R. M., and Lansbury, P. T. (2001). Kinetic stabilization of the α-synuclein protofibril by a dopamine-α-synuclein adduct. *Science* 294, 1346–1349. doi: 10.1126/science.1063522

Devos, D., Moreau, C., Devedjian, J., Kluza, J., Petrault, M., Laloux, C., et al. (2014). Targeting chelatable iron as a therapeutic modality in Parkinson's disease. *Antioxid. Redox Signal.* 21, 195–210. doi: 10.1089/ars.2013.5593

Dexter, D. T., Carayon, A., Javoy-Agid, F., Agid, Y., Wells, F. R., Daniel, S. E., et al. (1991). Alterations in the levels of iron, ferritin and other trace metals in Parkinson's disease and other neurodegenerative diseases affecting the basal ganglia. *Brain* 114, 1953–1975. doi: 10.1093/brain/114.4.1953

Dixon, S. J., and Stockwell, B. R. (2014). The role of iron and reactive oxygen species in cell death. *Nat. Chem. Biol.* 10, 9–17. doi: 10.1038/nchembio.1416

Donaldson, A. E., and Lamont, I. L. (2013). Biochemistry changes that occur after death: potential markers for determining post-mortem interval. *PLoS ONE* 8:e82011. doi: 10.1371/journal.pone.0082011

Double, K., Ben-Shachar, D., Youdim, M., Zecca, L., Riederer, P., and Gerlach, M. (2002). Influence of neuromelanin on oxidative pathways within the human substantia nigra. *Neurotoxicol. Teratol.* 24, 621–628. doi: 10.1016/S0892-0362(02)00218-0

El-Avaan, U., Herlinger, E., Jameson, R., and Linert, W. (1997). Anaerobic oxidation of dopamine by iron(III). *J. Chem. Soc. Dalton Trans.* 16, 2813–2818. doi: 10.1039/a701054k

Friedlich, A. L., Tanzi, R. E., and Rogers, J. T. (2007). The 5′-untranslated region of Parkinson's disease α-synuclein messengerRNA contains a predicted iron responsive element. *Mol. Psychiatry* 12, 222–223. doi: 10.1038/sj.mp.4001937

Garg, S., Ito, H., Rose, A. L., and Waite, T. D. (2013). Mechanism and kinetics of dark iron redox transformations in previously photolyzed acidic natural organic matter solutions. *Environ. Sci. Technol.* 47, 1861–1869. doi: 10.1021/es3035889

Gautier, C. A., Kitada, T., and Shen, J. (2008). Loss of PINK1 causes mitochondrial functional defects and increased sensitivity to oxidative stress. *Proc. Natl. Acad. Sci. U.S.A.* 105, 11364–11369. doi: 10.1073/pnas.0802076105

Genoud, S., Roberts, B. R., Gunn, A. P., Halliday, G. M., Lewis, S. J., Ball, H. J., et al. (2017). Subcellular compartmentalisation of copper, iron, manganese, and zinc in the Parkinson's disease brain. *Metallomics* 9, 1447–1455. doi: 10.1039/C7MT00244K

González-Davila, M., Santana-Casiano, J. M., and Millero, F. J. (2005). Oxidation of iron (II) nanomolar with H_2O_2 in seawater. *Geochim. Cosmochim. Acta* 69, 83–93. doi: 10.1016/j.gca.2004.05.043

Graham, D. G. (1978). Oxidative pathways for catecholamines in the genesis of neuromelanin and cytotoxic quinones. *Mol. Pharmacol.* 14, 633–643.

Graham, D. G., Tiffany, S. M., Bell, W. R., and Gutknecht, W. F. (1978). Autoxidation versus covalent binding of quinones as the mechanism of toxicity of dopamine, 6-hydroxydopamine, and related compounds toward C1300 neuroblastoma cells *in vitro*. *Mol. Pharmacol.* 14, 644–653.

Gustafsson, J. P. (2005). *Visual MINTEQ 3.0 User Guide*. Department of Land and Water Resources, KTH Royal Institute of Technolology, Stockhom.

Guttmacher, A. E., Collins, F. S., Nussbaum, R. L., and Ellis, C. E. (2003). Alzheimer's Disease and Parkinson's Disease. *N. Engl. J. Med.* 348, 1356–1364. doi: 10.1056/NEJM2003ra020003

Hagen, W. R., Hagedoorn, P., and Ebrahimi, K. (2017). The workings of ferritin: a crossroad of opinions. *Metallomics* 9, 595–605. doi: 10.1039/C7MT00124J

Halliwell, B., and Gutteridge, J. (1984). Oxygen toxicity, oxygen radicals, transition metals and disease. *Biochem. J.* 219:1. doi: 10.1042/bj2190001

Haque, E. M., Asanuma, M., Higashi, Y., Miyazaki, I., Tanaka, K.-I., and Ogawa, N. (2003). Apoptosis-inducing neurotoxicity of dopamine and its metabolites via reactive quinone generation in neuroblastoma cells. *Biochim. Biophys. Acta* 1619, 39–52. doi: 10.1016/S0304-4165(02)00440-3

Hardy, J., Wester, P., Winblad, B., Gezelius, C., Bring, G., and Eriksson, A. (1985). The patients dying after long terminal phase have acidotic brains; implications for biochemical measurements on autopsy tissue. *J. Neural Transm.* 61, 253–264. doi: 10.1007/BF01251916

Hare, D., Ayton, S., Bush, A., and Lei, P. (2013). A delicate balance: iron metabolism and diseases of the brain. *Front. Aging Neurosci.* 5:34. doi: 10.3389/fnagi.2013.00034

Hare, D. J., Arora, M., Jenkins, N. L., Finkelstein, D. I., Doble, P. A., and Bush, A. I. (2015). Is early-life iron exposure critical in neurodegeneration? *Nat. Rev. Neurol.* 11, 536–544. doi: 10.1038/nrneurol.2015.100

Hare, D. J., and Double, K. L. (2016). Iron and dopamine: a toxic couple. *Brain* 139, 1026–1035. doi: 10.1093/brain/aww022

Hare, D. J., Gerlach, M., and Riederer, P. (2012). Considerations for measuring iron in post-mortem tissue of Parkinson's disease patients. *J. Neural Transm.* 119, 1515–1521. doi: 10.1007/s00702-012-0898-4

Hare, D. J., Lei, P., Ayton, S., Roberts, B. R., Grimm, R., George, J. L., et al. (2014). An iron–dopamine index predicts risk of parkinsonian neurodegeneration in the substantia nigra pars compacta. *Chem. Sci.* 5, 2160–2169. doi: 10.1039/C3SC53461H

Harrison, F. E., and May, J. M. (2009). Vitamin C function in the brain: vital role of the ascorbate transporter SVCT2. *Free Radic. Biol. Med.* 46, 719–730. doi: 10.1016/j.freeradbiomed.2008.12.018

Harrison, P., Heath, P., Eastwood, S., Burnet, P., Mcdonald, B., and Pearson, R. (1995). The relative importance of premortem acidosis and postmortem interval for human brain gene expression studies: selective mRNA vulnerability and comparison with their encoded proteins. *Neurosci. Lett.* 200, 151–154. doi: 10.1016/0304-3940(95)12102-A

Hawley, M., Tatawawadi, S., Piekarski, S., and Adams, R. (1967). Electrochemical studies of the oxidation pathways of catecholamines. *J. Am. Chem. Soc.* 89, 447–450. doi: 10.1021/ja00978a051

He, N., Ling, H., Ding, B., Huang, J., Zhang, Y., Zhang, Z., et al. (2015). Region-specific disturbed iron distribution in early idiopathic Parkinson's disease measured by quantitative susceptibility mapping. *Hum. Brain Mapp.* 36, 4407–4420. doi: 10.1002/hbm.22928

Herlinger, E., Jameson, R. F., and Linert, W. (1995). Spontaneous autoxidation of dopamine. *J. Chem. Soc. Perkin Trans.* 2, 259–263. doi: 10.1039/p29950000259

Hermida-Ameijeiras, Á., Méndez-Álvarez, E. A., Sánchez-Iglesias, S. A., SanmartiN-Suárez, C., and Soto-Otero, R. (2004). Autoxidation and MAO-mediated metabolism of dopamine as a potential cause of oxidative stress: role of ferrous and ferric ions. *Neurochem. Int.* 45, 103–116. doi: 10.1016/j.neuint.2003.11.018

Herrera, A., Muñoz, P., Paris, I., Díaz-Veliz, G., Mora, S., Inzunza, J., et al. (2016). Aminochrome induces dopaminergic neuronal dysfunction: a new animal model for Parkinson's disease. *Cell. Mol. Life Sci.* 73, 3583–3597. doi: 10.1007/s00018-016-2182-5

Ianni, J. C. (2003). "A comparison of the Bader-Deuflhard and the Cash-Karp Runge-Kutta integrators for the GRI-MECH 3.0 model based on the chemical kinetics code Kintecus," in *Proceedings Second MIT Conference on Computational Fluid and Sold Mechanics,* ed K. J. Bathe (Cambridge, MA), 1368–1372.

Il'ichev, Y. V., and Simon, J. D. (2003). Building blocks of eumelanin: relative stability and excitation energies of tautomers of 5, 6-dihydroxyindole and 5, 6-indolequinone. *J. Phys. Chem. B* 107, 7162–7171. doi: 10.1021/jp034702x

Jameson, G. N., and Linert, W. (2001). The oxidation of 6-hydroxydopamine in aqueous solution. Part 3. 12 Kinetics and mechanism of the oxidation with iron (III). *J. Chem. Soc. Perkin Trans.* 4, 569–575. doi: 10.1039/B007203F

Jian, N., Dowle, M., Horniblow, R. D., Tselepis, C., and Palmer, R. E. (2016). Morphology of the ferritin iron core by aberration corrected scanning transmission electron microscopy. *Nanotechnology* 27:46LT02. doi: 10.1088/0957-4484/27/46/46LT02

Jiang, D., Shi, S., Zhang, L., Liu, L., Ding, B., Zhao, B., et al. (2013). Inhibition of the Fe(III)-catalyzed dopamine oxidation by ATP and its relevance to oxidative stress in Parkinson's disease. *ACS Chem. Neurosci.* 4, 1305–1313. doi: 10.1021/cn400105d

Johnson, K. A., Simpson, Z. B., and Blom, T. (2009). Global kinetic explorer: a new computer program for dynamic simulation and fitting of kinetic data. *Anal. Biochem.* 387, 20–29. doi: 10.1016/j.ab.2008.12.024

Koppenol, W., and Butler, J. (1985). Energetics of interconversion reactions of oxyradicals. *Adv. Free Radic. Biol. Med.* 1, 91–131. doi: 10.1016/8755-9668(85)90005-5

Kordower, J. H., Olanow, W. C., Dodiya, H. B., Chu, Y., Beach, T. G., Adler, C. H., et al. (2013). Disease duration and the integrity of the nigrostriatal system in Parkinson's disease. *Brain* 136, 2419–2431. doi: 10.1093/brain/awt192

Kowalchyk, W. K., Davis, K. L., and Morris, M. D. (1995). Surface-enhanced resonance Raman spectroscopy of iron-dopamine complexes. *Spectrochim. Acta Part A Mol. Biomol. Spectroscopy* 51, 145–151. doi: 10.1016/0584-8539(94)00153-3

La, A., Nguyen, T., Tran, K., Sauble, E., Tu, D., Gonzalez, A., et al. (2017). Mobilization of iron from ferritin: new steps and details. *Metallomics* 10, 154–168. doi: 10.1039/C7MT00284J

Land, E., Ito, S., Wakamatsu, K., and Riley, P. (2003). Rate constants for the first two chemical steps of eumelanogenesis. *Pigment Cell Res.* 16, 487–493. doi: 10.1034/j.1600-0749.2003.00082.x

Lhermitte, J., Kraus, W. M., and Mcalpine, D. (1924). Original papers: on the occurrence of abnormal deposits of iron in the brain in parkinsonism with special reference to its localisation. *J. Neurol. Psychopathol.* 5:195. doi: 10.1136/jnnp.s1-5.19.195

Li, W., Wu, B., Batrachenko, A., Bancroft-Wu, V., Morey, R. A., Shashi, V., et al. (2014). Differential developmental trajectories of magnetic susceptibility in human brain gray and white matter over the lifespan. *Hum. Brain Mapp.* 35, 2698–2713. doi: 10.1002/hbm.22360

Lin, M. T., and Beal, M. F. (2006). Mitochondrial dysfunction and oxidative stress in neurodegenerative diseases. *Nature* 443, 787–795. doi: 10.1038/nature05292

Lotharius, J., and Brundin, P. (2002a). Impaired dopamine storage resulting from α-synuclein mutations may contribute to the pathogenesis of Parkinson's disease. *Hum. Mol. Genet.* 11, 2395–2407. doi: 10.1093/hmg/11.20.2395

Lotharius, J., and Brundin, P. (2002b). Pathogenesis of Parkinson's disease: dopamine, vesicles and α-synuclein. *Nat. Rev. Neurosci.* 3, 932–942. doi: 10.1038/nrn983

Ludwig, C., Casey, W. H., and Rock, P. A. (1995). Prediction of ligand-promoted dissolution rates from the reactivities of aqueous complexes. *Nature* 375, 44–47. doi: 10.1038/375044a0

Martin-Bastida, A., Ward, R. J., Newbould, R., Piccini, P., Sharp, D., Kabba, C., et al. (2017). Brain iron chelation by deferiprone in a phase 2 randomised double-blinded placebo controlled clinical trial in Parkinson's disease. *Sci. Rep.* 7:1398. doi: 10.1038/s41598-017-01402-2

Miller, D. M., Buettner, G. R., and Aust, S. D. (1990). Transition metals as catalysts of "autoxidation" reactions. *Free Radic. Biol. Med.* 8, 95–108.

Monoranu, C. M., Apfelbacher, M., Grünblatt, E., Puppe, B., Alafuzoff, I., Ferrer, I., et al. (2009). pH measurement as quality control on human post mortem brain tissue: a study of the BrainNet Europe consortium. *Neuropathol. Appl. Neurobiol.* 35, 329–337. doi: 10.1111/j.1365-2990.2008.01003a.x

Moos, T., Nielsen, T., Skjørringe, T., and Morgan, E. H. (2007). Iron trafficking inside the brain. *J. Neurochem.* 103, 1730–1740. doi: 10.1111/j.1471-4159.2007.04976.x

Moreau, C., Duce, J. A., Rascol, O., Devedjian, J. C., Berg, D., Dexter, D., et al. (2018). Iron as a therapeutic target for Parkinson's disease. *Mov. Disord.* 33, 568–574. doi: 10.1002/mds.27275

Mosharov, E. V., Larsen, K. E., Kanter, E., Phillips, K. A., Wilson, K., Schmitz, Y., et al. (2009). Interplay between cytosolic dopamine, calcium, and α-synuclein causes selective death of substantia nigra neurons. *Neuron* 62, 218–229. doi: 10.1016/j.neuron.2009.01.033

Ndubuizu, O., and Lamanna, J. C. (2007). Brain tissue oxygen concentration measurements. *Antioxid. Redox Signal.* 9, 1207–1220. doi: 10.1089/ars.2007.1634

New, E. J., Wimmer, V. C., and Hare, D. J. (2018). Promises and Pitfalls of Metal Imaging in Biology. *Cell Chem. Biol.* 25, 7–18. doi: 10.1016/j.chembiol.2017.10.006

Norris, E. H., Giasson, B. I., Hodara, R., Xu, S., Trojanowski, J. Q., Ischiropoulos, H., et al. (2005). Reversible inhibition of α-synuclein fibrillization by dopaminochrome-mediated conformational alterations. *J. Biol. Chem.* 280, 21212–21219. doi: 10.1074/jbc.M412621200

Panicker, N., Saminathan, H., Jin, H., Neal, M., Harischandra, D. S., Gordon, R., et al. (2015). Fyn kinase regulates microglial neuroinflammatory responses in cell culture and animal models of Parkinson's disease. *J. Neurosci.* 35, 10058–10077. doi: 10.1523/JNEUROSCI.0302-15.2015

Pezzella, A., D'ischia, M., Napolitano, A., Misuraca, G., and Prota, G. (1997). Iron-mediated generation of the neurotoxin 6-hydroxydopamine quinone by reaction of fatty acid hydroperoxides with dopamine: a possible contributory mechanism for neuronal degeneration in Parkinson's disease. *J. Med. Chem.* 40, 2211–2216. doi: 10.1021/jm970099t

Pham, A. N., Rose, A. L., Feitz, A. J., and Waite, T. D. (2006). Kinetics of Fe(III) precipitation in aqueous solutions at pH 6.0–9.5 and 25°C. *Geochim. Cosmochim. Acta* 70, 640–650. doi: 10.1016/j.gca.2005.10.018

Pham, A. N., and Waite, T. D. (2014). Cu (II)-catalyzed oxidation of dopamine in aqueous solutions: mechanism and kinetics. *J. Inorg. Biochem.* 137, 74–84. doi: 10.1016/j.jinorgbio.2014.03.018

Phebus, L. A., Perry, K. W., Clemens, J. A., and Fuller, R. W. (1986). Brain anoxia releases striatal dopamine in rats. *Life Sci.* 38, 2447–2453. doi: 10.1016/0024-3205(86)90615-6

Pickrell, A. M., and Youle, R. J. (2015). The roles of PINK1, parkin, and mitochondrial fidelity in Parkinson's disease. *Neuron* 85, 257–273. doi: 10.1016/j.neuron.2014.12.007

Rose, A. L., and Waite, T. D. (2003). Effect of dissolved natural organic matter on the kinetics of ferrous iron oxygenation in seawater. *Environ. Sci. Technol.* 37, 4877–4886. doi: 10.1021/es034152g

Rush, J. D., and Bielski, B. (1985). Pulse radiolytic studies of the reactions of HO_2/O_2^- with Fe(II)/Fe(III) ions. the reactivity of HO_2/O_2^- with ferric ions and its implication on the occurrence of the Haber-Weiss reaction. *J. Phys. Chem.* 89, 5062–5066. doi: 10.1021/j100269a035

Sampson, T. R., Debelius, J. W., Thron, T., Janssen, S., Shastri, G. G., Ilhan, Z. E., et al. (2016). Gut microbiota regulate motor deficits and neuroinflammation in a model of Parkinson's disease. *Cell* 167, 1469–1480.e1412. doi: 10.1016/j.cell.2016.11.018

Schapira, A.H. V. (1994). Evidence for mitochondrial dysfunction in Parkinson's disease—a critical appraisal. *Mov. Disord.* 9, 125–138. doi: 10.1002/mds.870090202

Segura-Aguilar, J., and Huenchuguala, S. (2018). Aminochrome induces irreversible mitochondrial dysfunction by inducing autophagy dysfunction in Parkinson's disease. *Front. Neurosci.* 12:106. doi: 10.3389/fnins.2018.00106

Segura-Aguilar, J., and Lind, C. (1989). On the mechanism of the Mn 3+-induced neurotoxicity of dopamine: prevention of quinone-derived oxygen toxicity by DT diaphorase and superoxide dismutase. *Chem. Biol. Interact.* 72, 309–324. doi: 10.1016/0009-2797(89)90006-9

Segura-Aguilar, J., Paris, I., Muñoz, P., Ferrari, E., Zecca, L., and Zucca, F. A. (2014). Protective and toxic roles of dopamine in Parkinson's disease. *J. Neurochem.* 129, 898–915. doi: 10.1111/jnc.12686

Sever, M. J., and Wilker, J. J. (2004). Visible absorption spectra of metal–catecholate and metal–tironate complexes. *Dalton Trans.* 2004, 1061–1072. doi: 10.1039/B315811J

Solano, F., Hearing, V. J., and García-Borrón, J. C. (1999). Neurotoxicity due to o-Quinones: neuromelanin formation and possible mechanisms for o-Quinone detoxification. *Neurotox. Res.* 1, 153–169. doi: 10.1007/BF03033287

Stokes, A. H., Hastings, T. G., and Vrana, K. E. (1999). Cytotoxic and genotoxic potential of dopamine. *J. Neurosci. Res.* 55, 659–665. doi: 10.1002/(SICI)1097-4547(19990315)55:6<659::AID-JNR1>3.0.CO;2-C

Sun, Y., Pham, A. N., and Waite, T. D. (2015). Effect of chloride driven copper redox cycling on the kinetics of Fe(II) oxidation in aqueous solutions at pH 6.5–8.0. *Geochim. Cosmochim. Acta* 161, 118–127. doi: 10.1016/j.gca.2015.03.035

Sun, Y., Pham, A. N., and Waite, T. D. (2016). Elucidation of the interplay between Fe(II), Fe(III), and dopamine with relevance to iron solubilization and reactive oxygen species generation by catecholamines. *J. Neurochem.* 137, 955–968. doi: 10.1111/jnc.13615

Sun, Y., Pham, A. N., and Waite, T. D. (2018a). Effect of release of dopamine on iron transformations and reactive oxygen species (ROS) generation under conditions typical of coastal waters. *Environ. Sci.* 20, 232–244. doi: 10.1039/C7EM00497D

Sun, Y., Pham, A. N., and Waite, T. D. (2018b). The effect of vitamin C and iron on dopamine-mediated free radical generation: implications to Parkinson's disease. *Dalton Trans.* 47, 4059–4069. doi: 10.1039/C7DT04373B

Sun, Y., Pham, A. N., and Waite, T. D. (2018c). Mechanism underlying the effectiveness of deferiprone in alleviating Parkinson's disease symptoms. *ACS Chem. Neurosci.* 9, 1118–1127. doi: 10.1021/acschemneuro.7b00478

Surmeier, J. D., Obeso, J. A., and Halliday, G. M. (2017). Selective neuronal vulnerability in Parkinson disease. *Nat. Rev. Neurosci.* 18, 101–113. doi: 10.1038/nrn.2016.178

Thiel, T., Liczkowski, L., and Bissen, S. T. (1998). New zwitterionic butanesulfonic acids that extend the alkaline range of four families of good buffers: evaluation for use in biological systems. *J. Biochem. Biophys. Methods* 37, 117–129. doi: 10.1016/S0165-022X(98)00022-0

Trist, B., Davies, K., Cottam, V., Genoud, S., Ortega, R., Roudeau, S., et al. (2017). Amyotrophic lateral sclerosis-like superoxide dismutase 1 proteinopathy is associated with neuronal loss in Parkinson's disease brain. *Acta Neuropathol.* 134, 113–127. doi: 10.1007/s00401-017-1726-6

Trist, B., Hare, D., and Double, K. (2018). A proposed mechanism for neurodegeneration in movement disorders characterized by metal dyshomeostasis and oxidative stress. *Cell Chem. Biol.* 25, 807–816. doi: 10.1016/j.chembiol.2018.05.004.

Voelker, B. M., and Sulzberger, B. (1996). Effects of fulvic acid on Fe (II) oxidation by hydrogen peroxide. *Environ. Sci. Technol.* 30, 1106–1114. doi: 10.1021/es9502132

Wallis, L. I., Paley, M., Graham, J. M., Grünewald, R. A., Wignall, E. L., Joy, H. M., et al. (2008). MRI assessment of basal ganglia iron deposition in Parkinson's disease. *J. Magnet. Resonance Imaging* 28, 1061–1067. doi: 10.1002/jmri.21563

Wang, J.-Y., Zhuang, Q.-Q., Zhu, L.-B., Zhu, H., Li, T., Li, R., et al. (2016). Meta-analysis of brain iron levels of Parkinson's disease patients determined by postmortem and MRI measurements. *Sci. Rep.* 6:36669. doi: 10.1038/srep36669

Ward, R. J., Zucca, F. A., Duyn, J. H., Crichton, R. R., and Zecca, L. (2014). The role of iron in brain ageing and neurodegenerative disorders. *Lancet Neurol.* 13, 1045–1060. doi: 10.1016/S1474-4422(14)70117-6

Watt, G., Frankel, R. B., and Papaefthymiou, G. (1985). Reduction of mammalian ferritin. *Proc. Natl. Acad. Sci. U.S.A.* 82, 3640–3643. doi: 10.1073/pnas.82.11.3640

Yates, C. M., Butterworth, J., Tennant, M. C., and Gordon, A. (1990). Enzyme activities in relation to pH and lactate in postmortem brain in Alzheimer-type and other dementias. *J. Neurochem.* 55, 1624–1630. doi: 10.1111/j.1471-4159.1990.tb04948.x

Yu, Q., Kandegedara, A., Xu, Y., and Rorabacher, D. (1997). Avoiding interferences from Good's buffers: a contiguous series of noncomplexing tertiary amine buffers covering the entire range of pH 3–11. *Anal. Biochem.* 253, 50–56. doi: 10.1006/abio.1997.2349

Zafiriou, O. C. (1990). Chemistry of superoxide ion-radical (O_2^-) in seawater. I. pK*aswb (HOO) and uncatalyzed dismutation kinetics studied by pulse radiolysis. *Mar. Chem.* 30, 31–43. doi: 10.1016/0304-4203(90)90060-P

Zecca, L., Youdim, M. B., Riederer, P., Connor, J. R., and Crichton, R. R. (2004). Iron, brain ageing and neurodegenerative disorders. *Nat. Rev. Neurosci.* 5, 863–873. doi: 10.1038/nrn1537

Zhang, L., Yagnik, G., Jiang, D., Shi, S., Chang, P., and Zhou, F. (2012). Separation of intermediates of iron-catalyzed dopamine oxidation reactions using reversed-phase ion-pairing chromatography coupled in tandem with UV–visible and ESI-MS detections. *J. Chromatogr. B* 911, 55–58. doi: 10.1016/j.jchromb.2012.10.026

2

The Involvement of Iron in Traumatic Brain Injury and Neurodegenerative Disease

*Maria Daglas and Paul A. Adlard**

The Florey Institute of Neuroscience and Mental Health, The University of Melbourne, Parkville, VIC, Australia

***Correspondence:**
Paul A. Adlard
paul.adlard@florey.edu.au;
padlard@unimelb.edu.au

Traumatic brain injury (TBI) consists of acute and long-term pathophysiological sequelae that ultimately lead to cognitive and motor function deficits, with age being a critical risk factor for poorer prognosis. TBI has been recently linked to the development of neurodegenerative diseases later in life including Alzheimer's disease, Parkinson's disease, chronic traumatic encephalopathy, and multiple sclerosis. The accumulation of iron in the brain has been documented in a number of neurodegenerative diseases, and also in normal aging, and can contribute to neurotoxicity through a variety of mechanisms including the production of free radicals leading to oxidative stress, excitotoxicity and by promoting inflammatory reactions. A growing body of evidence similarly supports a deleterious role of iron in the pathogenesis of TBI. Iron deposition in the injured brain can occur via hemorrhage/microhemorrhages (heme-bound iron) or independently as labile iron (non-heme bound), which is considered to be more damaging to the brain. This review focusses on the role of iron in potentiating neurodegeneration in TBI, with insight into the intersection with neurodegenerative conditions. An important implication of this work is the potential for therapeutic approaches that target iron to attenuate the neuropathology/phenotype related to TBI and to also reduce the associated risk of developing neurodegenerative disease.

Keywords: iron, metals, traumatic brain injury, neurodegeneration, oxidative stress, inflammation

INTRODUCTION

Traumatic brain injury (TBI) is a leading cause of death and disability worldwide, particularly amongst young adults. Ten million individuals are affected by TBI annually, costing a staggering $9–10 billion/year (Gardner et al., 2017). The aged population have a greater risk of sustaining a TBI, with frequent falls being the major cause of injury, and they also have worse outcomes post-injury compared to other age groups (Stocchetti et al., 2012). Aging is also accompanied by a number of co-morbidities which may contribute to poorer outcomes in these individuals following TBI (Stocchetti et al., 2012). Common secondary events that follow the primary impact are neuronal cell death, oxidative stress, brain oedema, blood-brain barrier (BBB) breakdown, and inflammation (Toklu and Tumer, 2015). TBI often results in debilitating long-term cognitive and motor impairments, and there are currently no approved treatments available for TBI patients (Bramlett and Dietrich, 2015). This highlights the need for therapeutic agents that can alleviate brain damage and the deficits caused by the primary injury and more specifically the reversible secondary pathologies that develop after TBI.

Iron homeostasis appears to be an important process in the pathobiology of TBI. Iron is essential for normal brain functioning where it acts as an essential cofactor for several enzymatic/cellular processes (Ke and Qian, 2007). However, impaired regulation of iron can result in the production of reactive oxygen species (ROS) and the consequent promotion of oxidative stress, which can wreak havoc on an already compromised brain in the context of TBI (Nunez et al., 2012). Interestingly, the accumulation of iron in various tissues and cells in the body and brain is an inevitable consequence of aging (Hagemeier et al., 2012; Del et al., 2015). A concomitant increase in the iron storage protein (i.e., ferritin), which can scavenge any excess iron and prevent undesired production of ROS, is also evident with aging (Andersen et al., 2014). However, failed or weakened antioxidant defenses and mitochondrial dysfunction that progresses with aging can disrupt the balance and allow for excessive iron to be released (Venkateshappa et al., 2012a,b; Andersen et al., 2014). This can cause pathological iron overload resulting in cellular damage that is considered to be a contributing factor in several degenerative diseases that are more prevalent with age, such as cancer, liver fibrosis, cardiovascular disease, diabetes (type II), and particularly neurological conditions such as Alzheimer's disease (AD) (Smith et al., 1997; Kalinowski and Richardson, 2005; Ward et al., 2014; Hare et al., 2016). Abnormal brain iron deposition has also been discovered in other neurodegenerative diseases, such as Parkinson's disease (PD) (Griffiths et al., 1999; Zhang et al., 2010; Barbosa et al., 2015), multiple sclerosis (MS) (Bergsland et al., 2017), amyotrophic lateral sclerosis (ALS) (Oshiro et al., 2011), Huntington's disease (Agrawal et al., 2018), and Friedreich's ataxia (Martelli and Puccio, 2014), and there is now increasing evidence of altered iron levels in TBI patients (Raz et al., 2011; Lu et al., 2015). This raises the interesting proposition of an intersection between aging, iron, TBI and neurodegenerative disease. Whilst the role of iron in TBI is not well known, the literature suggests that the levels of iron (and other metals such as zinc) are abnormally regulated following injury, and that the pharmacological targeting (e.g., using chelators or chaperones) of these metals may be beneficial in improving outcomes. Iron chelation therapy has been approved for decades for the treatment of iron overload conditions, and there is a recent heightened interest for their use in neurodegenerative diseases (Kalinowski and Richardson, 2005; Dusek et al., 2016). Here, we review the role of iron dyshomeostasis in TBI and gain a deeper understanding of its involvement in neurodegeneration as well as neuroinflammation (**Figure 1**). We further examine the potential benefit of utilizing iron chelation therapy with the hope of limiting iron-induced neurotoxicity in TBI.

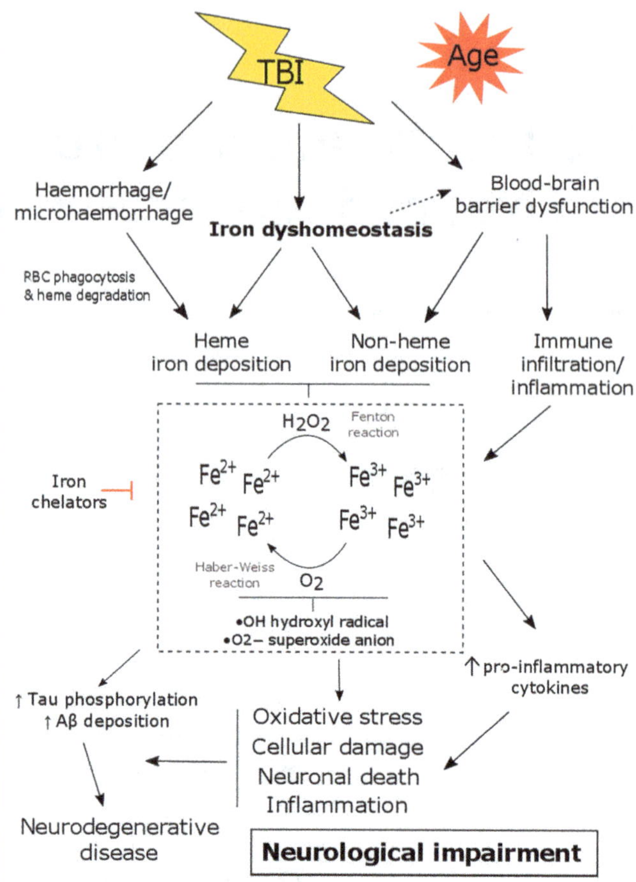

FIGURE 1 | The consequence of iron dyshomeostasis following TBI. TBI results in several secondary events including blood-brain barrier (BBB) breakdown, hemorrhage and iron dyshomeostasis. Together this leads to the accumulation of heme and/or non-heme bound iron in the brain. Iron can participate in Haber-Weiss/Fenton reactions and can promote oxidative stress, neuronal death, inflammation as well as tau phosphorylation/amyloid-β deposition. This contributes to the pathology of TBI, ultimately resulting in neurological decline and an increased risk of developing neurodegenerative disease.

IRON HOMEOSTASIS AND ITS ROLE IN NEUROLOGICAL FUNCTION

Iron is an important cofactor involved in a variety of bodily functions including cellular metabolism, energy production, cell growth and differentiation, and gene expression. It is primarily recognized for its ability to bind oxygen, contained within the hemoglobin complex, to transport oxygen throughout the body (Pantopoulos et al., 2012). Iron is also, however, fundamental for neuronal development, synaptic plasticity, neurotransmitter processing, and myelination (Ke and Qian, 2007; Ward et al., 2014). In the brain, iron, as well as other biometals, are found in numerous cell types including neurons, astrocytes, microglia, and most abundantly in oligodendrocytes (Burdo et al., 1999; Angelova and Brown, 2015). Astrocytes that are an integral part of the BBB have the ability to take up circulating iron and redistribute it to other cells in the CNS (Dringen et al., 2007). Iron is crucial for the maintenance of myelin, and therefore oligodendrocytes require a constant supply of iron (Connor and Menzies, 1996). Iron is also essential for optimal mitochondrial function (Urrutia et al., 2014), which is critical for neurons and other brain residing cells that have significant energy and metabolic requirements.

Iron homeostasis is carefully regulated in mammals by a plethora of proteins and enzymes produced in the liver such as hepcidin and ceruloplasmin, and other iron transporters (divalent metal transporter 1: DMT1, ferroportin, and transferrin) and their receptors (Ke and Qian, 2007). The expression levels of these proteins/receptors are in turn regulated by iron responsive elements (IRE) and iron regulatory proteins (IRP) especially when iron levels are low (Torben et al., 2007). Iron generally exists in an insoluble ferric (Fe^{3+}) or soluble ferrous (Fe^{2+}) state and is an active participant in electron transfer/redox reactions, which can drive oxidative stress-induced cellular toxicity (Graf et al., 1984; Nunez et al., 2012). Iron is solely absorbed through the diet, usually in its ferric form, and needs to be reduced to Fe^{2+} for its essential cellular uptake via transporter DMT1, with ferrous iron also released from cells via ferroportin (Gunshin et al., 1997; Donovan et al., 2000). In the circulation, iron is transported by binding to transferrin (ferric state; 2:1 ratio) whereas in tissues it is stored in a stable conformation by ferritin, a protein that consists of two subunits (i.e., ferritin heavy chain and light chain) (Ke and Qian, 2007; Nunez et al., 2012; Ward et al., 2014). The main regulator and inhibitor of iron release is hepcidin, which is secreted by the liver in response to stimulants (e.g., human hemochromatosis protein (HFE), inflammatory mediator IL-6, lipopolysaccharides (LPS) or high transferrin-Fe^{3+} complexes) ultimately to reduce levels of iron in the body (Ganz, 2003; Ward et al., 2014).

THE METABOLISM OF IRON IN THE BRAIN

The entry of iron into the brain parenchyma is restricted by the BBB due to its hydrophilic nature. Iron (ferric iron: Fe^{3+}) can enter through endothelial cells that line the BBB typically via endocytosis of transferrin/transferrin receptors and to a lesser extent either independently (non-transferrin bound iron) or as a low molecular weight complex (Ke and Qian, 2007; Torben et al., 2007; Ward et al., 2014). Iron is released from transferrin due to the acidic pH environment of the endosome, is then reduced to ferrous iron and thus contributes to the labile ferrous iron pool (Ke and Qian, 2007). Ferroportin is the only known iron exporter for almost all cell types including neurons and astrocytes (Donovan et al., 2000). Ceruloplasmin, which is primarily a copper containing α2-globulin (binds six copper ions) and mainly present as a GPI-linked membrane protein in the brain, is also an important regulator of iron-mediated transport via binding ferroportin and driving the conversion of Fe^{2+} to Fe^{3+} by its ferroxidase activity (Attieh et al., 1999). Amyloid precursor protein (APP), a key protein in AD pathology, stabilizes ferroportin to facilitate iron export in neurons, and its activity has recently been found to be regulated by iron (Rogers et al., 2008; Wong et al., 2014). Ceruloplasmin and APP expression are both increased alongside iron accumulation in the brain of TBI patients and brain injured mice, and were found to elicit neuroprotective effects (Ayton et al., 2014). **Figure 2** summarizes the proteins/receptors involved in iron metabolism in the brain.

Since iron is a transition metal, Fe^{2+} and Fe^{3+} can react with hydrogen peroxide and oxygen, respectively, catalyzing hydroxyl and superoxide radicals and can also react with lipids leading to the formation of alkoxy and peroxy radicals (Gutteridge, 1982). This is known as the Haber-Weiss and Fenton reaction. Hence, iron can increase ROS by participating in redox reactions and in turn lead to cellular oxidative stress and eventually cell death (Ke and Qian, 2007). Sufficient iron storage in the brain either by ferritin, neuromelanin (mainly in substantia nigra neurons) or hemosiderin is essential to prevent oxidative damage (Angelova and Brown, 2015).

Deficiency of iron or excessive iron, or changes in iron-regulating protein expression, can therefore be catastrophic to cells/tissues and are known to contribute to numerous disorders such as anemia, aceruloplasminemia, neuroferritinopathy, mitochondrial membrane protein-associated neurodegeneration (MPAN) and pantothenate kinase-associated neurodegeneration (PKAN) (Levi and Finazzi, 2014; Hogarth, 2015). Patients with inherited conditions that develop increased brain iron accumulation present with cognitive, motor and neuropsychiatric decline (Schröder et al., 2012; Hogarth, 2015). Excessive iron accumulation is harmful because it can promote the formation of free radicals resulting in oxidative stress, lipid peroxidation, protein aggregation and eventually cell/neuronal death (Nunez et al., 2012). On the other hand, iron deficiency can result in impaired myelin generation, neurotransmission and enzymatic processing. Iron deficiency anemia has been linked to the development of AD, and individuals with anemia are twice as likely to develop mild cognitive impairments over time (Faux et al., 2014). A recent study consisting of 939 patients with TBI found that anemia (i.e., presenting with low hemoglobin levels and low plasma iron), which affects approximately half of hospitalized TBI patients, is associated with poor outcomes following TBI (Litofsky et al., 2016). Taken together this shows that a delicate balance of iron metabolism needs to be achieved to protect the brain against its potentially harmful effects, in both healthy and diseased states.

IRON IN NEURODEGENERATIVE DISEASES

Iron dyshomeostasis appears to be a central factor in neurodegenerative conditions such as AD, PD, ALS, Huntington's disease, and Friedreich's ataxia (Oshiro et al., 2011; Agrawal et al., 2018). For decades, deposits of iron have been detected in brain lesions of patients with these neurodegenerative conditions (Hagemeier et al., 2012; Barbosa et al., 2015; Adlard and Bush, 2018). How iron accumulates in the diseased/injured brain is not known, however, heme-bound iron that is derived from the circulation and non-heme bound iron (i.e., all iron not bound to heme protein) are both present in affected tissue (Nisenbaum et al., 2014; Ward et al., 2014). It is likely that the deposition of iron into the brain parenchyma in these conditions is the result of either hemorrhage/microbleeds (i.e., heme-bound iron), damaged cells (i.e., neurons, oligodendrocytes and microglia),

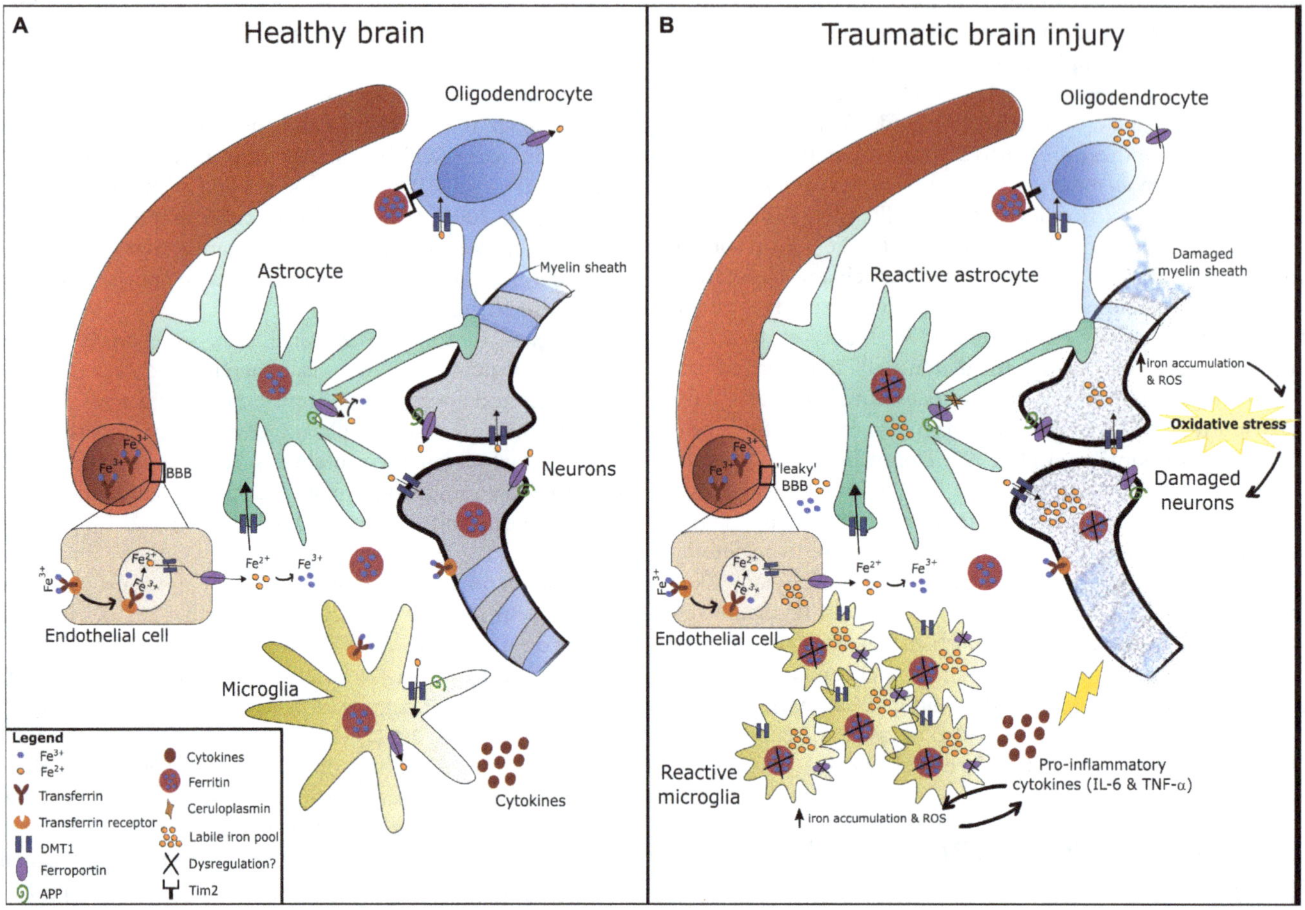

FIGURE 2 | Iron metabolism in the healthy and traumatically injured brain. **(A)** Circulating iron (Fe^{3+}) passes the blood-brain barrier (BBB) either bound to transferrin or independently, and is then taken up by endothelial cells expressing transferrin receptors via endocytosis. The acidic pH environment of the endosome detaches Fe^{3+} from transferrin and Fe^{3+} is then reduced to Fe^{2+} by ferric reductase (Ward et al., 2014). In the brain, Fe^{2+} is uptaken via DMT1 and distributed amongst astrocytes, neurons, oligodendrocytes, and microglia. Inside these cells, Fe^{2+} is converted to Fe^{3+} and stored by ferritin to prevent oxidative damage (Oshiro et al., 2011). Oligodendrocytes express Tim2 receptor that binds ferritin and iron can be imported through this mechanism, in addition to DMT1. Neurons and microglia can also uptake transferrin-bound iron via transferrin receptors (Ward et al., 2014). Ferrous iron is exported from cells via the iron exporter, ferroportin, which is present on all cell types. Fe^{2+} is rapidly oxidized to Fe^{3+} once outside the cell by ferroxidases such as hephaestin or ceruloplasmin (expressed on astrocytes mainly). Amyloid precursor protein (APP) is expressed on neurons, astrocytes and microglia, and has been found to facilitate iron export in neurons by stabilizing ferroportin (Wong et al., 2014). **(B)** Injury to the brain/neurovascular unit causes BBB damage, microglia activation, astrogliosis, and eventually damage to neurons and the myelin sheath surrounding axons. Dysregulation of iron metabolism in the brain following TBI can result in the accumulation of redox-active ferrous iron in various brain cells. This is possibly due to alterations in the expression/function of regulatory proteins such as ferroportin, ferritin and ceruloplasmin, which fail to export iron from cells and thereby increases the labile iron pool. Iron accumulation in microgia can cause increased pro-inflammatory cytokine production, and vice versa (Urrutia et al., 2014). Taken together, iron accumulation in the brain can promote oxidative stress that contributes to neurodegeneration.

and myelin, inflammatory processes, degradation of erythrocytes and heme proteins, and/or dysregulation of important iron-related proteins (e.g., ceruloplasmin, ferroportin) (Hametner et al., 2013; Hare et al., 2013; Nisenbaum et al., 2014). Excessive iron that is localized in affected neurons and glia can be found in brain regions such as the substantia nigra (dopaminergic neurons) in PD (Barbosa et al., 2015), and can also accompany regions of amyloid plaques and neurofibrillary tangles in AD (Smith et al., 1997). Similarly, patients with MS present with increased iron deposition in deep gray matter regions correlating with poor integrity of the white matter tissue (Bergsland et al., 2017). Increased brain iron accumulation in these neurological conditions have correlated with poorer functional outcomes and disease severity in patients (Zhang et al., 2010; van Duijn et al., 2017).

Although it is not yet clear whether iron is a causative or a contributing factor, its presence drives redox reactions, inflammatory processes as well as mitochondrial dysfunction (Urrutia et al., 2014). Iron accumulation in dopaminergic neurons, which are typically affected in PD, can exacerbate α-synuclein pathology and induce autophagy dysfunction (Wan et al., 2017). Ferric iron (Fe^{3+}) can cause the formation of neurofibrillary tangles by binding to aggregated hyperphosphorylated tau proteins and can also become reduced to its destructive redox-active form (free Fe^{2+}) during the process (Yamamoto et al., 2002; Oshiro et al., 2011). Iron can promote the toxicity of amyloid beta (Aß) by affecting aggregation, oligomerization, and amyloidosis of the peptide (Liu et al., 2011). It is also likely that the pathogenicity of Aß (e.g., in AD) is at least in part due to its interaction with iron and the potentiation of redox reactions (Rottkamp et al., 2001). In addition, expression of proteins that are involved in the regulation of iron are altered in these disease states; ceruloplasmin, ferroportin, and furin (regulates hepcidin) are decreased while DMT1 (iron importer) and transferrin are increased (Hare et al., 2013; Ward et al., 2014; Peters et al., 2015). The main iron storage protein in the brain, ferritin, is elevated in the cerebrospinal fluid (CSF) of patients with AD as well as areas containing amyloid plaques, and this protein also increases with age (Jellinger et al., 1990; Zecca et al., 2001; Ayton et al., 2018). These regulatory proteins in addition to iron are also associated with the production of Aß and hyperphosphorylated tau (Rogers et al., 2008). Together this reveals that the failure lies with various crucial proteins involved in the regulation of iron and is a possible explanation for the accumulation of iron in the brain.

Overall, increased iron accumulation in the brain, over and above the age-related changes, may be an indirect indicator of the progression and severity of AD and PD, and possibly other neurological conditions (van Duijn et al., 2017; Adlard and Bush, 2018). Elevated brain iron as measured by quantitative susceptibility mapping (via MRI) and increased CSF ferritin levels observed in patients with AD and mild cognitive impairment, were found to be predictive of cognitive decline over the long-term, and correlated with amyloid-β pathology (Ayton et al., 2017) and apolipoprotein E genotype (Ayton et al., 2015), respectively. Considering that brain iron content increases with age and that age is a major risk factor associated with neurodegenerative disease, the detection of iron using non-invasive imaging techniques may therefore prove to be a useful diagnostic tool as an early indicator of disease onset.

INTERPLAY OF IRON, INFLAMMATION AND NEURODEGENERATION

The immune system similarly plays an important role in the pathogenesis of neurodegenerative diseases although its interaction with biometals is unappreciated. Immune cells are also equipped with transferrin and ferroportin receptors to enable the influx/efflux of iron to meet their cellular needs. In particular, phagocytic immune cells such as microglia (brain-specific macrophages) have an important role in the regulation and distribution of iron since they function to engulf and recycle damaged/dying cells and thereby release iron into the brain interstitial space (Moos, 2002; Andersen et al., 2014). Intracellular iron accumulation is associated with macrophage infiltration/polarization and increased TNF-α expression (Kroner et al., 2014). Indeed, inflammatory cytokines (mainly IL-6 and TNF-α) and mediators such as LPS induce the expression of iron transporter receptors (e.g., DMT-1) and promote an increase in the accumulation of iron in neurons and microglia (Urrutia et al., 2014).

Iron can accumulate in myeloid cells including microglia and monocytes, causing oxidative damage to the cell and promoting chronic neuroinflammation. This is a typical feature observed in several neurological conditions including MS and AD (Andersen et al., 2014; Stuber et al., 2016). *In vitro* studies reveal that iron can directly increase NFκB activity and stimulate pro-inflammatory cytokine production in microglia (Saleppico et al., 1996). Indeed, hemosiderin-laden macrophages were present in the frontal and temporal lobes of a patient with mild TBI (Bigler, 2004). Damaged oligodendrocytes and myelin in neuroinflammatory conditions including MS were determined as the main sources of extracellular iron in the brain parenchyma (Hametner et al., 2013).

This interplay of iron deposition with phagocytic cells (macrophages) can lead to neuronal damage not only due to oxidative stress and free radical formation but also through the promotion of pro-inflammatory mediators that further contributes to secondary damage in TBI. There is also the hypothesis that the inflammatory cells that migrate to the site of injury in TBI (or plaque regions in neurodegenerative diseases) are largely responsible for depositing iron (Sastry and Arendash, 1995; Andersen et al., 2014). Hence, an unrecognized link between iron accumulation and the involvement of the immune response in TBI warrants investigation considering both these processes are persistently active in the brain from weeks to months following injury. Whether iron dyshomeostasis in the brain is the process that promotes glial reactivity and drives neuroinflammatory responses, or vice versa, is unknown. Perhaps both these processes are simultaneously contributing to brain damage and consequential neurological impairment following TBI. Supporting this, a recent review proposed a positive feedback cycle in which mitochondrial dysfunction, inflammation, and iron accumulation are critical synergistic mechanisms that induce and enhance one another, and eventually become responsible for neuronal/cell death in the pathogenesis of neurodegenerative diseases (Nunez et al., 2012; Urrutia et al., 2014).

THE ROLE OF IRON IN TBI

Iron deposits that accumulate in the brain can consist of both non-heme and heme iron sub-types. These features are more commonly observed in neurodegenerative conditions such as AD, although increasing evidence suggests that both these subtypes of iron are increased in the injured brain after TBI (Nisenbaum et al., 2014). Heme-bound iron is commonly found coinciding with intracranial hemorrhage, along with deposition of hemosiderin and ferritin due to the phagocytosis of erythrocytes by microglia/macrophages (Koeppen et al., 2008; Nisenbaum et al., 2014).

A feature seen in TBI as well as several neurodegenerative diseases is the formation of cerebral microhemorrhages. These have been observed at both the acute and chronic stages of TBI, in experimental models of single and repetitive TBI (Donovan et al., 2012; Glushakova et al., 2014) as well as in a subgroup of mild TBI patients (Park et al., 2009; Hasiloglu et al., 2011; Nisenbaum et al., 2014). The clinical relevance of cerebral microhemorrhages on TBI outcome is not yet clear (Scheid et al., 2006; Irimia et al., 2018; van der Horn et al., 2018) although the presence of microhemorrhages following TBI is a suggested predictor of injury severity (Huang et al., 2015; Lawrence et al., 2017). Microbleeds have been negatively associated with cognitive outcomes in patients with mild cognitive impairment, stroke and MS (Werring et al., 2004; Zivadinov et al., 2016; Li X. et al., 2017). Microhemorrhages are interestingly associated with areas of white matter damage, BBB breakdown, demyelination, and inflammation in experimental TBI (Glushakova et al., 2014). Microbleeds, which can be detected by Prussian blue iron staining, reveal an abnormal accumulation of iron and ferritin/hemosiderin that have been found to be toxic to brain-specific cells (neurons, astrocytes, and microglia) and endothelial cells (Glushakova et al., 2014). More importantly, non-heme bound iron and free iron are also elevated in the brain following TBI and are considered more problematic (Nisenbaum et al., 2014), as shown in **Figure 2**.

The origin of brain iron deposits independent of heme-bound iron in TBI is not yet known although several hypotheses exist. Dysregulation of ceruloplasmin (e.g., decreased levels) can lead to an increase in free copper ions and a concomitant decrease in ferroxidase activity, thereby reducing clearance of iron from the CNS (i.e., increasing iron deposition). Ceruloplasmin deficient mice subjected to TBI showed elevated brain iron levels and exacerbated infarct volume (Ayton et al., 2014). TBI (and specifically intracerebral hemorrhage: ICH) often accompanies hemorrhage, increased vascularisation and BBB breakdown, which likely results in heme-bound iron deposition in the brain initially. In this instance, the enzyme heme-oxygenase 1 (HO-1) is involved in the degradation of heme-bound iron into free iron or non-heme bound iron (Beschorner et al., 2000). HO-1 is also suggested to be involved in induction of antioxidants bilirubin and biliverdin, and can therefore protect against oxidative stress. Indeed, HO-1 expression is heightened following TBI in both experimental models (Fukuda et al., 1995; Okubo et al., 2013) and in humans over a long-term period (Beschorner et al., 2000). HO-1 is likely protective at the acute stage through its antioxidant properties and clearance of heme-bound iron but it also could be responsible for non-heme bound iron accumulation in the brain, thereby increasing labile iron content over time. Free iron released from the degradation of heme proteins is a main source of oxidative stress, particularly in the injured brain (Chang et al., 2005). Excessive quantities of labile iron (**Figure 2**) can be harmful by inducing excitotoxic-related neuronal death, impaired neurotransmission, and mitochondrial dysfunction (Nunez et al., 2012; Urrutia et al., 2014; Ward et al., 2014).

Literature characterizing the metal profile and spatiotemporal distribution of iron is relatively sparse in TBI of varying injury severities and repetitive injuries, as well as ICH and stroke, in both clinical (see **Table 1**) and animal studies (see **Table 2**). Importantly, the consequence of iron accumulation in the brain following TBI is currently unknown, although it is associated with the development of post-traumatic epilepsy (Willmore et al., 1978; Willmore and Ueda, 2009; Ueda et al., 2013). Brain-region specific accumulation of iron has been documented in patients with mild TBI, via magnetic resonance imaging (MRI) approaches such as Magnetic field correlation (MFC) and susceptibility weighted imaging (SWI) (Raz et al., 2011; Nisenbaum et al., 2014; Lu et al., 2015). Various regions of the brain are affected including the hippocampus, globus pallidus, thalamus, substantia nigra, and corpus callosum, as summarized in **Table 1**. Non-heme iron is more sensitively detected by MR imaging techniques although limitations do exist (e.g., tissue fluid content can affect iron quantitation) (Raz et al., 2011). However, it can be concluded that non-heme bound iron accumulates in deep gray matter areas of the brain and may contribute to pathological secondary injury (e.g., oxidative stress) following TBI since abnormal iron deposition correlated with poor cognitive outcome (Raz et al., 2011; Lu et al., 2015).

Recent studies (Portbury et al., 2016, 2017) thoroughly analyzed the time-dependent alteration in metals including iron, zinc, and copper, in the brain by laser ablation-inductively coupled plasma-mass spectrometry (LA-ICPMS) in a mouse controlled cortical impact (CCI) model. Elevated iron concentrations were detected at the impact site as early as 3 days and were persistently elevated up to 28 days in both young (Portbury et al., 2016) and aged mice (Portbury et al., 2017) following injury. Supporting this, histological staining revealed intracellular iron accumulated in the cortex and hippocampal regions of the injured hemisphere (Portbury et al., 2016). Another study subjected aged mice (21–24 month old) to the CCI model and found increased iron deposition using T2-weighted MRI in the ipsilateral thalamus that accompanied astrogliosis and microgliosis at 1 and 2 months post-TBI (Onyszchuk et al., 2009). The authors suggest that free iron may be elevated as a result of degenerating thalamic neurons (Onyszchuk et al., 2009). Therefore, the continued presence of both inflammation and iron accumulation in the lesion likely contributes to ongoing pathology following TBI, as summarized in **Figures 1, 2**.

IRON IN AGING, INJURY AND NEURODEGENERATION

It is well recognized that iron as well as iron-related proteins (e.g., ferritin and HO-1) progressively increase in the aging brain (Hirose et al., 2003; Stankiewicz et al., 2007). Microglia and astrocytes, but not oligodendrocytes, appear to accumulate iron more with age (Zecca et al., 2001; Angelova and Brown, 2015). Regions of the brain typically affected by age-related iron accumulation are the hippocampus, cortex, cerebellum, and most prominently the basal ganglia. Interestingly, these regions are commonly linked to neurodegenerative diseases (Angelova and Brown, 2015). Indeed, age remains one of the greatest risk factors associated with poor outcomes following TBI, and the development of neurodegenerative/neuroinflammatory conditions (Stocchetti et al., 2012; Ward et al., 2014). In aged individuals, iron accumulation in the brain could be caused by events that coincide with the aging process including increased permeability of the BBB, inflammation, dysregulation of iron-related proteins, mitochondrial dysfunction, and altered iron distribution within the CNS (Farrall and Wardlaw, 2009; Ward et al., 2014). Therefore, it is not clear whether age-related iron accumulation causes, or is rather a consequence of, neurodegeneration that commonly occurs with aging. Importantly, iron deposition in the aged brain has been linked

TABLE 1 | Brain iron accumulation in brain injury; evidence from clinical studies.

Brain injury	Patients	Detection method	Iron deposits/ region	Associated pathology	Outcome/prognosis	Study
Stroke	Ischemic stroke (*n* = 77) and transient ischemic attack (*n* = 74)	SWI	Lenticular nucleus	Correlated with cerebral microbleeds	N/A	Liu et al., 2016
	Unilateral ischemic stroke (*n* = 36)	T2-MRI	Thalamus	N/A	N/A	van Etten et al., 2015
	Ischemic stroke patients (*n* = 172)	R2 mapping, MRI	Thalamus, ipsilateral to infarct location	N/A	Associated with poor functional and cognitive outcome, and depression/anxiety at 1 year	Kuchcinski et al., 2017
ICH	Spontaneous ICH patients (*n* = 2, case study)	T2-MRI	Perihematoma, basal ganglia region (at 7 days)	N/A	N/A	Chaudhary et al., 2016
TBI	Mild TBI patients (*n* = 39)	SWI	Caudate nucleus, lenticular nucleus, hippocampus, thalamus, right substantia nigra, red nucleus, and the splenium of the corpus callosum	N/A	Negative correlation with Mini-Mental State Examination (MMSE) scores in mild TBI group compared to controls	Lu et al., 2015
	Mild TBI patients (*n* = 28)	MRI mapping/ MFC	Globus pallidus and thalamus	N/A	High MFC values (suggesting iron deposits) inversely correlated with cognitive function (i.e., Stroop color word test)	Raz et al., 2011
	TBI patients (*n* = 19)	PCR and IHC	Peri-contusional cortex (12 and 48 h post-injury)	Increased ferritin H-chain expression in neurons and iron in glial cells	N/A	Liu et al., 2013
Repetitive mild TBI/ CTE	CTE (Dementia Pugilistica)	Laser micro-probe mass analysis	Temporal cortex	Iron deposits in neuronal neurofibrillary tangles	More prominent in Dementia Pugilistica than AD	Bouras et al., 1997

CTE, chronic traumatic encephalopathy; IHC, immunohistochemistry; ICH, intracerebral hemorrhage; MRI, magnetic resonance imaging; MFC, magnetic field correlation; MMSE, Mini-Mental State Examination; N/A, not available; PCR, polymerase chain reaction; SWI, susceptibility weighted imaging.

to cognitive and motor deficits in the elderly (Pujol et al., 1992), and motor dysfunction in rhesus monkeys (Cass et al., 2007). Since aged individuals generally exhibit co-morbidities and present with systemic inflammation and altered neurovascular unit integrity among other age-related pathological processes (Stocchetti et al., 2012), this renders the brain vulnerable to iron-mediated oxidative damage (Stankiewicz et al., 2007). This can be particularly problematic for an already compromised brain following TBI. The extent of iron deposition between adults and elderly TBI patients has not yet been directly examined clinically. However, a recent study showed that aged (24 month old) mice have higher levels of iron (as well as other metals) in both the injured and contralateral (uninjured) hemisphere following TBI compared to young (3 month old) mice (Portbury et al., 2017). This heightened increase in brain iron levels can potentiate oxidative stress and neurotoxicity (as extensively covered in this review), and therefore is a possible explanation for the cognitive decline and overall worse outcomes observed in the aging TBI population. Further research is needed to better understand the role of iron in aging and its link to TBI and neurodegenerative disease.

THERAPEUTIC RELEVANCE AND FUTURE DIRECTIONS

Iron-mediated brain damage occurs in patients with TBI over a chronic time-period, and it is speculated that increasing iron deposition (with age) can predispose these individuals to the development of neurodegenerative diseases later in life or to post-traumatic epilepsy (see **Figure 1**). Hence, a targeted therapeutic approach to regulate iron levels in TBI patients will be an important advancement in limiting progressive neurodegeneration and neurological deficits that accompanies

TABLE 2 | Brain iron accumulation in brain injury; evidence from experimental studies.

Brain injury	Model	Iron deposits/ region	Time-period	Associated pathology	Outcome/ prognosis	Study
Stroke	Rat, middle cerebral artery occlusion (MCAO)	Thalamus; increased iron in microglia (at 3 wks), parenchyma (at 7 wks) and APP deposits (at 24 wks)	Over 24 weeks post-injury	Neuronal loss, increased microglia activation and HO-1 expression	Behavioral deficits up to 24 wks	Justicia et al., 2008
	Rat, permanent photo-thrombotic cortical vessel occlusion	Free (labile) iron and total iron increased in the ischemic lesion	1 h post-injury	N/A	Iron chelator 2,2'-dipyridyl (Bipyridine), injected 15 min or 1 h post-injury, improved BBB integrity	Millerot-Serrurot et al., 2008
ICH	Rat, ICH model – collagenase	Non-heme and total iron in injured striatum	3 days and 4 wks post-ICH	Increased lesion volume	N/A	Auriat et al., 2012
	Mice, ICH model – collagenase VII-S injected in the left striatum	Peri-hematomal region	Peaking at 3 days post-ICH	Increased lesion volume and neuronal degeneration	Neurological deficits up to 28 days. Iron chelator VK-28 reduced brain oedema, ROS and white matter injury yet promoted M2-microglia polarization and improved outcomes	Li Q. et al., 2017
	Rat, ICH, autologous whole blood injected into basal ganglia	Increased brain non-heme iron, transferrin/transferrin receptor and HO-1 levels	Over 4 weeks	N/A	N/A	Wu et al., 2003
TBI	Mice, CCI model	Ipsilateral parietal cortex (LA-ICPMS)	3–28 days post-CCI	N/A	N/A	Portbury et al., 2016; Portbury et al., 2017
	Mice, CCI model	Thalamus and internal capsule (T2-MRI)	1 and 2 months post-CCI	Reactive astrocytes and microglia	N/A	Onyszchuk et al., 2009
Repetitive mild TBI	Rat, mild CCI (2 impacts; 1, 3 or 7 days apart)	Extravascular iron deposits at lesion site (IHC)	14 days	Correlated with lesion volume and reactive glial cells	Behavioral and memory deficits at 1 month post-injury	Huang et al., 2013

APP, amyloid precursor protein; HO-1, heme oxygenase-1; LA-ICPMS, laser ablation-inductively coupled plasma-mass spectrometry; MRI, magnetic resonance imaging; MCAO, middle cerebral artery occlusion.

TBI of varying severities, and thereby reduce the risk of neurological disorders. Iron chelation therapies work by binding free iron and removing excess iron from the blood. Iron chelation not only works by scavenging labile free iron but some can also act as an antioxidant that neutralizes the radical reaction by donating hydrogen (e.g., deferiprone, HBED iron chelator) (Khalaf et al., 2018). They can also bind/remove other metals yet have a higher affinity for iron, and the absorption and tissue penetration properties of the different iron chelators can vary (e.g., desferrioxamine is poorly absorbed in the gut while deferiprone and deferasirox are orally active) thereby different routes of administration are needed (Kalinowski and Richardson, 2005; Dusek et al., 2016). Iron chelation therapy has only been investigated in a few pilot clinical trials of common neurological conditions including AD (Crapper McLachlan et al., 1991), PD (Devos et al., 2014; Martin-Bastida et al., 2017), and MS (Lynch et al., 1996). As yet, no compelling evidence has come to light with the use of iron chelators in these conditions, although they have proved relatively effective in attenuating disease progression in PD. The brain permeable iron chelator, deferiprone, decreased iron deposits in the substantia nigra, and slowed disease-severity progression in a small-scale study involving PD patients ($n = 40$) (Devos et al., 2014). However, another pilot clinical trial assessing deferiprone in PD patients only found a trending improvement in motor function over 6 months (Martin-Bastida et al., 2017); hence more extensive clinical and experimental studies are warranted. Baicalin and deferoxamine, which are iron chelating drugs that can (baicalin) or cannot (deferoxamine) pass through

TABLE 3 | The effectiveness of iron chelators in experimental TBI models.

Severity	Model	Iron chelator	Effect of treatment	Time-frame (post-injury)	Protective?	Study
Mild TBI	Mice, CCI model	HBED (N,N′-Di(2-hydroxybenzyl) ethylenediamine-N,N′-diacetic acid monohydrochloride)	Improved motor function and neurological deficits. Reduction in cortical injury volume, microgliosis and oxidative stress markers	3 days	Yes	Khalaf et al., 2018
Moderate TBI	Rats, CCI model	Deferoxamine	Improved spatial memory (Morris water maze) but no change in cortical tissue loss between deferoxamine and vehicle control	Up to 17 days	Yes, but only in spatial memory performance	Long et al., 1996
Moderate-severe TBI	Rats, fluid percussion injury model	Deferoxamine	Reduced hydrocephalus development after TBI and decreased heme oxygenase-1 expression	24 h	No outcome measures tested	Zhao et al., 2014
Severe TBI	Rats, weight drop model	Deferoxamine	Improved Morris water maze performance (spatial memory) and reduced brain atrophy	28 days	Yes	Zhang et al., 2013
	Mice, weight drop model (loss of consciousness)	Dextran-coupled deferoxamine	Improved grip-strength compared to mice treated with deferoxamine or dextran alone	1 h	Yes	Panter et al., 1992

the BBB, were assessed in a rat model of PD. Both these treatments inhibited iron deposition in the substantia nigra as well as the striatum, dentate gyrus, dentate-interpositus, and cerebellum, protected dopaminergic neurons from death (Xiong et al., 2012).

This strategy of chelating iron has yet to be trialed in patients with TBI, or chronic traumatic encephalopathy (CTE) patients with repetitive head injury, nor has it been greatly explored in animal models of TBI. However, it remains a potential treatment option based on the few promising experimental TBI studies that have assessed the effect of iron chelators (i.e., deferoxamine or dextran-coupled deferoxamine) in experimental models that will be described hereafter.

IRON CHELATION IN TBI

Only a handful of studies to date have investigated the therapeutic potential of chelating iron in experimental TBI models, mainly via the ferric iron chelator deferoxamine, as summarized in **Table 3**. However, deferoxamine has several limitations including its inability to cross the BBB, rapid elimination rate and it can theoretically generate superoxide radicals through binding Fe^{3+} leading to Fe^{2+} oxidation (Klebanoff et al., 1989; Hall et al., 2010).

In a recent study, the brain permeable iron chelator HBED was assessed in its effectiveness to attenuate iron-mediated brain damage in a mouse model of TBI (i.e., CCI) (Khalaf et al., 2018). They found that HBED improved locomotor function along with a reduction in lesion volumes and hippocampal swelling. Interestingly, HBED also limited microgliosis and the expression of immune markers in the corpus callosum (Khalaf et al., 2018). This pointed to a potential mechanism through which the drug mediates its protective effects. However, a limitation of this study is that HBED treatment did not significantly reduce iron in the brain as measured by Perls' staining (Khalaf et al., 2018). On the other hand, deferoxamine treatment reduced the levels of iron and iron-storage proteins (ferritin and transferrin) in the brain, which were elevated at 28 days post-TBI in rats. This was accompanied by a reduction in brain atrophy in the injured rats treated with deferoxamine as well as an improvement in spatial memory and learning, at 28 days after TBI (Zhang et al., 2013). A similar protective effect with deferoxamine treatment was also observed in earlier studies at an acute period following TBI (Panter et al., 1992; Long et al., 1996).

Several key limitations of these studies exist, including the short period of treatment, limited outcome measures and only one recent study assessed brain pathology at one time-point. Hence, there is a great need for long-term sequential analysis for the use of iron chelators (specifically those that are brain-permeable) in experimental TBI models, in which the influence of iron chelation on functional outcomes, pathology (e.g., oxidative stress, cell death, BBB breakdown), other biochemical alterations and also inflammation are essential before moving into clinical trials.

However, iron chelation therapy has been more thoroughly explored as a strategy for combating brain iron overload in ICH and to some degree in stroke (See **Table 2**), although these are still in the preclinical phase with only a few currently active clinical trials (Yeatts et al., 2013; Yu et al., 2015; Zeng et al., 2018). In particular, a small-scale clinical trial using deferoxamine in ICH patients ($n = 21$) showed improvement in oedema volume and hematoma absorption over a period of 30 days (Yu et al., 2015). Deferoxamine reduces odema, cell death, hippocampal degeneration and also inflammation following experimental ICH (Garton et al., 2016). Neuronal death and behavioral deficits were attenuated by deferoxamine treatment in aged rats with induced ICH (Hatakeyama et al., 2013). Deferiprone treatment has shown promise in reversing iron toxicity in the brain and improving outcome. Treatment was remarkably effective when deferiprone was combined with the antioxidant n-acetyl cysteine, in rats fed with a high iron-supplemented diet (Sripetchwandee et al., 2014, 2016). This combined treatment had a greater efficacy in improving learning and memory, long-term potentiation, mitochondrial function, BBB integrity and cell death, compared to individual treatment in iron-overloaded rats (Sripetchwandee et al., 2014, 2016). In addition, brain-related pathology including Aβ deposition, tau-hyperphosphorylation and dendritic spine loss were all significantly reduced to a greater extent with combined treatment (Sripetchwandee et al., 2016).

Most recently, the use of a ferroptosis (a form of iron-dependent cell death) inhibitor was shown to reduce iron deposition and result in a host of downstream benefits, including decreased neuronal degeneration and improved behavioral outcomes (motor and cognitive function) (Xie et al., 2018). Thus, ferroptosis may represent a new pathway of relevance for TBI, and such studies are currently underway in our lab.

CONCLUSION

Brain iron accumulation is a common feature of most neurodegenerative/neurological conditions including TBI. It is increasingly becoming clear that iron plays a detrimental role in the pathogenesis of various neurodegenerative diseases, however, its relationship to TBI pathobiology still requires consolidation. Although iron chelation with deferoxamine has shown limited potential in experimental TBI models, using a chelator that can penetrate the BBB (e.g., deferiprone, HBED, VK-28), with a known ability to lessen iron-induced neurotoxicity in ICH and neurodegenerative diseases, could prove to be superior than previously tested iron chelators in improving outcome after TBI. Whether a specified time-window for treatment is required (e.g., immediate vs delayed treatment) also needs to be addressed (as does the notion that a combination of iron and zinc-targeted treatments may have a synergistic benefit in TBI). Targeting both iron accumulation and subsequent oxidative damage and/or inflammation by proposed combined therapy (e.g., other antioxidants or anti-inflammatory agents) has not yet been assessed preclinically in TBI (Hall et al., 2010). This approach has the potential of limiting acute secondary injury and protecting against neurological deterioration, as well as attenuating long-term neurodegeneration thereby reducing the risk of neurodegenerative disease development. Lastly, there is a great need for experimental studies to focus on the long-term consequences of iron-mediated damage considering iron deposition progresses over time; as seen with age, neurodegenerative diseases as well as TBI.

AUTHOR CONTRIBUTIONS

MD and PA conceived and constructed the manuscript.

FUNDING

PA was supported by funding from the National Health and Medical Research Council of Australia, the Australian Research Council and the Department of Defense (United States). The funders played no role in the content of this review or in the decision to publish.

ACKNOWLEDGMENTS

The Florey Institute of Neuroscience and Mental Health acknowledge the strong support from the Victorian Government and in particular the funding from the Operational Infrastructure Support Grant.

REFERENCES

Adlard, P. A., and Bush, A. I. (2018). Metals and Alzheimer's disease: how far have we come in the clinic? *J. Alzheimers Dis.* 62, 1369–1379. doi: 10.3233/JAD-170662

Agrawal, S., Fox, J., Thyagarajan, B., and Fox, J. H. (2018). Brain mitochondrial iron accumulates in Huntington's disease, mediates mitochondrial dysfunction, and can be removed pharmacologically. *Free Radic. Biol. Med.* 120, 317–329. doi: 10.1016/j.freeradbiomed.2018.04.002

Andersen, H. H., Johnsen, K. B., and Moos, T. (2014). Iron deposits in the chronically inflamed central nervous system and contributes to neurodegeneration. *Cell. Mol. Life Sci.* 71, 1607–1622. doi: 10.1007/s00018-013-1509-8

Angelova, D., and Brown, D. (2015). Iron, aging, and neurodegeneration. *Metals* 5, 2070–2092. doi: 10.3390/met5042070

Attieh, Z. K., Mukhopadhyay, C. K., Seshadri, V., Tripoulas, N. A., and Fox, P. L. (1999). Ceruloplasmin ferroxidase activity stimulates cellular iron uptake by a trivalent cation-specific transport mechanism. *J. Biol. Chem.* 274, 1116–1123. doi: 10.1074/jbc.274.2.1116

Auriat, A. M., Silasi, G., Wei, Z., Paquette, R., Paterson, P., Nichol, H., et al. (2012). Ferric iron chelation lowers brain iron levels after intracerebral hemorrhage in rats but does not improve outcome. *Exp. Neurol.* 234, 136–143. doi: 10.1016/j.expneurol.2011.12.030

Ayton, S., Diouf, I., Bush, A. I., and Alzheimer's disease Neuroimaging Initiative (2018). Evidence that iron accelerates Alzheimer's pathology: a CSF biomarker study. *J. Neurol. Neurosurg. Psychiatry* 89, 456–460. doi: 10.1136/jnnp-2017-316551

Ayton, S., Faux, N. G., Bush, A. I., Alzheimer's Disease Neuroimaging Initiative, Weiner, M. W., Aisen, P., et al. (2015). Ferritin levels in the cerebrospinal fluid predict Alzheimer's disease outcomes and are regulated by APOE. *Nat. Commun.* 6:6760. doi: 10.1038/ncomms7760

Ayton, S., Fazlollahi, A., Bourgeat, P., Raniga, P., Ng, A., Lim, Y. Y., et al. (2017). Cerebral quantitative susceptibility mapping predicts amyloid-β-related cognitive decline. *Brain* 140, 2112–2119. doi: 10.1093/brain/awx137

Ayton, S., Zhang, M., Roberts, B. R., Lam, L. Q., Lind, M., McLean, C., et al. (2014). Ceruloplasmin and β-amyloid precursor protein confer neuroprotection in traumatic brain injury and lower neuronal iron. *Free Radic. Biol. Med.* 69, 331–337. doi: 10.1016/j.freeradbiomed.2014.01.041

Barbosa, J. H. O., Santos, A. C., Tumas, V., Liu, M., Zheng, W., Haacke, E. M., et al. (2015). Quantifying brain iron deposition in patients with Parkinson's disease using quantitative susceptibility mapping, R2 and R2*. *Magn. Reson. Imaging* 33, 559–565. doi: 10.1016/j.mri.2015.02.021

Bergsland, N., Tavazzi, E., Laganà, M. M., Baglio, F., Cecconi, P., Viotti, S., et al. (2017). White matter tract injury is associated with deep gray matter iron deposition in multiple sclerosis. *J. Neuroimaging* 27, 107–113. doi: 10.1111/jon.12364

Beschorner, R., Adjodah, D., Schwab, J. M., Mittelbronn, M., Pedal, I., Mattern, R., et al. (2000). Long-term expression of heme oxygenase-1 (HO-1, HSP-32) following focal cerebral infarctions and traumatic brain injury in humans. *Acta Neuropathol.* 100, 377–384. doi: 10.1007/s004010000202

Bigler, E. D. (2004). Neuropsychological results and neuropathological findings at autopsy in a case of mild traumatic brain injury. *J. Int. Neuropsychol. Soc.* 10, 794–806. doi: 10.1017/s1355617704105146

Bouras, C., Giannakopoulos, P., Good, P. F., Hsu, A., Hof, P. R., and Perl, D. P. (1997). A laser microprobe mass analysis of brain aluminum and iron in dementia pugilistica: comparison with Alzheimer's disease. *Eur. Neurol.* 38, 53–58. doi: 10.1159/000112903

Bramlett, H. M., and Dietrich, W. D. (2015). Long-term consequences of traumatic brain injury: current status of potential mechanisms of injury and neurological outcomes. *J. Neurotrauma* 32, 1834–1848. doi: 10.1089/neu.2014.3352

Burdo, J. R., Martin, J., Menzies, S. L., Dolan, K. G., Romano, M. A., Fletcher, R. J., et al. (1999). Cellular distribution of iron in the brain of the Belgrade rat. *Neuroscience* 93, 1189–1196. doi: 10.1016/S0306-4522(99)00207-9

Cass, W. A., Grondin, R., Andersen, A. H., Zhang, Z., Hardy, P. A., Hussey-Andersen, L. K., et al. (2007). Iron accumulation in the striatum predicts aging-related decline in motor function in rhesus monkeys. *Neurobiol. Aging* 28, 258–271. doi: 10.1016/j.neurobiolaging.2005.12.010

Chang, E. F., Claus, C. P., Vreman, H. J., Wong, R. J., and Noble-Haeusslein, L. J. (2005). Heme regulation in traumatic brain injury: relevance to the adult and developing brain. *J. Cereb. Blood Flow Metab.* 25, 1401–1417. doi: 10.1038/sj.jcbfm.9600147

Chaudhary, N., Pandey, A. S., Merchak, K., Gemmete, J. J., Chenevert, T., and Xi, G. (2016). "Perihematomal cerebral tissue iron quantification on MRI following intracerebral hemorrhage in two human subjects: proof of principle," in *Brain Edema XVI: Translate Basic Science into Clinical Practice*, eds R. L. Applegate, G. Chen, H. Feng, and J. H. Zhang (Cham: Springer International Publishing), 179–183.

Connor, J. R., and Menzies, S. L. (1996). Relationship of iron to oligodendrocytes and myelination. *Glia* 17, 83–93. doi: 10.1002/(SICI)1098-1136(199606)17:2<83::AID-GLIA1>3.0.CO;2-7

Crapper McLachlan, D. R., Dalton, A. J., Kruck, T. P., Bell, M. Y., Smith, W. L., Kalow, W., et al. (1991). Intramuscular desferrioxamine in patients with Alzheimer's disease. *Lancet* 337, 1304–1308. doi: 10.1016/0140-6736(91)92978-B

Del, C., Valdés Hernández, M., Ritchie, S., Glatz, A., Allerhand, M., Muñoz Maniega, S., et al. (2015). Brain iron deposits and lifespan cognitive ability. *Age* 37:100. doi: 10.1007/s11357-015-9837-2

Devos, D., Moreau, C., Devedjian, J. C., Kluza, J., Petrault, M., Laloux, C., et al. (2014). Targeting chelatable iron as a therapeutic modality in Parkinson's disease. *Antioxid. Redox Signal.* 21, 195–210. doi: 10.1089/ars.2013.5593

Donovan, A., Brownlie, A., Zhou, Y., Shepard, J., Pratt, S. J., Moynihan, J., et al. (2000). Positional cloning of zebrafish ferroportin1 identifies a conserved vertebrate iron exporter. *Nature* 403, 776–781. doi: 10.1038/35001596

Donovan, V., Bianchi, A., Hartman, R., Bhanu, B., Carson, M. J., and Obenaus, A. (2012). Computational analysis reveals increased blood deposition following repeated mild traumatic brain injury. *Neuroimage Clin.* 1, 18–28. doi: 10.1016/j.nicl.2012.08.001

Dringen, R., Bishop, G. M., Koeppe, M., Dang, T. N., and Robinson, S. R. (2007). The pivotal role of astrocytes in the metabolism of iron in the brain. *Neurochem. Res.* 32, 1884–1890. doi: 10.1007/s11064-007-9375-0

Dusek, P., Schneider, S. A., and Aaseth, J. (2016). Iron chelation in the treatment of neurodegenerative diseases. *J. Trace Elem. Med. Biol.* 38, 81–92. doi: 10.1016/j.jtemb.2016.03.010

Farrall, A. J., and Wardlaw, J. M. (2009). Blood-brain barrier: ageing and microvascular disease–systematic review and meta-analysis. *Neurobiol. Aging* 30, 337–352. doi: 10.1016/j.neurobiolaging.2007.07.015

Faux, N. G., Rembach, A., Wiley, J., Ellis, K. A., Ames, D., Fowler, C. J., et al. (2014). An anemia of Alzheimer's disease. *Mol. Psychiatry* 19, 1227–1234. doi: 10.1038/mp.2013.178

Fukuda, K., Panter, S. S., Sharp, F. R., and Noble, L. J. (1995). Induction of heme oxygenase-1 (HO-1) after traumatic brain injury in the rat. *Neurosci. Lett.* 199, 127–130. doi: 10.1016/0304-3940(95)12042-3

Ganz, T. (2003). Hepcidin, a key regulator of iron metabolism and mediator of anemia of inflammation. *Blood* 102, 783–788. doi: 10.1182/blood-2003-03-0672

Gardner, A. J., Shih, S. L., Adamov, E. V., and Zafonte, R. D. (2017). Research frontiers in traumatic brain injury: defining the injury. *Phys. Med. Rehabil. Clin. N. Am.* 28, 413–431. doi: 10.1016/j.pmr.2016.12.014

Garton, T., Keep, R. F., Hua, Y., and Xi, G. (2016). Brain iron overload following intracranial haemorrhage. *Stroke Vasc. Neurol.* 1, 172–184. doi: 10.1136/svn-2016-000042

Glushakova, O. Y., Johnson, D., and Hayes, R. L. (2014). Delayed increases in microvascular pathology after experimental traumatic brain injury are associated with prolonged inflammation, blood-brain barrier disruption, and progressive white matter damage. *J. Neurotrauma* 31, 1180–1193. doi: 10.1089/neu.2013.3080

Graf, E., Mahoney, J. R., Bryant, R. G., and Eaton, J. W. (1984). Iron-catalyzed hydroxyl radical formation. Stringent requirement for free iron coordination site. *J. Biol. Chem.* 259, 3620–3624.

Griffiths, P. D., Dobson, B. R., Jones, G. R., and Clarke, D. T. (1999). Iron in the basal ganglia in Parkinson's disease: an in vitro study using extended X-ray absorption fine structure and cryo-electron microscopy. *Brain* 122, 667–673. doi: 10.1093/brain/122.4.667

Gunshin, H., Mackenzie, B., Berger, U. V., Gunshin, Y., Romero, M. F., Boron, W. F., et al. (1997). Cloning and characterization of a mammalian proton-coupled metal-ion transporter. *Nature* 388, 482–488. doi: 10.1038/41343

Gutteridge, J. M. (1982). The role of superoxide and hydroxyl radicals in phospholipid peroxidation catalysed by iron salts. *FEBS Lett.* 150, 454–458. doi: 10.1016/0014-5793(82)80788-6

Hagemeier, J., Geurts, J. J., and Zivadinov, R. (2012). Brain iron accumulation in aging and neurodegenerative disorders. *Expert Rev. Neurother.* 12, 1467–1480. doi: 10.1586/ern.12.128

Hall, E. D., Vaishnav, R. A., and Mustafa, A. G. (2010). Antioxidant therapies for traumatic brain injury. *Neurotherapeutics* 7, 51–61. doi: 10.1016/j.nurt.2009.10.021

Hametner, S., Wimmer, I., Haider, L., Pfeifenbring, S., Brück, W., and Lassmann, H. (2013). Iron and neurodegeneration in the multiple sclerosis brain. *Ann. Neurol.* 74, 848–861. doi: 10.1002/ana.23974

Hare, D., Ayton, S., Bush, A., and Lei, P. (2013). A delicate balance: iron metabolism and diseases of the brain. *Front. Aging Neurosci.* 5:34. doi: 10.3389/fnagi.2013.00034

Hare, D. J., Raven, E. P., Roberts, B. R., Bogeski, M., Portbury, S. D., McLean, C. A., et al. (2016). Laser ablation-inductively coupled plasma-mass spectrometry imaging of white and gray matter iron distribution in Alzheimer's disease frontal cortex. *Neuroimage* 137, 124–131. doi: 10.1016/j.neuroimage.2016.05.057

Hasiloglu, Z. I., Albayram, S., Selcuk, H., Ceyhan, E., Delil, S., Arkan, B., et al. (2011). Cerebral microhemorrhages detected by susceptibility-weighted imaging in amateur boxers. *Am. J. Neuroradiol.* 32, 99–102. doi: 10.3174/ajnr.A2250

Hatakeyama, T., Okauchi, M., Hua, Y., Keep, R. F., and Xi, G. (2013). Deferoxamine reduces neuronal death and hematoma lysis after intracerebral hemorrhage in aged rats. *Transl. Stroke Res.* 4, 546–553. doi: 10.1007/s12975-013-0270-5

Hirose, W., Ikematsu, K., and Tsuda, R. (2003). Age-associated increases in heme oxygenase-1 and ferritin immunoreactivity in the autopsied brain. *Leg. Med.* 5(Suppl. 1), S360–S366. doi: 10.1016/S1344-6223(02)00133-5

Hogarth, P. (2015). Neurodegeneration with brain iron accumulation: diagnosis and management. *J. Mov. Disord.* 8, 1–13. doi: 10.14802/jmd.14034

Huang, L., Coats, J. S., Mohd-Yusof, A., Yin, Y., Assaad, S., Muellner, M. J., et al. (2013). Tissue vulnerability is increased following repetitive mild traumatic brain injury in the rat. *Brain Res.* 1499, 109–120. doi: 10.1016/j.brainres.2012.12.038

Huang, Y. L., Kuo, Y. S., Tseng, Y. C., Chen, D. Y., Chiu, W. T., and Chen, C. J. (2015). Susceptibility-weighted MRI in mild traumatic brain injury. *Neurology* 84, 580–585. doi: 10.1212/wnl.0000000000001237

Irimia, A., Van Horn, J. D., and Vespa, P. M. (2018). Cerebral microhemorrhages due to traumatic brain injury and their effects on the aging human brain. *Neurobiol. Aging* 66, 158–164. doi: 10.1016/j.neurobiolaging.2018.02.026

Jellinger, K., Paulus, W., Grundke-Iqbal, I., Riederer, P., and Youdim, M. B. (1990). Brain iron and ferritin in Parkinson's and Alzheimer's diseases. *J. Neural Transm. Park. Dis. Dement. Sect.* 2, 327–340. doi: 10.1007/BF02252926

Justicia, C., Ramos-Cabrer, P., and Hoehn, M. (2008). MRI detection of secondary damage after stroke: chronic iron accumulation in the thalamus of the rat brain. *Stroke* 39, 1541–1547. doi: 10.1161/strokeaha.107.503565

Kalinowski, D. S., and Richardson, D. R. (2005). The evolution of iron chelators for the treatment of iron overload disease and cancer. *Pharmacol. Rev.* 57, 547–583. doi: 10.1124/pr.57.4.2

Ke, Y., and Qian, Z. M. (2007). Brain iron metabolism: neurobiology and neurochemistry. *Prog. Neurobiol.* 83, 149–173. doi: 10.1016/j.pneurobio.2007.07.009

Khalaf, S., Ahmad, A. S., Chamara, K., and Dore, S. (2018). Unique properties associated with the brain penetrant iron chelator HBED reveal remarkable beneficial effects after brain trauma. *J. Neurotrauma* doi: 10.1089/neu.2017.5617 [Epub ahead of print].

Klebanoff, S. J., Waltersdorph, A. M., Michel, B. R., and Rosen, H. (1989). Oxygen-based free radical generation by ferrous ions and deferoxamine. *J. Biol. Chem.* 264, 19765–19771.

Koeppen, A. H., Michael, S. C., Li, D., Chen, Z., Cusack, M. J., Gibson, W. M., et al. (2008). The pathology of superficial siderosis of the central nervous system. *Acta Neuropathol.* 116, 371–382. doi: 10.1007/s00401-008-0421-z

Kroner, A., Greenhalgh, A. D., Zarruk, J. G., Passos Dos Santos, R., Gaestel, M., and David, S. (2014). TNF and increased intracellular iron alter macrophage polarization to a detrimental M1 phenotype in the injured spinal cord. *Neuron* 83, 1098–1116. doi: 10.1016/j.neuron.2014.07.027

Kuchcinski, G., Munsch, F., Lopes, R., Bigourdan, A., Su, J., Sagnier, S., et al. (2017). Thalamic alterations remote to infarct appear as focal iron accumulation and impact clinical outcome. *Brain* 140, 1932–1946. doi: 10.1093/brain/awx114

Lawrence, T. P., Pretorius, P. M., Ezra, M., Cadoux-Hudson, T., and Voets, N. L. (2017). Early detection of cerebral microbleeds following traumatic brain injury using MRI in the hyper-acute phase. *Neurosci. Lett.* 655, 143–150. doi: 10.1016/j.neulet.2017.06.046

Levi, S., and Finazzi, D. (2014). Neurodegeneration with brain iron accumulation: update on pathogenic mechanisms. *Front. Pharmacol.* 5:99. doi: 10.3389/fphar.2014.00099

Li, Q., Wan, J., Lan, X., Han, X., Wang, Z., and Wang, J. (2017). Neuroprotection of brain-permeable iron chelator VK-28 against intracerebral hemorrhage in mice. *J. Cereb. Blood Flow Metab.* 37, 3110–3123. doi: 10.1177/0271678X17709186

Li, X., Yuan, J., Yang, L., Qin, W., Yang, S., Li, Y., et al. (2017). The significant effects of cerebral microbleeds on cognitive dysfunction: an updated meta-analysis. *PLoS One* 12:e0185145. doi: 10.1371/journal.pone.0185145

Litofsky, N. S., Martin, S., Diaz, J., Ge, B., Petroski, G., Miller, D. C., et al. (2016). The negative impact of anemia in outcome from traumatic brain injury. *World Neurosurg.* 90, 82–90. doi: 10.1016/j.wneu.2016.02.076

Liu, B., Moloney, A., Meehan, S., Morris, K., Thomas, S. E., Serpell, L. C., et al. (2011). Iron promotes the toxicity of amyloid β peptide by impeding its ordered aggregation. *J. Biol. Chem.* 286, 4248–4256. doi: 10.1074/jbc.M110.158980

Liu, H.-D., Li, W., Chen, Z.-R., Zhou, M.-L., Zhuang, Z., Zhang, D.-D., et al. (2013). Increased expression of ferritin in cerebral cortex after human traumatic brain injury. *Neurol. Sci.* 34, 1173–1180. doi: 10.1007/s10072-012-1214-7

Liu, Y., Liu, J., Liu, H., Liao, Y., Cao, L., Ye, B., et al. (2016). Investigation of cerebral iron deposition in aged patients with ischemic cerebrovascular disease using susceptibility-weighted imaging. *Ther. Clin. Risk Manag.* 12, 1239–1247. doi: 10.2147/TCRM.S107783

Long, D. A., Ghosh, K., Moore, A. N., Dixon, C. E., and Dash, P. K. (1996). Deferoxamine improves spatial memory performance following experimental brain injury in rats. *Brain Res.* 717, 109–117. doi: 10.1016/0006-8993(95)01500-0

Lu, L., Cao, H., Wei, X., Li, Y., and Li, W. (2015). Iron deposition is positively related to cognitive impairment in patients with chronic mild traumatic brain injury: assessment with susceptibility weighted imaging. *Biomed Res. Int.* 2015:470676. doi: 10.1155/2015/470676

Lynch, S. G., Peters, K., and LeVine, S. M. (1996). Desferrioxamine in chronic progressive multiple sclerosis: a pilot study. *Mult. Scler.* 2, 157–160. doi: 10.1177/135245859600200306

Martelli, A., and Puccio, H. (2014). Dysregulation of cellular iron metabolism in Friedreich ataxia: from primary iron-sulfur cluster deficit to mitochondrial iron accumulation. *Front. Pharmacol.* 5:130. doi: 10.3389/fphar.2014.00130

Martin-Bastida, A., Ward, R. J., Newbould, R., Piccini, P., Sharp, D., Kabba, C., et al. (2017). Brain iron chelation by deferiprone in a phase 2 randomised double-blinded placebo controlled clinical trial in Parkinson's disease. *Sci. Rep.* 7:1398. doi: 10.1038/s41598-017-01402-2

Millerot-Serrurot, E., Bertrand, N., Mossiat, C., Faure, P., Prigent-Tessier, A., Garnier, P., et al. (2008). Temporal changes in free iron levels after brain ischemia: relevance to the timing of iron chelation therapy in stroke. *Neurochem. Int.* 52, 1442–1448. doi: 10.1016/j.neuint.2008.04.002

Moos, T. (2002). Brain iron homeostasis. *Dan. Med. Bull.* 49, 279–301.

Nisenbaum, E. J., Novikov, D. S., and Lui, Y. W. (2014). The presence and role of iron in mild traumatic brain injury: an imaging perspective. *J. Neurotrauma* 31, 301–307. doi: 10.1089/neu.2013.3102

Nunez, M. T., Urrutia, P., Mena, N., Aguirre, P., Tapia, V., and Salazar, J. (2012). Iron toxicity in neurodegeneration. *Biometals* 25, 761–776. doi: 10.1007/s10534-012-9523-0

Okubo, S., Xi, G., Keep, R. F., Muraszko, K. M., and Hua, Y. (2013). Cerebral hemorrhage, brain edema, and heme oxygenase-1 expression after experimental traumatic brain injury. *Acta Neurochir. Suppl.* 118, 83–87. doi: 10.1007/978-3-7091-1434-6_14

Onyszchuk, G., LeVine, S. M., Brooks, W. M., and Berman, N. E. J. (2009). Post-acute pathological changes in the thalamus and internal capsule in aged mice following controlled cortical impact injury: a magnetic resonance imaging, iron histochemical, and glial immunohistochemical study. *Neurosci. Lett.* 452, 204–208. doi: 10.1016/j.neulet.2009.01.049

Oshiro, S., Morioka, M. S., and Kikuchi, M. (2011). Dysregulation of iron metabolism in Alzheimer's disease, Parkinson's disease, and amyotrophic lateral sclerosis. *Adv. Pharmacol. Sci.* 2011:378278. doi: 10.1155/2011/378278

Panter, S. S., Braughler, J. M., and Hall, E. D. (1992). Dextran-coupled deferoxamine improves outcome in a murine model of head injury. *J. Neurotrauma* 9, 47–53. doi: 10.1089/neu.1992.9.47

Pantopoulos, K., Porwal, S. K., Tartakoff, A., and Devireddy, L. (2012). Mechanisms of mammalian iron homeostasis. *Biochemistry* 51, 5705–5724. doi: 10.1021/bi300752r

Park, J.-H., Park, S.-W., Kang, S.-H., Nam, T.-K., Min, B.-K., and Hwang, S.-N. (2009). Detection of traumatic cerebral microbleeds by susceptibility-weighted image of MRI. *J. Korean Neurosurg. Soc.* 46, 365–369. doi: 10.3340/jkns.2009.46.4.365

Peters, D. G., Connor, J. R., and Meadowcroft, M. D. (2015). The relationship between iron dyshomeostasis and amyloidogenesis in Alzheimer's disease: two sides of the same coin. *Neurobiol. Dis.* 81, 49–65. doi: 10.1016/j.nbd.2015.08.007

Portbury, S. D., Hare, D. J., Sgambelloni, C., Finkelstein, D. I., and Adlard, P. A. (2016). A time-course analysis of changes in cerebral metal levels following a controlled cortical impact. *Metallomics* 8, 193–200. doi: 10.1039/c5mt00234f

Portbury, S. D., Hare, D. J., Sgambelloni, C. J., Bishop, D. P., Finkelstein, D. I., Doble, P. A., et al. (2017). Age modulates the injury-induced metallomic profile in the brain. *Metallomics* 9, 402–410. doi: 10.1039/c6mt00260a

Pujol, J., Junqué, C., Vendrell, P., Grau, J. M., Martí-Vilalta, J. L., Olivé, C., et al. (1992). Biological significance of iron-related magnetic resonance imaging changes in the brain. *Arch. Neurol.* 49, 711–717. doi: 10.1001/archneur.1992.00530310053012

Raz, E., Jensen, J. H., Ge, Y., Babb, J. S., Miles, L., Reaume, J., et al. (2011). Brain iron quantification in mild traumatic brain injury: a magnetic field correlation study. *AJNR Am. J. Neuroradiol.* 32, 1851–1856. doi: 10.3174/ajnr.A2637

Rogers, J., Bush, A., Cho, H.-H., Smith, D., Thomson, A., Friedlich, A., et al. (2008). Iron and the translation of the amyloid precursor protein (APP) and ferritin: riboregulation against neural oxidative damage in Alzheimer's disease. *Biochem. Soc. Trans.* 36(Pt 6), 1282–1287. doi: 10.1042/BST0361282

Rottkamp, C. A., Raina, A. K., Zhu, X., Gaier, E., Bush, A. I., Atwood, C. S., et al. (2001). Redox-active iron mediates amyloid-β toxicity. *Free Radic. Biol. Med.* 30, 447–450. doi: 10.1016/S0891-5849(00)00494-9

Saleppico, S., Mazzolla, R., Boelaert, J. R., Puliti, M., Barluzzi, R., Bistoni, F., et al. (1996). Iron regulates microglial cell-mediated secretory and effector functions. *Cell. Immunol.* 170, 251–259. doi: 10.1006/cimm.1996.0159

Sastry, S., and Arendash, G. W. (1995). Time-dependent changes in iron levels and associated neuronal loss within the *Substantia nigra* following lesions within the neostriatum/globus pallidus complex. *Neuroscience* 67, 649–666. doi: 10.1016/0306-4522(94)00618-F

Scheid, R., Walther, K., Guthke, T., Preul, C., and von Cramon, D. Y. (2006). Cognitive sequelae of diffuse axonal injury. *Arch. Neurol.* 63, 418–424. doi: 10.1001/archneur.63.3.418

Schröder, N., Figueiredo, L., and Martins de Lima, M. N. (2012). Role of brain iron accumulation in cognitive dysfunction: evidence from animal models and human studies. *J. Alzheimers Dis.* 34, 797–812. doi: 10.3233/JAD-121996

Smith, M. A., Harris, P. L., Sayre, L. M., and Perry, G. (1997). Iron accumulation in Alzheimer disease is a source of redox-generated free radicals. *Proc. Natl. Acad. Sci. U.S.A.* 94, 9866–9868. doi: 10.1073/pnas.94.18.9866

Sripetchwandee, J., Pipatpiboon, N., Chattipakorn, N., and Chattipakorn, S. (2014). Combined therapy of iron chelator and antioxidant completely restores brain dysfunction induced by iron toxicity. *PLoS One* 9:e85115. doi: 10.1371/journal.pone.0085115

Sripetchwandee, J., Wongjaikam, S., Krintratun, W., Chattipakorn, N., and Chattipakorn, S. C. (2016). A combination of an iron chelator with an antioxidant effectively diminishes the dendritic loss, Tau-hyperphosphorylation, amyloids-beta accumulation and brain mitochondrial dynamic disruption in rats with chronic iron-overload. *Neuroscience* 332, 191–202. doi: 10.1016/j.neuroscience.2016.07.003

Stankiewicz, J., Panter, S. S., Neema, M., Arora, A., Batt, C. E., and Bakshi, R. (2007). Iron in chronic brain disorders: imaging and neurotherapeutic implications. *Neurotherapeutics* 4, 371–386. doi: 10.1016/j.nurt.2007.05.006

Stocchetti, N., Paternò, R., Citerio, G., Beretta, L., and Colombo, A. (2012). Traumatic brain injury in an aging population. *J. Neurotrauma* 29, 1119–1125. doi: 10.1089/neu.2011.1995

Stuber, C., Pitt, D., and Wang, Y. (2016). Iron in multiple sclerosis and its noninvasive imaging with quantitative susceptibility mapping. *Int. J. Mol. Sci.* 17:E100. doi: 10.3390/ijms17010100

Toklu, H. Z., and Tumer, N. (2015). "Oxidative stress, brain edema, blood-brain barrier permeability, and autonomic dysfunction from traumatic brain injury," in *Brain Neurotrauma: Molecular, Neuropsychological, and Rehabilitation Aspects*, ed. F. H. Kobeissy (Boca Raton, FL: CRC Press).

Torben, M., Rosengren, N. T., Skjørringe, T., and Morgan, E. H. (2007). Iron trafficking inside the brain. *J. Neurochem.* 103, 1730–1740. doi: 10.1111/j.1471-4159.2007.04976.x

Ueda, Y., Kitamoto, A., Willmore, L. J., and Kojima, T. (2013). Hippocampal gene expression profiling in a rat model of posttraumatic epilepsy reveals temporal upregulation of lipid metabolism-related genes. *Neurochem. Res.* 38, 1399–1406. doi: 10.1007/s11064-013-1037-9

Urrutia, P. J., Mena, N. P., and Nunez, M. T. (2014). The interplay between iron accumulation, mitochondrial dysfunction, and inflammation during the execution step of neurodegenerative disorders. *Front. Pharmacol.* 5:38. doi: 10.3389/fphar.2014.00038

van der Horn, H. J., de Haan, S., Spikman, J. M., de Groot, J. C., and van der Naalt, J. (2018). Clinical relevance of microhemorrhagic lesions in subacute mild traumatic brain injury. *Brain Imaging Behav.* 12, 912–916. doi: 10.1007/s11682-017-9743-6

van Duijn, S., Bulk, M., van Duinen, S. G., Nabuurs, R. J. A., van Buchem, M. A., van der Weerd, L., et al. (2017). Cortical iron reflects severity of Alzheimer's disease. *J. Alzheimers Dis.* 60, 1533–1545. doi: 10.3233/JAD-161143

van Etten, E. S., van der Grond, J., Dumas, E. M., van den Bogaard, S. J., van Buchem, M. A., and Wermer, M. J. (2015). MRI susceptibility changes suggestive of iron deposition in the thalamus after ischemic stroke. *Cerebrovasc. Dis.* 40, 67–72. doi: 10.1159/000433560

Venkateshappa, C., Harish, G., Mahadevan, A., Srinivas Bharath, M. M., and Shankar, S. K. (2012a). Elevated oxidative stress and decreased antioxidant function in the human hippocampus and frontal cortex with increasing age: implications for neurodegeneration in Alzheimer's disease. *Neurochem. Res.* 37, 1601–1614. doi: 10.1007/s11064-012-0755-8

Venkateshappa, C., Harish, G., Mythri, R. B., Mahadevan, A., Bharath, M. M., and Shankar, S. K. (2012b). Increased oxidative damage and decreased antioxidant function in aging human *Substantia nigra* compared to striatum: implications for Parkinson's disease. *Neurochem. Res.* 37, 358–369. doi: 10.1007/s11064-011-0619-7

Wan, W., Jin, L., Wang, Z., Wang, L., Fei, G., Ye, F., et al. (2017). Iron deposition leads to neuronal α-synuclein pathology by inducing autophagy dysfunction. *Front. Neurol.* 8:1. doi: 10.3389/fneur.2017.00001

Ward, R. J., Zucca, F. A., Duyn, J. H., Crichton, R. R., and Zecca, L. (2014). The role of iron in brain ageing and neurodegenerative disorders. *Lancet Neurol.* 13, 1045–1060. doi: 10.1016/S1474-4422(14)70117-6

Werring, D. J., Frazer, D. W., Coward, L. J., Losseff, N. A., Watt, H., Cipolotti, L., et al. (2004). Cognitive dysfunction in patients with cerebral microbleeds on T2*-weighted gradient-echo MRI. *Brain* 127, 2265–2275. doi: 10.1093/brain/awh253

Willmore, L. J., Sypert, G. W., and Munson, J. B. (1978). Recurrent seizures induced by cortical iron injection: a model of posttraumatic epilepsy. *Ann. Neurol.* 4, 329–336. doi: 10.1002/ana.410040408

Willmore, L. J., and Ueda, Y. (2009). Posttraumatic epilepsy: hemorrhage, free radicals and the molecular regulation of glutamate. *Neurochem. Res.* 34, 688–697. doi: 10.1007/s11064-008-9841-3

Wong, B. X., Tsatsanis, A., Lim, L. Q., Adlard, P. A., Bush, A. I., and Duce, J. A. (2014). β-amyloid precursor protein does not possess ferroxidase activity but does stabilize the cell surface ferrous iron exporter ferroportin. *PLoS One* 9:e114174. doi: 10.1371/journal.pone.0114174

Wu, J., Hua, Y., Keep, R. F., Nakamura, T., Hoff, J. T., and Xi, G. (2003). Iron and iron-handling proteins in the brain after intracerebral hemorrhage. *Stroke* 34, 2964–2969. doi: 10.1161/01.Str.0000103140.52838.45

Xie, B. S., Wang, Y. Q., Lin, Y., Mao, Q., Feng, J. F., Gao, G. Y., et al. (2018). Inhibition of ferroptosis attenuates tissue damage and improves long-term outcomes after traumatic brain injury in mice. *CNS Neurosci. Ther.* doi: 10.1111/cns.13069 [Epub ahead of print].

Xiong, P., Chen, X., Guo, C., Zhang, N., and Ma, B. (2012). Baicalin and deferoxamine alleviate iron accumulation in different brain regions of Parkinson's disease rats. *Neural Regen. Res.* 7, 2092–2098. doi: 10.3969/j.issn.1673-5374.2012.27.002

Yamamoto, A., Shin, R. W., Hasegawa, K., Naiki, H., Sato, H., Yoshimasu, F., et al. (2002). Iron (III) induces aggregation of hyperphosphorylated tau and its reduction to iron (II) reverses the aggregation: implications in the formation of neurofibrillary tangles of Alzheimer's disease. *J. Neurochem.* 82, 1137–1147. doi: 10.1046/j.1471-4159.2002.t01-1-01061.x

Yeatts, S. D., Palesch, Y. Y., Moy, C. S., and Selim, M. (2013). High dose deferoxamine in intracerebral hemorrhage (Hi-Def) trial: rationale, design, and methods. *Neurocrit. Care* 19, 257–266. doi: 10.1007/s12028-013-9861-y

Yu, Y., Zhao, W., Zhu, C., Kong, Z., Xu, Y., Liu, G., et al. (2015). The clinical effect of deferoxamine mesylate on edema after intracerebral hemorrhage. *PLoS One* 10:e0122371. doi: 10.1371/journal.pone.0122371

Zecca, L., Gallorini, M., Schunemann, V., Trautwein, A. X., Gerlach, M., Riederer, P., et al. (2001). Iron, neuromelanin and ferritin content in the *Substantia nigra* of normal subjects at different ages: consequences for iron storage and neurodegenerative processes. *J. Neurochem.* 76, 1766–1773. doi: 10.1046/j.1471-4159.2001.00186.x

Zeng, L., Tan, L., Li, H., Zhang, Q., Li, Y., and Guo, J. (2018). Deferoxamine therapy for intracerebral hemorrhage: a systematic review. *PLoS One* 13:e0193615. doi: 10.1371/journal.pone.0193615

Zhang, J., Zhang, Y., Wang, J., Cai, P., Luo, C., Qian, Z., et al. (2010). Characterizing iron deposition in Parkinson's disease using susceptibility-weighted imaging: an in vivo MR study. *Brain Res.* 1330, 124–130. doi: 10.1016/j.brainres.2010.03.036

Zhang, L., Hu, R., Li, M., Li, F., Meng, H., Zhu, G., et al. (2013). Deferoxamine attenuates iron-induced long-term neurotoxicity in rats with traumatic brain injury. *Neurol. Sci.* 34, 639–645. doi: 10.1007/s10072-012-1090-1

Zhao, J., Chen, Z., Xi, G., Keep, R. F., and Hua, Y. (2014). Deferoxamine attenuates acute hydrocephalus after traumatic brain injury in rats. *Transl. Stroke Res.* 5, 586–594. doi: 10.1007/s12975-014-0353-y

Zivadinov, R., Ramasamy, D. P., Benedict, R. R., Polak, P., Hagemeier, J., Magnano, C., et al. (2016). Cerebral microbleeds in multiple sclerosis evaluated on susceptibility-weighted images and quantitative susceptibility maps: a case-control study. *Radiology* 281, 884–895. doi: 10.1148/radiol.2016160060

3

Oxidative Stress Related to Iron Metabolism in Relapsing Remitting Multiple Sclerosis Patients with Low Disability

Mariacristina Siotto[1], Maria Maddalena Filippi[2], Ilaria Simonelli[3], Doriana Landi[4], Anna Ghazaryan[2,5], Stefano Vollaro[5], Mariacarla Ventriglia[2], Patrizio Pasqualetti[3], Mauro Ciro Antonio Rongioletti[6], Rosanna Squitti[7] and Fabrizio Vernieri[5]*

[1] IRCCS Fondazione Don Carlo Gnocchi, Milan, Italy, [2] Fatebenefratelli Foundation for Health Research and Education, AFaR Division, Rome, Italy, [3] Service of Medical Statistics and Information Technology, Fatebenefratelli Foundation for Health Research and Education, AFaR Division, Rome, Italy, [4] Multiple Sclerosis Clinical and Research Unit, Department of Systems Medicine, Tor Vergata University, Rome, Italy, [5] Neurology Unit, Campus Bio-Medico University of Rome, Rome, Italy, [6] Department of Laboratory Medicine, Research and Development Division, "San Giovanni Calibita", Fatebenefratelli Hospital, Rome, Italy, [7] IRCCS Istituto Centro San Giovanni di Dio Fatebenefratelli, Brescia, Italy

***Correspondence:**
Mariacristina Siotto
mary.siotto@gmail.com
orcid.org/0000-0003-0837-0594

Oxidative status may play a role in chronic inflammation and neurodegeneration which are considered critical etiopathogenetic factors in Multiple Sclerosis (MS), both in the early phase of the disease and in the progressive one. The aim of this study is to explore oxidative status related to iron metabolism in peripheral blood of stable Relapsing-Remitting MS with low disability. We studied 60 Relapsing-Remitting MS patients (age 37.2 ± 9.06, EDSS median 1.0), and 40 healthy controls (age 40.3 ± 10.86). We measured total hydroperoxides (dROMs test) and Total Antioxidant Status (TAS), along with the iron metabolism biomarkers: Iron (Fe), ferritin (Ferr), transferrin (Tf), transferrin saturation (Tfsat), and ceruloplasmin (Cp) panel biomarkers [concentration (iCp) and enzymatic activity (eCp), copper (Cu), ceruloplasmin specific activity (eCp:iCp), copper to ceruloplasmin ratio (Cu:Cp), non-ceruloplasmin copper (nCp-Cu)]. We computed also the Cp:Tf ratio as an index of oxidative stress related to iron metabolism. We found lower TAS levels in MS patients than in healthy controls (CTRL) and normal reference level and higher dROMs and Cp:Tf ratio in MS than in healthy controls. Cp and Cu were higher in MS while biomarkers of iron metabolism were not different between patients and controls. Both in controls and MS, dROMs correlated with iCp (CTRL $r = 0.821$, $p < 0.001$; MS $r = 0.775$ $p < 0.001$) and eCp (CTRL $r = 0.734$, $p < 0.001$; MS $r = 0.820$ $p < 0.001$). Moreover, only in MS group iCp correlated negatively with Tfsat ($r = -0.257$, $p = 0.047$). Dividing MS patients in "untreated" group and "treated" group, we found a significant difference in Fe values [$F(2, 97) = 10.136$, $p < 0.001$]; in particular "MS untreated" showed higher mean values (mean = 114.5, $SD = 39.37$ μg/dL) than CTRL (mean 78.6, $SD = 27.55$ μg/dL $p = 0.001$) and "MS treated" (mean = 72.4, $SD = 38.08$ μg/dL; $p < 0.001$). Moreover, "MS untreated" showed significantly higher values of Cp:Tf (mean = 10.19, $SD = 1.77*10^{-2}$; $p = 0.015$), than CTRL (mean = 9.03,

$SD = 1.46 * 10^{-2}$). These results suggest that chronic oxidative stress is relevant also in the remitting phase of the disease in patients with low disability and short disease duration. Therefore, treatment with antioxidants may be beneficial also in the early stage of the disease to preserve neuronal reserve.

Keywords: multiple sclerosis, oxidative stress, iron metabolism, total antioxidant status, hydroperoxides, ceruloplasmin:transferrin ratio, ceruloplasmin

INTRODUCTION

Multiple sclerosis (MS) is a chronic immune-mediated condition that can affect the brain and the spinal cord and is characterized by a relapsing remitting (RRMS) course eventually followed by secondary progression (SPMS) or gradual progression of disability since the beginning (primary progressive MS – PPMS). MS has been traditionally considered a focal inflammatory demyelinating disease of the white matter, while today the role of chronic and diffuse gray matter neurodegeneration in the disability accrual is well established (Stys et al., 2012). Neurodegeneration accompanies demyelination since the early phases of the disease and becomes the main pathological feature in the secondary and primary progressive forms.

Inflammation and neurodegeneration are mutually dependent phenomena. Inflammation, in fact, induces degeneration, likely through excitotoxicity mechanisms (Centonze et al., 2009); on the other hand neurodegeneration can induce inflammatory response, both in the central nervous system (CNS) and in peripheral blood (Träger and Tabrizi, 2013), as demonstrated also in other neurodegenerative conditions (i.e., amyotrophic lateral sclerosis, Alzheimer's disease, Parkinson's disease, and Huntington's disease) (Träger and Tabrizi, 2013). Nevertheless, consolidated biomarkers of chronic inflammation in MS are lacking, although many studies have identified oxidative stress markers as particularly promising to estimate peripheral inflammation in MS since inflammation leads to oxidative stress and vice-versa (Naidoo and Knapp, 1992; Karg et al., 1999; Besler and Comoğlu, 2003; Ferretti et al., 2005; Koch et al., 2006; Alimonti et al., 2007; Ortiz et al., 2009, 2013; Ghabaee et al., 2010; Ristori et al., 2011; Miller et al., 2012; Oliveira et al., 2012; Tasset et al., 2012). The majority of these studies have demonstrated an increase of peripheral inflammation in the progressive forms of MS or during a relapse; few of them have suggested that oxidative stress and antioxidant capacity are elevated also in RRMS during the remitting phase (Ferretti et al., 2005; Koch et al., 2006; Miller et al., 2012; Oliveira et al., 2012).

Oxidative status is considered to be related to iron (Fe) metabolism. This metal might play a role in the pathogenesis of inflammation and neurodegeneration in MS, causing microglia activation, induction of mitochondria dysfunction and free radicals in the body and in the CNS (Drayer et al., 1987; Bizzi et al., 1990; Zivadinov et al., 2010, 2018; Sheykhansari et al., 2018). Ceruloplasmin (Cp) is an acute phase protein (Hellman and Gitlin, 2002), playing a fundamental role in copper (Cu) and Fe metabolism and holding a strong antioxidant function due to its ferroxidase activity (Gutteridge, 1995): indeed, the Cp:Transferrin (Tf) system (measured by the Cp:Tf ratio) is reported to be the main antioxidant system in peripheral blood (Kozlov et al., 1984). Cp has also been recognized as marker of inflammation in systemic pathologies (Göçmen et al., 2008; Tang et al., 2012) and we found that the Cp:Tf ratio is elevated in Alzheimer's disease (Squitti et al., 2010; Siotto et al., 2016), in stroke (Altamura et al., 2009; Squitti et al., 2018b) and in subacute post-stroke patients affected by neuropathic pain (Siotto et al., 2017), where it correlates with the clinical status.

Our study aimed to identify possible and easy to test markers of peripheral inflammation and to explore Fe metabolism in relation to the clinical status in MS patients with low disability in the remitting phase. For this purpose, we used two commercially available biomarker of oxidative stress, along with a panel of biomarkers related to Fe metabolism, strictly associated with oxidative stress.

MATERIALS AND METHODS

Subjects

The study was performed at Neuroscience Department of the Fatebenefratelli Hospital, Isola Tiberina, Rome and at Neurology Unit of the Campus Bio-Medico University of Rome.

Sixty Relapsing-Remitting MS patients (45 females, age 37.2 ± 9.06) fulfilling the 2010 revision of diagnostic criteria of MS (Polman et al., 2011) were recruited. Forty healthy unrelated volunteers (22 females, age 40.3 ± 10.86) of comparable age were also selected as control group (CTRL). All the included patients were free from relapses for at least 6 months before the blood sampling.

Exclusion criteria were the following: therapy with corticosteroids or ACTH in the month before the blood sampling, pregnancy, anemia, alcohol, and drug abuse, use of dietary supplements, chronic diseases potentially inducing systemic inflammation (heart or pulmonary diseases, diabetes, autoimmune diseases, etc.), primary or secondary hepatic diseases, hemochromatosis, aceruloplasminemia and any other diseases with known or presumable effect on Cu/Fe metabolism.

Local institutional ethics committees approved the study and all participating subjects gave written informed consent to be included in the study, in line with the Code of Ethics of the World Medical Association (Declaration of Helsinki) and the standards established by the Authors' Institutional Review Board.

Blood Sampling and Biochemical Assay

Fasting blood samples were collected in the morning and sera fractions were separated by centrifugation (3000 rpm, 10 min, and 4°C). They were then aliquoted and rapidly stored at −80°C.

The subject's aliquots and the reference samples were thawed just before the assay.

All the serum analyses were performed in duplicate on the biochemical analyzer Horiba Pentra 400 (ABX Diagnostic, Montpellier, France).

Total antioxidant blood capacity (TAS) was measured using the TAS kit (Randox Laboratories, Crumlin, United Kingdom) (Rice-Evans and Miller, 1994). Hydroperoxide content was assessed by d-ROMs test (Diacron, Italy) and expressed in arbitrary units (U.CARR) where 1 U.CARR corresponding to 0.08 mg/100 ml of hydrogen peroxide (Alberti et al., 2000).

Iron (Fe) was measured by the photometric test using Ferene (Higgins, 1981) (Horiba ABX, Montpellier, France). Transferrin (Tf) levels were measured by immunoturbidimetric assay (Skikne et al., 1990) and Ferritin was measured by latex-enhanced turbidimetric immunoassay (Simó et al., 1994) (Horiba ABX, Montpellier, France). Concentration of immunological Cp (iCp) was measured by immunoturbidimetric assay (Wolf, 1982) (Futura System SRL, Rome, Italy). The enzymatic activity of Cp (eCp) was tested with an automated version of the manual Schosinsky *o*-dianisidine eCp assay (Lehmann et al., 1974; Schosinsky et al., 1974), adapted by our laboratory (Siotto et al., 2014). The serum copper (Cu) concentration was measured using the colorimetric assay of Abe et al. (1989) (Randox Laboratories, Crumlin, United Kingdom).

For each sample, we also computed the specific activity of Cp (enzymatic activity *per* mg of Cp concentration in IU/mg$*10^{-1}$), as the ratio between the Cp enzymatic activity and immunoturbidimetric Cp concentration (eCp/iCp) (Siotto et al., 2014) and the ratio between Cp and Tf serum concentrations (Cp:Tf $*10^{-2}$) (Nobili et al., 2013). nCp-Cu was calculated by means of the equation provided by Walshe [appendix of Walshe (2003)] on the basis of total copper and iCp concentrations in serum. For each serum copper and ceruloplasmin pair, we computed the amount of copper bound to ceruloplasmin (CB) and the amount of nCp-Cu, following standard procedures (Appendix 1: "Calculation of 'free copper' concentration"). The Cu:Cp ratio (Twomey et al., 2006; Squitti et al., 2014) was calculated as reported in Twomey et al. (2006). Moreover, Tf saturation (Tf-sat) was calculated by dividing serum Fe (μg/dL) by the total iron binding capacity (TBC = TF in mg/dL*1.25) and multiplying by 100.

Statistical Analysis

Smirnov test was applied to test the normality distribution of continuous variables. To test difference in age and clinical characteristics between two groups was applied the Student's *t*-test or, when necessary, non-parametric Mann-Whitney test. A logarithmic transformation was applied to minimize the variability and to better approximate the data distribution to normality.

Correlation between all biochemical variables were calculated by the Pearson's correlation coefficient separately in the MS and CTRL groups to look for any differences in the reciprocal behavior of the variables between the two groups. Non-parametric Spearman's correlation was calculated to test the correlation between the biochemical variables and the clinical variables (EDSS, disease duration). Analysis of variance (ANOVA) model was applied to evaluate the difference in the biochemical variables between CTRL and MS patients and between CTRL and MS divided in "untreated MS" and "treated MS," adjusting for sex and age. The results were presented as mean and standard deviation (*SD*). Benjamini-Hochberg procedure was applied to adjust the *p*-value in multiple comparisons. A *p*-value < 0.05 has been considered statistically significant. The statistical analysis was performed using IBM SPSS Statistics for Windows version 19.0.0.

RESULTS

All patients had a low disability [Expanded Disability Status Scale, EDSS 1.0 (0.0–4.5)], except for a single male patient with EDSS 4.5. Patients on disease modifying therapy (DMT) were 78%, of which 85% treated with interferon-beta (Significant demographic and clinical data are listed in **Table 1**). Patients and controls did not diverge for age but were different for sex distribution ($p = 0.018$, see **Table 1**).

Differences in biochemical variables, adjusted for sex and age in ANOVA analyses, between MS patients and CTRL were reported in **Table 2**. TAS was significantly lower in patients than in controls (MS mean = 1.24, *SD* = 0.14 vs. CTRL mean = 1.39, *SD* = 0.13 mmol/L; $p = 0.001$) and lower than normal reference range indicated by the manufacturer (1.30–1.77 mmol/L). The total hydroperoxides in circulation were higher in MS patients than in healthy volunteers (MS mean = 329.6, *SD* = 75.15 vs. CTRL mean = 295.2, *SD* = 61.38 UCarr; $p = 0.032$). Moreover, the Cp:Tf ratio was higher in MS patients than in controls (MS mean = 9.89, *SD* = $1.48*10^{-2}$ vs. CTRL mean = 9.03, *SD* = 1.46 $*10^{-2}$; $p = 0.005$) (**Table 2** and **Figure 1**).

The iCp values were higher in patients with respect to healthy controls (MS mean = 26.9, *SD* = 3.86 vs. CTRL mean = 24.8, *SD* = 3.28 mg/dL; $p = 0.006$) and coherently the Cu values were a slightly higher in patients (MS mean = 13.7, *SD* = 0.29 vs. CTRL mean = 12.8, *SD* = 0.33 μmol/L; $p = 0.043$; **Figure 1**).

The following biological variables correlated both in healthy controls and MS patients: dROMs with iCp (CTRL: $r = 0.821$, $p < 0.001$; MS: $r = 0.775$ $p < 0.001$) and eCp (CTRL: $r = 0.734$, $p < 0.001$; MS: $r = 0.820$ $p < 0.001$). Moreover, in MS patients iCp correlated negatively with Tfsat ($r = -0.257$, $p = 0.047$) but it not survived after the adjustment for multiple comparisons (B-H adjusted $p = 0.094$) (**Figure 2**). No additional correlations were found among any of the other biochemical parameters and EDSS, disease duration (all $p > 0.2$).

Considering untreated MS patients and treated MS as two separate groups, we did not observe differences in disease duration (Mann Whitney test $p = 0.10$) and EDSS (Mann Whitney test $p = 0.448$).

We performed the ANOVA analyses comparing the two groups of MS patients with CTRL. All analyses were adjusted for sex and age. TAS was significantly lower in both patients' groups than in controls ("untreated MS" mean = 1.25, *SD* = 0.14 mmol/L and "treated MS" mean = 1.23, *SD* = 0.15 mmol/L vs. CTRL mean = 1.39 *SD* = 0.15 mmol/L; $p = 0.015$ and

TABLE 1 | Demographic of multiple sclerosis patients (MS) and healthy volunteers (CTRL).

	n	Age Mean (*SD*)	Disease duration Median (range)	EDSS Median (IQR)	Patients on Disease Modifying Therapy (DMT) (*n*)
MS patients	**60**	**37.2 (9.06)**	**2.39 (0.01–19.86)**	**1.0 (1–2)**	**41 (78%)**
Females	45	36.0 (9.08)	3.9 (0.2–20.1)	1.0 (0.0–1.75)	32
Controls	**42**	**40.3 (10.86)**			
Females	22	40.4 (11.05)			

In non-bold are reported data of Female MS and Female CTRL.

TABLE 2 | Biological variable differences in multiple sclerosis patients (MS) and in healthy volunteers (CTRL).

Biochemical variables		MS *n* = 60	CTRL *n* = 42	ANOVA[a] *p*-value
Total antioxidant capacity (TAS, mmol/L)	Mean (*SD*)	1.24 (0.14)	1.39 (0.13)	**0.001**
Hydroperoxides, dROMs (UCarr)	Mean (*SD*)	329.6 (75.15)	295.2 (61.38)	**0.032**
Iron (Fe, μg/dL)	Mean (*SD*)	85.7 (42.97)	78.6 (27.55)	0.268
Ferritin (Ferr, ng/mL)	Median (25–75)	42.2 (22.8–110.17)	39.6 (26.23–112.47)	0.236[b]
Transferrin (Tf, g/L)	Mean (*SD*)	2.75 (0.05)	2.79 (0.05)	0.616
Ceruloplasmin (iCp, mg/dL)	Mean (*SD*)	26.9 (3.86)	24.8 (3.28)	**0.006**
Copper (Cu, μmol/L)	Mean (*SD*)	13.74 (0.29)	12.84 (0.33)	**0.043**
Ceruloplasmin activity (eCp, IU/L)	Mean (*SD*)	105.5 (21.94)	97.6 (19.14)	0.142
Cp:Tf ratio ($*10^{-2}$)	Mean (*SD*)	9.89 (1.485)	9.03 (1.463)	**0.005**
Transferrin saturation (Tf sat, %)	Mean (*SD*)	25.2 (13.96)	22.7 (8.43)	0.192
Ceruloplasmin specific activity (eCp/iCp IU/mg$*10^{-1}$)	Mean (*SD*)	3.85 (0.09)	3.91 (0.10)	0.667
Copper not bound to ceruloplasmin (nCp-Cu, μmol/L)	Mean (*SD*)	1.05 (0.2)	1.12 (0.22)	0.832
Cu:Cp ratio	Mean (*SD*)	6.76 (0.11)	6.85 (0.12)	0.589

[a]*ANOVA model was applied to evaluated the difference in the biochemical variables between healthy controls and SM patients adjusting for sex and age.*
[b]*ANOVA model was applied considered the logarithmic transformation of the variable.*
Bold indicates $p < 0.05$.

$p = 0.005$, respectively) which is consistent with our previous observations. The total hydroperoxides in circulation were no longer significantly different between the three groups ($p = 0.081$). Dividing MS patients in "untreated" group and "treated" group, we found a significant difference in Fe values [$F(2, 97) = 10.136$, $p < 0.001$]; in particular "untreated MS" showed higher mean values (mean = 114.5, $SD = 39.37$ μg/dL) than CTRL (mean 78.6, $SD = 27.55$ μg/dL $p = 0.001$) and "treated MS" (mean = 72.4, $SD = 38.08$ μg/dL; $p < 0.001$). Moreover, "untreated MS" presented significantly higher values of Cp:Tf (mean = 10.19, $SD = 1.77*10^{-2}$; $p = 0.015$), than CTRL (mean = 9.03, $SD = 1.46*10^{-2}$) (**Figure 3**).

DISCUSSION

The main result of this study is that in RRMS patients with low disability in the early phase of disease, the oxidative stress status is altered, as it is revealed by low levels of TAS, and high levels of total hydroperoxides and of Cp:Tf (**Table 2** and **Figure 1**). In fact, even though EDSS scores were low, suggesting a low rate of neurodegeneration, all the serum biomarkers of oxidative status analyzed revealed a marked imbalance in systemic oxidative stress.

Another interesting result is that dividing MS patients in "treated" and "untreated," we found increased level of Fe and Cp:Tf ratio in "MS untreated," suggesting a role of therapy in oxidative stress related to Fe levels (**Figure 3**).

We employed TAS and dROMs as oxidative stress markers, two easy to use and common laboratory assays to test general oxidative stress status of the body, and the Cp: Tf ratio which is an index optimized from our laboratory to explore oxidative stress mediated by Fe.

The TAS is a measure of the total antioxidant capacity of general circulation. The biochemical assay is based on the principle of inducing the antioxidant defense of serum; this is achieved by introducing a radical reagent opportunely and previously formed in the sample; the serum sample is then added. Serum can exert a suppression of the radical in a way that is directly proportional to the ability of all antioxidant components in serum to counteract the radical oxidation. We found that serum samples of MS patients were not able to counteract the induced oxidative stress, as revealed by TAS values lower than healthy control and reference range (**Table 2** and **Figure 1**). No differences in TAS levels were found between "treated MS" and "untreated MS"; TAS values were significantly lower in both patients' group and under the reference range.

The dROMs is a test that measures directly the hydroperoxides circulating in serum (Cesarone et al., 1999; Alberti et al., 2000). High dROMs have been found in patients with different chronic conditions, correlating with the clinical outcome (Daniil et al., 2008; Capone et al., 2012; Vassalle et al., 2012; Taguchi et al., 2013) and with C reactive protein (Kotani and Taniguchi, 2012; Taguchi et al., 2013). Moreover, antioxidant administration has been demonstrated to reduce dROMs (Cornelli et al., 2001). In this study we noticed a very strong positive correlation

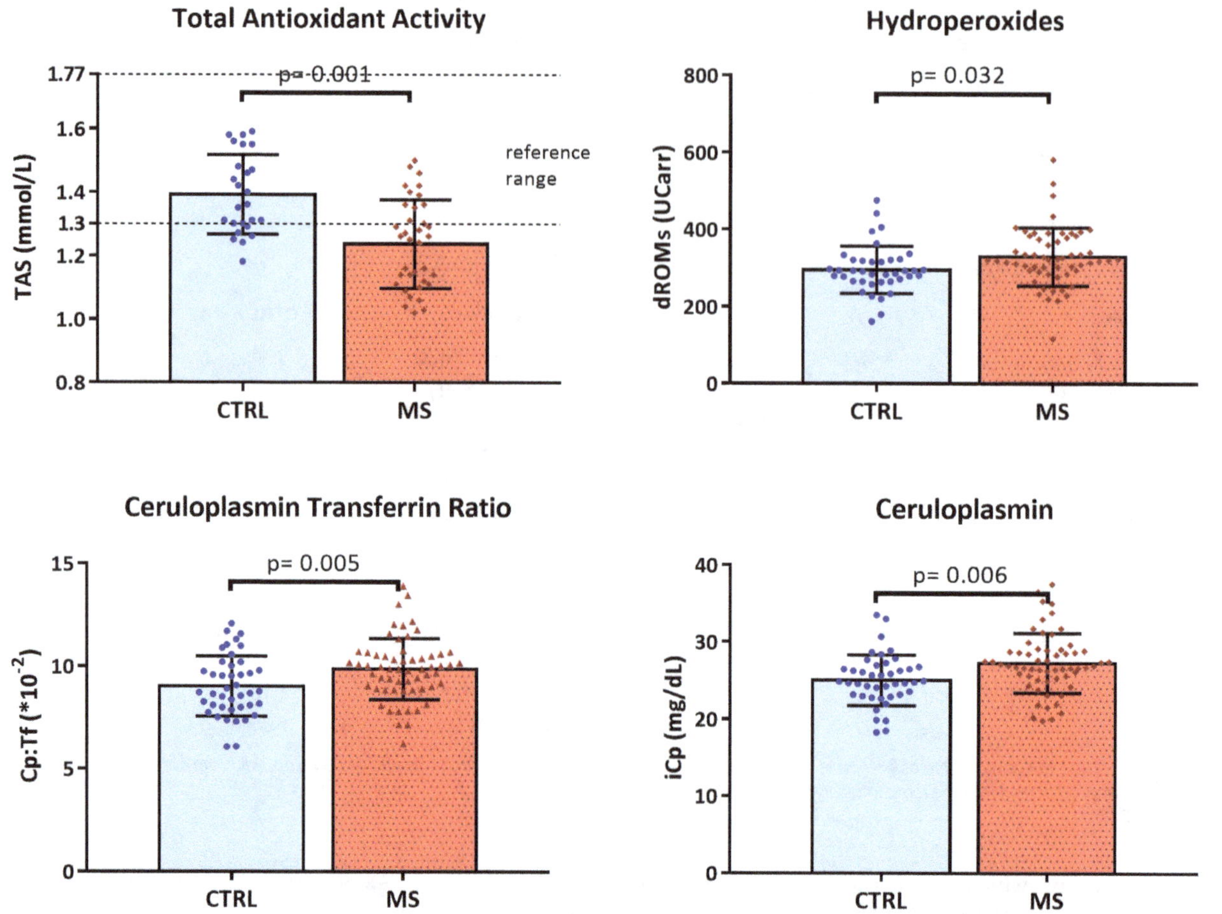

FIGURE 1 | Scattered dot plot with bar plot (mean with *SD*) of total antioxidant status (TAS), hydroperoxides (dROMs), ceruloplasmin transferrin ratio (Cp:Tf), and ceruloplasmin (iCp) in CTRL and MS.

between iCp and eCp and dROMs (both in healthy CTRL and in MS with a Spearman's rho close to 0.8, **Figure 2**). On this basis, dROMs test appears as an alternative measurement of Cp enzymatic activity, or related to the antioxidant activity of Cp. Erel et al. (Harma, 2006) sustained that the chromogen employed in dROMs test was a substrate of the ferroxidase Cp while another study asserted that there is no correlation between ceruloplasmin and dROMs (Colombini et al., 2016). Nevertheless, the hypothesis that enzymatic *o*-dianisidine assays such as *e*Cp might in turn be influenced by the presence of blood hydroperoxides cannot be excluded. Whether measuring oxidative stress or the ferroxidase activity of Cp (as sustained by Erel), dROMs is a reliable method to detect a peripheral response to a systemic stress.

In this study we found dROMs levels higher in MS compared to healthy controls (**Table 2** and **Figure 1**) but no differences were found dividing patients in treated or not.

In order to further explore the oxidative stress status in MS, we also measured the Cp:Tf ratio and we found higher values in MS than in CTRL (**Table 1** and **Figure 1**) and in the group of "untreated MS" (**Figure 3**). This ratio is reported to be the main antioxidant system in serum, and it was measured with Electron Paramagnetic Resonance Spectroscopy by Kozlov et al. (1984). The Cp:Tf variable analyzed in this study, is a calculated index that provides a good quantification of this antioxidant system (Altamura et al., 2009; Nobili et al., 2013). In fact, it quantifies the existing ratio between Cp and Tf. A correct "handling" and distribution of Fe is evinced by a correct stoichiometry between these two proteins. When this occurs, there is consequently a lower probability to develop oxidative stress because the two proteins work in concert reducing levels of ferrous ions, Fe^{2+}, the Fe ion more toxic (Singh et al., 2012) that reacts with hydrogen peroxides initiating oxidative stress chain reactions via Fenton's and Heber Weiss reactions and generating reactive oxygen species.

According to the hypothesis of cerebrospinal venous insufficiency (Zamboni et al., 2009; Zivadinov et al., 2010) abnormality in blood drainage from the brain and spinal cord may contribute to nervous system damage in MS through Fe overload and deposition (Singh and Zamboni, 2009; Singh, 2010). In 2018 a clinical trial study showed no efficacy of venous percutaneous transluminal angioplasty (Zamboni et al., 2018); in fact, the treatment did not increase the proportion of patients who improved functionally nor did it reduce the mean

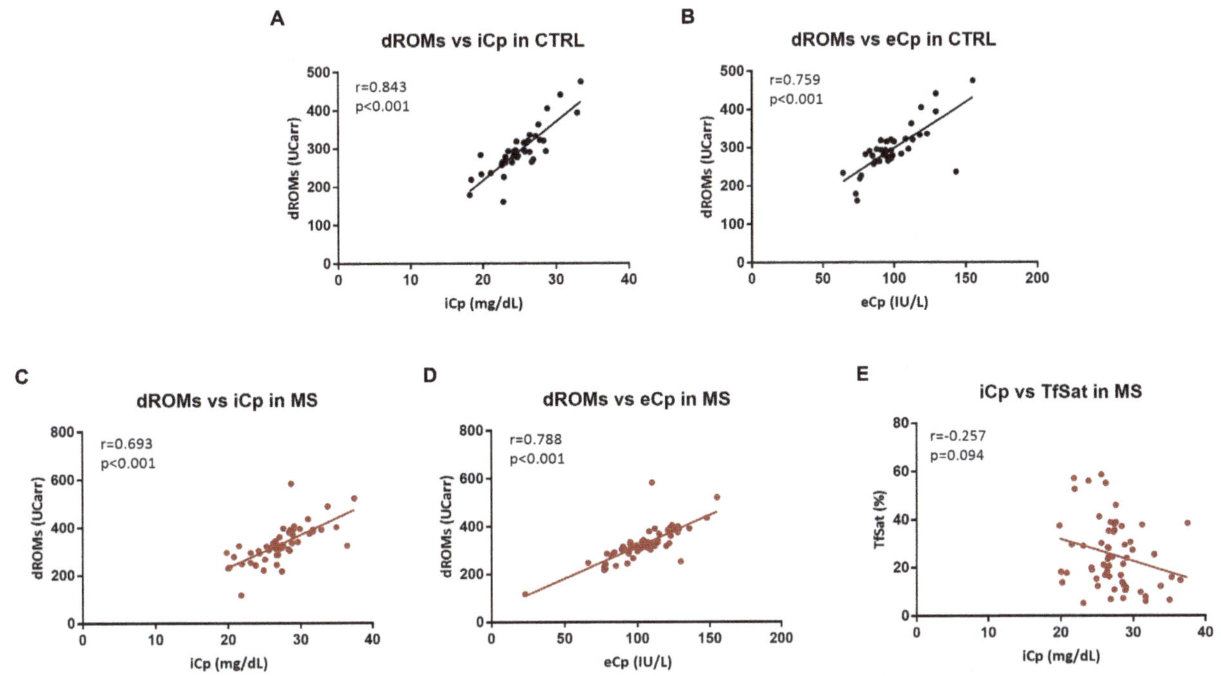

FIGURE 2 | (A,B) Correlation between hydroperoxides (dROMs) and ceruloplasmin (iCp and eCp, respectively) in CTRL. **(C,D)** Correlation between hydroperoxides (dROMs) and ceruloplasmin (iCp and eCp, respectively) in MS. **(E)** Correlation between ceruloplasmin (iCp) vs. transferrin saturation (TfSat %) in MS. A *p*-value < 0.05 was considered statistically significant.

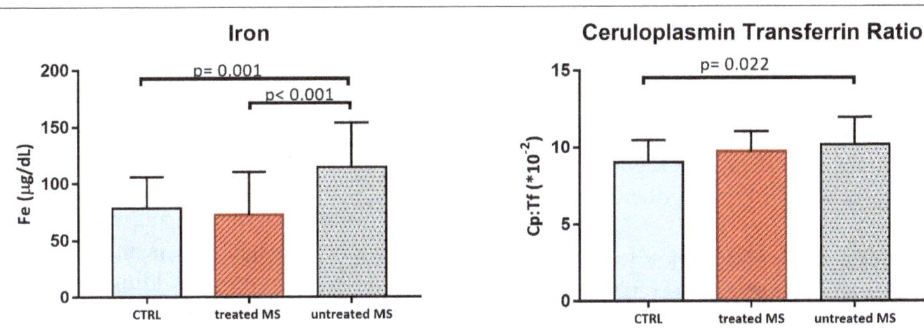

FIGURE 3 | Bar plot (mean with *SD*) of iron (Fe) and ceruloplasmin transferrin ratio (Cp:Tf) in CTRL, MS in disease modifying therapy (treated MS), and in MS not in disease modifying therapy (untreated MS).

number of new combined brain lesions on magnetic resonance imaging (MRI) at 12 months. However, the CCSVI hypothesis has been linked with the potential effects of Fe deposition in the brain parenchyma. Together with radiological data which suggest excessive Fe accumulation in the brain of MS patients (Drayer et al., 1987; Bizzi et al., 1990; Zivadinov et al., 2010), this hypothesis drove researchers attention upon the Fe as a possible cause of neurodegeneration, although the reasons of Fe overload are not clear yet and presumably they do not depend on CCSVI. The brain Fe accumulation could lead to chronic cell stress, with consequent axonal and neuronal death. Moreover, there are some heme-involved processes that caused lipid oxidation. During de-myelinization, Fe could be released from myelin sheath (for an extensive review see Adamczyk and Adamczyk-Sowa, 2016).

However, we did not find any significant difference between MS group and controls in the markers strictly related to Fe as Fe itself, Ferr, and Tf. On the other hand, we found significant higher level of Fe in "untreated MS" respect to both control and "treated MS" (**Table 2** and **Figure 3**). Despite preliminary and limited by the small sample size, these results are quite interesting as they highlight the importance of better investigating the role of treatment in Fe metabolism.

Looking at the other variables, we also found iCp and Cu higher in MS patients compared to healthy controls. Cp is acute-phase reactant in inflammation processes (such as infection, chronic diseases, arthritis and several neoplasia) and Cu follows the same trend being structurally bound to Cp. Holo-Cp biosynthesis occurs in liver where the Cu is charged in the apo-form of the protein. The Cu in the Cp is not exchangeable, being part of the protein structure. So, in MS, the rise of Cp can explain also the rise of Cu due to an inflammation status. Recently, a study from De Riccardis et al. (2018) on 38 MS patients with EDSS scores under 3.5 reported that Cp and Cu values were higher in MS than in controls of an age and sex matched group of 39 subjects, according to our results. Moreover, they found a significant increase in dROMs values in MS patients.

In our study we found no significative difference in other important markers of Cu status like nCp-Cu that measures the portion of Cu not structurally bound to Cp, and Cu:Cp ratio which is an index of the correct stoichiometry between Cu and Cp (**Table 2**). Conversely, in various study on different neurological diseases, such as Alzheimer's or Wilson's disease (Siotto et al., 2016; Squitti et al., 2018a) or stroke (Siotto et al., 2017; Squitti et al., 2018b) we found these specific markers of Cu status altered, with a clear indication of Cu dishomeostasis.

In our opinion, in our MS group iCp and Cu were higher due to systemic inflammation and not as a result of an imbalance systemic Cu management.

Cp is involved in the metabolism of Fe being the main ferroxidase of the serum, as it oxidizes Fe from Fe^{2+} to Fe^{3+}, which could be charged from Tf for being transported into the circulation. The increase of iCp in MS and its negative correlation with TfSat stands for an impairment in the Fe handling, being that in MS the more circulating Cp correlates with less TfSat (Letendre and Holbein, 1984; Hellman and Gitlin, 2002). Transferrin itself showed no differences between MS and CTRL as reported also in a study on CSF samples (LeVine et al., 1999).

Summarizing our results, the oxidative stress is clearly an evidence in MS patients, but while the values of TAS and dROMs appeared not to be influenced by therapy, underlining the general systemic oxidative stress in MS, Cp:Tf ratio is a good index to detect oxidative stress strictly related to Fe and potentially related with therapy.

Cp:Tf ratio values is an easy and good marker to investigate the mismanagement of Fe. A higher Cp:Tf ratio has been observed in two studies on stroke patients during acute phase (Altamura et al., 2009; Squitti et al., 2018b). Moreover, we recently found an increase of Cp:Tf ratio in subacute stroke patients affected by neuropathic pain (Siotto et al., 2017). In this group of patients, TAS levels were lower than normal, whereas the Cp:Tf ratio was higher. Decreased TAS levels indicated depletion of the antioxidant system compounds and a reduced ability to counteract the increased oxidative stress generated by stroke injury. The parallel increase of Cp:Tf ratio revealed the activation of systemic processes leading to the cellular internalization of Fe in order to contain oxidative stress in subacute post-stroke patients with neuropathic pain (Carbonell and Rama, 2007).

Similarly, TAS levels, being lower in our group of MS patients, than both in healthy controls and in the reference range, reveal an inability to counteract oxidative stress in patients with early MS. In the meantime, the Cp:Tf system responds to a general status of oxidation (as depicted also from higher levels of hydroperoxides) and is activated to exert a cellular internalization of Fe, especially in patients with higher levels of Fe.

In a study by Oliveira et al. (2012) oxidative stress in MS was evaluated by measuring various oxidative biomarkers. Compared to controls, MS patients with EDSS > 3.5 exhibited higher plasma levels of tert-butyl hydroperoxide-initiated chemiluminescence and carbonyl protein, as well as lower plasma levels of nitric oxide, total radical-trapping antioxidant parameter (measured by the same test we used in current study). In agreement with our results, Oliveira et al. (2012) demonstrated that oxidative stress is important in the physiopathology of MS progression. Is it well known that reactive oxygen species are generated in excess by macrophages which have been implicated as mediators of demyelination and axonal damage in both MS and experimental autoimmune animal models (Gilgun-Sherki et al., 2004).

Another study exploring the value of oxidative stress biomarkers in MS patients reported that plasmatic advanced oxidation protein products were significantly higher while ferric reducing ability and thiol group levels were lower in MS patients in comparison with healthy controls (Pasquali et al., 2015).

Our results underline the importance to monitor oxidative stress and Fe in patients, both at the beginning of the disease and during the DMT. The blood tests employed in this study are easier to perform and cheaper than other serum and radiological biomarkers. MRI is a very well-established method for qualitative and quantitative assessment of MS related damage, but it needs clinical expertise and cumbersome instrumentation set up.

CONCLUSION

An altered status of oxidative stress and/or antioxidant response is detectable in MS patients with low disability analyzed during a relapse-free period, suggesting the occurrence of a systemic subclinical inflammation that accompanies MS even in the early stages and in the remitting phase. Assessment of the oxidative stress biomarkers and particularly of Cp:Tf ratio, which is strictly related to Fe management, is an easy way to monitor oxidative stress in MS. Moreover, adding antioxidants to conventional immunotherapy in MS may be reasonable and highly beneficial for MS patients due to their ability to reduce oxidative stress. Further research should be performed to test new antioxidants, and to develop new methods to monitor oxidative stress.

AUTHOR CONTRIBUTIONS

MMF, DL, AG, SV, and FV contributed to patient enrolment and clinical evaluation. MS, RS, and MV contributed to blood sample collection and biochemical evaluation. MS, IS, MMF, PP, MCAR, RS, and FV contributed to study design, statistical analysis, data interpretation, and manuscript preparation.

FUNDING

The research leading to these results has received funding from: Grant Merck Serono SPC0188 "Impact of systemic metal homeostasis and oxidative status on clinical and radiological parameters of disease severity in Multiple Sclerosis."

REFERENCES

Abe, A., Yamashita, S., and Noma, A. (1989). Sensitive, direct colorimetric assay for copper in serum. *Clin. Chem.* 35, 552–554.

Adamczyk, B., and Adamczyk-Sowa, M. (2016). New insights into the role of oxidative stress mechanisms in the pathophysiology and treatment of multiple sclerosis. *Oxid. Med. Cell. Longev.* 2016:1973834. doi: 10.1155/2016/1973834

Alberti, A., Bolognini, L., Macciantelli, D., and Caratelli, M. (2000). The radical cation of N,N-Diethyl-para-phenylendiamine: a possible indicator of oxidative stress in biological samples. *Res. Chem. Intermed.* 26, 253–267. doi: 10.1163/156856700X00769

Alimonti, A., Ristori, G., Giubilei, F., Stazi, M. A., Pino, A., Visconti, A., et al. (2007). Serum chemical elements and oxidative status in Alzheimer's disease, Parkinson disease and multiple sclerosis. *Neurotoxicology* 28, 450–456. doi: 10.1016/j.neuro.2006.12.001

Altamura, C., Squitti, R., Pasqualetti, P., Gaudino, C., Palazzo, P., Tibuzzi, F., et al. (2009). Ceruloplasmin/Transferrin system is related to clinical status in acute stroke. *Stroke* 40, 1282–1288. doi: 10.1161/STROKEAHA.108.536714

Besler, H. T., and Comoğlu, S. (2003). Lipoprotein oxidation, plasma total antioxidant capacity and homocysteine level in patients with multiple sclerosis. *Nutr. Neurosci.* 6, 189–196. doi: 10.1080/1028415031000115945

Bizzi, A., Brooks, R. A., Brunetti, A., Hill, J. M., Alger, J. R., Miletich, R. S., et al. (1990). Role of iron and ferritin in MR imaging of the brain: a study in primates at different field strengths. *Radiology* 177, 59–65. doi: 10.1148/radiology.177.1.2399339

Capone, F., Guerriero, E., Sorice, A., Maio, P., Colonna, G., Castello, G., et al. (2012). Characterization of metalloproteinases, oxidative status and inflammation levels in the different stages of fibrosis in HCV patients. *Clin. Biochem.* 45, 525–529. doi: 10.1016/j.clinbiochem.2012.02.004

Carbonell, T., and Rama, R. (2007). Iron, oxidative stress and early neurological deterioration in ischemic stroke. *Curr. Med. Chem.* 14, 857–874. doi: 10.2174/092986707780363014

Centonze, D., Muzio, L., Rossi, S., Furlan, R., Bernardi, G., and Martino, G. (2009). The link between inflammation, synaptic transmission and neurodegeneration in multiple sclerosis. *Cell Death Differ.* 17, 1083–1091. doi: 10.1038/cdd.2009.179

Cesarone, M. R., Belcaro, G., Carratelli, M., Cornelli, U., De Sanctis, M. T., Incandela, L., et al. (1999). A simple test to monitor oxidative stress. *Int. Angiol.* 18, 127–130.

Colombini, F., Carratelli, M., and Alberti, A. (2016). Oxidative stress, d-ROMs test, and ceruloplasmin. *Free Radic. Res.* 50, 447–453. doi: 10.3109/10715762.2015.1136063

Cornelli, U., Terranova, R., Luca, S., Cornelli, M., and Alberti, A. (2001). Bioavailability and antioxidant activity of some food supplements in men and women using the d-Roms test as a marker of oxidative stress. *J. Nutr.* 131, 3208–3211. doi: 10.1093/jn/131.12.3208

Daniil, Z. D., Papageorgiou, E., Koutsokera, A., Kostikas, K., Kiropoulos, T., Papaioannou, A. I., et al. (2008). Serum levels of oxidative stress as a marker of disease severity in idiopathic pulmonary fibrosis. *Pulm. Pharmacol. Ther.* 21, 26–31. doi: 10.1016/j.pupt.2006.10.005

De Riccardis, L., Buccolieri, A., Muci, M., Pitotti, E., De Robertis, F., Trianni, G., et al. (2018). Copper and ceruloplasmin dyshomeostasis in serum and cerebrospinal fluid of multiple sclerosis subjects. *Biochim. Biophys. Acta Mol. Basis Dis.* 1864(5 Pt A), 1828–1838. doi: 10.1016/j.bbadis.2018.03.007

Drayer, B., Burger, P., Hurwitz, B., Dawson, D., and Cain, J. (1987). Reduced signal intensity on MR images of thalamus and putamen in multiple sclerosis: increased iron content? *AJR Am. J. Roentgenol.* 149, 357–363. doi: 10.2214/ajr.149.2.357

Ferretti, G., Bacchetti, T., Principi, F., Di Ludovico, F., Viti, B., Angeleri, V. A., et al. (2005). Increased levels of lipid hydroperoxides in plasma of patients with multiple sclerosis: a relationship with paraoxonase activity. *Mult. Scler.* 11, 677–682. doi: 10.1191/1352458505ms1240oa

Ghabaee, M., Jabedari, B., Al-E-Eshagh, N., Ghaffarpour, M., and Asadi, F. (2010). Serum and cerebrospinal fluid antioxidant activity and lipid peroxidation in guillain-barre syndrome and multiple sclerosis patients. *Int. J. Neurosci.* 120, 301–304. doi: 10.3109/00207451003695690

Gilgun-Sherki, Y., Melamed, E., and Offen, D. (2004). The role of oxidative stress in the pathogenesis of multiple sclerosis: the need for effective antioxidant therapy. *J. Neurol.* 251, 261–268. doi: 10.1007/s00415-004-0348-9

Göçmen, A. Y., Sahin, E., Semiz, E., and Gümuşlü, S. (2008). Is elevated serum ceruloplasmin level associated with increased risk of coronary artery disease? *Can. J. Cardiol.* 24, 209–212.

Gutteridge, J. M. C. (1995). Lipid peroxidation and antioxidants as biomarkers of tissue damage. *Clin. Chem.* 41, 1819–1828.

Harma, M. I. (2006). d-ROMs Test Detects Ceruloplasmin, Not Oxidative Stress. *CHEST J.* 130:1276. doi: 10.1378/chest.130.4.1276

Hellman, N. E., and Gitlin, J. D. (2002). Ceruloplasmin metabolism and function. *Annu. Rev. Nutr.* 22, 439–458. doi: 10.1146/annurev.nutr.22.012502.114457

Higgins, T. (1981). Novel chromogen for serum iron determinations. *Clin. Chem.* 27, 1619–1620.

Karg, E., Klivényi, P., Németh, I., Bencsik, K., Pintér, S., and Vécsei, L. (1999). Nonenzymatic antioxidants of blood in multiple sclerosis. *J. Neurol.* 246, 533–539. doi: 10.1007/s004150050399

Koch, M., Ramsaransing, G. S. M., Arutjunyan, A. V., Stepanov, M., Teelken, A., Heersema, D. J., et al. (2006). Oxidative stress in serum and peripheral blood leukocytes in patients with different disease courses of multiple sclerosis. *J. Neurol.* 253, 483–487. doi: 10.1007/s00415-005-0037-3

Kotani, K., and Taniguchi, N. (2012). Correlation between high-sensitivity C-reactive protein and reactive oxygen metabolites during a one-year period among asymptomatic subjects. *J. Clin. Med. Res.* 4, 52–55. doi: 10.4021/jocmr755w

Kozlov, A. V., Sergienko, V. I., Vladimirov, Iu. A, and Azizova, O. A. (1984). The antioxidant system of transferrin-ceruloplasmin in experimental hypercholesterolemia. *Biull. Eksp. Biol. Med.* 98, 668–671.

Lehmann, H. P., Schosinsky, K. H., and Beeler, M. F. (1974). Standardization of serum ceruloplasmin concentrations in international enzyme units with o dianisidine dihydrochloride as substrate. *Clin. Chem.* 20, 1564–1567.

Letendre, E. D., and Holbein, B. E. (1984). Ceruloplasmin and regulation of transferrin iron during *Neisseria meningitidis* infection in mice. *Infect. Immun.* 45, 133–138.

LeVine, S. M., Lynch, S. G., Ou, C. N., Wulser, M. J., Tam, E., and Boo, N. (1999). Ferritin, transferrin and iron concentrations in the cerebrospinal fluid of multiple sclerosis patients. *Brain Res.* 821, 511–515. doi: 10.1016/S0006-8993(98)01360-2

Miller, E., Walczak, A., Saluk, J., Ponczek, M. B., and Majsterek, I. (2012). Oxidative modification of patient's plasma proteins and its role in pathogenesis of multiple sclerosis. *Clin. Biochem.* 45, 26–30. doi: 10.1016/j.clinbiochem.2011.09.021

Naidoo, R., and Knapp, M. L. (1992). Studies of lipid peroxidation products in cerebrospinal fluid and serum in multiple sclerosis and other conditions. *Clin. Chem.* 38, 2449–2454.

Nobili, V., Siotto, M., Bedogni, G., Ravà, L., Pietrobattista, A., Panera, N., et al. (2013). Levels of serum ceruloplasmin associate with pediatric nonalcoholic fatty liver disease. *J. Pediatr. Gastroenterol. Nutr.* 56, 370–375. doi: 10.1097/MPG.0b013e31827aced4

Oliveira, S. R., Kallaur, A. P., Simão, A. N. C., Morimoto, H. K., Lopes, J., Panis, C., et al. (2012). Oxidative stress in multiple sclerosis patients in clinical remission: association with the expanded disability status scale. *J. Neurol. Sci.* 321, 49–53. doi: 10.1016/j.jns.2012.07.045

Ortiz, G. G., Macías-Islas, M. A., Pacheco-Moisés, F. P., Cruz-Ramos, J. A., Sustersik, S., Barba, E. A., et al. (2009). Oxidative stress is increased in serum from mexican patients with relapsing-remitting multiple sclerosis. *Dis. Markers* 26, 35–39. doi: 10.3233/DMA-2009-0602

Ortiz, G. G., Pacheco-Moisés, F. P., Bitzer-Quintero, O. K., Ramírez-Anguiano, A. C., Flores-Alvarado, L. J., Ramírez-Ramírez, V., et al. (2013). Immunology and oxidative stress in multiple sclerosis: clinical and basic approach. *Clin. Dev. Immunol.* 2013:708659. doi: 10.1155/2013/708659

Pasquali, L., Pecori, C., Lucchesi, C., LoGerfo, A., Iudice, A., Siciliano, G., et al. (2015). Plasmatic oxidative stress biomarkers in multiple sclerosis: relation with clinical and demographic characteristics. *Clin. Biochem.* 48, 19–23. doi: 10.1016/j.clinbiochem.2014.09.024

Polman, C. H., Reingold, S. C., Banwell, B., Clanet, M., Cohen, J. A., Filippi, M., et al. (2011). Diagnostic criteria for multiple sclerosis: 2010 revisions to the McDonald criteria. *Ann. Neurol.* 69, 292–302. doi: 10.1002/ana.22366

Rice-Evans, C., and Miller, N. (1994). Total antioxidant status in plasma and body fluids. *Methods Enzym.* 234, 274–279. doi: 10.1016/0076-6879(94)34095-1

Ristori, G., Brescianini, S., Pino, A., Visconti, A., Vittori, D., Coarelli, G., et al. (2011). Serum elements and oxidative status in clinically isolated syndromes: imbalance and predictivity. *Neurology* 76, 549–555. doi: 10.1212/WNL.0b013e31820af7de

Schosinsky, K. H., Lehmann, H. P., and Beeler, M. F. (1974). Measurement of ceruloplasmin from its oxidase activity in serum by use of o-dianisidine dihydrochloride. *Clin. Chem.* 20, 1556–1563.

Sheykhansari, S., Kozielski, K., Bill, J., Sitti, M., Gemmati, D., Zamboni, P., et al. (2018). Redox metals homeostasis in multiple sclerosis and amyotrophic lateral sclerosis: a review review. *Cell Death Dis.* 9:348. doi: 10.1038/s41419-018-0379-2

Simó, J., Joven, J., Clivillé, X., and Sans, T. (1994). Automated latex agglutination immunoassay of serum ferritin with a centrifugal analyzer. *Clin. Chem.* 40, 625–629.

Singh, A., Vyas, V., Montani, E., Cartelli, D., Parazzoli, D., Oldani, A., et al. (2012). Investigation of in vitro cytotoxicity of the redox state of ionic iron in neuroblastoma cells. *J. Neurosci. Rural Pract.* 3, 301–310. doi: 10.4103/0976-3147.102611

Singh, A. V. (2010). Multiple sclerosis takes venous route: CCSVI and liberation therapy. *Indian J. Med. Sci.* 64, 337–340. doi: 10.4103/0019-5359.99879

Singh, A. V., and Zamboni, P. (2009). Anomalous venous blood flow and iron deposition in multiple sclerosis. *J. Cereb. Blood Flow Metab.* 29, 1867–1878. doi: 10.1038/jcbfm.2009.180

Siotto, M., Aprile, I., Simonelli, I., Pazzaglia, C., Ventriglia, M., Santoro, M., et al. (2017). An exploratory study of BDNF and oxidative stress marker alterations in subacute and chronic stroke patients affected by neuropathic pain. *J. Neural Transm.* 124, 1557–1566. doi: 10.1007/s00702-017-1805-9

Siotto, M., Pasqualetti, P., Marano, M., and Squitti, R. (2014). Automation of o-dianisidine assay for ceruloplasmin activity analyses: usefulness of investigation in Wilson's disease and in hepatic encephalopathy. *J. Neural Transm.* 121, 1281–1286. doi: 10.1007/s00702-014-1196-0

Siotto, M., Simonelli, I., Pasqualetti, P., Mariani, S., Caprara, D., Bucossi, S., et al. (2016). Association between serum ceruloplasmin specific activity and risk of Alzheimer's disease. *J. Alzheimers. Dis.* 50, 1181–1189. doi: 10.3233/JAD-150611

Skikne, B. S., Flowers, C. H., and Cook, J. D. (1990). Serum transferrin receptor: a quantitative measure of tissue iron deficiency. *Blood* 75, 1870–1876.

Squitti, R., Ghidoni, R., Simonelli, I., Ivanova, I. D., Colabufo, N. A., Zuin, M., et al. (2018a). Copper dyshomeostasis in Wilson disease and Alzheimer's disease as shown by serum and urine copper indicators. *J. Trace Elem. Med. Biol.* 45, 181–188. doi: 10.1016/j.jtemb.2017.11.005

Squitti, R., Siotto, M., Assenza, G., Giannantoni, N. M., Rongioletti, M., Zappasodi, F., et al. (2018b). Prognostic value of serum copper for post-stroke clinical recovery: a pilot study. *Front. Neurol.* 9:333. doi: 10.3389/fneur.2018.00333

Squitti, R., Salustri, C., Siotto, M., Ventriglia, M., Vernieri, F., Lupoi, D., et al. (2010). Ceruloplasmin/Transferrin ratio changes in Alzheimer's disease. *Int. J. Alzheimers Dis.* 2011:231595. doi: 10.4061/2011/231595

Squitti, R., Simonelli, I., Ventriglia, M., Siotto, M., Pasqualetti, P., Rembach, A., et al. (2014). Meta-analysis of serum non-ceruloplasmin copper in Alzheimer's disease. *J. Alzheimers. Dis.* 38, 809–822. doi: 10.3233/JAD-131247

Stys, P. K., Zamponi, G. W., Van Minnen, J., and Geurts, J. J. G. (2012). Will the real multiple sclerosis please stand up? *Nat. Rev. Neurosci.* 13, 507–514. doi: 10.1038/nrn3275

Taguchi, I., Toyoda, S., Takano, K., Arikawa, T., Kikuchi, M., Ogawa, M., et al. (2013). Irbesartan, an angiotensin receptor blocker, exhibits metabolic, anti-inflammatory and antioxidative effects in patients with high-risk hypertension. *Hypertens. Res.* 36, 608–613. doi: 10.1038/hr.2013.3

Tang, W. H. W., Wu, Y., Hartiala, J., Fan, Y., Stewart, A. F. R., Roberts, R., et al. (2012). Clinical and genetic association of serum ceruloplasmin with cardiovascular risk. *Arterioscler. Thromb. Vasc. Biol.* 32, 516–522. doi: 10.1161/ATVBAHA.111.237040

Tasset, I., Agüera, E., Sánchez-López, F., Feijóo, M., Giraldo, A. I., Cruz, A. H., et al. (2012). Peripheral oxidative stress in relapsing-remitting multiple sclerosis. *Clin. Biochem.* 45, 440–444. doi: 10.1016/j.clinbiochem.2012.01.023

Träger, U., and Tabrizi, S. J. (2013). Peripheral inflammation in neurodegeneration. *J. Mol. Med.* 91, 673–681. doi: 10.1007/s00109-013-1026-0

Twomey, P. J., Viljoen, A., House, I. M., Reynolds, T. M., and Wierzbicki, A. S. (2006). Copper:caeruloplasmin ratio. *J. Clin. Pathol.* 60, 441–442. doi: 10.1136/jcp.2006.041756

Vassalle, C., Bianchi, S., Battaglia, D., Landi, P., Bianchi, F., and Carpeggiani, C. (2012). Elevated levels of oxidative stress as a prognostic predictor of major adverse cardiovascular events in patients with coronary artery disease. *J. Atheroscler. Thromb.* 19, 712–717. doi: 10.5551/jat.12740

Walshe, J. M. (2003). Wilson's disease: the importance of measuring serum caeruloplasmin non-immunologically. *Ann. Clin. Biochem.* 40, 115–121. doi: 10.1258/000456303763046021

Wolf, P. (1982). Ceruloplasmin: methods and clinical use. *Crit. Rev. Clin. Lab. Sci.* 17, 229–245. doi: 10.3109/10408368209107037

Zamboni, P., Galeotti, R., Menegatti, E., Malagoni, A. M., Tacconi, G., Dall'ara, S., et al. (2009). Chronic cerebrospinal venous insufficiency in patients with multiple sclerosis. *J. Neurol. Neurosurg. Psychiatry* 80, 392–399. doi: 10.1136/jnnp.2008.157164

Zamboni, P., Tesio, L., Galimberti, S., Massacesi, L., Salvi, F., D'Alessandro, R., et al. (2018). Efficacy and safety of extracranial vein angioplasty in multiple sclerosis: a randomized clinical trial. *JAMA Neurol.* 75, 35–43. doi: 10.1001/jamaneurol.2017.3825

Zivadinov, R., Schirda, C., Dwyer, M. G., Haacke, M. E., Weinstock-Guttman, B., Menegatti, E., et al. (2010). Chronic cerebrospinal venous insufficiency and iron deposition on susceptibility-weighted imaging in patients with multiple sclerosis: a pilot case-control study. *Int. Angiol.* 29, 158–175.

Zivadinov, R., Tavazzi, E., Bergsland, N., Hagemeier, J., Lin, F., Dwyer, M. G., et al. (2018). Brain iron at quantitative mri is associated with disability in multiple sclerosis. *Radiology* 289, 487–496. doi: 10.1148/radiol.2018180136

4

The Role of Iron in Friedreich's Ataxia: Insights from Studies in Human Tissues and Cellular and Animal Models

José Vicente Llorens[1,2*], *Sirena Soriano*[3,4], *Pablo Calap-Quintana*[1,2], *Pilar Gonzalez-Cabo*[5,6,7] *and María Dolores Moltó*[1,2,8*]

[1] Department of Genetics, Faculty of Biological Sciences, University of Valencia, Valencia, Spain, [2] Unit for Psychiatry and Neurodegenerative Diseases, Biomedical Research Institute INCLIVA, Valencia, Spain, [3] Department of Molecular and Human Genetics, Baylor College of Medicine, Houston, TX, United States, [4] Jan and Dan Duncan Neurological Research Institute, Texas Children's Hospital, Houston, TX, United States, [5] Department of Physiology, Faculty of Medicine and Dentistry, University of Valencia, Valencia, Spain, [6] Center of Biomedical Network Research on Rare Diseases CIBERER, Valencia, Spain, [7] Associated Unit for Rare Diseases INCLIVA-CIPF, Biomedical Research Institute INCLIVA, Valencia, Spain, [8] Center of Biomedical Network Research on Mental Health CIBERSAM, Valencia, Spain

***Correspondence:**
José Vicente Llorens
j.vicente.llorens@uv.es
María Dolores Moltó
dmolto@uv.es

Friedreich's ataxia (FRDA) is a rare early-onset degenerative disease that affects both the central and peripheral nervous systems, and other extraneural tissues, mainly the heart and endocrine pancreas. This disorder progresses as a mixed sensory and cerebellar ataxia, primarily disturbing the proprioceptive pathways in the spinal cord, peripheral nerves and nuclei of the cerebellum. FRDA is an inherited disease with an autosomal recessive pattern caused by an insufficient amount of the nuclear-encoded mitochondrial protein frataxin, which is an essential and highly evolutionary conserved protein whose deficit results in iron metabolism dysregulation and mitochondrial dysfunction. The first experimental evidence connecting frataxin with iron homeostasis came from *Saccharomyces cerevisiae*; iron accumulates in the mitochondria of yeast with deletion of the frataxin ortholog gene. This finding was soon linked to previous observations of iron deposits in the hearts of FRDA patients and was later reported in animal models of the disease. Despite advances made in the understanding of FRDA pathophysiology, the role of iron in this disease has not yet been completely clarified. Some of the questions still unresolved include the molecular mechanisms responsible for the iron accumulation and iron-mediated toxicity. Here, we review the contribution of the cellular and animal models of FRDA and relevance of the studies using FRDA patient samples to gain knowledge about these issues. Mechanisms of mitochondrial iron overload are discussed considering the potential roles of frataxin in the major mitochondrial metabolic pathways that use iron. We also analyzed the effect of iron toxicity on neuronal degeneration in FRDA by reactive oxygen species (ROS)-dependent and ROS-independent mechanisms. Finally, therapeutic strategies based on the control of iron toxicity are considered.

Keywords: Friedreich's ataxia, frataxin, iron, animal models, oxidative stress, lipid deregulation, iron chelators

INTRODUCTION

Nicholaus Friedreich, a German neurologist among a family of professors of medicine, had described a new disease entity in successive papers published between 1863 and 1877 (Koeppen, 2013). The new disease, named later Friedreich's ataxia (FRDA), was characterized by degenerative atrophy of the posterior columns of the spinal cord, leading to the development of progressive ataxia, sensory loss and muscle weakness in patients and was associated with cardiomyopathy in many cases. Clear diagnostic criteria for FRDA were established by Anita Harding in the 1980s (Harding, 1981), who specified the hereditary nature of the disease with an autosomal recessive pattern, an onset during puberty, progressive ataxia of the limbs and gait with the absence of tendon reflexes in the legs, extensor plantar responses, and dysarthria. In 1996, the identification of the causative gene of FRDA and expansion of a trinucleotide repeat as the most frequent mutation (Campuzano et al., 1996) led to the development of a molecular tool for a definitive diagnosis of the disease. It was crucial to address the differential diagnosis with respect to other peripheral neuropathies and ataxias with similar clinical features, as well as the clinical heterogeneity in FRDA, including atypical phenotypes (Bidichandani and Delatycki, 2017). Moreover, the availability of this molecular approach allowed for appropriate genetic counseling.

Epidemiological, Pathophysiological and Molecular Aspects of FRDA

Friedreich's ataxia (OMIM #229300; ORPHA:95) is a rare neurodegenerative disease affecting 1:20,000–1:50,000 people of Indo-European and North African descendent (Vankan, 2013), and with a carrier frequency of 1:60–1:100, FRDA is the most frequently inherited ataxia in these populations. The neurological signs and symptoms in FRDA are the results of pathological changes that disturb both the central and peripheral nervous systems (NSs) (reviewed in Marmolino, 2011; Koeppen and Mazurkiewicz, 2013). The dorsal root ganglia (DRG) are particularly vulnerable and have been identified as the first site of neuropathology with the degeneration of the large sensory neurons and posterior columns, leading to the loss of position and vibration senses. Next, affectation of the corticospinal and spinocerebellar tracts of the spinal cord occurs, with loss of myelinated fibers. In the cerebellum, dentate nuclei (DN) also show progressive atrophy. Cerebral abnormalities are being progressively reported with the application of neuroimaging techniques (Selvadurai et al., 2018). Non-neurological phenotypes of FRDA mainly include hypertrophic cardiomyopathy, which is the leading cause of mortality (Raman R. et al., 2011; Payne and Wagner, 2012; Weidemann et al., 2013; Koeppen et al., 2015). The heart typically maintains adequate systolic function (Kipps et al., 2009) in FRDA patients who develop a severe hypertrophic cardiomyopathy until shortly before death (Rajagopalan et al., 2010). Additionally, diabetes mellitus and skeletal abnormalities are also present in this disease (Parkinson et al., 2013; Bidichandani and Delatycki, 2017).

Friedreich's ataxia is caused by loss-of-function mutations in the frataxin gene (*FXN*) (Campuzano et al., 1996). The most common mutation appears in homozygosis in most patients and consists of an abnormally expanded GAA trinucleotide repeat (usually between 600 and 900 repeats) in the first intron of the gene *FXN* (Campuzano et al., 1996; Monrós et al., 1997). The remaining patients (approximately 4%) are compound heterozygous with the expanded GAA repeat on one allele and another pathogenic variant (point mutation, deletion or insertion) on the other allele (Galea et al., 2016). The pathological GAA expansion affects the expression of *FXN* by blocking the transcription of mRNA through the formation of sticky DNA triplexes and R-loop structures (reviewed in Kumari and Usdin, 2012) and/or inducing abnormal heterochromatinization (Saveliev et al., 2003). Thus, the level of frataxin is strongly reduced from 5 to 30% of the physiological level (Campuzano et al., 1997). This reduction is related to the disease severity and length of the GAA repeat. In general, longer expansions are present in patients with a more severe phenotype such as earlier onset, faster progression and/or presence of non-neurological features (Parkinson et al., 2013). Although most of the pathogenic point mutations also decrease the level of functional protein, some lead to the production of a less active protein (De Castro et al., 2000; Bridwell-Rabb et al., 2011).

Protein Frataxin

Frataxin is a small acidic protein, synthetized in the cytoplasm as a 210-residue polypeptide that is then imported into the mitochondria, where it is proteolytically processed to the mature and most abundant form of 130 residues [frataxin (81–210)] (Condò et al., 2007). Although frataxin has historically been considered a protein exclusively confined to the mitochondrial matrix, several studies have reported the existence of an extramitochondrial pool of frataxin in different human cell types (Acquaviva et al., 2005; Condò et al., 2006; Lu and Cortopassi, 2007). Extramitochondrial frataxin corresponds to the (81–210) mature form of the protein (Condò et al., 2010) and earlier studies suggested that after the initial transport and processing in the mitochondria, mature frataxin was transported back to the cytosol (Acquaviva et al., 2005; Condò et al., 2006). However, a recent study describes an N-terminal acetylated extramitochondrial form of frataxin in erythrocytes. This (76–210) isoform does not contain the mitochondrial targeting sequence, and remains in the cytosol where it is cleaved to produce an (81–210) protein identical to the mitochondrial mature form (Guo et al., 2018).

The three-dimensional structure of frataxin shows seven antiparallel β-sheets flanked by two α-helices, producing a characteristic globular αβ fold (Dhe-Paganon et al., 2000). The protein is ubiquitously expressed (Campuzano et al., 1996, 1997), but different cells types show distinct susceptibility to its deficiency. This could be explained by frataxin reduction in different tissues being associated with distinct transcriptomic profiles, as described recently (Chandran et al., 2017). Frataxin is a highly conserved protein through evolution, and its cellular function is critical for life in multicellular organisms. A strong reduction of frataxin in *Drosophila melanogaster* seriously affects viability (Anderson et al., 2005; Llorens et al., 2007). Knockout of the frataxin gene causes embryonic lethality in mice (Cossée et al., 2000) and in the plant *Arabidopsis thaliana* (Vazzola et al., 2007). In line with this, FRDA patients with non-GAA-repeat mutations in both frataxin alleles, resulting in totally deficient frataxin function, have not been reported.

At the time of *FXN* identification, there was no evidence about the function of frataxin. Experiments in yeast *Saccharomyces cerevisiae* promptly suggested a potential role for frataxin in iron homeostasis regulation. Deletion of the ortholog of frataxin in yeast (*Yfh1*) causes iron accumulation in the mitochondria (Babcock et al., 1997; Foury and Cazzalini, 1997) that was initially suggested at the expense of the cytosolic iron pool (Knight et al., 1998). However, measurements of cytosolic iron in frataxin-deficient yeast cells show that the cytosolic iron levels are not affected by the reduction of the frataxin synthesis (Li et al., 2012). Also associated with frataxin deficiency are reduced activities of mitochondrial iron-sulfur cluster (ISC) enzymes and aconitase, mitochondrial dysfunction and oxidative stress (reviewed in Calabrese et al., 2005; Lupoli et al., 2018). Since then, efforts have been made to answer several questions about iron in FRDA, including whether its accumulation is a primary or secondary event in the disease, what is the mechanism causing the deregulation and buildup of iron, and the role of this metal in the neuropathology of FRDA. Here, we review the contribution of the cellular and animal models of this disease and relevance of the studies using patient samples to gain knowledge about these issues.

IRON ACCUMULATION IN FRDA

Iron accumulation is a hallmark in FRDA and initially was suggested to be a primary pathogenic event triggered by frataxin deficiency. Tissues in which iron overload has been reported in FRDA patients are showed in **Supplementary Table S1**. The first observations linking iron and FRDA were made in postmortem heart samples from a few patients, where dense intracytoplasmic deposits of iron particles were detected in the cardiac fibers (Sanchez-Casis et al., 1976; Lamarche et al., 1980). These findings were later corroborated in subsequent studies that use different techniques for iron quantitation, such as Perls Prussian blue staining for histological detection or atomic absorption spectroscopy to measure total iron levels in tissue. The excess iron in the heart of FRDA patients appears as multifocal aggregates highly localized rather than as a diffuse pattern (Ramirez et al., 2012; Koeppen et al., 2015). This regional distribution of the excess of iron could be responsible for the findings of iron levels equivalent to healthy controls in bulk extracts or from random biopsied cardiac samples (Michael et al., 2006; Koeppen et al., 2015; Kruger et al., 2016). In addition to the heart, positive iron staining was observed in the liver and spleen of patients, showing a distribution consistent with a mitochondrial location (Bradley et al., 2000) as has been described in the frataxin-deficient yeast model (Babcock et al., 1997; Foury and Cazzalini, 1997).

In regions of the NS, such as DN and DRG, several scenarios regarding the iron content in FRDA have been reported: normal levels (Bradley et al., 2000; Koeppen et al., 2007, 2013; Solbach et al., 2014), accumulation (Bonilha da Silva et al., 2014; Harding et al., 2016), and limited and regional increases of this metal (Koeppen et al., 2009). These diverse results could be partly due to the technique used for iron measurements and their capability to discriminate between the accumulation and redistribution of iron. In most of these studies, the iron content has been quantified from a small number of patient samples, a situation that could also contribute to the different results reported. A more recent study with a higher number of FRDA subjects analyzed used magnetic resonance imaging, which allows *in vivo* iron quantitation (Harding et al., 2016). The authors found a significant increase in the iron concentration in the FRDA cohort compared with that in controls, in the DN and Red nucleus in the midbrain. However, the technical approach used in this study did not allow the authors to discriminate between deposition and redistribution or whether the location of the iron was extracellular or intracellular. Changes in the distribution of iron and other metals, such as copper and zinc, in the DN of FRDA patients have also been reported (Koeppen et al., 2012), although the total amount of these metals was similar to that of controls. It is worth highlighting that copper can also generate oxygen radicals and, in the context of FRDA, may exacerbate the oxidative injury caused by the increased amount of iron. Mitochondrial iron accumulation has also been documented in fibroblasts and lymphoblasts of FRDA patients. Although some authors have found an increase in the total iron content (Delatycki et al., 1999) or labile iron fraction (Tan et al., 2001), normal levels of iron have been reported in other studies (Wong et al., 1999; Sturm et al., 2005).

Several mouse models of FRDA have been obtained using different experimental strategies, and most of them show iron overload because of frataxin reduction (**Supplementary Table S2**). However, no iron accumulation was detected in embryonic samples of the frataxin knockout (KO) mice (Cossée et al., 2000), and the conditional model of frataxin deficiency in striated muscle (MCK-KO mice) showed heart intramitochondrial iron buildup only in late stages of the disease (Puccio et al., 2001). This led to the hypothesis that the increase in iron is not the causative pathological mechanism in FRDA and is a secondary effect.

Iron accumulation has been studied, particularly in muscle creatine kinase (MCK) conditional *Fxn* knockout mice (MCK-KO). This mutant develops a severe cardiac phenotype associated with almost ablation of frataxin in heart and skeletal muscle (Puccio et al., 2001). Different studies on this mouse line have reported distinct ages of onset for the iron overload despite using the same iron detection methodology (**Supplementary Table S2**). Some authors (Puccio et al., 2001) found iron deposits in 10-week-old mice, whereas animals 7 weeks of age did not present iron accumulation but showed deficits in ISC enzyme activities. By contrast, other authors (Huang et al., 2013) observed progressive iron accumulation from 5 to 10 weeks of age, with the presence of the iron deposits being the first observable histological change in the MCK-KO hearts. Therefore, there is no consensus about when iron starts to accumulate and whether the presence of iron deposits is relevant for the development of heart pathology in FRDA.

An interesting result found in the MCK-KO model is that iron levels increase in other tissues besides the heart (**Supplementary Table S2**), such as the liver, kidney and spleen, as well as serum (Huang et al., 2009; Whitnall et al., 2012). Because the amount of frataxin in these non-muscular tissues is within the normal range in the MCK-KO model (Huang et al., 2009; Whitnall et al., 2012), the iron increase was explained as an alteration of systemic iron metabolism orchestrated by the frataxin reduction in heart and skeletal muscle. It could be operated through a signaling mechanism involving hepcidin (Huang et al., 2009; Whitnall et al., 2012), a key regulator of systemic iron metabolism in mammals. These explanations indicate that excess iron plays a significant role in the disease. The mitochondrial iron in the heart of MCK-KO mutants is in the form of biomineral iron, which aggregates with phosphorus and sulfur (Whitnall et al., 2012). This is important because excess of iron that is not bound to ferritin, the main cellular protein that stores iron, can be very toxic by generating reactive oxygen species (ROS).

In the liver of mice with hepatic Fxn deficiency (Fxn^{Alb} mice), a fivefold increase in the mitochondrial iron level has been observed at 28 days of age compared with that in control mice. Meanwhile, 14-day-old mutant showed deficits in ISC enzymes in the liver but normal levels of iron (Martelli et al., 2015), suggesting that iron accumulation is a secondary event also in the liver. As in FRDA patients, iron deposition in the NS of FRDA mouse models has not been clarified yet. In conditional knockout models with frataxin reduction in neurons and other tissues (Puccio et al., 2001) or in parvalbumin-positive cells in the DRG, cerebellum and brain (Piguet et al., 2018), no iron accumulation has been observed. Other studies have reported few iron deposits in NS late in disease progression (Simon et al., 2004) or that iron accumulates both intracellularly and extracellularly in the brain following the loss of Fxn (Chen et al., 2016a). To understand these diverse findings, the authors have indicated that the different sensitivities of the techniques used to measure iron could be an explanation, or that, in some mouse models, cells loss may occur before sufficient iron is accumulated to be detected.

Other animal models of FRDA have also shown an increase in iron levels in the mitochondria (**Supplementary Table S2**), as is the case of *D. melanogaster* (Soriano et al., 2013). In this species, severe loss of frataxin function results in iron accumulation in multiple tissues, including the brain (Chen et al., 2016b). This was the first FRDA model clearly demonstrating that iron can accumulate in the NS. Additionally, frataxin-deficient flies also showed increased levels of other transition metals, such as zinc, copper and manganese, suggesting that frataxin reduction affects the homeostasis of other metals besides iron (Soriano et al., 2016). In the plant *A. thaliana*, frataxin is localized in both the mitochondria and chloroplasts, where it is suggested to have similar functions; its deficiency alters the iron content, and this metal accumulates in the two organelles (Martin et al., 2009; Turowski et al., 2015). These results indicate that frataxin-defective organisms show a common propensity to accumulate Fe into organelles where this protein is located. Although many studies have suggested that iron deposits are not instrumental and represent a late event in the pathogenesis of FRDA, the role of Fe in the disease pathophysiology is not fully understood. Recently, frataxin function has been nicely discussed (Alsina et al., 2018), and it can offer some insight into the mechanisms underlying iron accumulation in FRDA tissues and in model organisms. We review this subject in the following section.

FRATAXIN FUNCTION AND POTENTIAL MECHANISMS OF MITOCHONDRIAL IRON ACCUMULATION

Iron is vital for the cell because it participates in essential biological processes such as DNA synthesis, gene regulation, cellular respiration, and energy production. The mitochondria play a major role in the cellular metabolism of this element and synthesis of heme and ISCs, which are needed for the function of many proteins involved in such cellular processes (Napier et al., 2005; Richardson et al., 2010). Iron homeostasis must be highly controlled because the depletion of its level can produce cellular death, and an increased level of iron promotes the production of ROS. In its Fe^{+2} state, iron can interact with oxygen via the Fenton and Haber-Weiss reactions to catalyze the production of ROS, which oxidize and damage proteins, lipids and nucleic acids (Eaton and Qian, 2002). Therefore, precise regulatory systems are needed to ensure the proper amount and oxidative state of iron in the cell and its different compartments.

Although frataxin has been proven to be a mitochondrial iron-binding protein (Foury et al., 2007) involved in the homeostasis of iron, its role remains unclear. Many studies have indicated that this protein could play roles related to iron storage (Park et al., 2003; Huang et al., 2011), heme (Yoon and Cowan, 2004; Napier et al., 2005) and ISC synthesis (Foury et al., 2007; Richardson et al., 2010; Lane et al., 2015) and could function as an iron sensor (Adinolfi et al., 2009) and a metabolic switch (Becker et al., 2002). Some of these possible roles have been more thoroughly tested and proven that others, with the involvement in ISC synthesis being the most accepted one thus far. We discuss these functions next and its possible relationship with mitochondrial iron accumulation in FRDA.

Iron Storage

The observation that yeast frataxin (Yfh1), under aerobic conditions and an excess of iron, can form spheroidal oligomers that have ferroxidase activity (Adamec et al., 2000; Gakh et al., 2002; Park et al., 2002) promptly suggested that frataxin could function as an iron storage protein, similar to ferritin (Pandolfo and Pastore, 2009). These Yfh1 multimers have the capacity to bind up to 50 atoms of iron per monomer and maintain it in a redox-inactive state through the ferroxidase activity, which converts redox-active Fe^{+2} to Fe^{+3} (Gakh et al., 2006). On this line, frataxin could store iron in a bioavailable form in the mitochondria, thus its deficit would lead to iron loading in this organelle.

Frataxins are proteins capable of binding iron. Nuclear magnetic resonance (NMR) studies predominantly mapped the iron-binding sites in the conserved acidic $\alpha 1$ and $\beta 1$ regions, which contain a clustering of negatively charged aspartate and glutamate residues (reviewed in Bencze et al., 2006;

Pandolfo and Pastore, 2009). However, the hypothesis of frataxin as an iron storage protein presents several problems. Perhaps, one of most serious questions is that, in the case of human frataxin (FXN), the mature form of the protein is not prone to oligomerization. Only the precursor and intermediate forms of FXN can form oligomers and in an iron-independent manner (Adinolfi et al., 2002; O'Neill et al., 2005). Nevertheless, it has lately reported that the mature form of FXN, under specific experimental conditions can form oligomers, but they are unstable (Ahlgren et al., 2017). Other important caveat to this hypothesis is the redundant role that FXN would play with mitochondrial ferritin. In addition, it has been reported that oligomerization-deficient mutant Yfh1 is able to substitute functionally wild-type Yfh1 (Aloria et al., 2004), indicating that oligomerization is not required for frataxin function.

Heme Biosynthesis

Frataxin can bind iron directly without forming oligomers (Bencze et al., 2006; Cook et al., 2006). Depending on the organism (bacteria, yeast or human) and state of iron (Fe^{+2} or Fe^{+3}), different possible iron-binding sites in the protein have been described (Yoon and Cowan, 2003; Bou-Abdallah et al., 2004; Cook et al., 2006; Yoon et al., 2007; Huang et al., 2008). The primary site that binds Fe^{+2} involves the residues 18, 19 and 22 of CyaY (and corresponding ones in Yfh1 and FXN) at the acidic ridge in the $\alpha 1$ helix of frataxin. This raised the possibility of new functions for frataxin in iron-dependent processes, in which some of the involved machinery components seem to interact with FXN. Frataxin interactions have been reported with mitochondrial aconitase, ferrochelatase (Fech), succinate dehydrogenase and the components of the ISC synthesis machinery (Gerber et al., 2003; Yoon and Cowan, 2003; Bulteau et al., 2004; Bencze et al., 2006). Among these interactions, the binding of frataxin with components of the ISC complex has been reproduced and characterized in independent studies (reviewed in Martelli and Puccio, 2014).

The heme biosynthetic pathway is carried out in mitochondria. This pathway includes several enzymes (Sassa, 2006; Furuyama et al., 2007; Chung et al., 2012; Dailey and Meissner, 2013; Chiabrando et al., 2014), with the 5-aminolevulinic acid synthase (ALAS) being the first one in that pathway and the rate-limiting enzyme. ALAS has two isoenzymes, ALAS1 and ALAS2. Whereas ALAS1 expression is negatively regulated by heme directly bound to a cysteine-proline dipeptide motif (Furuyama et al., 2007), the ALAS2 gene contains an iron-responsive element (IRE) that interacts with iron regulatory proteins (IRPs) regulating its expression at the posttranscriptional level. Under iron deficiency conditions, the binding of IRP to ALAS2 mRNA inhibits its translation; by contrast, under iron sufficiency conditions, IRPs detach from the IRE, resulting in increased ALAS2 translation. In this manner, the cytosolic iron availability regulates the rate of heme synthesis (Ponka, 1997).

The final enzyme in the heme biosynthetic pathway is Fech, which inserts ferrous iron into protoporphyrin IX. This enzyme contains a [2Fe-2S] cluster that is necessary for enzymatic activity (Wu et al., 2001). The disruption in ISC synthesis could adversely affect the rate of heme synthesis (Richardson et al., 2010; Huang et al., 2011). It has been shown that mitoferrin (Mfrnl) is responsible for iron transport into mitochondria, allowing the direct transfer of ferrous iron for heme and/or ISC synthesis (Fleming, 2011). The role of frataxin in heme synthesis is not clear, although a reduction of heme synthesis was observed in yeast and mouse frataxin mutants (Lesuisse et al., 2003; Huang et al., 2009). Different studies have suggested a direct role of frataxin in the heme synthesis pathway by binding directly to Fech and acting as an iron donor (Yoon and Cowan, 2004; Napier et al., 2005). Thus, this metal would accumulate because of frataxin deficiency.

ISC Biogenesis Chaperone

Iron-sulfur clusters are protein cofactors present in almost all living organisms. They play a critical role in several cellular functions, from electron transport in mitochondrial respiratory complexes to DNA repair or metabolism. The *de novo* synthesis of ISC occurs in the mitochondria (Lill, 2009; Beilschmidt and Puccio, 2014). The components of the ISC synthesis machinery are the cysteine desulfurase (NFS1), which converts L-cysteine to L-alanine with the generation of sulfur, an accessory protein (ISD11), a reductant (ferredoxin), a scaffold protein (ISCU) and an iron delivery protein that is at the core of the debate (Lill and Mühlenhoff, 2006; Py and Barras, 2010). Besides ISD11, recent findings showed that human NFS1 needs another accessory protein, the mitochondrial acyl carrier protein (ACP), making the cysteine desulfurase complex (NFS1-ISD11-ACP) (Van Vranken et al., 2016). In addition, NFS1 requires FXN for its full function (Tsai and Barondeau, 2010; Fox et al., 2015). Regarding the role of FXN in the ISC synthesis, there are two main hypothesis. It was first suggested that frataxin could be the iron donor (Gerber et al., 2003; Yoon and Cowan, 2003; Layer et al., 2006). Using a combination of different techniques based on isothermal titration calorimetry and multinuclear NMR spectroscopy, Cai et al. (2018) have recently showed that FXN can function as an iron donor *in vitro*. They found that FXN-Fe^{2+} interacts weakly to the NFS1-ISD11-ACP complex, but the presence of ISCU largely improves this interaction and that dissociation of Fe^{2+} from FXN occurs when the L-cysteine and ferredoxin enters into the equation. These results suggest that FXN is the proximal source of iron for ISC assembly, but *in vivo* characterization is required to confirm this role for frataxin.

Other studies have proposed that frataxin could actually act as a regulator in the synthesis of ISC (Adinolfi et al., 2009; Tsai and Barondeau, 2010; Bridwell-Rabb et al., 2012). The binding of frataxin to the ISCU/NFS1/ISD11 complex can stabilize it, activates the cysteine desulfurase activity and control the entry of iron to the complex (Tsai and Barondeau, 2010; Colin et al., 2013; Pandey et al., 2013).

Mutation of specific aspartate and glutamate residues in the acidic ridge of frataxin, where iron-binding sites were previously mapped, alters the interaction of frataxin with ISCU. Unexpectedly, these mutations does not reduce the total number of iron-binding sites (Schmucker et al., 2011). These results suggested that some of these residues might be critical for frataxin interaction with the core components of the ISC complex, but not for binding iron. Consequently, some authors (Gentry et al., 2013) proposed that frataxin might have unknown binding sites for this metal. Using different spectroscopic and structural methodologies, a new iron-binding site was identified at His86 in the N-terminus of the mature FXN form, therefore not positioned in the acidic ridge. Interestingly, this residue was essential for iron binding and for *in vitro* productive synthesis of ISC by ISCU, without showing a direct interaction with the scaffold protein (Gentry et al., 2013). These results support the proposal that frataxin is the iron donor for ISC assembly.

Extramitochondrial frataxin has been shown to physically interact with IscU1, the cytosolic isoform of the human ISC, indicating a role for frataxin in the Fe/S cluster assembly in the cytosol (Acquaviva et al., 2005). The cytosolic form of frataxin has also been reported to interact and possibly regulate the function of the cytosolic aconitase/iron regulatory protein-1 (IRP1) (Condò et al., 2010). Other functions suggested for frataxin in the cytosol include preventing oxidative stress and apoptosis (Condò et al., 2006); and in the nucleus, frataxin could promote DNA repair and telomere stability (Lill et al., 2015).

Iron Sensor and Metabolic Switch

As indicate above, frataxin could act as an iron sensor to tightly regulate ISC synthesis (Adinolfi et al., 2009). In *E. coli*, CyaY, far from facilitating iron delivery, can inhibit the ISC synthesis process. With normal iron levels, CyaY has a low affinity for the IscS-IscU system (the bacterial ISC synthesis machinery), and ISC is loaded to the final acceptor. However, under conditions of iron excess, the affinity of CyaY for IscS would increase, slowing the rate of ISC synthesis and avoiding an overproduction of ISC. This would avoid the degradation of ISC not inserted into an acceptor protein and the release of free iron that could catalyze the production of ROS. However, the consequence of frataxin deficiency in FRDA patients is a decrease in ISC protein function, suggesting that FXN might operate as an activator of the ISC synthesis. *In vitro* studies also support the role of FXN as an allosteric activator of the ISC assembly (Tsai and Barondeau, 2010). In contrast, both FXN and CyaY can complement a yeast strain with deletion of *Yfh1*, indicating that eukaryotic and bacterial frataxins can at least partially conserve their functions (Cavadini et al., 2000; Bedekovics et al., 2007). To clarify this controversial results, Bridwell-Rabb et al. (2012) conducted enzyme kinetic assays in which analogous components of the human and *E. coli* ISC complex were interchanged. Interestingly, they found that CyaY could substitute FXN as an activator of the cysteine desulfurase in the human ISC complex. Conversely, FXN could also replace CyaY as an inhibitor in the assembly of the bacterial ISC. Therefore, both frataxin proteins have the property to modulate the ISC formation, but the mechanism of action of any of them, as an activator or inhibitor of ISC biogenesis, depends on another component of the ISC assembly machinery. This component was found to be the cysteine desulfurase, which controls how the frataxin protein operates in the ISC complex (Bridwell-Rabb et al., 2012). Differences between the human and bacteria cysteine desulfurase might explain the different role of frataxin in humans with respect to *E. coli* and by extension in eukaryotes vs prokaryotes. Further studies are needed to define the nature of these differences that dictate how frataxin acts in the process of the ISC synthesis.

Examination of the role of frataxin in ISC and heme metabolism in differentiating erythroid cells has suggested that frataxin acts as a metabolic switch in the diversion of iron from one metabolic pathway to another. This was supported by the observation that an increased level of protoporphyrin IX (PPIX) leads to the downregulation of frataxin expression and potential diversion of iron from ISC synthesis toward heme synthesis (Becker et al., 2002). The molar ratio between frataxin and Fech affects the rate of heme synthesis (Yoon and Cowan, 2004), and these findings have suggested that frataxin could function as a metabolic switch in regulating mitochondrial iron metabolism, independently of the expression levels of PPIX or Fech. This metabolic switch allows the mitochondria to favor heme or ISC syntheses, depending on the frataxin levels. The possible mechanism behind this switching may be the relative affinities of frataxin for Fech vs ISCU. This may result in the preferential binding of frataxin to Fech over ISCU at relatively lower frataxin levels (Richardson et al., 2010).

When the frataxin level is reduced, there would be no control in the rate of ISC formation, causing iron accumulation (Adinolfi et al., 2009). Regarding the metabolic switch role of frataxin, its depletion would provoke the enhancement in the reduction of ISC formation at the ISCU machinery level and at the end, subjecting the cell to increased iron accumulation and ROS production (Yoon and Cowan, 2004).

Dysregulation of Iron Homeostasis in FRDA

Although the mechanisms responsible for mitochondrial iron loading in FRDA are not fully understood, there are several reasonable hypotheses that could explain this alteration. In the MCK-KO mouse, Huang et al. reported altered heme and ISC synthesis and mitochondrial iron storage. Significantly diminished activity and expression of ISC enzymes, such as NFS1 and ISCU1/2, were observed that agreed with the reduction in the expression of succinate dehydrogenase complex, subunit A (Sdha) (Huang et al., 2009). At the same time, other studies have shown a downregulation in the number of key heme synthesis enzymes and decreased heme levels in the heart of the MCK KO model (Schoenfeld et al., 2005; Huang et al., 2009). A decrease in the synthesis of different products that require iron in the mitochondria could explain the accumulation of this metal because it cannot be exported from the organelle being part of those products. However, frataxin deficiency can also affect the expression of several other proteins, some of them critical for the proper control of iron metabolism (**Figure 1**). In DN, Koeppen et al. (2007) observed modification of the expression of proteins such as transferrin receptor 1 (TFR1), ferritins (FRTs) and ferroportin (FPN), alterations shared among animal models of FRDA. In the MCK-KO mouse (Martelli and Puccio, 2014), has been described marked TFR1 upregulation, leading to increased iron uptake, and the downregulation of FPN, decreasing cellular iron release from the cytosol. There are also decreased levels of ferritin light chain 1 (FRTL1)

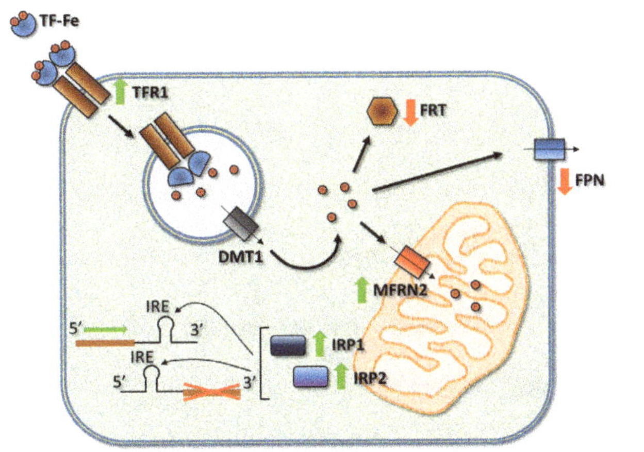

FIGURE 1 | Frataxin deficiency leads to a series of alterations in the activity and/or expression of different iron-related proteins. Among the most relevant changes observed in humans and FRDA models, there is an increase in the activity of the iron regulatory proteins IRP1 and IRP2, upregulation of TFR1 (transferrin receptor 1) and the mitochondrial iron importer MFRN2 (mitoferrin-2), and downregulation of the iron exporter FPN (ferroportin) and iron storage proteins FRTs (ferritins, light and heavy chains). TF, transferrin; DMT1, divalent metal transporter 1.

and heavy chain 1 (FRTH), implying reduced cytosolic iron incorporation and storage. Finally, an increased expression of Sec15l1 (an exocyst complex protein) and the mitochondrial iron importer mitoferrin-2 (MFRN2) in the mutant could facilitate mitochondrial iron influx, which was seen to be enhanced in this model (Whitnall et al., 2008).

The link between frataxin deficiency and alteration in the expression of some of these proteins could be IRP1 and IRP2. Both proteins bind to IRE elements in the 5′ and 3′ UTR of the mRNAs of iron metabolism-related proteins (Chiang et al., 2016). When bound to a 5′ IRE, IRP1 and IRP2 repress the translation of the mRNAs while binding of the IRPs to a 3′ IRE increases the stability and translation of the mRNAs. The activity of both IRPs is increased by the low levels of cellular iron by different mechanisms. Interestingly, IRP1 activity is controlled by the insertion of an ISC, which converts the protein into a cytosolic aconitase and makes it unable to bind to IRE elements. Since frataxin depletion reduces ISC synthesis, it is reasonable to suggest a role for IRP1 in the deregulation of iron metabolism. Nevertheless, the activity of IRP2, which is controlled by iron-dependent controlled ubiquitination and degradation, is also increased in MCK-KO mouse, possibly due to cytosolic iron depletion (Whitnall et al., 2008). More recently, Martelli et al. (2015) studied a double KO mouse with complete ablation of *Irp1* and liver-specific deletion of *Fxn*. In these mice, the authors observed that alterations in the expression of proteins such as TFR1 and divalent metal transporter 1 (DMT1) were indeed due, a least partially, to IRP1, while the regulatory protein seemed to exert little effect on the expression of other proteins such as FRTL and FPN. Other models of the disease also manifest similar alterations in the expression of proteins involved in iron metabolism. Frataxin depletion in *D. melanogaster* produces alterations in the expression of mitoferrin, IRP-1A and ferritin, while genetic modifiers for *Malvolio*, *Tsf1* and *Tsf3* (*Drosophila* homologs of DMT1 and transferrins) and *IRP-1A* and *IRP-1B* could correct the motor deficiency phenotype of frataxin-deficient flies (Soriano et al., 2016; Calap-Quintana et al., 2018; Monnier et al., 2018). Although some hints point to the possible causes of iron dysregulation in FRDA, more research is needed to propose a more precise and final hypothesis.

MECHANISMS OF IRON NEUROTOXICITY IN FRDA

Initially, it was postulated that iron overload in FRDA activates the formation of ROS via the Fenton reaction, which would arbitrate the pathogenesis of the disease. The highly redox active environment in the mitochondria could promote ROS generation when the free iron content increases. Nevertheless, an ROS independent mechanism mediated by iron has recently been proposed for FRDA neurodegeneration. These two mechanisms are described in the following paragraphs (**Figure 2**).

ROS-Dependent Mechanism of Iron Neurotoxicity

Iron accumulation in the NS is a common feature in neurodegenerative diseases, including Alzheimer's disease (Connor et al., 1992), Parkinson's disease (Gorell et al., 1995), Huntington's disease (Dumas et al., 2012) or amyotrophic lateral sclerosis (Kwan et al., 2012). In these disorders, iron deposits are observed in specific regions of the NS. As indicated previously, in Friedreich ataxia patients, deposits of iron have not been clearly reported in NS, and the increment of iron levels in the DN remains controversial (Waldvogel et al., 1999; Koeppen et al., 2007; Harding et al., 2016). This region is interesting because the patients develop neuronal atrophy and abnormal proliferation of the synaptic terminal, called grumose degeneration. The Koeppen's group confirmed the presence of iron metabolism alteration in the NS of FRDA patients by changes in the expression of proteins related to iron, such as FPN, FRT and TFR1, in the DN (Koeppen et al., 2012) and DRG (Koeppen et al., 2009). They observed a relocation of iron from the affected neurons to the microglia, in the case of DN, or from neurons to the satellite cells in the DRGs. The increment of iron levels correlates with the production of ROS in these areas, suggesting that alterations of iron homeostasis could contribute to the pathogenesis of the disease through ROS production. Additionally, frataxin deficiency is related to low antioxidant defenses (Chantrel-Groussard et al., 2001; Paupe et al., 2009), making the nervous cells have an oxidative stress-prone phenotype.

The toxicity of iron may be due to its localization, biochemical form or cell ability to prevent the generation and propagation of iron. In living organisms, iron can be found in its reduced form, ferrous iron (Fe^{2+}), and its oxidized form, ferric iron (Fe^{3+}). Most iron binds, as a prosthetic group, to proteins such as hemoglobin, myoglobin, cytochromes or storage proteins; only less than 5% of iron in the cell is in the labile iron pool

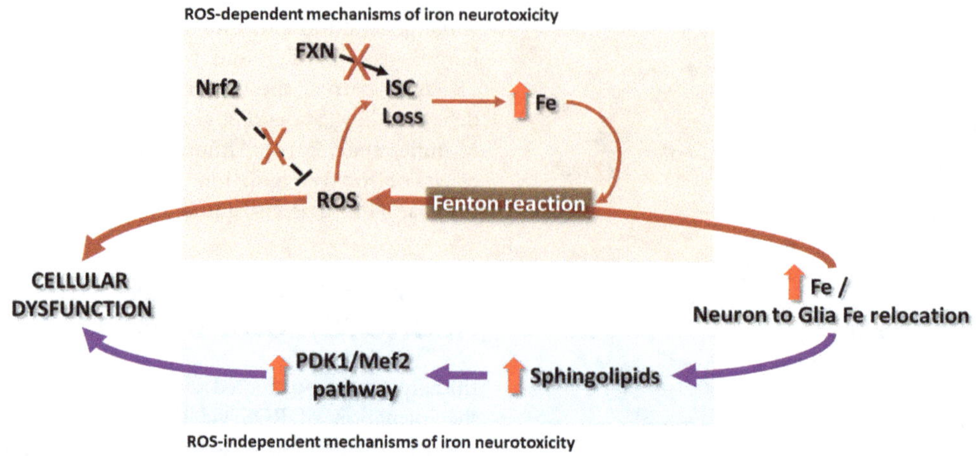

FIGURE 2 | In Friedreich ataxia patients, deposits of iron in NS have not been clearly reported and it remains a controversial topic, while some evidences point to a relocation of iron from neurons to glial cells. So far there are some hypotheses that explain the possible mechanisms of iron toxicity that lead to cellular dysfunction. The ROS-dependent hypothesis proposes the iron-mediated catalysis of ROS by Fenton reaction. Besides the impairment in ISC synthesis due to frataxin deficiency, the radical species can in turn damage the ISC of proteins generating new free iron that will participate in the Fenton reaction. Contributing to this cycle is the observation that the Nrf2 signaling is defective in some cells and models of the disease. Another recent hypothesis, independent of ROS production, was explored in *Drosophila* and mouse models. It suggests that the cellular dysfunction can be due to the activation of the PDK1/Mef2 (3-phosphoinositide dependent protein kinase-1/myocyte enhancer factor-2) pathway by means of an increase in sphingolipids synthesis. Both hypothesis as well as the relevance of ROS in the pathology of FRDA have partial support, since the evidence pointing to them vary depending on the study.

(LIP) (Li and Reichmann, 2016). The cellular LIP is defined as a pool of chelatable and redox-active iron complexes (Kakhlon and Cabantchik, 2002). LIP has the capacity to participate in the formation of harmful free radicals including the hydroxyl radical. Fe^{2+} is catalyzed to Fe^{3+} in a chemical reaction mediated by hydrogen peroxide (H_2O_2), which leads to the formation of hydroxide radical (OH•). Cytotoxic events are started in the cell via the Fenton reaction. To avoid the negative effects of excess free iron, it is coupled to proteins such as FRT, which is responsible for iron storage inside the cell. In the satellite cells of DRG from FRDA patients, an increment of cytosolic FRT (Koeppen et al., 2009) was observed; in DN, ferritin is expressed mostly in oligodendrocytes, satellite cells around the neurons. As the disease progresses, the neurons begin to undergo atrophy, and these cells disappear, producing microglia FRT-positive cells (Koeppen et al., 2007). Noteworthy, mitochondrial FRT has not been detected in DRG neurons, a protein responsible to store free mitochondrial iron and with a very important role in antioxidant activity (Koeppen et al., 2007; Campanella et al., 2009). FPN is a transmembrane protein that exports iron and is expressed in the central NS and DRG. Interestingly, in the DRG from FRDA patients, the expression of FPN is exclusive to satellite cells (Koeppen et al., 2009), probably as a response to the iron release from DRG neurons to these cells (Koeppen et al., 2016). In the synaptic terminals of neurons from the DN of FRDA patients, is observed an increment of the ferroportin levels (Koeppen et al., 2007). The nerve endings present an elevated number of mitochondria, suggesting a response in the biosynthesis of this protein due to the dyshomeostasis of iron. Thus, the toxicity of this metal could be an important factor in grumose degeneration.

Because mitochondria are an important generator of ROS, the continuous presence of iron in the mitochondrial matrix makes it susceptible to new production of ROS. Proteins with ISC clusters, such as complex I, II and III of the electron transport chain, can be damaged by ROS. These complexes show reduced activity in FRDA patients (Rötig et al., 1997), probably because of iron toxicity. Moreover, these proteins will generate new free iron that will participate in the Fenton reaction and carry out new oxidative processes. In plasma and urine from FRDA patients (Emond et al., 2000; Schulz et al., 2000), similar to in all the disease models generated (González-Cabo and Palau, 2013), oxidative stress markers have been detected.

In the last years, neuronal models of the disease have been developed to better understand the neurodegenerative process. Oxidative stress, mitochondrial dysfunction, and iron dyshomeostasis are features shared among the neuronal models. For example, the granulate cells of the cerebellum from YG8R mice show an increment of ROS, lipid peroxidation and reduced glutathione levels (Bradshaw et al., 2016); the neurons of DRG from YG8R mice present an increment of ROS, dysfunctional mitochondria, and calcium dyshomeostasis (Mollá et al., 2017); the motor neuron cell line (NSC34) with reduced expression of the frataxin gene shows an increment in the GSSG/GSH ratio and more production of ROS (Piermarini et al., 2016) and alteration in complex I activity of the electron transport chain (Carletti et al., 2014); reduction of *Drosophila* frataxin (fh) expression in glial cells produces massive accumulation of fatty acids and increased sensitivity to oxidative stress (Navarro et al., 2010).

Under oxidative stress, the transcription factor Nrf2 binds to antioxidant response element (ARE) and modulates the expression of many genes involved in the antioxidant defense. It has been reported that Nrf2 signaling is defective in fibroblasts from FRDA patients (Paupe et al., 2009), the DRG and cerebellum of YG8R mice (Shan et al., 2013) and motor neuron and

Schwann cell models (D'Oria et al., 2013; Shan et al., 2013), making these cells and tissues more vulnerable to oxidative stress damage and the neurodegeneration process. Concretely, frataxin deficiency in neurons promotes axonal dystrophy with multiple axonal spheroid formation mainly due to Ca^{2+} imbalance and oxidative stress (Mollá et al., 2017). The axonal swellings are associated with specific cytoskeletal changes (Mincheva-Tasheva et al., 2014; Piermarini et al., 2016; Mollá et al., 2017), improper axonal transport and autophagic flux (Shidara and Hollenbeck, 2010; Mollá et al., 2017). Moreover, the oxidative stress damage effects to the neurites growth leads to shorter dendrites due to alterations in the dynamics of the microtubules (Shan et al., 2013; Carletti et al., 2014; Piermarini et al., 2016). When oxidative stress is reduced in these neurons, either by direct addition of antioxidants (Piermarini et al., 2016) or through drugs that increase the expression of Nrf2 (Petrillo et al., 2017), axonal growth is improved. In any case, these alterations affect the cellular viability of both neurons and glia, triggering cell death processes either by apoptosis (Mincheva-Tasheva et al., 2014; Igoillo-Esteve et al., 2015; Katsu-Jiménez et al., 2016) or autophagy (Bolinches-Amorós et al., 2014; Edenharter et al., 2018). It has been shown that iron is a key element in the induction of cell death (Dixon et al., 2012). This new process, called ferroptosis, is dependent on iron and is accompanied by an increase in ROS and lipid peroxidation and a decrease in GSH. As we have reviewed previously, these characteristics are observed in frataxin-deficient cells; therefore, new studies are needed to determine the possible cell death due to a ferroptosis process.

ROS-Independent Mechanisms of Iron Neurotoxicity

The extent to which oxidative stress is necessary for the pathogenesis of FRDA is, however, controversial. The deficit in ISC enzymes and increase in iron levels were not paired with an increase in ROS in the MCK-KO mouse (Seznec et al., 2005), in Fxn^{Alb} mice with specific depletion of Fxn in liver (Martelli et al., 2015), and in the inducible and reversible FRDAkd mouse model (Chandran et al., 2017). Similarly, increased oxidative stress was not detected in several *Drosophila* knockdown models, and overexpression of ROS scavengers did not rescue the viability, heart dysfunction or neurodegeneration phenotypes (Anderson et al., 2005; Shidara and Hollenbeck, 2010; Tricoire et al., 2014; Chen et al., 2016b). Moreover, FRDA neural tissue did not show differences in the susceptibility to oxidative stress in a study using patient samples (Macevilly and Muller, 1997). The absence of ROS markers in these studies might be attributed to differences in methodology or the distinctive features of each of the animal models or tissues employed. Alternatively, it was suggested that the discrepancies in the presence of ROS would be explained by differences in the timepoints studied, in a scenario where oxidative stress would be a secondary effect rather than a primary cause, occurring later in the progression of FRDA (discussed in Lupoli et al., 2018). Recent findings in the fly and mouse models of FRDA actually support a mechanism that is independent of ROS that links neurodegeneration and iron accumulation via the sphingolipid pathway (Chen et al., 2016a,b).

Alterations in the homeostasis of lipids are not exclusive of FRDA (Huang et al., 1978; Filla et al., 1980; Thurman and Draper, 1989; Raman S.V. et al., 2011; Worth et al., 2014) and have been reported in neurodegenerative disorders, including Parkinson's, Alzheimer's, Huntington's, multiple sclerosis and Niemann–Pick diseases (reviewed in Shamim et al., 2018). In the case of FRDA, lipid droplet accumulation was first described in the cardiac muscle of the NSE-KO mouse model (Puccio et al., 2001) and was further characterized as pathological in a glial frataxin knockdown model in *Drosophila* (Navarro et al., 2010). The accumulation and dyshomeostasis of lipids have been reported as well in several other cellular and animal models of the disease (Martelli et al., 2012; Schiavi et al., 2013; Obis et al., 2014). More recently, the expression of a mutant allele of the *Drosophila fh* in mosaic clones produced an age-dependent degeneration of photoreceptor neurons with impaired mitochondrial function, increased levels of Fe^{2+} and Fe^{3+} in multiple tissues and dramatic lipid droplet accumulation in glial cells (Chen et al., 2016b), consistent with the work from Navarro et al. (2010). Because the Fenton reaction can induce lipid peroxidation, oxidative stress has been classically proposed to be the link between abnormal lipid homeostasis and neurodegeneration in FRDA. However, Chen et al. did not observe an increase in free radical production and, neither providing the antioxidant AD4 nor overexpressing the ROS scavengers catalase, SOD1 and SOD2, suppressed neurodegeneration (Chen et al., 2016b). Moreover, reducing the number of lipid droplets by overexpressing brummer lipase or lipase 4 was insufficient to improve the neurodegeneration defect in the knockout photoreceptors. Because high iron conditions increase sphingolipid synthesis in wild-type yeast (Lee et al., 2012), Chen et al. (2016b) pursued the characterization of this pathway in their fly model. The synthesis of sphingolipids, including dihydrosphingosine, dihydroceramide and sphingosine, was actually increased in the *fh* mutants. Both the genetic knockdown and chemical inhibition of the fly serine palmitoyltransferase, an enzyme essential for the *de novo* synthesis of sphingolipids, rescued neurodegeneration. Additionally, they found that downstream targets of the transcription factor Mef2 were upregulated in response to the increase in sphingolipids in *fh* mutants and knocking down the Pdk1/Mef2 pathway led to the suppression of photoreceptor degeneration. To ask whether this novel pathway described in *Drosophila* was conserved in vertebrates, Chen et al. (2016a) developed a mouse model with reduced *Fxn* levels in the NS. Both ferrous and ferric iron were found to be increased in the cerebral cortex and, consistent with their observation in the fly model, they could not find increased ROS production measured as levels of lipid peroxidation. Loss of *Fxn* in the NS led to the activation of the PDK1/Mef2 pathway in the mouse before the appearance of the neurological manifestations. Sphingolipids and PDK1 activation were also found to be increased in cardiac tissue from FRDA patients (Chen et al., 2016a). Nevertheless, alterations in the PDK1/Mef2 pathway were not replicated in the FRDAkd-inducible mouse model of FRDA (Chandran et al., 2017). In this study, the authors did not find changes in PDK phosphorylation in the brain, muscle, heart or liver in the chronic adult knockdown mice. The levels in the cerebellum and heart of five target genes of *Mef2* were analyzed as well and displayed changes that were inconsistent across tissues. Alternatively, other biochemical pathways could be altered in relation to iron under frataxin-deficient conditions. In line, several genes involved in hemochromatosis, an iron-overload disorder, are upregulated in the FRDAkd-inducible mouse model, in which no increase in ROS and no strong evidence of Pdkl/Mef2 activation were observed (Chandran et al., 2017).

POTENTIAL TREATMENT OF FRDA BY REDUCING IRON TOXICITY

An optimal therapy in FRDA could consist of providing patients with sufficient frataxin amount to restore the functions of this protein. Several strategies are being developed to obtain this objective, such as gene therapy (Perdomini et al., 2014; Piguet et al., 2018), transplanting hematopoietic stem and progenitor cells (Rocca et al., 2017) or improving *FXN* transcription (Soragni and Gottesfeld, 2016). While advancing the development of such strategies for its application to patients, rational treatment could be considered to remove excess iron.

The utilization of iron chelators is one of the first strategies proposed to treat FRDA patients to eliminate excess iron accumulation in the mitochondria. To that end, an iron chelator should be able to cross the cell membranes, access mitochondria and redistribute the excess labile iron. Deferiprone (DFP, 1, 2 dimethyl-3-hydroxy-pyrid-4-one), an orally administered lipid soluble iron chelator can easily cross the blood–brain barrier and cellular membranes. DFP shows relatively low affinity for iron and can transfer this metal to circulating transferrin, as well as to cellular acceptors—e.g., for heme synthesis (Sohn et al., 2008). Therefore, its use is less probable to produce iron depletion than other known chelators. For all these reasons, DFP has been considered as the prototypic compound for iron redeployment (Cabantchik et al., 2013). It is also used to treat iron-overloaded patients with β-thalassemia who need continuous blood transfusions (Totadri et al., 2015), and their properties make it an interesting therapeutic compound for FRDA.

The use of DFP in cellular and animal models of FRDA has beneficial results, e.g., frataxin-deficient HEK-293 cells could restore mitochondrial dysfunction after DFP treatment. It was attributed to the ability of this compound to make available the iron accumulated into mitochondria (Kakhlon et al., 2008). These conclusions were also supported by our group using a *Drosophila* FRDA model, in which DFP improved the survival and climbing ability phenotypes because of the removal of excess free mitochondrial iron, thereby preventing its toxic effects (Soriano et al., 2013). Recently, it has been reported that DFP is effective to reduce ROS production and improve calcium handling kinetics in an FRDA human-induced pluripotent stem cell-derived cardiomyocyte model (Lee et al., 2016).

The efficacy of DFP has already been assessed in clinical trials in FRDA patients, but the results are inconclusive. However, considering these studies, DFP has shown beneficial effects on cardiac parameters achieved at low doses of the compound, while treatment with higher doses of DFP could aggravate the disorder by affecting the ataxia phenotype (Pandolfo et al., 2014). A high dose of DFP could remove too much iron, provoking a deficiency of this metal, which could affect the cellular functions that require iron. On the other hand, the positive action of this drug on the heart compared with NS has also been related to the initiation of treatment before cardiac dysfunction is present (Elincx-Benizri et al., 2016). Overall, DFP seems to have therapeutic value in FRDA and is quite safe at lower doses, but systematic, large scale, placebo controlled longer studies are needed to evaluate its usefulness (Strawser et al., 2017). In line with these issues, our results using a *Drosophila* model of the disease indicate that DFP treatments at the larval stage recover FRDA-like phenotypes in flies, but no improvement was observed when the drug is administered to adults (Soriano et al., 2013). Additionally, we found that reducing the excess of iron accumulating into mitochondria through a genetic strategy has benefit in this FRDA model (Navarro et al., 2015; Soriano et al., 2016). These results show a causal relationship between iron and frataxin deficiency. Thus, iron is a critical factor in the pathophysiology of FRDA and appears not be a simple epiphenomenal event in the disease. Consequently, research on how to deal with the iron excess and eradicate the iron toxicity is still an area of great interest.

In the last decades, some small molecules with pharmacophore characteristics for iron chelation are being explored for treatment in neurodegenerative diseases with regional increase of iron levels (reviewed in Singh et al., 2018). These compounds are derivatives of the 8-hydroxyquinoline, hydroxypyridone, and arylhydrazones, and some of them are able to reduce selectively the iron excess in the mitochondria (Mena et al., 2015). The use of pro-chelating compounds, which are activated in the target region, have the benefit to remove the excess of iron in the affected regions. Thus, this strategy would protect cells in non-affected areas from the risk of iron subtraction. Novel pro-chelators triggered by H_2O_2 were obtained as promising candidates for management of Parkinson's disease (Perez et al., 2008). Similarly, this approach might be useful in FRDA since H_2O_2 is a critical pathogenic agent associated to frataxin deficiency (Anderson et al., 2008). Finally, new compounds with multifunctional actions, as previously indicated for DFP, are also being examined for effective treatment of neurodegenerative diseases (Singh et al., 2018). Several of these diseases, including FRDA, share some pathological features such as regional iron increase, oxidative stress and dysregulation of calcium signaling. Recently, a novel compound, named CT51 (N-(1,3-dihydroxy-2-(hydroxymethyl)propan-2-yl)-2-(7-hydroxy-2-oxo-2H-chromen-4 yl) acetamide), has been synthesized that seems to suppress these cellular impairments (García-Beltrán et al., 2017). CT51 can easily permeate the cell membrane and distribute to both mitochondria and the cytoplasm. It works as a highly selective iron chelator and possesses significant capability for free radical quenching, protecting cells against oxidative damage. The use of CT51 in primary hippocampal neurons decreases the continuous release of calcium provoked by an agonist of ryanodine receptor-calcium channels, supporting a protective role of this compound in neuronal function. Although developments of this kind of drugs are not a curative strategy, because the frataxin deficiency will persist, they might improve the current pharmacological treatments and might produce increases in quality of life and slowing of disease progression.

CONCLUSION

The relationship between neurodegeneration and iron accumulation is well established. However, in Friedreich's ataxia, it remains unclear whether iron loading is the cause or consequence of the pathophysiology. The studies in model organisms suggested both hypotheses in relation to the role of iron in this disease: a key role in the pathophysiologic mechanisms or a secondary event that appeared late in the disease progression. It was also debated the extent to which oxidative stress is crucial to explain the pathogenesis of FRDA. Indeed, additional pathways might be involved in the toxicity of iron independent of ROS production. Differences in the distinctive features of each of the FRDA models studied, vulnerability of the different tissues and cells to frataxin deficit and timepoints analyzed could partially explain the contradictory results. Nevertheless, from the therapeutic point of view, it is interesting to explore whether new iron chelators showing protective properties on cellular function could improve the mitochondrial dysfunction in FRDA.

AUTHOR CONTRIBUTIONS

JL and MM planned the manuscript. JL, SS, PC-Q, PG-C, and MM wrote the manuscript and agreed on the finally submitted version of the manuscript.

FUNDING

Financial support of this work came from Generalitat Valenciana, Spain (PROMETEOII/2014/067) to MM, the Spanish Ministry of Economy and Competitiveness [SAF2015-66625-R] within the framework of the National R+D+I Plan to PG-C, Fundación Ramón Areces, Spain (CIVP18A3899) to PG-C and MM. PC-Q was a recipient of a fellowship from Generalitat Valenciana, Spain, and JL is supported by a research contract from FARA and FARA Ireland.

REFERENCES

Acquaviva, F., De Biase, I., Nezi, L., Ruggiero, G., Tatangelo, F., Pisano, C., et al. (2005). Extra-mitochondrial localisation of frataxin and its association with IscU1 during enterocyte-like differentiation of the human colon adenocarcinoma cell line Caco-2. *J. Cell Sci.* 118, 3917–3924. doi: 10.1242/jcs.02516

Adamec, J., Rusnak, F., Owen, W. G., Naylor, S., Benson, L. M., Gacy, A. M., et al. (2000). Iron-dependent self-assembly of recombinant yeast frataxin: implications for Friedreich ataxia. *Am. J. Hum. Genet.* 67, 549–562. doi: 10.1086/303056

Adinolfi, S., Iannuzzi, C., Prischi, F., Pastore, C., Iametti, S., Martin, S. R., et al. (2009). Bacterial frataxin CyaY is the gatekeeper of iron-sulfur cluster formation catalyzed by IscS. *Nat. Struct. Mol. Biol.* 16, 390–396. doi: 10.1038/nsmb.1579

Adinolfi, S., Trifuoggi, M., Politou, A. S., Martin, S., and Pastore, A. (2002). A structural approach to understanding the iron-binding properties of phylogenetically different frataxins. *Hum. Mol. Genet.* 11, 1865–1877. doi: 10.1093/hmg/11.16.1865

Ahlgren, E.-C., Fekry, M., Wiemann, M., Söderberg, C. A., Bernfur, K., Gakh, O., et al. (2017). Iron-induced oligomerization of human FXN81-210 and bacterial CyaY frataxin and the effect of iron chelators. *PLoS One* 12:e0188937. doi: 10.1371/journal.pone.0188937

Aloria, K., Schilke, B., Andrew, A., and Craig, E. A. (2004). Iron-induced oligomerization of yeast frataxin homologue Yfh1 is dispensable in vivo. *EMBO Rep.* 5, 1096–1101. doi: 10.1038/sj.embor.7400272

Alsina, D., Purroy, R., Ros, J., and Tamarit, J. (2018). Iron in Friedreich ataxia: a central role in the pathophysiology or an epiphenomenon? *Pharmaceuticals* 11:E89. doi: 10.3390/ph11030089

Anderson, P. R., Kirby, K., Hilliker, A. J., and Phillips, J. P. (2005). RNAi-mediated suppression of the mitochondrial iron chaperone, frataxin, in *Drosophila. Hum. Mol. Genet.* 14, 3397–3405. doi: 10.1093/hmg/ddi367

Anderson, P. R., Kirby, K., Orr, W. C., Hilliker, A. J., and Phillips, J. P. (2008). Hydrogen peroxide scavenging rescues frataxin deficiency in a *Drosophila* model of Friedreich's ataxia. *Proc. Natl. Acad. Sci. U.S.A.* 105, 611–616. doi: 10.1073/pnas.0709691105

Babcock, M., de Silva, D., Oaks, R., Davis-Kaplan, S., Jiralerspong, S., Montermini, L., et al. (1997). Regulation of mitochondrial iron accumulation by Yfh1p, a putative homolog of frataxin. *Science* 276, 1709–1712. doi: 10.1126/science.276.5319.1709

Becker, E. M., Greer, J. M., Ponka, P., and Richardson, D. R. (2002). Erythroid differentiation and protoporphyrin IX down-regulate frataxin expression in Friend cells: characterization of frataxin expression compared to molecules involved in iron metabolism and hemoglobinization. *Blood* 99, 3813–3822. doi: 10.1182/blood.V99.10.3813

Bedekovics, T., Gajdos, G. B., Kispal, G., and Isaya, G. (2007). Partial conservation of functions between eukaryotic frataxin and the *Escherichia coli* frataxin homolog CyaY. *FEMS Yeast Res.* 7, 1276–1284. doi: 10.1111/j.1567-1364.2007.00296.x

Beilschmidt, L. K., and Puccio, H. M. (2014). Mammalian Fe-S cluster biogenesis and its implication in disease. *Biochimie* 100, 48–60. doi: 10.1016/j.biochi.2014.01.009

Bencze, K. Z., Kondapalli, K. C., Cook, J. D., McMahon, S., Millán-Pacheco, C., Pastor, N., et al. (2006). The structure and function of frataxin. *Crit. Rev. Biochem. Mol. Biol.* 41, 269–291. doi: 10.1080/10409230600846058

Bidichandani, S. I., and Delatycki, M. B. (2017). *Friedreich Ataxia.* Available at: http://www.ncbi.nlm.nih.gov/pubmed/20301458

Bolinches-Amorós, A., Mollá, B., Pla-Martín, D., Palau, F., and González-Cabo, P. (2014). Mitochondrial dysfunction induced by frataxin deficiency is associated with cellular senescence and abnormal calcium metabolism. *Front. Cell. Neurosci.* 8:124. doi: 10.3389/fncel.2014.00124

Bonilha da Silva, C., Bergo, F. P. G., D'Abreu, A., Cendes, F., Lopes-Cendes, I., and França, M. C. (2014). Dentate nuclei T2 relaxometry is a reliable neuroimaging marker in Friedreich's ataxia. *Eur. J. Neurol.* 21, 1131–1136. doi: 10.1111/ene.12448

Bou-Abdallah, F., Adinolfi, S., Pastore, A., Laue, T. M., and Dennis Chasteen, N. (2004). Iron binding and oxidation kinetics in frataxin CyaY of *Escherichia coli*. *J. Mol. Biol.* 341, 605–615. doi: 10.1016/j.jmb.2004.05.072

Bradley, J. L., Blake, J. C., Chamberlain, S., Thomas, P. K., Cooper, J. M., and Schapira, A. H. (2000). Clinical, biochemical and molecular genetic correlations in Friedreich's ataxia. *Hum. Mol. Genet.* 9, 275–282. doi: 10.1093/hmg/9.2.275

Bradshaw, T. Y., Romano, L. E. L., Duncan, E. J., Nethisinghe, S., Abeti, R., Michael, G. J., et al. (2016). A reduction in Drp1-mediated fission compromises mitochondrial health in autosomal recessive spastic ataxia of Charlevoix Saguenay. *Hum. Mol. Genet.* 25, 3232–3244. doi: 10.1093/hmg/ddw173

Bridwell-Rabb, J., Iannuzzi, C., Pastore, A., and Barondeau, D. P. (2012). Effector role reversal during evolution: the case of frataxin in Fe-S cluster biosynthesis. *Biochemistry* 51, 2506–2514. doi: 10.1021/bi201628j

Bridwell-Rabb, J., Winn, A. M., and Barondeau, D. P. (2011). Structure-function analysis of Friedreich's ataxia mutants reveals determinants of frataxin binding and activation of the Fe-S assembly complex. *Biochemistry* 50, 7265–7274. doi: 10.1021/bi200895k

Bulteau, A.-L., O'Neill, H. A., Kennedy, M. C., Ikeda-Saito, M., Isaya, G., and Szweda, L. I. (2004). Frataxin acts as an iron chaperone protein to modulate mitochondrial aconitase activity. *Science* 305, 242–245. doi: 10.1126/science.1098991

Cabantchik, Z. I., Munnich, A., Youdim, M. B., and Devos, D. (2013). Regional siderosis: a new challenge for iron chelation therapy. *Front. Pharmacol.* 4:167. doi: 10.3389/fphar.2013.00167

Cai, K., Frederick, R. O., Tonelli, M., and Markley, J. L. (2018). Interactions of iron-bound frataxin with ISCU and ferredoxin on the cysteine desulfurase complex leading to Fe-S cluster assembly. *J. Inorg. Biochem.* 183, 107–116. doi: 10.1016/j.jinorgbio.2018.03.007

Calabrese, V., Lodi, R., Tonon, C., D'Agata, V., Sapienza, M., Scapagnini, G., et al. (2005). Oxidative stress, mitochondrial dysfunction and cellular stress response in Friedreich's ataxia. *J. Neurol. Sci.* 233, 145–162. doi: 10.1016/j.jns.2005.03.012

Calap-Quintana, P., Navarro, J. A., González-Fernández, J., Martínez-Sebastián, M. J., Moltó, M. D., and Llorens, J. V. (2018). *Drosophila melanogaster* models of Friedreich's ataxia. *Biomed. Res. Int.* 2018:5065190. doi: 10.1155/2018/5065190

Campanella, A., Rovelli, E., Santambrogio, P., Cozzi, A., Taroni, F., and Levi, S. (2009). Mitochondrial ferritin limits oxidative damage regulating mitochondrial iron availability: hypothesis for a protective role in Friedreich ataxia. *Hum. Mol. Genet.* 18, 1–11. doi: 10.1093/hmg/ddn308

Campuzano, V., Montermini, L., Lutz, Y., Cova, L., Hindelang, C., Jiralerspong, S., et al. (1997). Frataxin is reduced in Friedreich ataxia patients and is associated with mitochondrial membranes. *Hum. Mol. Genet.* 6, 1771–1780. doi: 10.1093/hmg/6.11.1771

Campuzano, V., Montermini, L., Moltò, M. D., Pianese, L., Cossée, M., Cavalcanti, F., et al. (1996). Friedreich's ataxia: autosomal recessive disease caused by an intronic GAA triplet repeat expansion. *Science* 271, 1423–1427. doi: 10.1126/science.271.5254.1423

Carletti, B., Piermarini, E., Tozzi, G., Travaglini, L., Torraco, A., Pastore, A., et al. (2014). Frataxin silencing inactivates mitochondrial Complex I in NSC34 motoneuronal cells and alters glutathione homeostasis. *Int. J. Mol. Sci.* 15, 5789–5806. doi: 10.3390/ijms15045789

Cavadini, P., Gellera, C., Patel, P. I., and Isaya, G. (2000). Human frataxin maintains mitochondrial iron homeostasis in *Saccharomyces cerevisiae*. *Hum. Mol. Genet.* 9, 2523–2530. doi: 10.1093/hmg/9.17.2523

Chandran, V., Gao, K., Swarup, V., Versano, R., Dong, H., Jordan, M. C., et al. (2017). Inducible and reversible phenotypes in a novel mouse model of Friedreich's Ataxia. *eLife* 6:e30054. doi: 10.7554/eLife.30054

Chantrel-Groussard, K., Geromel, V., Puccio, H., Koenig, M., Munnich, A., Rötig, A., et al. (2001). Disabled early recruitment of antioxidant defenses in Friedreich's ataxia. *Hum. Mol. Genet.* 10, 2061–2067. doi: 10.1093/hmg/10.19.2061

Chen, K., Ho, T. S.-Y., Lin, G., Tan, K. L., Rasband, M. N., and Bellen, H. J. (2016a). Loss of Frataxin activates the iron/sphingolipid/PDK1/Mef2 pathway in mammals. *eLife* 5:e20732. doi: 10.7554/eLife.20732

Chen, K., Lin, G., Haelterman, N. A., Ho, T. S.-Y., Li, T., Li, Z., et al. (2016b). Loss of Frataxin induces iron toxicity, sphingolipid synthesis, and Pdk1/Mef2 activation, leading to neurodegeneration. *eLife* 5:e16043. doi: 10.7554/eLife.16043

Chiabrando, D., Mercurio, S., and Tolosano, E. (2014). Heme and erythropoieis: more than a structural role. *Haematologica* 99, 973–983. doi: 10.3324/haematol.2013.091991

Chiang, S., Kovacevic, Z., Sahni, S., Lane, D. J. R., Merlot, A. M., Kalinowski, D. S., et al. (2016). Frataxin and the molecular mechanism of mitochondrial iron-loading in Friedreich's ataxia. *Clin. Sci.* 130, 853–870. doi: 10.1042/CS20160072

Chung, J., Chen, C., and Paw, B. H. (2012). Heme metabolism and erythropoiesis. *Curr. Opin. Hematol.* 19, 156–162. doi: 10.1097/MOH.0b013e328351c48b

Colin, F., Martelli, A., Clémancey, M., Latour, J.-M., Gambarelli, S., Zeppieri, L., et al. (2013). Mammalian frataxin controls sulfur production and iron entry during de novo Fe4S4 cluster assembly. *J. Am. Chem. Soc.* 135, 733–740. doi: 10.1021/ja308736e

Condò, I., Malisan, F., Guccini, I., Serio, D., Rufini, A., and Testi, R. (2010). Molecular control of the cytosolic aconitase/IRP1 switch by extramitochondrial frataxin. *Hum. Mol. Genet.* 19, 1221–1229. doi: 10.1093/hmg/ddp592

Condò, I., Ventura, N., Malisan, F., Rufini, A., Tomassini, B., and Testi, R. (2007). In vivo maturation of human frataxin. *Hum. Mol. Genet.* 16, 1534–1540. doi: 10.1093/hmg/ddm102

Condò, I., Ventura, N., Malisan, F., Tomassini, B., and Testi, R. (2006). A pool of extramitochondrial frataxin that promotes cell survival. *J. Biol. Chem.* 281, 16750–16756. doi: 10.1074/jbc.M511960200

Connor, J. R., Snyder, B. S., Beard, J. L., Fine, R. E., and Mufson, E. J. (1992). Regional distribution of iron and iron-regulatory proteins in the brain in aging and Alzheimer's disease. *J. Neurosci. Res.* 31, 327–335. doi: 10.1002/jnr.490310214

Cook, J. D., Bencze, K. Z., Jankovic, A. D., Crater, A. K., Busch, C. N., Bradley, P. B., et al. (2006). Monomeric yeast frataxin is an iron-binding protein. *Biochemistry* 45, 7767–7777. doi: 10.1021/bi060424r

Cossée, M., Puccio, H., Gansmuller, A., Koutnikova, H., Dierich, A., LeMeur, M., et al. (2000). Inactivation of the Friedreich ataxia mouse gene leads to early embryonic lethality without iron accumulation. *Hum. Mol. Genet.* 9, 1219–1226. doi: 10.1093/hmg/9.8.1219

Dailey, H. A., and Meissner, P. N. (2013). Erythroid heme biosynthesis and its disorders. *Cold Spring Harb. Perspect. Med.* 3:a011676. doi: 10.1101/cshperspect.a011676

De Castro, M., García-Planells, J., Monrós, E., Cañizares, J., Vázquez-Manrique, R., Vílchez, J. J., et al. (2000). Genotype and phenotype analysis of Friedreich's ataxia compound heterozygous patients. *Hum. Genet.* 106, 86–92. doi: 10.1007/s004399900201

Delatycki, M. B., Camakaris, J., Brooks, H., Evans-Whipp, T., Thorburn, D. R., Williamson, R., et al. (1999). Direct evidence that mitochondrial iron accumulation occurs in Friedreich ataxia. *Ann. Neurol.* 45, 673–675. doi: 10.1002/1531-8249(199905)45:5<673::AID-ANA20>3.0.CO;2-Q

Dhe-Paganon, S., Shigeta, R., Chi, Y. I., Ristow, M., and Shoelson, S. E. (2000). Crystal structure of human frataxin. *J. Biol. Chem.* 275, 30753–30756. doi: 10.1074/jbc.C000407200

Dixon, S. J., Lemberg, K. M., Lamprecht, M. R., Skouta, R., Zaitsev, E. M., Gleason, C. E., et al. (2012). Ferroptosis: an iron-dependent form of nonapoptotic cell death. *Cell* 149, 1060–1072. doi: 10.1016/j.cell.2012.03.042

D'Oria, V., Petrini, S., Travaglini, L., Priori, C., Piermarini, E., Petrillo, S., et al. (2013). Frataxin deficiency leads to reduced expression and impaired translocation of NF-E2-related factor (Nrf2) in cultured motor neurons. *Int. J. Mol. Sci.* 14, 7853–7865. doi: 10.3390/ijms14047853

Dumas, E. M., Versluis, M. J., van den Bogaard, S. J. A., van Osch, M. J. P., Hart, E. P., van Roon-Mom, W. M. C., et al. (2012). Elevated brain iron is independent from atrophy in Huntington's Disease. *Neuroimage* 61, 558–564. doi: 10.1016/j.neuroimage.2012.03.056

Eaton, J. W., and Qian, M. (2002). Molecular bases of cellular iron toxicity. *Free Radic. Biol. Med.* 32, 833–840. doi: 10.1016/S0891-5849(02)00772-4

Edenharter, O., Schneuwly, S., and Navarro, J. A. (2018). Mitofusin-dependent ER stress triggers glial dysfunction and nervous system degeneration in a drosophila model of Friedreich's ataxia. *Front. Mol. Neurosci.* 11:38. doi: 10.3389/fnmol.2018.00038

Elincx-Benizri, S., Glik, A., Merkel, D., Arad, M., Freimark, D., Kozlova, E., et al. (2016). Clinical experience with deferiprone treatment for friedreich ataxia. *J. Child Neurol.* 31, 1036–1040. doi: 10.1177/0883073816636087

Emond, M., Lepage, G., Vanasse, M., and Pandolfo, M. (2000). Increased levels of plasma malondialdehyde in Friedreich ataxia. *Neurology* 55, 1752–1753. doi: 10.1212/WNL.55.11.1752

Filla, A., Postiglione, A., Rubba, P., Patti, L., De Michele, G., Palma, V., et al. (1980). Plasma lipoprotein concentration and erythrocyte membrane lipids in patients with Friedreich's ataxia. *Acta Neurol.* 2, 382–389.

Fleming, M. D. (2011). Congenital sideroblastic anemias: iron and heme lost in mitochondrial translation. *Hematol. Am. Soc. Hematol. Educ. Progr.* 2011, 525–531. doi: 10.1182/asheducation-2011.1.525

Foury, F., and Cazzalini, O. (1997). Deletion of the yeast homologue of the human gene associated with Friedreich's ataxia elicits iron accumulation in mitochondria. *FEBS Lett.* 411, 373–377. doi: 10.1016/S0014-5793(97)00734-5

Foury, F., Pastore, A., and Trincal, M. (2007). Acidic residues of yeast frataxin have an essential role in Fe-S cluster assembly. *EMBO Rep.* 8, 194–199. doi: 10.1038/sj.embor.7400881

Fox, N. G., Das, D., Chakrabarti, M., Lindahl, P. A., and Barondeau, D. P. (2015). Frataxin accelerates [2Fe-2S] cluster formation on the human Fe-S assembly complex. *Biochemistry* 54, 3880–3889. doi: 10.1021/bi5014497

Furuyama, K., Kaneko, K., and Vargas, P. D. (2007). Heme as a magnificent molecule with multiple missions: heme determines its own fate and governs cellular homeostasis. *Tohoku J. Exp. Med.* 213, 1–16. doi: 10.1620/tjem.213.1

Gakh, O., Adamec, J., Gacy, A. M., Twesten, R. D., Owen, W. G., and Isaya, G. (2002). Physical evidence that yeast frataxin is an iron storage protein. *Biochemistry* 41, 6798–6804. doi: 10.1021/bi025566+

Gakh, O., Park, S., Liu, G., Macomber, L., Imlay, J. A., Ferreira, G. C., et al. (2006). Mitochondrial iron detoxification is a primary function of frataxin that limits oxidative damage and preserves cell longevity. *Hum. Mol. Genet.* 15, 467–479. doi: 10.1093/hmg/ddi461

Galea, C. A., Huq, A., Lockhart, P. J., Tai, G., Corben, L. A., Yiu, E. M., et al. (2016). Compound heterozygous FXN mutations and clinical outcome in friedreich ataxia. *Ann. Neurol.* 79, 485–495. doi: 10.1002/ana.24595

García-Beltrán, O., Mena, N. P., Aguirre, P., Barriga-González, G., Galdámez, A., Nagles, E., et al. (2017). Development of an iron-selective antioxidant probe with protective effects on neuronal function. *PLoS One* 12:e0189043. doi: 10.1371/journal.pone.0189043

Gentry, L. E., Thacker, M. A., Doughty, R., Timkovich, R., and Busenlehner, L. S. (2013). His86 from the N-terminus of frataxin coordinates iron and is required for Fe-S cluster synthesis. *Biochemistry* 52, 6085–6096. doi: 10.1021/bi400443n

Gerber, J., Mühlenhoff, U., and Lill, R. (2003). An interaction between frataxin and Isu1/Nfs1 that is crucial for Fe/S cluster synthesis on Isu1. *EMBO Rep.* 4, 906–911. doi: 10.1038/sj.embor.embor918

González-Cabo, P., and Palau, F. (2013). Mitochondrial pathophysiology in Friedreich's ataxia. *J. Neurochem.* 126(Suppl.), 53–64. doi: 10.1111/jnc.12303

Gorell, J. M., Ordidge, R. J., Brown, G. G., Deniau, J. C., Buderer, N. M., and Helpern, J. A. (1995). Increased iron-related MRI contrast in the *Substantia nigra* in Parkinson's disease. *Neurology* 45, 1138–1143. doi: 10.1212/WNL.45.6.1138

Guo, L., Wang, Q., Weng, L., Hauser, L. A., Strawser, C. J., Mesaros, C., et al. (2018). Characterization of a new N-terminally acetylated extra-mitochondrial isoform of frataxin in human erythrocytes. *Sci. Rep.* 8:17043. doi: 10.1038/s41598-018-35346-y

Harding, A. E. (1981). Early onset cerebellar ataxia with retained tendon reflexes: a clinical and genetic study of a disorder distinct from Friedreich's ataxia. *J. Neurol. Neurosurg. Psychiatry* 44, 503–508. doi: 10.1136/jnnp.44.6.503

Harding, I. H., Raniga, P., Delatycki, M. B., Stagnitti, M. R., Corben, L. A., Storey, E., et al. (2016). Tissue atrophy and elevated iron concentration in the extrapyramidal motor system in Friedreich ataxia: the IMAGE-FRDA study. *J. Neurol. Neurosurg. Psychiatry* 87, 1261–1263. doi: 10.1136/jnnp-2015-312665

Huang, J., Dizin, E., and Cowan, J. A. (2008). Mapping iron binding sites on human frataxin: implications for cluster assembly on the ISU Fe-S cluster scaffold protein. *J. Biol. Inorg. Chem.* 13, 825–836. doi: 10.1007/s00775-008-0369-4

Huang, M. L.-H., Becker, E. M., Whitnall, M., Suryo Rahmanto, Y., Ponka, P., and Richardson, D. R. (2009). Elucidation of the mechanism of mitochondrial iron loading in Friedreich's ataxia by analysis of a mouse mutant. *Proc. Natl. Acad. Sci. U.S.A.* 106, 16381–16386. doi: 10.1073/pnas.0906784106

Huang, M. L.-H., Lane, D. J. R., and Richardson, D. R. (2011). Mitochondrial mayhem: the mitochondrion as a modulator of iron metabolism and its role in disease. *Antioxid. Redox Signal.* 15, 3003–3019. doi: 10.1089/ars.2011.3921

Huang, M. L.-H., Sivagurunathan, S., Ting, S., Jansson, P. J., Austin, C. J. D., Kelly, M., et al. (2013). Molecular and functional alterations in a mouse cardiac model of Friedreich ataxia: activation of the integrated stress response, eIF2α phosphorylation, and the induction of downstream targets. *Am. J. Pathol.* 183, 745–757. doi: 10.1016/j.ajpath.2013.05.032

Huang, Y. S., Nestruck, A. C., Barbeau, A., Bouchard, J. P., and Davignon, J. (1978). Plasma lipids and lipoproteins in Friedreich's ataxia and familial spastic ataxia–evidence for an abnormal composition of high density lipoproteins. *Can. J. Neurol. Sci.* 5, 149–156.

Igoillo-Esteve, M., Gurgul-Convey, E., Hu, A., Romagueira Bichara Dos Santos, L., Abdulkarim, B., Chintawar, S., et al. (2015). Unveiling a common mechanism of apoptosis in β-cells and neurons in Friedreich's ataxia. *Hum. Mol. Genet.* 24, 2274–2286. doi: 10.1093/hmg/ddu745

Kakhlon, O., and Cabantchik, Z. I. (2002). The labile iron pool: characterization, measurement, and participation in cellular processes(1). *Free Radic. Biol. Med.* 33, 1037–1046. doi: 10.1016/S0891-5849(02)01006-7

Kakhlon, O., Manning, H., Breuer, W., Melamed-Book, N., Lu, C., Cortopassi, G., et al. (2008). Cell functions impaired by frataxin deficiency are restored by drug-mediated iron relocation. *Blood* 112, 5219–5227. doi: 10.1182/blood-2008-06-161919

Katsu-Jiménez, Y., Loría, F., Corona, J. C., and Díaz-Nido, J. (2016). Gene transfer of brain-derived neurotrophic factor (BDNF) prevents neurodegeneration triggered by FXN deficiency. *Mol. Ther.* 24, 877–889. doi: 10.1038/mt.2016.32

Kipps, A., Alexander, M., Colan, S. D., Gauvreau, K., Smoot, L., Crawford, L., et al. (2009). The longitudinal course of cardiomyopathy in Friedreich's ataxia during childhood. *Pediatr. Cardiol.* 30, 306–310. doi: 10.1007/s00246-008-9305-1

Knight, S. A., Sepuri, N. B., Pain, D., and Dancis, A. (1998). Mt-Hsp70 homolog, Ssc2p, required for maturation of yeast frataxin and mitochondrial iron homeostasis. *J. Biol. Chem.* 273, 18389–18393. doi: 10.1074/jbc.273.29.18389

Koeppen, A. H. (2013). Nikolaus Friedreich and degenerative atrophy of the dorsal columns of the spinal cord. *J. Neurochem.* 126, 4–10. doi: 10.1111/jnc.12218

Koeppen, A. H., Kuntzsch, E. C., Bjork, S. T., Ramirez, R. L., Mazurkiewicz, J. E., and Feustel, P. J. (2013). Friedreich ataxia: metal dysmetabolism in dorsal root ganglia. *Acta Neuropathol. Commun.* 1:26. doi: 10.1186/2051-5960-1-26

Koeppen, A. H., and Mazurkiewicz, J. E. (2013). Friedreich ataxia: neuropathology revised. *J. Neuropathol. Exp. Neurol.* 72, 78–90. doi: 10.1097/NEN.0b013e31827e5762

Koeppen, A. H., Michael, S. C., Knutson, M. D., Haile, D. J., Qian, J., Levi, S., et al. (2007). The dentate nucleus in Friedreich's ataxia: the role of iron-responsive proteins. *Acta Neuropathol.* 114, 163–173. doi: 10.1007/s00401-007-0220-y

Koeppen, A. H., Morral, J. A., Davis, A. N., Qian, J., Petrocine, S. V., Knutson, M. D., et al. (2009). The dorsal root ganglion in Friedreich's ataxia. *Acta Neuropathol.* 118, 763–776. doi: 10.1007/s00401-009-0589-x

Koeppen, A. H., Ramirez, R. L., Becker, A. B., Bjork, S. T., Levi, S., Santambrogio, P., et al. (2015). The pathogenesis of cardiomyopathy in Friedreich ataxia. *PLoS One* 10:e0116396. doi: 10.1371/journal.pone.0116396

Koeppen, A. H., Ramirez, R. L., Becker, A. B., and Mazurkiewicz, J. E. (2016). Dorsal root ganglia in Friedreich ataxia: satellite cell proliferation and inflammation. *Acta Neuropathol. Commun.* 4:46. doi: 10.1186/s40478-016-0288-5

Koeppen, A. H., Ramirez, R. L., Yu, D., Collins, S. E., Qian, J., Parsons, P. J., et al. (2012). Friedreich's ataxia causes redistribution of iron, copper, and zinc in the dentate nucleus. *Cerebellum* 11, 845–860. doi: 10.1007/s12311-012-0383-5

Kruger, P. C., Yang, K. X., Parsons, P. J., Becker, A. B., Feustel, P. J., and Koeppen, A. H. (2016). Abundance and significance of iron, zinc, copper, and calcium in the hearts of patients with friedreich ataxia. *Am. J. Cardiol.* 118, 127–131. doi: 10.1016/j.amjcard.2016.04.024

Kumari, D., and Usdin, K. (2012). Is Friedreich ataxia an epigenetic disorder? *Clin. Epigenetics* 4:2. doi: 10.1186/1868-7083-4-2

Kwan, J. Y., Meoded, A., Danielian, L. E., Wu, T., and Floeter, M. K. (2012). Structural imaging differences and longitudinal changes in primary lateral sclerosis and amyotrophic lateral sclerosis. *Neuroimage Clin.* 2, 151–160. doi: 10.1016/j.nicl.2012.12.003

Lamarche, J. B., Côté, M., and Lemieux, B. (1980). The cardiomyopathy of Friedreich's ataxia morphological observations in 3 cases. *Can. J. Neurol. Sci.* 7, 389–396. doi: 10.1017/S0317167100022927

Lane, D. J. R., Merlot, A. M., Huang, M. L.-H., Bae, D.-H., Jansson, P. J., Sahni, S., et al. (2015). Cellular iron uptake, trafficking and metabolism: key molecules and mechanisms and their roles in disease. *Biochim. Biophys. Acta* 1853, 1130–1144. doi: 10.1016/j.bbamcr.2015.01.021

Layer, G., Ollagnier-de Choudens, S., Sanakis, Y., and Fontecave, M. (2006). Iron-sulfur cluster biosynthesis: characterization of *Escherichia coli* CYaY as an iron donor for the assembly of [2Fe-2S] clusters in the scaffold IscU. *J. Biol. Chem.* 281, 16256–16263. doi: 10.1074/jbc.M513569200

Lee, Y.-J., Huang, X., Kropat, J., Henras, A., Merchant, S. S., Dickson, R. C., et al. (2012). Sphingolipid signaling mediates iron toxicity. *Cell Metab.* 16, 90–96. doi: 10.1016/j.cmet.2012.06.004

Lee, Y.-K., Lau, Y.-M., Ng, K.-M., Lai, W.-H., Ho, S.-L., Tse, H.-F., et al. (2016). Efficient attenuation of Friedreich's ataxia (FRDA) cardiomyopathy by modulation of iron homeostasis-human induced pluripotent stem cell (hiPSC) as a drug screening platform for FRDA. *Int. J. Cardiol.* 203, 964–971. doi: 10.1016/j.ijcard.2015.11.101

Lesuisse, E., Santos, R., Matzanke, B. F., Knight, S. A. B., Camadro, J.-M., and Dancis, A. (2003). Iron use for haeme synthesis is under control of the yeast frataxin homologue (Yfh1). *Hum. Mol. Genet.* 12, 879–889. doi: 10.1093/hmg/ddg096

Li, K., and Reichmann, H. (2016). Role of iron in neurodegenerative diseases. *J. Neural Transm.* 123, 389–399. doi: 10.1007/s00702-016-1508-7

Li, L., Miao, R., Bertram, S., Jia, X., Ward, D. M., and Kaplan, J. (2012). A role for iron-sulfur clusters in the regulation of transcription factor Yap5-dependent high iron transcriptional responses in yeast. *J. Biol. Chem.* 287, 35709–35721. doi: 10.1074/jbc.M112.395533

Lill, R. (2009). Function and biogenesis of iron-sulphur proteins. *Nature* 460, 831–838. doi: 10.1038/nature08301

Lill, R., Dutkiewicz, R., Freibert, S. A., Heidenreich, T., Mascarenhas, J., Netz, D. J., et al. (2015). The role of mitochondria and the CIA machinery in the maturation of cytosolic and nuclear iron–sulfur proteins. *Eur. J. Cell Biol.* 94, 280–291. doi: 10.1016/j.ejcb.2015.05.002

Lill, R., and Mühlenhoff, U. (2006). Iron-sulfur protein biogenesis in eukaryotes: components and mechanisms. *Annu. Rev. Cell Dev. Biol.* 22, 457–486. doi: 10.1146/annurev.cellbio.22.010305.104538

Llorens, J. V., Navarro, J. A., Martínez-Sebastián, M. J., Baylies, M. K., Schneuwly, S., Botella, J. A., et al. (2007). Causative role of oxidative stress in a *Drosophila* model of Friedreich ataxia. *FASEB J.* 21, 333–344. doi: 10.1096/fj.05-5709com

Lu, C., and Cortopassi, G. (2007). Frataxin knockdown causes loss of cytoplasmic iron-sulfur cluster functions, redox alterations and induction of heme transcripts. *Arch. Biochem. Biophys.* 457, 111–122. doi: 10.1016/j.abb.2006.09.010

Lupoli, F., Vannocci, T., Longo, G., Niccolai, N., and Pastore, A. (2018). The role of oxidative stress in Friedreich's ataxia. *FEBS Lett.* 592, 718–727. doi: 10.1002/1873-3468.12928

Macevilly, C. J., and Muller, D. P. (1997). Oxidative stress does not appear to be involved in the aetiology of Friedreich's ataxia. *Restor. Neurol. Neurosci.* 11, 131–137. doi: 10.3233/RNN-1997-11303

Marmolino, D. (2011). Friedreich's ataxia: past, present and future. *Brain Res. Rev.* 67, 311–330. doi: 10.1016/j.brainresrev.2011.04.001

Martelli, A., Friedman, L. S., Reutenauer, L., Messaddeq, N., Perlman, S. L., Lynch, D. R., et al. (2012). Clinical data and characterization of the liver conditional mouse model exclude neoplasia as a non-neurological manifestation associated with Friedreich's ataxia. *Dis. Model. Mech.* 5, 860–869. doi: 10.1242/dmm.009829

Martelli, A., and Puccio, H. (2014). Dysregulation of cellular iron metabolism in Friedreich ataxia: from primary iron-sulfur cluster deficit to mitochondrial iron accumulation. *Front. Pharmacol.* 5:130. doi: 10.3389/fphar.2014.00130

Martelli, A., Schmucker, S., Reutenauer, L., Mathieu, J. R. R., Peyssonnaux, C., Karim, Z., et al. (2015). Iron regulatory protein 1 sustains mitochondrial iron loading and function in frataxin deficiency. *Cell Metab.* 21, 311–323. doi: 10.1016/j.cmet.2015.01.010

Martin, M., Colman, M. J. R., Gómez-Casati, D. F., Lamattina, L., and Zabaleta, E. J. (2009). Nitric oxide accumulation is required to protect against iron-mediated oxidative stress in frataxin-deficient Arabidopsis plants. *FEBS Lett.* 583, 542–548. doi: 10.1016/j.febslet.2008.12.039

Mena, N. P., García-Beltrán, O., Lourido, F., Urrutia, P. J., Mena, R., Castro-Castillo, V., et al. (2015). The novel mitochondrial iron chelator 5-((methylamino)methyl)-8-hydroxyquinoline protects against mitochondrial-induced oxidative damage and neuronal death. *Biochem. Biophys. Res. Commun.* 463, 787–792. doi: 10.1016/j.bbrc.2015.06.014

Michael, S., Petrocine, S. V., Qian, J., Lamarche, J. B., Knutson, M. D., Garrick, M. D., et al. (2006). Iron and iron-responsive proteins in the cardiomyopathy of Friedreich's ataxia. *Cerebellum* 5, 257–267. doi: 10.1080/14734220600913246

Mincheva-Tasheva, S., Obis, E., Tamarit, J., and Ros, J. (2014). Apoptotic cell death and altered calcium homeostasis caused by frataxin depletion in dorsal root ganglia neurons can be prevented by BH4 domain of Bcl-xL protein. *Hum. Mol. Genet.* 23, 1829–1841. doi: 10.1093/hmg/ddt576

Mollá, B., Muñoz-Lasso, D. C., Riveiro, F., Bolinches-Amorós, A., Pallardó, F. V., Fernandez-Vilata, A., et al. (2017). Reversible axonal dystrophy by calcium modulation in frataxin-deficient sensory neurons of YG8R mice. *Front. Mol. Neurosci.* 10:264. doi: 10.3389/fnmol.2017.00264

Monnier, V., Llorens, J. V., and Navarro, J. A. (2018). Impact of *Drosophila* models in the study and treatment of Friedreich's Ataxia. *Int. J. Mol. Sci.* 19:E1989. doi: 10.3390/ijms19071989

Monrós, E., Moltó, M. D., Martínez, F., Cañizares, J., Blanca, J., Vílchez, J. J., et al. (1997). Phenotype correlation and intergenerational dynamics of the Friedreich ataxia GAA trinucleotide repeat. *Am. J. Hum. Genet.* 61, 101–110. doi: 10.1086/513887

Napier, I., Ponka, P., and Richardson, D. R. (2005). Iron trafficking in the mitochondrion: novel pathways revealed by disease. *Blood* 105, 1867–1874. doi: 10.1182/blood-2004-10-3856

Navarro, J. A., Botella, J. A., Metzendorf, C., Lind, M. I., and Schneuwly, S. (2015). Mitoferrin modulates iron toxicity in a *Drosophila* model of Friedreich's ataxia. *Free Radic. Biol. Med.* 85, 71–82. doi: 10.1016/j.freeradbiomed.2015.03.014

Navarro, J. A., Ohmann, E., Sanchez, D., Botella, J. A., Liebisch, G., Moltó, M. D., et al. (2010). Altered lipid metabolism in a *Drosophila* model of Friedreich's ataxia. *Hum. Mol. Genet.* 19, 2828–2840. doi: 10.1093/hmg/ddq183

Obis, È., Irazusta, V., Sanchís, D., Ros, J., and Tamarit, J. (2014). Frataxin deficiency in neonatal rat ventricular myocytes targets mitochondria and lipid metabolism. *Free Radic. Biol. Med.* 73, 21–33. doi: 10.1016/j.freeradbiomed.2014.04.016

O'Neill, H. A., Gakh, O., Park, S., Cui, J., Mooney, S. M., Sampson, M., et al. (2005). Assembly of human frataxin is a mechanism for detoxifying redox-active iron. *Biochemistry* 44, 537–545. doi: 10.1021/bi048459j

Pandey, A., Gordon, D. M., Pain, J., Stemmler, T. L., Dancis, A., and Pain, D. (2013). Frataxin directly stimulates mitochondrial cysteine desulfurase by exposing substrate-binding sites, and a mutant Fe-S cluster scaffold protein with frataxin-bypassing ability acts similarly. *J. Biol. Chem.* 288, 36773–36786. doi: 10.1074/jbc.M113.525857

Pandolfo, M., Arpa, J., Delatycki, M. B., Le Quan Sang, K. H., Mariotti, C., Munnich, A., et al. (2014). Deferiprone in Friedreich ataxia: a 6-month randomized controlled trial. *Ann. Neurol.* 76, 509–521. doi: 10.1002/ana.24248

Pandolfo, M., and Pastore, A. (2009). The pathogenesis of Friedreich ataxia and the structure and function of frataxin. *J. Neurol.* 256(Suppl.), 9–17. doi: 10.1007/s00415-009-1003-2

Park, S., Gakh, O., Mooney, S. M., and Isaya, G. (2002). The ferroxidase activity of yeast frataxin. *J. Biol. Chem.* 277, 38589–38595. doi: 10.1074/jbc.M206711200

Park, S., Gakh, O., O'Neill, H. A., Mangravita, A., Nichol, H., Ferreira, G. C., et al. (2003). Yeast frataxin sequentially chaperones and stores iron by coupling protein assembly with iron oxidation. *J. Biol. Chem.* 278, 31340–31351. doi: 10.1074/jbc.M303158200

Parkinson, M. H., Boesch, S., Nachbauer, W., Mariotti, C., and Giunti, P. (2013). Clinical features of Friedreich's ataxia: classical and atypical phenotypes. *J. Neurochem.* 126(Suppl.), 103–117. doi: 10.1111/jnc.12317

Paupe, V., Dassa, E. P., Goncalves, S., Auchère, F., Lönn, M., Holmgren, A., et al. (2009). Impaired nuclear Nrf2 translocation undermines the oxidative stress response in Friedreich ataxia. *PLoS One* 4:e4253. doi: 10.1371/journal.pone.0004253

Payne, R. M., and Wagner, G. R. (2012). Cardiomyopathy in Friedreich ataxia: clinical findings and research. *J. Child Neurol.* 27, 1179–1186. doi: 10.1177/0883073812448535

Perdomini, M., Belbellaa, B., Monassier, L., Reutenauer, L., Messaddeq, N., Cartier, N., et al. (2014). Prevention and reversal of severe mitochondrial cardiomyopathy by gene therapy in a mouse model of Friedreich's ataxia. *Nat. Med.* 20, 542–547. doi: 10.1038/nm.3510

Perez, C. A., Tong, Y., and Guo, M. (2008). Iron chelators as potential therapeutic agents for Parkinson's disease. *Curr. Bioact. Compd.* 4, 150–158. doi: 10.2174/157340708786305952

Petrillo, S., Piermarini, E., Pastore, A., Vasco, G., Schirinzi, T., Carrozzo, R., et al. (2017). Nrf2-inducers counteract neurodegeneration in frataxin-silenced motor neurons: disclosing new therapeutic targets for Friedreich's ataxia. *Int. J. Mol. Sci.* 18:E2173. doi: 10.3390/ijms18102173

Piermarini, E., Cartelli, D., Pastore, A., Tozzi, G., Compagnucci, C., Giorda, E., et al. (2016). Frataxin silencing alters microtubule stability in motor neurons: implications for Friedreich's ataxia. *Hum. Mol. Genet.* 25, 4288–4301. doi: 10.1093/hmg/ddw260

Piguet, F., de Montigny, C., Vaucamps, N., Reutenauer, L., Eisenmann, A., and Puccio, H. (2018). Rapid and complete reversal of sensory ataxia by gene therapy in a novel model of friedreich ataxia. *Mol. Ther.* 26, 1940–1952. doi: 10.1016/j.ymthe.2018.05.006

Ponka, P. (1997). Tissue-specific regulation of iron metabolism and heme synthesis: distinct control mechanisms in erythroid cells. *Blood* 89, 1–25.

Puccio, H., Simon, D., Cossée, M., Criqui-Filipe, P., Tiziano, F., Melki, J., et al. (2001). Mouse models for Friedreich ataxia exhibit cardiomyopathy, sensory nerve defect and Fe-S enzyme deficiency followed by intramitochondrial iron deposits. *Nat. Genet.* 27, 181–186. doi: 10.1038/84818

Py, B., and Barras, F. (2010). Building Fe-S proteins: bacterial strategies. *Nat. Rev. Microbiol.* 8, 436–446. doi: 10.1038/nrmicro2356

Rajagopalan, B., Francis, J. M., Cooke, F., Korlipara, L. V. P., Blamire, A. M., Schapira, A. H. V., et al. (2010). Analysis of the factors influencing the cardiac phenotype in Friedreich's ataxia. *Mov. Disord.* 25, 846–852. doi: 10.1002/mds.22864

Raman, R., Vaitheeswaran, K., Vinita, K., and Sharma, T. (2011). Is prevalence of retinopathy related to the age of onset of diabetes? Sankara nethralaya diabetic retinopathy epidemiology and molecular genetic report No. 5. *Ophthalmic Res.* 45, 36–41. doi: 10.1159/000314720

Raman, S. V., Phatak, K., Hoyle, J. C., Pennell, M. L., McCarthy, B., Tran, T., et al. (2011). Impaired myocardial perfusion reserve and fibrosis in Friedreich ataxia: a mitochondrial cardiomyopathy with metabolic syndrome. *Eur. Heart J.* 32, 561–567. doi: 10.1093/eurheartj/ehq443

Ramirez, R. L., Qian, J., Santambrogio, P., Levi, S., and Koeppen, A. H. (2012). Relation of cytosolic iron excess to cardiomyopathy of Friedreich's ataxia. *Am. J. Cardiol.* 110, 1820–1827. doi: 10.1016/j.amjcard.2012.08.018

Richardson, D. R., Lane, D. J. R., Becker, E. M., Huang, M. L.-H., Whitnall, M., Suryo Rahmanto, Y., et al. (2010). Mitochondrial iron trafficking and the integration of iron metabolism between the mitochondrion and cytosol. *Proc. Natl. Acad. Sci. U.S.A.* 107, 10775–10782. doi: 10.1073/pnas.0912925107

Rocca, C. J., Goodman, S. M., Dulin, J. N., Haquang, J. H., Gertsman, I., Blondelle, J., et al. (2017). Transplantation of wild-type mouse hematopoietic stem and progenitor cells ameliorates deficits in a mouse model of Friedreich's ataxia. *Sci. Transl. Med.* 9:eaaj2347. doi: 10.1126/scitranslmed.aaj2347

Rötig, A., de Lonlay, P., Chretien, D., Foury, F., Koenig, M., Sidi, D., et al. (1997). Aconitase and mitochondrial iron-sulphur protein deficiency in Friedreich ataxia. *Nat. Genet.* 17, 215–217. doi: 10.1038/ng1097-215

Sanchez-Casis, G., Cote, M., and Barbeau, A. (1976). Pathology of the heart in Friedreich's ataxia: review of the literature and report of one case. *Can. J. Neurol. Sci.* 3, 349–354. doi: 10.1017/S0317167100025580

Sassa, S. (2006). Modern diagnosis and management of the porphyrias. *Br. J. Haematol.* 135, 281–292. doi: 10.1111/j.1365-2141.2006.06289.x

Saveliev, A., Everett, C., Sharpe, T., Webster, Z., and Festenstein, R. (2003). DNA triplet repeats mediate heterochromatin-protein-1-sensitive variegated gene silencing. *Nature* 422, 909–913. doi: 10.1038/nature01596

Schiavi, A., Torgovnick, A., Kell, A., Megalou, E., Castelein, N., Guccini, I., et al. (2013). Autophagy induction extends lifespan and reduces lipid content in response to frataxin silencing in *C. elegans*. *Exp. Gerontol.* 48, 191–201. doi: 10.1016/j.exger.2012.12.002

Schmucker, S., Martelli, A., Colin, F., Page, A., Wattenhofer-Donzé, M., Reutenauer, L., et al. (2011). Mammalian frataxin: an essential function for cellular viability through an interaction with a preformed ISCU/NFS1/ISD11 iron-sulfur assembly complex. *PLoS One* 6:e16199. doi: 10.1371/journal.pone.0016199

Schoenfeld, R. A., Napoli, E., Wong, A., Zhan, S., Reutenauer, L., Morin, D., et al. (2005). Frataxin deficiency alters heme pathway transcripts and decreases mitochondrial heme metabolites in mammalian cells. *Hum. Mol. Genet.* 14, 3787–3799. doi: 10.1093/hmg/ddi393

Schulz, J. B., Dehmer, T., Schöls, L., Mende, H., Hardt, C., Vorgerd, M., et al. (2000). Oxidative stress in patients with Friedreich ataxia. *Neurology* 55, 1719–1721. doi: 10.1212/WNL.55.11.1719

Selvadurai, L. P., Harding, I. H., Corben, L. A., and Georgiou-Karistianis, N. (2018). Cerebral abnormalities in Friedreich ataxia: a review. *Neurosci. Biobehav. Rev.* 84, 394–406. doi: 10.1016/j.neubiorev.2017.08.006

Seznec, H., Simon, D., Bouton, C., Reutenauer, L., Hertzog, A., Golik, P., et al. (2005). Friedreich ataxia: the oxidative stress paradox. *Hum. Mol. Genet.* 14, 463–474. doi: 10.1093/hmg/ddi042

Shamim, A., Mahmood, T., Ahsan, F., Kumar, A., and Bagga, P. (2018). Lipids: an insight into the neurodegenerative disorders. *Clin. Nutr. Exp.* 20, 1–19. doi: 10.1016/j.yclnex.2018.05.001

Shan, Y., Schoenfeld, R. A., Hayashi, G., Napoli, E., Akiyama, T., Iodi Carstens, M., et al. (2013). Frataxin deficiency leads to defects in expression of antioxidants and Nrf2 expression in dorsal root ganglia of the Friedreich's ataxia YG8R mouse model. *Antioxid. Redox Signal.* 19, 1481–1493. doi: 10.1089/ars.2012.4537

Shidara, Y., and Hollenbeck, P. J. (2010). Defects in mitochondrial axonal transport and membrane potential without increased reactive oxygen species production in a Drosophila model of Friedreich ataxia. *J. Neurosci.* 30, 11369–11378. doi: 10.1523/JNEUROSCI.0529-10.2010

Simon, D., Seznec, H., Gansmuller, A., Carelle, N., Weber, P., Metzger, D., et al. (2004). Friedreich ataxia mouse models with progressive cerebellar and sensory ataxia reveal autophagic neurodegeneration in dorsal root ganglia. *J. Neurosci.* 24, 1987–1995. doi: 10.1523/JNEUROSCI.4549-03.2004

Singh, Y. P., Pandey, A., Vishwakarma, S., and Modi, G. (2018). A review on iron chelators as potential therapeutic agents for the treatment of Alzheimer's and Parkinson's diseases. *Mol. Divers.* doi: 10.1007/s11030-018-9878-4 [Epub ahead of print].

Sohn, Y.-S., Breuer, W., Munnich, A., and Cabantchik, Z. I. (2008). Redistribution of accumulated cell iron: a modality of chelation with therapeutic implications. *Blood* 111, 1690–1699. doi: 10.1182/blood-2007-07-102335

Solbach, K., Kraff, O., Minnerop, M., Beck, A., Schöls, L., Gizewski, E. R., et al. (2014). Cerebellar pathology in Friedreich's ataxia: atrophied dentate nuclei with normal iron content. *Neuroimage Clin.* 6, 93–99. doi: 10.1016/j.nicl.2014.08.018

Soragni, E., and Gottesfeld, J. M. (2016). Translating HDAC inhibitors in Friedreich's ataxia. *Expert Opin. Orphan Drugs* 4, 961–970. doi: 10.1080/21678707.2016.1215910

Soriano, S., Calap-Quintana, P., Llorens, J. V., Al-Ramahi, I., Gutiérrez, L., Martínez-Sebastián, M. J., et al. (2016). Metal homeostasis regulators suppress FRDA phenotypes in a *Drosophila* model of the disease. *PLoS One* 11:e0159209. doi: 10.1371/journal.pone.0159209

Soriano, S., Llorens, J. V., Blanco-Sobero, L., Gutiérrez, L., Calap-Quintana, P., Morales, M. P., et al. (2013). Deferiprone and idebenone rescue frataxin depletion phenotypes in a *Drosophila* model of Friedreich's ataxia. *Gene* 521, 274–281. doi: 10.1016/j.gene.2013.02.049

Strawser, C., Schadt, K., Hauser, L., McCormick, A., Wells, M., Larkindale, J., et al. (2017). Pharmacological therapeutics in Friedreich ataxia: the present state. *Expert Rev. Neurother.* 17, 895–907. doi: 10.1080/14737175.2017.1356721

Sturm, B., Bistrich, U., Schranzhofer, M., Sarsero, J. P., Rauen, U., Scheiber-Mojdehkar, B., et al. (2005). Friedreich's ataxia, no changes in mitochondrial labile iron in human lymphoblasts and fibroblasts: a decrease in antioxidative capacity? *J. Biol. Chem.* 280, 6701–6708. doi: 10.1074/jbc.M408717200

Tan, G., Chen, L. S., Lonnerdal, B., Gellera, C., Taroni, F. A., and Cortopassi, G. A. (2001). Frataxin expression rescues mitochondrial dysfunctions in FRDA cells. *Hum. Mol. Genet.* 10, 2099–2107. doi: 10.1093/hmg/10.19.2099

Thurman, P., and Draper, P. (1989). Biosynthesis of phenolic glycolipids in *M. microti*. *Acta Leprol.* 7(Suppl. 1):74.

Totadri, S., Bansal, D., Bhatia, P., Attri, S. V., Trehan, A., and Marwaha, R. K. (2015). The deferiprone and deferasirox combination is efficacious in iron overloaded patients with β-thalassemia major: a prospective, single center, open-label study. *Pediatr. Blood Cancer* 62, 1592–1596. doi: 10.1002/pbc.25533

Tricoire, H., Palandri, A., Bourdais, A., Camadro, J.-M., and Monnier, V. (2014). Methylene blue rescues heart defects in a Drosophila model of Friedreich's ataxia. *Hum. Mol. Genet.* 23, 968–979. doi: 10.1093/hmg/ddt493

Tsai, C.-L., and Barondeau, D. P. (2010). Human frataxin is an allosteric switch that activates the Fe-S cluster biosynthetic complex. *Biochemistry* 49, 9132–9139. doi: 10.1021/bi1013062

Turowski, V. R., Aknin, C., Maliandi, M. V., Buchensky, C., Leaden, L., Peralta, D. A., et al. (2015). Frataxin is localized to both the chloroplast and mitochondrion and is involved in chloroplast Fe-S protein function in Arabidopsis. *PLoS One* 10:e0141443. doi: 10.1371/journal.pone.0141443

Van Vranken, J. G., Jeong, M.-Y., Wei, P., Chen, Y.-C., Gygi, S. P., Winge, D. R., et al. (2016). The mitochondrial acyl carrier protein (ACP) coordinates mitochondrial fatty acid synthesis with iron sulfur cluster biogenesis. *eLife* 5:e17828. doi: 10.7554/eLife.17828

Vankan, P. (2013). Prevalence gradients of Friedreich's ataxia and R1b haplotype in Europe co-localize, suggesting a common Palaeolithic origin in the Franco-Cantabrian ice age refuge. *J. Neurochem.* 126(Suppl.), 11–20. doi: 10.1111/jnc.12215

Vazzola, V., Losa, A., Soave, C., and Murgia, I. (2007). Knockout of frataxin gene causes embryo lethality in *Arabidopsis*. *FEBS Lett.* 581, 667–672. doi: 10.1016/j.febslet.2007.01.030

Waldvogel, D., van Gelderen, P., and Hallett, M. (1999). Increased iron in the dentate nucleus of patients with Friedrich's ataxia. *Ann. Neurol.* 46, 123–125. doi: 10.1002/1531-8249(199907)46:1<123::AID-ANA19>3.0.CO;2-H

Weidemann, F., Störk, S., Liu, D., Hu, K., Herrmann, S., Ertl, G., et al. (2013). Cardiomyopathy of Friedreich ataxia. *J. Neurochem.* 126(Suppl.), 88–93. doi: 10.1111/jnc.12217

Whitnall, M., Suryo Rahmanto, Y., Huang, M. L.-H., Saletta, F., Lok, H. C., Gutiérrez, L., et al. (2012). Identification of nonferritin mitochondrial iron deposits in a mouse model of Friedreich ataxia. *Proc. Natl. Acad. Sci. U.S.A.* 109, 20590–20595. doi: 10.1073/pnas.1215349109

Whitnall, M., Suryo Rahmanto, Y., Sutak, R., Xu, X., Becker, E. M., Mikhael, M. R., et al. (2008). The MCK mouse heart model of Friedreich's ataxia: alterations in iron-regulated proteins and cardiac hypertrophy are limited by iron chelation. *Proc. Natl. Acad. Sci. U.S.A.* 105, 9757–9762. doi: 10.1073/pnas.0804261105

Wong, A., Yang, J., Cavadini, P., Gellera, C., Lonnerdal, B., Taroni, F., et al. (1999). The Friedreich's ataxia mutation confers cellular sensitivity to oxidant stress which is rescued by chelators of iron and calcium and inhibitors of apoptosis. *Hum. Mol. Genet.* 8, 425–430. doi: 10.1093/hmg/8.3.425

Worth, A. J., Basu, S. S., Snyder, N. W., Mesaros, C., and Blair, I. A. (2014). Inhibition of neuronal cell mitochondrial complex I with rotenone increases lipid β-oxidation, supporting acetyl-coenzyme A levels. *J. Biol. Chem.* 289, 26895–26903. doi: 10.1074/jbc.M114.591354

Wu, C. K., Dailey, H. A., Rose, J. P., Burden, A., Sellers, V. M., and Wang, B. C. (2001). The 2.0 A structure of human ferrochelatase, the terminal enzyme of heme biosynthesis. *Nat. Struct. Biol.* 8, 156–160. doi: 10.1038/84152

Yoon, T., and Cowan, J. A. (2003). Iron-sulfur cluster biosynthesis. Characterization of frataxin as an iron donor for assembly of [2Fe-2S] clusters in ISU-type proteins. *J. Am. Chem. Soc.* 125, 6078–6084. doi: 10.1021/ja027967i

Yoon, T., and Cowan, J. A. (2004). Frataxin-mediated iron delivery to ferrochelatase in the final step of heme biosynthesis. *J. Biol. Chem.* 279, 25943–25946. doi: 10.1074/jbc.C400107200

Yoon, T., Dizin, E., and Cowan, J. A. (2007). N-terminal iron-mediated self-cleavage of human frataxin: regulation of iron binding and complex formation with target proteins. *J. Biol. Inorg. Chem.* 12, 535–542. doi: 10.1007/s00775-007-0205-2

5

The Contribution of Iron to Protein Aggregation Disorders in the Central Nervous System

Karina Joppe[1], Anna-Elisa Roser[1], Fabian Maass[1] and Paul Lingor[1,2,3,4]**

[1] Department of Neurology, University Medical Center Göttingen, Göttingen, Germany, [2] Center for Biostructural Imaging of Neurodegeneration, Göttingen, Germany, [3] German Center for Neurodegenerative Diseases, Göttingen, Germany, [4] Rechts der Isar Hospital, Technical University of Munich, Munich, Germany

***Correspondence:**
Karina Joppe
Karina.Joppe@med.uni-goettingen.de
Paul Lingor
plingor@gwdg.de

The homeostasis of iron is of fundamental importance in the central nervous system (CNS) to ensure biological processes such as oxygen transport, mitochondrial respiration or myelin synthesis. Dyshomeostasis and accumulation of iron can be observed during aging and both are shared characteristics of several neurodegenerative diseases. Iron-mediated generation of reactive oxygen species (ROS) may lead to protein aggregation and cellular toxicity. The process of misfolding and aggregation of neuronal proteins such as α-synuclein, Tau, amyloid beta (Aβ), TDP-43 or SOD1 is a common hallmark of many neurodegenerative disorders and iron has been shown to facilitate protein aggregation. Thus, both, iron and aggregating proteins are proposed to amplify their detrimental effects in the disease state. In this review, we give an overview on effects of iron on aggregation of different proteins involved in neurodegeneration. Furthermore, we discuss the proposed mechanisms of iron-mediated toxicity and protein aggregation emphasizing the red-ox chemistry and protein-binding properties of iron. Finally, we address current therapeutic approaches harnessing iron chelation as a disease-modifying intervention in neurodegenerative disorders, such as Parkinson's disease, Alzheimer's disease, and amyotrophic lateral sclerosis.

Keywords: iron, protein aggregation, neurodegeneration, disease mechanism, iron chelator

INTRODUCTION

Neurodegenerative disorders (NDDs) rapidly gain importance due to their age-related prevalence and the resulting socio-economic burden (Hindle, 2010; Abbott, 2011). Aging is one of the main risk factors for NDDs (Ashraf et al., 2018) and the constantly growing life expectancy will result in their increased prevalence (Oeppen and Vaupel, 2002). Although different NDDs present a variety of symptoms ranging from cognitive, motor, sensory and/or autonomic failure, neuronal loss is the shared characteristic. Therefore, it is of great relevance to identify common pathophysiological features that are present in multiple NDDs to elucidate general mechanisms of neurodegeneration and potential pathways for intervention.

Iron does not only play a main role in cellular senescence but also in NDDs such as Parkinson's disease (PD), Alzheimer's disease (AD), amyotrophic lateral sclerosis (ALS) or prion diseases (PrD) (Ashraf et al., 2018). As protein aggregation is another shared hallmark among many NDDs

(Iadanza et al., 2018), it is suggestive to assume a mutual interplay of iron and protein aggregation amplifying their detrimental effects. In addition to iron, other transition metals such as copper and manganese are also considered in the pathogenesis of NDDs. This review, however, is focusing on the role of iron in protein aggregation disorders and the reader is referred to alternative publications on the role of other metals (e.g., Carboni and Lingor, 2015; Kim et al., 2018).

In this review, we discuss the mode of action of iron in NDDs and proposed mechanisms of iron-mediated protein aggregation. Finally, we outline recent therapeutic approaches targeting iron as promising treatment option for NDDs.

IRON DYSHOMEOSTASIS AND ACCUMULATION

Iron is the most abundant trace metal in the human brain, present in neuronal and glial cells. It acts as a catalytic center for multiple enzymes and supports the synthesis of DNA, neurotransmitters and myelin in the brain. Furthermore, it participates in oxygen transport, neurotransmitter metabolism and mitochondrial respiration (Ward R.J. et al., 2014; Ashraf et al., 2018).

Iron metabolism is tightly regulated by iron responsive elements (IREs). In the presence of iron, binding of the iron regulatory protein (IRP) to IREs controls the translation of mRNAs related to proteins of iron metabolism, e.g., iron import, export and storage proteins. Under physiological conditions, extracellular ferric iron (Fe^{3+}) is mainly bound to the glycoprotein transferrin (Tf), being delivered to cells by transferrin receptors (TfR). Non-transferrin-bound ferrous iron (Fe^{2+}) is mainly transported into the cell via the divalent metal-ion transporter 1 (DMT1) (Hider and Kong, 2013; Jiang et al., 2017). DMT1 is also an important player in mitochondrial uptake of Fe^{2+} (Wolff et al., 2018). Intracellularly, ferritin is the major iron storage protein complex. Before storage in both H- or L-ferritins, Fe^{2+} is oxidized by H-ferritin to Fe^{3+}. Under normal conditions, the labile Fe^{2+} pool and ferritin molecules are at an equilibrium. The export of Fe^{2+} is regulated by ferroportin-1 (FPN1) being controlled by hepcidin (Hider and Kong, 2013; Ashraf et al., 2018).

Impaired iron metabolism coupled with its accumulation in various brain regions are hallmarks of physiological aging. H-and L-ferritins also are more abundant with age (Zecca et al., 2001). During life, both ferritin subunits increase in their concentration within the SN but stay constant within the locus coeruleus. Both regions are important target areas for PD whereas the locus coeruleus is also affected in AD (Zecca et al., 2004a). Brains of patients suffering from NDDs, e.g., PD and AD, are lacking the age-associated rise of both ferritins. In PD, reduced ferritin levels in SN and pathological iron accumulation were found (Dexter et al., 1991; Connor et al., 1995).

Excessive ROS production resulting in oxidative stress is a common feature of NDDs and accumulated redox-active iron triggers ROS formation by the *Fenton* and *Haber-Weiss* reactions, providing the basis for catalyzed oxidation processes. Accordingly, iron reacts with hydrogen peroxide, which is a by-product of the mitochondrial respiration and intracellularly abundant, resulting in hydroxyl free radicals (HO•). Therefore, iron fosters the formation of ROS that lead to oxidative stress, inducing mitochondrial dysfunction and cell death (Zecca et al., 2004b).

This said, the reasons for iron accumulation and its precise effects on pathomechanisms in neurodegeneration remain still incompletely understood. Its contribution to the aggregation of disease-relevant proteins may be a major effector of its toxicity in NDDs.

PROTEIN AGGREGATION

A shared hallmark of numerous NDDs is protein aggregation. For example, α-synuclein aggregates are the main components of Lewy bodies in PD (Spillantini et al., 1998), whereas neurofibrillary tangles and plaques in AD are composed of Tau and Amyloid beta (Aβ), respectively (Glenner and Wong, 1984; Brion, 1998). Aggregation of TDP-43 or SOD1 are observed in ALS (Brown, 1998; Neumann et al., 2006). Recent data demonstrate, however, that aggregation of one particular protein is not specific for one disease (e.g., Cisbani et al., 2017; Trist et al., 2018). Under physiological conditions, the ubiquitin proteasome system (UPS), autophagosomes and chaperone activity ensure the clearance of protein aggregates (Stroo et al., 2017). However, genetic or environmental factors can disturb the balance of aggregate formation and clearance, so that native soluble proteins or peptides start misfolding and assemble into insoluble beta-sheet oligomers and protofibrils. This filamentous aggregation results in amyloid fibrils and protein inclusion formation. For different disease-dependent proteins this aggregation process is likely to follow similar pathways (Soto and Pritzkow, 2018).

Whereas for protein inclusions a possible neuroprotective role is still discussed, oligomers and protofibrils of the above-mentioned species are very likely neurotoxic. Amyloid structures are believed to impair axonal transport, DNA transcription and the UPS, and trigger mitochondrial dysfunction, synaptic dysfunction and oxidative stress (Dhouafli et al., 2018; Iadanza et al., 2018). Furthermore, oligomers increase the lipid bilayer conductance and, therefore, induce calcium dyshomeostasis (Verma et al., 2015). Altogether, these mechanisms contribute to cellular dysfunction and cytotoxicity.

IRON AND PROTEIN AGGREGATION

Via interaction with redox-active metal ions, amyloidogenic forms of, e.g., Aβ or α-synuclein triggered ROS production and oxidative cytotoxicity (Liu et al., 2011; Deas et al., 2016). Especially iron was shown to enhance aggregation processes of α-synuclein (Ostrerova-Golts et al., 2000), Aβ (Rottkamp et al., 2001) or Tau (Sayre et al., 2000). How iron enhances protein aggregation is not fully understood, but two distinct mechanisms are considered as relevant. First, the direct binding of iron to amyloidogenic proteins, and second, an indirect iron-mediated

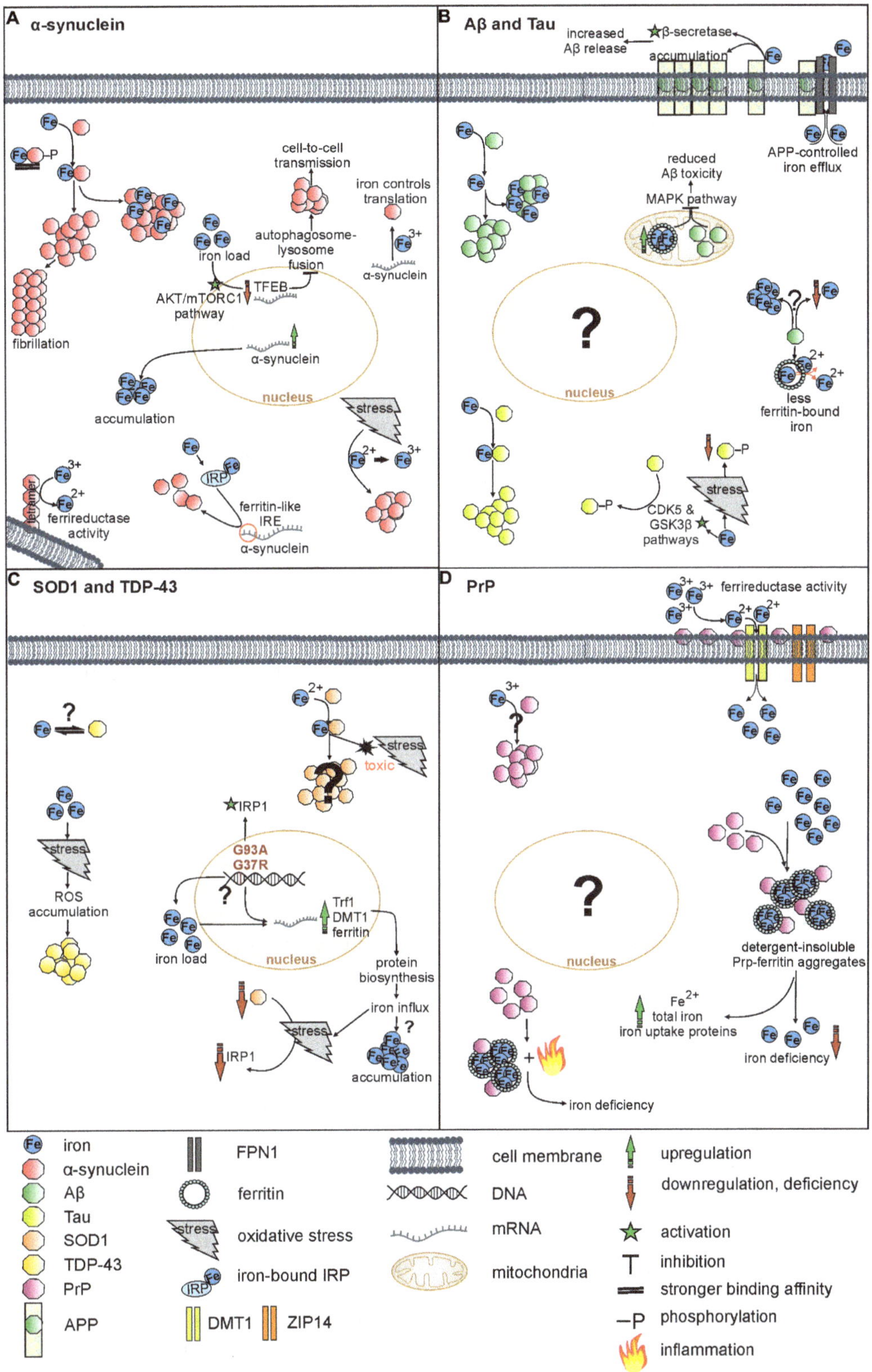

FIGURE 1 | Overview on relevant interactions of iron and NDDs-associated proteins. **(A)** Iron induces α-synuclein aggregation by direct binding or via oxidation. Indirectly, iron also influences α-synuclein on its transcriptional and translational level. α-synuclein acts as a ferrireductase and can induce iron accumulation by overexpression. **(B)** Iron fosters aggregation of both Aβ und Tau by binding. Whereas Aβ reduces levels of ferritin-bound iron, an overexpression of mitochondrial ferritin reduces Aβ toxicity. APP controls iron efflux and together with iron it affects the Aβ release. Furthermore, there is evidence for both, Aβ-induced iron

(Continued)

FIGURE 1 | Continued
accumulation and Aβ-induced iron depletion. Whereas iron increases Tau-phosphorylation via CDK5 and GSK3ß pathways, iron-induced oxidative stress reduces Tau-phosphorylation. **(C)** Iron binds SOD1, inducing oxidative stress and toxicity. Mutations of SOD1 lead to an upregulation of iron metabolism proteins followed by iron influx. Iron is suggested to affect TDP-43 aggregation indirectly via oxidative stress-mediated ROS accumulation. An interaction of iron and TDP-43 has not been objectified so far. **(D)** PrP operates as a ferrireductase partner of ZIP14 and DMT1 increasing Fe^{3+} uptake. Furthermore, PrP-ferritin aggregates induce iron deficiency and an upregulation of total iron, Fe^{2+} and iron uptake proteins. Inflammation processes may contribute to iron deficiency. Vice versa, Fe^{3+} triggers PrP accumulation within the cell.

process, where the above-mentioned *Fenton* and *Haber-Weiss* reaction of Fe^{2+} triggers aggregation by ROS production and resulting oxidative stress. An overview on relevant interactions of iron and below-mentioned proteins is shown in **Figure 1**.

α-Synuclein

α-Synuclein is a 140 amino acid protein expressed in neuronal cytosol and presynaptic terminals that is thought to participate in vesicle packaging, release and trafficking as well as in membrane remodeling. Furthermore, interactions of α-synuclein with histones as well as with nuclear DNA are suspected, but its concrete function in the nucleus and presynaptic terminals needs to be further investigated (Bendor et al., 2013; Rocha et al., 2018). α-Synuclein is intensively studied in regard to the pathophysiology of PD, since some inherited forms of PD can result from point mutations and from overproduction of α-synuclein through multiplications of the SNCA gene encoding the human α-synuclein protein. In total, six point mutations (A30P, E46K, H50Q, G51D, A53T, and A53E) of the SNCA gene were identified so far leading to a biophysical change of amino acid substitutions (Uchihara and Giasson, 2016). Therefore, models overexpressing α-synuclein or a mutated form are used to understand the role of α-synuclein and its interaction with iron (e.g., Zhu et al., 2016; Carboni et al., 2017).

Analyzing the interaction of iron and α-synuclein, different studies could show that α-synuclein fibrillation can be induced by iron (Uversky et al., 2001; Golts et al., 2002; Kostka et al., 2008). *In vitro*, using BE-M17 neuroblastoma cells iron had stronger effects on aggregation of A53T and A30P mutant compared to wild-type α-synuclein (Ostrerova-Golts et al., 2000). *In vivo*, iron treatment showed reduced survival of α-synuclein mutant (A53T, A30P) and α-synuclein wild-type flies compared to w1118 wild-type controls, but only the mutant flies showed a strong motor decline (Zhu et al., 2016). Transmission electron microscopy resolved that *ex vivo* Fe^{3+} addition to wild-type and mutant (A53T, A30P, E46K) α-synuclein generates fibrils, resembling fibril conformations formed without iron incubation, whereas copper addition to mutant α-synuclein led to the formation of amorphous aggregates. These results indicate that the fibril morphology is metal-specific (Bharathi et al., 2007).

Even micromolar concentrations of Fe^{3+} increased α-synuclein aggregation and produced larger SDS-resistant oligomers. Since H_2O_2 treatment did not lead to the same effects as iron treatment, oxidation of α-synuclein *per se* cannot be the reason for the oligomerization, showing that trivalent ions play a relevant role (Kostka et al., 2008). However, further *in vitro* studies showed that Fe^{2+} also promoted α-synuclein aggregation, transmission and affected viability of SK-N-SH and SN4741 cells (Li et al., 2011; Xiao et al., 2018). Specifically, in SK-N-SH cells α-synuclein aggregation was increased around the nucleus (Li et al., 2011). Under aerobic conditions *in vitro*, Fe^{2+} treatment caused a polymerization into antiparallel soluble α-synuclein oligomers, whereas under anaerobic conditions both Fe^{2+} and Fe^{3+} induced parallel ß-sheet aggregates (Abeyawardhane et al., 2018).

How iron influences α-synuclein aggregation is not completely understood. However, α-synuclein has a high metal binding affinity and it is known that both Fe^{2+} and Fe^{3+} can bind α-synuclein, revealing a binding constant of $1.2 \times 10^{13}\ M^{-1}$ for Fe^{3+} and $5.8 \times 10^{3}\ M^{-1}$ for Fe^{2+} (Peng et al., 2010). Fe^{2+} binds at the C-terminus, specifically at Asp-121, Asn-122, and Glu-123 (Binolfi et al., 2006) and the binding affinity is increased in phosphorylated (pY125 or pS129) α-synuclein (Lu et al., 2011). Additionally, Fe^{3+} can bind α-synuclein, having two binding sites, which are likely at the C-terminus (Davies et al., 2011).

Interestingly, there is a close homology in the 5′-UTR of human α-synuclein mRNA to the IRE of the ferritin mRNA, which could explain the regulation of α-synuclein levels by intracellular iron (Friedlich et al., 2007). Fe^{3+} was suggested to control the translation of α-synuclein mRNA since the iron chelator deferoxamine (DFO) highly decreased the polysome-associated endogenous α-synuclein mRNA in HEK293 cells (Febbraro et al., 2012). Furthermore, a knockdown of the IRP in SK-N-SH cells enhanced α-synuclein aggregation by upregulation of α-synuclein transcription, indicating that iron partially controls the aggregation process through the IRE/IRP system (Li et al., 2011). In addition to its direct binding there is thus evidence that iron also influences α-synuclein on a transcriptional and translational level.

Iron also promotes α-synuclein aggregation indirectly by regulating the nuclear transcription factor EB (TFEB), which is a transcriptional regulator of the autophagosome-lysosome pathway. Iron enrichment decreased the TFEB expression and inhibited its nuclear translocation through the activation of the Akt/mTORC1 pathway resulting in increased α-synuclein aggregation in cell lysates by the inhibition of TFEB-mediated autophagosome-lysosome fusion. Furthermore, iron increased α-synuclein cell-to-cell transmission, which was attenuated by TFEB overexpression (Xiao et al., 2018). As an indirect pathway, oxidative stress contributes to the iron-induced aggregation. This was further supported by the finding that supplementation of the antioxidative vitamin E attenuated aggregation in SK-N-SH cells (Li et al., 2011). Additionally, an *ex vivo* study indicated that oxidative stress enhances α-synuclein aggregation indirectly via oxidation of iron from Fe^{2+} to Fe^{3+} (Levin et al., 2011).

Vice versa, iron levels were increased by the overexpression of α-synuclein itself in primary midbrain neurons and PC12 cells which were analyzed with particle induced X-ray emission. Iron accumulation quantified by X-ray fluorescence was specifically observed within the perinuclear regions of PC12 cells (Ortega et al., 2016).

Furthermore, α-synuclein was also found to act as a ferrireductase, reducing Fe^{3+} to Fe^{2+} (Davies et al., 2011). The ferrireductase active form of α-synuclein is suggested to be a membrane-associated helical-rich tetramer (McDowall et al., 2017; Angelova and Brown, 2018). Previous studies suggest a resistance of the tetramer to fibril and aggregate formation, making the tetramer to an interesting subspecies *in vivo* (Bartels et al., 2011; Wang W. et al., 2011; Dettmer et al., 2015).

Regarding treatment strategies to reduce or prevent α-synuclein aggregation, iron seems to be a promising target. Iron recycling by Nramp1 (Soe-Lin et al., 2009) was shown to degrade microglial α-synuclein oligomers *in vitro* and *in vivo*, highlighting natural defense mechanisms in iron overload conditions (Wu et al., 2017). Furthermore, different iron chelators showed various beneficial effects in preclinical cell or animal PD models (e.g., Sangchot et al., 2002; Mandel et al., 2004; Billings et al., 2016; Finkelstein et al., 2016, 2017; Carboni et al., 2017; Das et al., 2017).

Iron and α-synuclein thus influence each other mutually: whereas iron contributes to α-synuclein aggregation by direct binding and indirectly via oxidative stress and transcription factors, α-synuclein shows ferrireductase activity influencing iron homeostasis.

Aβ and Tau

Aβ is a metalloprotein consisting of 39–43 residues that is derived from the transmembrane amyloid precursor protein (APP) by proteolytic cleavage. Aβ aggregates are found as amyloid plaques in AD and Aβ plays a role in metal sequestration and homeostasis, synaptic activity and neuronal plasticity (Smith et al., 2007; Rajasekhar et al., 2015). Aβ was found to be strongly colocalized with brain iron in risk patients for AD measured by magnetic resonance imaging and positron emission tomography (Van Bergen et al., 2016). X-ray studies analyzing Aβ plaques in cortex tissue of transgenic mice and Aβ plaque cores of AD patients confirmed a direct correlation of iron and Aβ localization, suggesting the formation of an iron-Aβ complex (Telling et al., 2017; Everett et al., 2018). *Ex vivo*, Fe^{3+} was found to promote aggregation of Aβ1-40 and Aβ1-42 visualized by fluorescence spectroscopy and atomic force microscopy (Tahmasebinia and Emadi, 2017). Fe^{3+} was also shown to bind Aβ using the phenolic oxygen of tyrosine 10 as binding site (Miura et al., 2001). Fe^{3+}-mediated generation of Aβ aggregates was also reported *in vitro*. However, these aggregates were shorter and less ordered than in iron-free Aβ incubation (Liu et al., 2011). In drosophila, the affinity of Aβ for iron is mediated by three N-terminal histidines enhancing Aβ dimerization and leading to histidine-dependent oxidative damage (Ott et al., 2015).

Furthermore, treatment with iron chelators (clioquinol, YM-F24) increased survival and locomotor function of flies expressing Aβ1-42 compared to control wild-type flies, highlighting the relevance of oxidative stress for neurotoxicity of Aβ (Rival et al., 2009; Liu et al., 2011). Iron chelation also showed beneficial effects in mammalian models (Fine et al., 2015; Zhao et al., 2017) and reduced Aβ1-42 aggregation in an *ex vivo* study (Tahmasebinia and Emadi, 2017). Other studies showed that the presence of the important iron storage protein ferritin has beneficial effects on Aβ pathology. Accordingly, *in vitro* and *in vivo*, mitochondrial ferritin reduced neurotoxic effects exerted by Aβ (Wu et al., 2013; Wang P. et al., 2017). The overexpression of mitochondrial ferritin in SHSY5Y cells prevented the activation of the MAPK signaling pathway, which is related to oxidative stress-induced cell death (Wu et al., 2013).

Iron also strongly influences APP. Treating SHSY5Y cells with Fe^{3+} caused APP accumulation in membrane-enriched cellular fraction and increased activity of β-secretase that both triggered increased release of Aβ1-42 (Banerjee et al., 2014). Another study using SHSY5Y cells confirmed increased APP steady state levels and APP production after iron treatment (Rogers et al., 2016).

Furthermore, APP influences iron export by controlling the persistence of FPN1 on the neuronal surface, even if it does not function as a ferroxidase (Wong et al., 2014). There is evidence that Aβ induces iron accumulation in a cell-free *ex vivo* study (Everett et al., 2014b). Other studies suggest that Aβ controls the redox-activity of iron and reduces iron chemically *in vivo* (Everett et al., 2018). Accordingly, Aβ was able to inhibit ascorbate-dependent hydroxyl radical generation by free Fe^{3+} (Nakamura et al., 2007). Furthermore, interaction with Aβ led to a reduction of ferrihydrite (ferritin-bound iron) to pure redox-active Fe^{2+} (Everett et al., 2014a).

Iron was not only shown to modulate the aggregation of Aβ but also of Tau (Kim et al., 2018). Tau is a microtubule-associated protein that is the main component of neurofibrillary tangles in AD. Mostly, it is located in axons and sometimes in dendrites (Nisbet et al., 2015). So far, little is known about the interplay of iron and Tau and present studies are not consistent. Iron treatment enhanced Tau aggregation in iron-enriched hippocampal regions and iron was shown to bind Tau (Sayre et al., 2000). Some studies showed that only trivalent metal ions, as Fe^{3+}, trigger Tau aggregation but not divalent ions (Yamamoto et al., 2002; Bader et al., 2011). Fe^{3+}-generated Tau oligomers were even more stable than DMSO-generated ones (Nübling et al., 2012). However, a recent electrochemical study showed that both, Fe^{3+} and Fe^{2+}, bind Tau at different binding sites, inducing a structural change, which was more pronounced with Fe^{2+} (Ahmadi et al., 2017).

Iron-induced oxidative stress reduced Tau phosphorylation by interfering with the function of the CDK5/p25 system of hippocampal neurons (Egaña et al., 2003). Another study using primary cultures of rat cortical neurons showed iron-induced Tau phosphorylation by activation of GSK3 (Lovell et al., 2004). Ebselen, an organo-selenium compound with antioxidant activity, inhibits the CDK5 and GSK3β pathway leading to less Tau phosphorylation. These effects were not only caused by the antioxidant effects of Ebselen, but rather by the inhibition of DMT1 in SHSY5Y cells (Xie et al., 2012). The same effects on CDK5 and GSK3β as well as on Tau phosphorylation were shown with the iron chelator DFO analyzing APP/PS1 transgenic mouse brains (Guo et al., 2013).

In summary, iron binds both, Aβ and Tau, partially modifying their structure and fostering their aggregation process. Furthermore, the Aβ and Tau phenotypes can be partially rescued by iron chelation.

SOD1 and TDP-43

SOD1 is an abundant antioxidant protein predominantly located within the cytosol. Its aggregation leads to, e.g., neuronal degeneration and changes in DNA/RNA metabolism, neurofilament and axonal transport (Pasinelli and Brown, 2006). An NMR study showed binding of iron to SOD1 with binding sites closely located to Cu/Zn binding pockets leading to Fe^{2+}-bound SOD1 complexes, which are likely toxic (Lim and Song, 2015). Even if there is no direct evidence for iron-induced SOD1 aggregation, several studies emphasize a coherence of iron load and SOD1 pathology.

Therapeutic approaches showed that in SOD1 mouse models (G93A, G37R, G86R) iron chelators [VK-28, M30, HLA20, VAR-ced, deferiprone (DFP)] extended lifespan, increased locomotor function and motoneuron survival and decreased oxygen free radicals, iron levels and TfR expression (Jeong et al., 2009; Kupershmidt et al., 2009; Wang Q. et al., 2011; Golko-Perez et al., 2016; Moreau et al., 2018).

Furthermore, several studies observed an impact of SOD1 on iron metabolism. Accordingly, *in vivo* studies with SOD1.G93A mutant mice showed increased mRNA expression of ferritin, TfR1 and DMT1. These results indicate enhanced iron load, since iron is known to regulate ferritin expression (Jeong et al., 2009; Wang Q. et al., 2011). *In vitro* studies analyzing cell lysates showed an increased iron content and altered iron metabolism mediated by an impaired Akt signaling pathway. Accordingly, SOD1.G93A overexpression triggered an inactivation of Akt, activation of the transcription factor FOXO3a and subsequently increased ferritin synthesis and iron accumulation (Hadzhieva et al., 2013; Halon-Golabek et al., 2018). SOD1.G37R mutants showed *in vivo* and *in vitro* increased mRNA levels of TfR1, ferritin, DMT1 but also of mitochondrial ferritin (Jeong et al., 2009). The above-mentioned results of an increased iron content and increased TfR levels suggest an iron dyshomeostasis, which is not primarily controlled by IRE/IRP1 mechanisms (Lovejoy and Guillemin, 2014). Other studies showed diverse effects of SOD1 on the cytosolic iron sensor IRP1. SOD1 activation in G93A mutant mice showed no changes of IRP1 expression but more activated IRP1 (Jeong et al., 2009; Gajowiak et al., 2016). *In vivo*, SOD1 deficiency and the resulting oxidative stress caused IRP1 downregulation (Milczarek et al., 2017). Furthermore, in SOD1.G93A mutant mice ROS induction led to an upregulated iron import, triggering oxidative stress (Hadzhieva et al., 2013).

SOD1 is also thought to interact with the ALS-relevant protein TDP-43 (Higashi et al., 2010). Aggregates of the RNA-binding protein TDP-43 are incorporated in ubiquitinated inclusions within the neuronal cytoplasm found in ALS and in syndromes jointly named 'neurodegeneration with brain iron accumulation' (NBIA) (Neumann et al., 2006; Haraguchi et al., 2011). SOD1 was shown to initiate modification and accumulation of TDP-43 (Zeineddine et al., 2017; Jeon et al., 2018). In SOD1 mutant mice, iron chelators reduced TDP-43 aggregation, whereas vehicle-treated animals showed TDP-43 aggregates located in the cytoplasm of motor neurons (Wang Q. et al., 2011). Since oxidative stress-mediated accumulation of ROS fosters the TDP-43 aggregation *in vitro* (Cohen et al., 2012), iron chelator effects on TDP-43 aggregation suggest an indirect effect of iron by oxidative stress induction.

In conclusion, proteins of the iron metabolism are altered in SOD1 mutants, which partially could explain enhanced iron loading. Iron chelator effects in SOD1 models indicate an impact of iron on SOD1 pathology. Even if iron accumulation is a common feature of ALS (e.g., Moreau et al., 2018), a contribution of iron to aggregation of SOD1 or TDP-43 is yet unproven.

Prion Protein

The prion protein (PrP) is located intracellularly and is also an important membrane-bound protein at the cell surface. Therefore, PrP is involved in exocytotic and endocytic synaptic vesicle processing as well as in signaling pathways, but also in myelination and neurogenesis (Liebert et al., 2014; Legname, 2017; Watts et al., 2018).

By using PrP knockout or PrP-overexpressing mouse models, studies showed that upregulation or downregulation of PrP levels, respectively, affect the iron homeostasis (Singh et al., 2009a,b; Pushie et al., 2011; Ashok et al., 2018). Accordingly, iron deficiency is a crucial characteristic in brains of humans, hamster and mice affected with prion pathology. Analyzing pathological brain tissue as well as scrapie-infected ScN2a and SMB cells, iron dyshomeostasis was supposedly caused by the iron sequestration in detergent-insoluble PrP-scrapie-ferritin aggregates, resulting in a decreased bio-available iron pool and a state of cellular iron deficiency. These results also explain increased amounts of total iron and Fe^{2+} as well as iron uptake proteins (Singh et al., 2009a). Another study investigated PrP-mediated iron deficiency in retinas of scrapie-injected hamsters and demonstrated an accumulation of detergent-insoluble ferritin. Furthermore, they showed a correlation of the ferritin accumulation with microglia activity. These results suggested a contribution of chronic inflammation as a side effect of PrP accumulation to functional iron deficiency (Asthana et al., 2017).

Another explanation for the influence of PrP on the iron homeostasis is that PrP operates as a plasma membrane ferrireductase. Accordingly, PrP-expressing neuroblastoma cells showed a significant increase in ferrireductase activity compared to non-transfected cells. Furthermore, mutant PrP forms showed that for an optimal ferrireductase function of PrP the presence of NADH, the copper binding octa-peptide repeat region and the linkage to the plasma membrane is needed (Singh et al., 2013). Also in HepG2-cells, expressing PrP, ferrireductase activity was indicated by an increased uptake of Fe^{3+} but not of Fe^{2+}. Since Fe^{3+} uptake was significantly increased after a co-expression of PrP with metal transporter ZIP14 and DMT1, PrP is suggested to be the ferrireductase partner of both metal transporter (Tripathi et al., 2015).

So far, there is not much evidence for the influence of iron on the PrP pathology. One study using PrP-deficient HpL3-4 cells showed that Fe^{3+} but not Fe^{2+} induced accumulation of internalized PrP after iron exposure and PrP treatment of cells (Choi et al., 2013). However, it is not clarified if a direct binding to the PrP protein or indirect mechanisms triggered by iron foster the aggregation of PrP.

Vice versa, PrP was shown to influence the iron homeostasis via its ferrireductase activity and PrP-ferritin aggregates but it needs further investigation to explain if these two modes of action or indirect mechanisms such as the activation of inflammation processes lead to iron deficiency.

CLINICAL APPLICATION

Iron accumulation in NDDs argues for a clinical evaluation of iron chelators as symptomatic or neuroprotective agents. Iron chelation by DFO, DFP or deferasirox (DFX) is clinically approved by the FDA for systemic conditions like acute iron intoxication and chronic iron overload[1]. DFO application is problematic due to the required continuous injection (short plasma half-life period) and dose-dependent neurotoxicity. DFX and DFP can be administered orally. DFX must be especially monitored for renal failure and DFP for agranulocytosis and neutropenia (Mobarra et al., 2016). With its ability to relocate iron and to cross the blood brain barrier, DFP presents the most promising candidate for targeting iron load in the CNS, being tested in NDDs with regional iron overload, e.g., Friedreich ataxia (e.g., Velasco-Sánchez et al., 2011; Pandolfo et al., 2014) and NBIA (e.g., Lim et al., 2018; Rohani et al., 2018).

In PD patients (*FAIR-PARK-I*, NCT00943748), DFP treatment showed benefits in motor performance and reduced MR-quantified substantia nigra iron content (Devos et al., 2014). In another trial (*DeferipronPD*, NCT01539837), administration of a lower dosage resulted in a reduced T2* MRI iron content in the dentate and caudate nucleus (Martin-Bastida et al., 2017). Based on these results, a European multicenter, parallel-group, placebo-controlled, randomized phase III trial is ongoing to assess disease-modifying effects of DFP in PD patients (*FAIRPARKII*, NCT02655315).

In a pilot trial (*SAFEFAIRALS*, NCT02164253), DFP treatment of ALS patients reduced R2* iron content in the cervical spinal cord, medulla oblongata and motor cortex. Additionally, patients showed a smaller decrease in the ALS function rating scale and in the body mass index in the first 3 months of treatment compared to the first treatment-free period (Moreau et al., 2018). Based on these results, a phase II/phase III study with a larger sample size has been initiated testing DFP (*FAIR-ALSII*, NCT03293069).

In AD, intramuscular application of DFO significantly reduced the decline of daily living skills (Crapper McLachlan et al., 1991). Besides, cognition of AD patients benefited from treatment with the metal-attenuating compound clioquinol or its derivate (Ritchie et al., 2003; Lannfelt et al., 2008). Now, AD patients are recruited for an ongoing phase II study investigating effects of DFP (*The 3D Study*, NCT03234686).

Details of the mentioned studies can be found in **Supplementary Table 1**. Summing up, iron chelators already showed promising results in smaller trials and this advocates for further assessment in larger studies.

[1] www.fda.gov

CONCLUSION

Current investigations focus on iron accumulation and protein aggregation as two pathological hallmarks of multiple NDDs. The interaction of both features appears to be an essential part of common neurodegeneration mechanisms. So far, iron was found to bind amyloidogenic proteins like α-synuclein, Aβ and Tau fostering their aggregation. Indirectly, iron influences disease-related proteins via oxidative stress or manipulation of their transcription and translation. On the other hand, α-synuclein, Aβ and SOD1 were found to affect iron metabolism and iron accumulation, proposing a mutual interplay and an amplification of their detrimental effects in the disease state. Even if precise effects of iron on neurodegenerative pathomechanisms remain incompletely understood, translational trials in human patients already showed beneficial effects of iron chelation as a treatment strategy for NDDs. Thus, iron may be a substantial contributor to neurodegeneration and merits further investigation as molecular and therapeutic target.

AUTHOR CONTRIBUTIONS

KJ developed the idea under the lead of PL, performed literature research, wrote and finalized the manuscript, and prepared the figure. A-ER and FM were involved in literature research and writing of the manuscript. PL developed the idea for this review and revised the manuscript. All authors have seen and approved the final version.

FUNDING

We acknowledge support by the German Research Foundation and the Open Access Publication Funds of the Göttingen University.

ACKNOWLEDGMENTS

The support of the SFB 1286 "Quantitative Synaptology" was greatly acknowledged.

REFERENCES

Abbott, A. (2011). Dementia: a problem for our age. *Nature* 475, S2–S4. doi: 10.1038/475S2a

Abeyawardhane, D. L., Fernández, R. D., Murgas, C. J., Heitger, D. R., Forney, A. K., Crozier, M. K., et al. (2018). Iron redox chemistry promotes antiparallel oligomerization of α-synuclein. *J. Am. Chem. Soc.* 140, 5028–5032. doi: 10.1021/jacs.8b02013

Ahmadi, S., Ebralidze, I. I., She, Z., and Kraatz, H.-B. (2017). Electrochemical studies of tau protein-iron interactions—Potential implications for Alzheimer's disease. *Electrochim. Acta* 236, 384–393. doi: 10.1016/J.ELECTACTA.2017.03.175

Angelova, D. M., and Brown, D. R. (2018). Model senescent microglia induce disease related changes in α-synuclein expression and activity. *Biomolecules* 8:67. doi: 10.3390/biom8030067

Ashok, A., Karmakar, S., Chandel, R., Ravikumar, R., Dalal, S., Kong, Q., et al. (2018). Prion protein modulates iron transport in the anterior segment: implications for ocular iron homeostasis and prion transmission. *Exp. Eye Res.* 175, 1–13. doi: 10.1016/j.exer.2018.05.031

Ashraf, A., Clark, M., and So, P.-W. (2018). The aging of iron man. *Front. Aging Neurosci.* 10:65. doi: 10.3389/fnagi.2018.00065

Asthana, A., Baksi, S., Ashok, A., Karmakar, S., Mammadova, N., Kokemuller, R., et al. (2017). Prion protein facilitates retinal iron uptake and is cleaved at the β-site: implications for retinal iron homeostasis in prion disorders. *Sci. Rep.* 7, 1–14. doi: 10.1038/s41598-017-08821-1

Bader, B., Nübling, G., Mehle, A., Nobile, S., Kretzschmar, H., and Giese, A. (2011). Single particle analysis of tau oligomer formation induced by metal ions and organic solvents. *Biochem. Biophys. Res. Commun.* 411, 190–196. doi: 10.1016/j.bbrc.2011.06.135

Banerjee, P., Sahoo, A., Anand, S., Ganguly, A., Righi, G., Bovicelli, P., et al. (2014). Multiple mechanisms of iron-induced amyloid beta-peptide accumulation in SHSY5Y cells: protective action of negletein. *Neuro Mol. Med.* 16, 787–798. doi: 10.1007/s12017-014-8328-4

Bartels, T., Choi, J. G., and Selkoe, D. J. (2011). α-Synuclein occurs physiologically as a helically folded tetramer that resists aggregation. *Nature* 477, 107–111. doi: 10.1038/nature10324

Bendor, J. T., Logan, T. P., and Edwards, R. H. (2013). The function of α-synuclein. *Neuron* 79, 1044–1066. doi: 10.1016/j.neuron.2013.09.004

Bharathi, Indi, S. S., and Rao, K. S. J. (2007). Copper- and iron-induced differential fibril formation in α-synuclein: TEM study. *Neurosci. Lett.* 424, 78–82. doi: 10.1016/j.neulet.2007.06.052

Billings, J. L., Hare, D. J., Nurjono, M., Volitakis, I., Cherny, R. A., Bush, A. I., et al. (2016). Effects of neonatal iron feeding and chronic clioquinol administration on the parkinsonian human A53T transgenic mouse. *ACS Chem. Neurosci.* 7, 360–366. doi: 10.1021/acschemneuro.5b00305

Binolfi, A., Rasia, R. M., Bertoncini, C. W., Ceolin, M., Zweckstetter, M., Griesinger, C., et al. (2006). Interaction of α-synuclein with divalent metal ions reveals key differences: a link between structure, binding specificity and fibrillation enhancement. *J. Am. Chem. Soc.* 128, 9893–9901. doi: 10.1021/ja0618649

Brion, J.-P. (1998). Neurofibrillary tangles and alzheimer's disease. *Eur. Neurol.* 40, 130–140. doi: 10.1159/000007969

Brown, R. H. (1998). SOD1 aggregates in ALS: cause, correlate or consequence? *Nat. Med.* 4, 1362–1364. doi: 10.1038/3945

Carboni, E., and Lingor, P. (2015). Insights on the interaction of alpha-synuclein and metals in the pathophysiology of Parkinson's disease. *Metallomics* 7, 395–404. doi: 10.1039/C4MT00339J

Carboni, E., Tatenhorst, L., Tönges, L., Barski, E., Dambeck, V., Bähr, M., et al. (2017). Deferiprone rescues behavioral deficits induced by mild iron exposure in a mouse model of alpha-synuclein aggregation. *Neuro Mol. Med.* 19, 309–321. doi: 10.1007/s12017-017-8447-9

Choi, B. R., Lee, J., Kim, S. Y., Yim, I., Kim, E. H., and Woo, H. J. (2013). Prion protein conversion induced by trivalent iron in vesicular trafficking. *Biochem. Biophys. Res. Commun.* 432, 539–544. doi: 10.1016/j.bbrc.2013.02.021

Cisbani, G., Maxan, A., Kordower, J. H., Planel, E., Freeman, T. B., and Cicchetti, F. (2017). Presence of tau pathology within foetal neural allografts in patients with Huntington's and Parkinson's disease. *Brain* 140, 2982–2992. doi: 10.1093/brain/awx255

Cohen, T. J., Hwang, A. W., Unger, T., Trojanowski, J. Q., and Lee, V. M. (2012). Redox signalling directly regulates TDP-43 via cysteine oxidation and disulphide cross-linking. *EMBO J.* 31, 1241–1252. doi: 10.1038/emboj.2011.471

Connor, J. R., Snyder, B. S., Arosio, P., Loeffler, D. A., and Lewitt, P. (1995). A quantitative analysis of isoferritins in select regions of aged, parkinsonian, and Alzheimer's diseased brains. *J. Neurochem.* 65, 717–724. doi: 10.1046/j.1471-4159.1995.65020717.x

Crapper, McLachlan, D. R., Dalton, A. J., Kruck, T. P., Bell, M. Y., Smith, W. L., et al. (1991). Intramuscular desferrioxamine in patients with Alzheimer's disease. *Lancet (London, England)* 337, 1304–1308. doi: 10.1016/0140-6736(91)92978-B

Das, B., Rajagopalan, S., Joshi, G. S., Xu, L., Luo, D., Andersen, J. K., et al. (2017). A novel iron (II) preferring dopamine agonist chelator D-607 significantly suppresses α-syn- and MPTP-induced toxicities in vivo. *Neuropharmacology* 123, 88–99. doi: 10.1016/J.NEUROPHARM.2017.05.019

Davies, P., Moualla, D., and Brown, D. R. (2011). Alpha-synuclein is a cellular ferrireductase. *PLoS One* 6:e015814. doi: 10.1371/journal.pone.0015814

Deas, E., Cremades, N., Angelova, P. R., Ludtmann, M. H. R., Yao, Z., Chen, S., et al. (2016). Alpha-synuclein oligomers interact with metal ions to induce oxidative stress and neuronal death in Parkinson's disease. *Antioxid. Redox Signal.* 24, 376–391. doi: 10.1089/ars.2015.6343

Dettmer, U., Newman, A. J., von Saucken, V. E., Bartels, T., and Selkoe, D. (2015). KTKEGV repeat motifs are key mediators of normal α-synuclein tetramerization: their mutation causes excess monomers and neurotoxicity. *Proc. Natl. Acad. Sci. U.S.A.* 112, 9596–9601. doi: 10.1073/pnas.1505953112

Devos, D., Moreau, C., Devedjian, J. C., Kluza, J., Petrault, M., Laloux, C., et al. (2014). Targeting chelatable iron as a therapeutic modality in Parkinson's disease. *Antioxid. Redox Signal.* 21, 195–210. doi: 10.1089/ars.2013.5593

Dexter, D. T., Carayon, A., Javoy-Agid, F., Agid, Y., Wells, F. R., Daniel, S. E., et al. (1991). Alterations in the levels of iron, ferritin and other trace metals in Parkinson's disease and other neurodegenerative. *Brain* 114, 1953–1975. doi: 10.1093/brain/114.4.1953

Dhouafli, Z., Cuanalo-Contreras, K., Hayouni, E. A., Mays, C. E., Soto, C., and Moreno-Gonzalez, I. (2018). Inhibition of protein misfolding and aggregation by natural phenolic compounds. *Cell. Mol Life Sci.* 75, 3521–3538. doi: 10.1007/s00018-018-2872-2

Egaña, J. T., Zambrano, C., Nuñez, M. T., Gonzalez-Billault, C., and Maccioni, R. B. (2003). Iron-induced oxidative stress modify tau phosphorylation patterns in hippocampal cell cultures. *BioMetals* 16, 215–223. doi: 10.1023/A:1020727218493

Everett, J., Céspedes, E., Shelford, L. R., Exley, C., Collingwood, J. F., Dobson, J., et al. (2014a). Evidence of redox-active iron formation following aggregation of ferrihydrite and the Alzheimer's disease peptide β-amyloid. *Inorg. Chem.* 53, 2803–2809. doi: 10.1021/ic402406g

Everett, J., Céspedes, E., Shelford, L. R., Exley, C., Collingwood, J. F., Dobson, J., et al. (2014b). Ferrous iron formation following the co-aggregation of ferric iron and the Alzheimer's disease peptide-amyloid (1-42). *J. R. Soc. Interface* 11:20140165. doi: 10.1098/rsif.2014.0165

Everett, J., Collingwood, J. F., Tjendana-Tjhin, V., Brooks, J., Lermyte, F., Plascencia-Villa, G., et al. (2018). Nanoscale synchrotron X-ray speciation of iron and calcium compounds in amyloid plaque cores from Alzheimer's disease subjects. *Nanoscale* 10, 11782–11796. doi: 10.1039/C7NR06794A

Febbraro, F., Giorgi, M., Caldarola, S., Loreni, F., and Romero-ramos, M. (2012). α-Synuclein expression is modulated at the translational level by iron. *Neuroreport* 23, 576–580. doi: 10.1097/WNR.0b013e328354a1f0

Fine, J. M., Renner, D. B., Forsberg, A. C., Cameron, R. A., Galick, B. T., Le, C., et al. (2015). Intranasal deferoxamine engages multiple pathways to decrease memory loss in the APP/PS1 model of amyloid accumulation. *Neurosci. Lett.* 584, 362–367. doi: 10.1016/j.neulet.2014.11.013

Finkelstein, D. I., Billings, J. L., Adlard, P. A., Ayton, S., Sedjahtera, A., Masters, C. L., et al. (2017). The novel compound PBT434 prevents iron mediated neurodegeneration and alpha-synuclein toxicity in multiple models of Parkinson's disease. *Acta Neuropathol. Commun.* 5:53. doi: 10.1186/s40478-017-0456-2

Finkelstein, D. I., Hare, D. J., Billings, J. L., Sedjahtera, A., Nurjono, M., Arthofer, E., et al. (2016). Clioquinol improves cognitive, motor function, and microanatomy of the alpha-synuclein hA53T transgenic mice. *ACS Chem. Neurosci.* 7, 119–129. doi: 10.1021/acschemneuro.5b00253

Friedlich, A. L., Tanzi, R. E., and Rogers, J. T. (2007). The 5′-untranslated region of Parkinson's disease α-synuclein messenger RNA contains a predicted iron responsive element. *Mol. Psychiatry* 12, 222–223. doi: 10.1038/sj.mp.4001937

Gajowiak, A., Styś, A., Starzyński, R. R., Bednarz, A., Lenartowicz, M., Staroń, R., et al. (2016). Mice overexpressing both non-mutated human SOD1 and mutated SOD1G93A genes: a competent experimental model for studying iron metabolism in amyotrophic lateral sclerosis. *Front. Mol. Neurosci.* 8:82. doi: 10.3389/fnmol.2015.00082

Glenner, G. G., and Wong, C. W. (1984). Alzheimer's disease: initial report of the purification and characterization of a novel cerebrovascular amyloid protein. *Biochem. Biophys. Res. Commun.* 120, 885–890. doi: 10.1016/S0006-291X(84)80190-4

Golko-Perez, S., Amit, T., Youdim, M. B., and Weinreb, O. (2016). Beneficial effects of multitarget iron chelator on central nervous system and gastrocnemius muscle in SOD1(G93A) transgenic ALS mice. *J. Mol. Neurosci.* 59, 504–510. doi: 10.1007/s12031-016-0763-2

Golts, N., Snyder, H., Frasier, M., Theisler, C., Choi, P., and Wolozin, B. (2002). Magnesium inhibits spontaneous and iron-induced aggregation of α-synuclein. *J. Biol. Chem.* 277, 16116–16123. doi: 10.1074/jbc.M107866200

Guo, C., Wang, P., Zhong, M. L., Wang, T., Huang, X. S., Li, J. Y., et al. (2013). Deferoxamine inhibits iron induced hippocampal tau phosphorylation in the Alzheimer transgenic mouse brain. *Neurochem. Int.* 62, 165–172. doi: 10.1016/j.neuint.2012.12.005

Hadzhieva, M., Kirches, E., Wilisch-Neumann, A., Pachow, D., Wallesch, M., Schoenfeld, P., et al. (2013). Dysregulation of iron protein expression in the G93A model of amyotrophic lateral sclerosis. *Neuroscience* 230, 94–101. doi: 10.1016/j.neuroscience.2012.11.021

Halon-Golabek, M., Borkowska, A., Kaczor, J. J., Ziolkowski, W., Flis, D. J., Knap, N., et al. (2018). hmSOD1 gene mutation-induced disturbance in iron metabolism is mediated by impairment of Akt signalling pathway. *J. Cachexia Sarcopenia Muscle* 9, 557–569. doi: 10.1002/jcsm.12283

Haraguchi, T., Terada, S., Ishizu, H., Yokota, O., Yoshida, H., Takeda, N., et al. (2011). Coexistence of TDP-43 and tau pathology in neurodegeneration with brain iron accumulation type 1 (NBIA-1, formerly Hallervorden-Spatz syndrome). *Neuropathology* 31, 531–539. doi: 10.1111/j.1440-1789.2010.01186.x

Hider, R. C., and Kong, X. (2013). "Iron: effect of overload and deficiency," in *Interrelations between Essential Metal Ions and Human Diseases*, eds A. Sigel, H. Sigel, and R. K. O. Sigel (Dordrecht: Springer Netherlands), 1–535.

Higashi, S., Tsuchiya, Y., Araki, T., Wada, K., and Kabuta, T. (2010). TDP-43 physically interacts with amyotrophic lateral sclerosis-linked mutant CuZn superoxide dismutase. *Neurochem. Int.* 57, 906–913. doi: 10.1016/J.NEUINT.2010.09.010

Hindle, J. V. (2010). Ageing, neurodegeneration and Parkinson's disease. *Age Ageing* 39, 156–161. doi: 10.1093/ageing/afp223

Iadanza, M. G., Jackson, M. P., Hewitt, E. W., Ranson, N. A., and Radford, S. E. (2018). A new era for understanding amyloid structures and disease. *Nat. Rev. Mol. Cell Biol.* 19, 755–773. doi: 10.1038/s41580-018-0060-8

Jeon, G. S., Shim, Y. M., Lee, D. Y., Kim, J. S., Kang, M. J., Ahn, S. H., et al. (2018). Pathological modification of TDP-43 in amyotrophic lateral sclerosis with SOD1 mutations. *Mol. Neurobiol.* doi: 10.1007/s12035-018-1218-2 [Epub ahead of print].

Jeong, S. Y., Rathore, K. I., Schulz, K., Ponka, P., Arosio, P., and David, S. (2009). Dysregulation of iron homeostasis in the CNS contributes to disease progression in a mouse model of amyotrophic lateral sclerosis. *J. Neurosci.* 29, 610–619. doi: 10.1523/JNEUROSCI.5443-08.2009

Jiang, H., Wang, J., Rogers, J., and Xie, J. (2017). Brain iron metabolism dysfunction in Parkinson's disease. *Mol. Neurobiol.* 54, 3078–3101. doi: 10.1007/s12035-016-9879-1

Kim, A. C., Lim, S., and Kim, Y. K. (2018). Metal ion effects on A β and tau aggregation. *Int. J. Mol. Sci.* 19:128. doi: 10.3390/ijms19010128

Kostka, M., Högen, T., Danzer, K. M., Levin, J., Habeck, M., Wirth, A., et al. (2008). Single particle characterization of iron-induced pore-forming α-synuclein oligomers. *J. Biol. Chem.* 283, 10992–11003. doi: 10.1074/jbc.M709634200

Kupershmidt, L., Weinreb, O., Amit, T., Mandel, S., Carri, M. T., and Youdim, M. B. (2009). Neuroprotective and neuritogenic activities of novel multimodal iron-chelating drugs in motor-neuron-like NSC-34 cells and transgenic mouse model of amyotrophic lateral sclerosis. *FASEB J.* 23, 3766–3779. doi: 10.1096/fj.09-130047

Lannfelt, L., Blennow, K., Zetterberg, H., Batsman, S., Ames, D., Harrison, J., et al. (2008). Safety, efficacy, and biomarker findings of PBT2 in targeting Abeta as a modifying therapy for Alzheimer's disease: a phase IIa, double-blind, randomised, placebo-controlled trial. *Lancet Neurol.* 7, 779–786. doi: 10.1016/S1474-4422(08)70167-4

Legname, G. (2017). Elucidating the function of the prion protein. *PLoS Pathog.* 13:e1006458. doi: 10.1371/journal.ppat.1006458

Levin, J., Högen, T., Hillmer, A. S., Bader, B., Schmidt, F., Kamp, F., et al. (2011). Generation of ferric iron links oxidative stress to α-synuclein oligomer formation. *J. Parkinsons. Dis.* 1, 205–216. doi: 10.3233/JPD-2011-11040

Li, W., Jiang, H., Song, N., and Xie, J. (2011). Oxidative stress partially contributes to iron-induced alpha-synuclein aggregation in SK-N-SH cells. *Neurotox. Res.* 19, 435–442. doi: 10.1007/s12640-010-9187-x

Liebert, A., Bicknell, B., and Adams, R. (2014). Prion protein signaling in the nervous system—a review and perspective. *Sign. Transduct. Insights* 3:STI.S12319. doi: 10.4137/STI.S12319

Lim, L. Z., and Song, J. (2015). A novel SOD1-dependent mechanism for the iron-induced production of toxic SOD1 and oxidative stress that initiates ALS. *bioRxiv* [Preprint]. doi: 10.1101/018846

Lim, S.-Y., Tan, A. H., Ahmad-Annuar, A., Schneider, S. A., Bee, P. C., Lim, J. L., et al. (2018). A patient with beta-propeller protein-associated neurodegeneration: treatment with iron chelation therapy. *J. Mov. Disord.* 11, 89–92. doi: 10.14802/jmd.17082

Liu, B., Moloney, A., Meehan, S., Morris, K., Thomas, S. E., Serpell, L. C., et al. (2011). Iron promotes the toxicity of amyloid β peptide by impeding its ordered aggregation. *J. Biol. Chem.* 286, 4248–4256. doi: 10.1074/jbc.M110.158980

Lovejoy, D. B., and Guillemin, G. J. (2014). The potential for transition metal-mediated neurodegeneration in amyotrophic lateral sclerosis. *Front. Aging Neurosci.* 6:173. doi: 10.3389/fnagi.2014.00173

Lovell, M. A., Xiong, S., Xie, C., Davies, P., and Markesbery, W. R. (2004). Induction of hyperphosphorylated tau in primary rat cortical neuron cultures mediated by oxidative stress and glycogen synthase kinase-3. *JAD* 6, 659–671. doi: 10.3233/JAD-2004-6610

Lu, Y., Prudent, M., Fauvet, B., Lashuel, H. A., and Girault, H. H. (2011). Phosphorylation of alpha-synuclein at Y125 and S129 alters its metal binding properties: implications for understanding the role of alpha-synuclein in the pathogenesis of Parkinson's disease and related disorders. *ACS Chem. Neurosci.* 2, 667–675. doi: 10.1021/cn200074d

Mandel, S., Maor, G., and Youdim, M. B. H. (2004). Iron and α-synuclein in the substantia nigra of MPTP-treated mice. *J. Mol. Neurosci.* 24, 401–416. doi: 10.1385/JMN:24:3:401

Martin-Bastida, A., Ward, R. J., Newbould, R., Piccini, P., Sharp, D., Kabba, C., et al. (2017). Brain iron chelation by deferiprone in a phase 2 randomised double-blinded placebo controlled clinical trial in Parkinson's disease. *Sci. Rep.* 7, 1–9. doi: 10.1038/s41598-017-01402-2

McDowall, J. S., Ntai, I., Hake, J., Whitley, P. R., Mason, J. M., Pudney, C. R., et al. (2017). Steady-state kinetics of α-synuclein ferrireductase activity identifies the catalytically competent species. *Biochemistry* 56, 2497–2505. doi: 10.1021/acs.biochem.7b00257

Milczarek, A., Starzyński, R. R., Styś, A., Jończy, A., Staroń, R., Grzelak, A., et al. (2017). A drastic superoxide-dependent oxidative stress is prerequisite for the down-regulation of IRP1: insights from studies on SOD1-deficient mice and macrophages treated with paraquat. *PLoS One* 12:e0176800. doi: 10.1371/journal.pone.0176800

Miura, T., Suzuki, K., and Takeuchi, H. (2001). Binding of iron (III) to the single tyrosine residue of amyloid b-peptide probed by Raman spectroscopy. *J. Mol. Liq.* 598, 79–84. doi: 10.1016/S0022-2860(01)00807-9

Mobarra, N., Shanaki, M., Ehteram, H., Nasiri, H., Sahmani, M., Saeidi, M., et al. (2016). A review on iron chelators in treatment of iron overload syndromes. *Int. J. Hematol. Stem Cell Res.* 10, 239–247.

Moreau, C., Danel, V., Devedjian, J. C., Grolez, G., Timmerman, K., Laloux, C., et al. (2018). Could conservative iron chelation lead to neuroprotection in amyotrophic lateral sclerosis? *Antioxid. Redox Signal.* 29, 742–748. doi: 10.1089/ars.2017.7493

Nakamura, M., Shishido, N., Nunomura, A., Smith, M. A., Perry, G., Hayashi, Y., et al. (2007). Three histidine residues of amyloid-β peptide control the redox activity of copper and iron. *Biochemistry* 46, 12737–12743. doi: 10.1021/bi701079z

Neumann, M., Sampathu, D. M., Kwong, L. K., Truax, A. C., Micsenyi, M. C., Chou, T. T., et al. (2006). Ubiquitinated TDP-43 in frontotemporal lobar degeneration and amyotrophic lateral sclerosis. *Science (80-)* 314, 130–134. doi: 10.1126/science.1134108

Nisbet, R. M., Polanco, J. C., Ittner, L. M., and Götz, J. (2015). Tau aggregation and its interplay with amyloid-β. *Acta Neuropathol.* 129, 207–220. doi: 10.1007/s00401-014-1371-2

Nübling, G., Bader, B., Levin, J., Hildebrandt, J., Kretzschmar, H., and Giese, A. (2012). Synergistic influence of phosphorylation and metal ions on tau oligomer formation and coaggregation with α-synuclein at the single molecule level. *Mol. Neurodegener.* 7, 1–13. doi: 10.1186/1750-1326-7-35

Oeppen, J., and Vaupel, J. W. (2002). Demography: broken limits to life expectancy. *Science (80-)* 296, 1029–1031. doi: 10.1126/science.1069675

Ortega, R., Carmona, A., Roudeau, S., Perrin, L., Dučić, T., Carboni, E., et al. (2016). α-Synuclein over-expression induces increased iron accumulation and redistribution in iron-exposed neurons. *Mol. Neurobiol.* 53, 1925–1934. doi: 10.1007/s12035-015-9146-x

Ostrerova-Golts, N., Petrucelli, L., Hardy, J., Lee, J. M., Farer, M., and Wolozin, B. (2000). The A53T alpha-synuclein mutation increases iron-dependent aggregation and toxicity. *J. Neurosci.* 20, 6048–6054. doi: 10.1523/JNEUROSCI.20-16-06048.2000

Ott, S., Dziadulewicz, N., and Crowther, D. C. (2015). Iron is a specific cofactor for distinct oxidation- and aggregation- dependent Aβ toxicity mechanisms in a *Drosophila* model. *Dis. Model. Mech.* 8, 657–667. doi: 10.1242/dmm.019042

Pandolfo, M., Arpa, J., Delatycki, M. B., Le Quan, Sang, K. H., Mariotti, C., et al. (2014). Deferiprone in Friedreich ataxia: a 6-month randomized controlled trial. *Ann. Neurol.* 76, 509–521. doi: 10.1002/ana.24248

Pasinelli, P., and Brown, R. H. (2006). Molecular biology of amyotrophic lateral sclerosis: insights from genetics. *Nat. Rev. Neurosci.* 7, 710–723. doi: 10.1038/nrn1971

Peng, Y., Wang, C., Xu, H., Liu, Y.-N., and Zhou, F. (2010). Binding of α-synuclein with Fe(III) and with Fe(II) and biological implications of the resultant complexes. *J. Inorg. Biochem.* 104, 365–370. doi: 10.1016/j.jinorgbio.2009.11.005.Binding

Pushie, M. J., Pickering, I. J., Martin, G. R., Tsutsui, S., Jirik, F. R., and George, G. N. (2011). Prion protein expression level alters regional copper, iron and zinc content in the mouse brain. *Metallomics* 3, 206–214. doi: 10.1039/c0mt00037j

Rajasekhar, K., Chakrabarti, M., and Govindaraju, T. (2015). Function and toxicity of amyloid beta and recent therapeutic interventions targeting amyloid beta in Alzheimer's disease. *Chem. Commun.* 51, 13434–13450. doi: 10.1039/c5cc05264e

Ritchie, C., Bush, A. L., Mackinnon, A., Macfarlane, S., Mastwyk, MacGregor L, M., et al. (2003). Metal-protein attenuation with iodochlorhydroxyquin (clioquinol) targeting aβ amyloid deposition and toxicity in alzheimer disease: a pilot phase 2 clinical trial. *Arch. Neurol.* 60, 1685–1691. doi: 10.1001/archneur.60.12.1685

Rival, T., Page, R. M., Chandraratna, D. S., Sendall, T. J., Ryder, E., Liu, B., et al. (2009). Fenton chemistry and oxidative stress mediate the toxicity of the beta-amyloid peptide in a *Drosophila* model of Alzheimer's disease. *Eur. J. Neurosci.* 29, 1335–1347. doi: 10.1111/j.1460-9568.2009.06701.x

Rocha, E. M., De Miranda, B., and Sanders, L. H. (2018). Alpha-synuclein: pathology, mitochondrial dysfunction and neuroinflammation in Parkinson's disease. *Neurobiol. Dis.* 109, 249–257. doi: 10.1016/j.nbd.2017.04.004

Rogers, J. T., Venkataramani, V., Washburn, C., Liu, Y., Tummala, V., Jiang, H., et al. (2016). A role for amyloid precursor protein translation to restore iron homeostasis and ameliorate lead (Pb) neurotoxicity. *J. Neurochem.* 138, 479–494. doi: 10.1111/jnc.13671

Rohani, M., Razmeh, S., Shahidi, G. A., and Orooji, M. (2018). A pilot trial of deferiprone in pantothenate kinase-associated neurodegeneration patients. *Neurol. Int.* 9, 79–81. doi: 10.4081/ni.2017.7279

Rottkamp, C. A., Raina, A. K., Zhu, X., Gaier, E., Bush, A. I., Atwood, C. S., et al. (2001). Redox-active iron mediates amyloid-beta toxicity. *Free Radic. Biol. Med.* 30, 447–450. doi: 10.1016/S0891-5849(00)00494-9

Sangchot, P., Sharma, S., Chetsawang, B., Porter, J., Govitrapong, P., and Ebadi, M. (2002). Deferoxamine attenuates iron-induced oxidative stress and prevents mitochondrial aggregation and α-synuclein translocation in SK-N-SH cells in culture. *Dev. Neurosci.* 24, 143–153. doi: 10.1159/000065700

Sayre, L. M., Perry, G., Harris, P. L. R., Liu, Y., Schubert, K. A., and Smith, M. A. (2000). In situ oxidative catalysis by neurofibrillary tangles and senile plaques in Alzheimer's disease. *J. Neurochem.* 74, 270–279. doi: 10.1046/j.1471-4159.2000.0740270.x

Singh, A., Haldar, S., Horback, K., Tom, C., Zhou, L., Meyerson, H., et al. (2013). Prion protein regulates iron transport by functioning as a ferrireductase. *J. Alzheimer's Dis.* 35, 541–552. doi: 10.3233/JAD-130218

Singh, A., Isaac, A. O., Luo, X., Mohan, M. L., Cohen, M. L., Chen, F., et al. (2009a). Abnormal brain iron homeostasis in human and animal prion disorders. *PLoS Pathog.* 5:e1000336. doi: 10.1371/journal.ppat.1000336

Singh, A., Kong, Q., Luo, X., Petersen, R. B., Meyerson, H., and Singh, N. (2009b). Prion protein (PrP) knock-out mice show altered iron metabolism: a functional role for PrP in iron uptake and transport. *PLoS One* 4:e6115. doi: 10.1371/journal.pone.0006115

Smith, D. G., Cappai, R., and Barnham, K. J. (2007). The redox chemistry of the Alzheimer's disease amyloid β peptide. *Biochim. Biophys. Acta – Biomembr.* 1768, 1976–1990. doi: 10.1016/j.bbamem.2007.02.002

Soe-Lin, S., Apte, S. S., Andriopoulos, B., Andrews, M. C., Schranzhofer, M., Kahawita, T., et al. (2009). Nramp1 promotes efficient macrophage recycling of iron following erythrophagocytosis in vivo. *Proc. Natl. Acad. Sci. U.S.A.* 106, 5960–5965. doi: 10.1073/pnas.0900808106

Soto, C., and Pritzkow, S. (2018). Protein misfolding, aggregation, and conformational strains in neurodegenerative diseases. *Nat. Neurosci.* 21, 1332–1340. doi: 10.1038/s41593-018-0235-9

Spillantini, M. G., Crowther, R. A., Jakes, R., Hasegawa, M., and Goedert, M. (1998). alpha-Synuclein in filamentous inclusions of Lewy bodies from Parkinson' s disease and dementia with Lewy bodies. *Proc. Natl. Acad. Sci. U.S.A.* 95, 6469–6473. doi: 10.1073/pnas.95.11.6469

Stroo, E., Koopman, M., Nollen, E. A. A., and Mata-Cabana, A. (2017). Cellular regulation of amyloid formation in aging and disease. *Front. Neurosci.* 11:64. doi: 10.3389/fnins.2017.00064

Tahmasebinia, F., and Emadi, S. (2017). Effect of metal chelators on the aggregation of beta-amyloid peptides in the presence of copper and iron. *BioMetals* 30, 285–293. doi: 10.1007/s10534-017-0005-2

Telling, N. D., Everett, J., Collingwood, J. F., Gallagher, J. J., Wang, J., Hitchcock, A. P., et al. (2017). Iron Biochemistry is correlated with amyloid plaque morphology in an established mouse model of alzheimer' s disease article iron biochemistry is correlated with amyloid plaque morphology in an established mouse model of alzheimer' s disease. *Cell Chem. Biol.* 24, 1205.e3–1215.e3. doi: 10.1016/j.chembiol.2017.07.014

Tripathi, A. K., Haldar, S., Qian, J., Beserra, A., Suda, S., Singh, A., et al. (2015). Prion protein functions as a ferrireductase partner for ZIP14 and DMT1. *Free Radic. Biol. Med.* 84, 322–330. doi: 10.2144/000114329.Functional

Trist, B. G., Fifita, J. A., Freckleton, S. E., Hare, D. J., Lewis, S. J. G., Halliday, G. M., et al. (2018). Accumulation of dysfunctional SOD1 protein in Parkinson's disease is not associated with mutations in the SOD1 gene. *Acta Neuropathol.* 135, 155–156. doi: 10.1007/s00401-017-1779-6

Uchihara, T., and Giasson, B. I. (2016). Propagation of alpha-synuclein pathology: hypotheses, discoveries, and yet unresolved questions from experimental and human brain studies. *Acta Neuropathol.* 131, 49–73. doi: 10.1007/s00401-015-1485-1

Uversky, V. N., Li, J., and Fink, A. L. (2001). Metal-triggered structural transformations, aggregation, and fibrillation of human α-synuclein: a possible molecular link between parkinson's disease and heavy metal exposure. *J. Biol. Chem.* 276, 44284–44296. doi: 10.1074/jbc.M105343200

Van Bergen, J. M. G., Li, X., Hua, J., Schreiner, S. J., Steininger, S. C., Quevenco, F. C., et al. (2016). Colocalization of cerebral iron with amyloid beta in mild cognitive impairment. *Sci. Rep.* 6, 1–9. doi: 10.1038/srep35514

Velasco-Sánchez, D., Aracil, A., Montero, R., Mas, A., Jiménez, L., O'Callaghan, M., et al. (2011). Combined therapy with idebenone and deferiprone in patients with Friedreich's ataxia. *Cerebellum* 10, 1–8. doi: 10.1007/s12311-010-0212-7

Verma, M., Vats, A., and Taneja, V. (2015). Toxic species in amyloid disorders: oligomers or mature fibrils. *Ann. Indian Acad. Neurol.* 18, 138–145. doi: 10.4103/0972-2327.144284

Wang, P., Wu, Q., Wu, W., Li, H., Guo, Y., Yu, P., et al. (2017). Mitochondrial ferritin deletion exacerbates ß-amyloid-induced neurotoxicity in mice. *Oxid. Med. Cell Longev.* 2017:1020357. doi: 10.1155/2017/1020357

Wang, Q., Zhang, X., Chen, S., Zhang, X., Zhang, S., Youdium, M., et al. (2011). Prevention of motor neuron degeneration by novel iron chelators in SOD1(G93A) transgenic mice of amyotrophic lateral sclerosis. *Neurodegener. Dis.* 8, 310–321. doi: 10.1159/000323469

Wang, W., Perovic, I., Chittuluru, J., Kaganovich, A., Nguyen, L. T. T., Liao, J., et al. (2011). A soluble -synuclein construct forms a dynamic tetramer. *Proc. Natl. Acad. Sci. U.S.A.* 108, 17797–17802. doi: 10.1073/pnas.1113260108

Ward, R. J., Zucca, F. A., Duyn, J. H., Crichton, R. R., and Zecca, L. (2014). The role of iron in brain ageing and neurodegenerative disorders. *Lancet Neurol.* 13, 1045–1060. doi: 10.1016/j.cogdev.2010.08.003.Personal

Watts, J. C., Bourkas, M. E. C., and Arshad, H. (2018). The function of the cellular prion protein in health and disease. *Acta Neuropathol.* 135, 159–178. doi: 10.1007/s00401-017-1790-y

Wolff, N. A., Garrick, M. D., Zhao, L., Garrick, L. M., Ghio, A. J., and Thévenod, F. (2018). A role for divalent metal transporter (DMT1) in mitochondrial uptake of iron and manganese. *Sci. Rep.* 8, 1–12. doi: 10.1038/s41598-017-18584-4

Wong, B. X., Tsatsanis, A., Lim, L. Q., Adlard, P. A., Bush, A. I., and Duce, J. A. (2014). B-Amyloid precursor protein does not possess ferroxidase activity but does stabilize the cell surface ferrous iron exporter ferroportin. *PLoS One* 9:e114174. doi: 10.1371/journal.pone.0114174

Wu, K. C., Liou, H. H., Kao, Y. H., Lee, C. Y., and Lin, C. J. (2017). The critical role of Nramp1 in degrading α-synuclein oligomers in microglia under iron overload condition. *Neurobiol. Dis.* 104, 61–72. doi: 10.1016/j.nbd.2017.05.001

Wu, W.-S., Zhao, Y.-S., Shi, Z.-H., Chang, S.-Y., Nie, G.-J., Duan, X.-L., et al. (2013). Mitochondrial ferritin attenuates β-Amyloid-induced neurotoxicity: reduction in oxidative damage through the Erk/P38 mitogen-activated protein kinase pathways. *Antioxid. Redox Signal.* 18, 158–169. doi: 10.1089/ars.2011.4285

Xiao, Y., Chen, X., Huang, S., Li, G., Mo, M., Zhang, L., et al. (2018). Iron promotes α-synuclein aggregation and transmission by inhibiting TFEB-mediated autophagosome-lysosome fusion. *J. Neurochem.* 145, 34–50. doi: 10.1111/jnc.14312

Xie, L., Zheng, W., Xin, N., Xie, J. W., Wang, T., and Wang, Z. Y. (2012). Ebselen inhibits iron-induced tau phosphorylation by attenuating DMT1 up-regulation and cellular iron uptake. *Neurochem. Int.* 61, 334–340. doi: 10.1016/j.neuint.2012.05.016

Yamamoto, A., Shin, R., and Hasegawa, K. (2002). Iron (III) induces aggregation of hyperphosphorylated s and its reduction to iron (II) reverses the aggregation: implications in the formation of neurofibrillary tangles of Alzheimer' s disease. *J. Neurochem.* 82, 1137–1147. doi: 10.1046/j.1471-4159.2003.02066.x

Zecca, L., Gallorini, M., Schünemann, V., Trautwein, A. X., Gerlach, M., Riederer, P., et al. (2001). Iron, neuromelanin and ferritin content in the substantia nigra of normal subjects at different ages: consequences for iron storage and neurodegenerative processes. *J. Neurochem.* 76, 1766–1773. doi: 10.1046/j.1471-4159.2001.00186.x

Zecca, L., Stroppolo, A., Gatti, A., Tampellini, D., Toscani, M., Gallorini, M., et al. (2004a). The role of iron and copper molecules in the neuronal vulnerability of locus coeruleus and substantia nigra during aging. *Proc. Natl. Acad. Sci. U.S.A.* 101, 9843–9848. doi: 10.1073/pnas.0403495101

Zecca, L., Youdim, M. B. H., Riederer, P., Connor, J. R., and Crichton, R. R. (2004b). Iron, brain ageing and neurodegenerative disorders. *Nat. Rev. Neurosci.* 5, 863–873. doi: 10.1038/nrn1537

Zeineddine, R., Farrawell, N. E., Lambert-Smith, I. A., and Yerbury, J. J. (2017). Addition of exogenous SOD1 aggregates causes TDP-43 mislocalisation and aggregation. *Cell Stress Chaperones* 22, 893–902. doi: 10.1007/s12192-017-0804-y

Zhao, Y., Sun, P., Chen, B., Lun, P., Dou, Y., and Cao, W. W. (2017). A study on the effect of ion chelating agent on Alzheimer disease. *Biomed. Res.* 28, 8022–8026.

Zhu, Z. J., Wu, K. C., Yung, W. H., Qian, Z. M., and Ke, Y. (2016). Differential interaction between iron and mutant alpha-synuclein causes distinctive Parkinsonian phenotypes in *Drosophila. Biochim. Biophys. Acta – Mol. Basis Dis.* 1862, 518–525. doi: 10.1016/j.bbadis.2016.01.002

6

Noxious Iron–Calcium Connections in Neurodegeneration

Marco Tulio Núñez[1] and Cecilia Hidalgo[2,3]*

[1] *Iron and Neuroregeneration Laboratory, Department of Biology, Faculty of Sciences, Universidad de Chile, Santiago, Chile,* [2] *Calcium Signaling Laboratory, Biomedical Research Institute, CEMC, Physiology and Biophysics Program, Institute of Biomedical Sciences, Faculty of Medicine, Universidad de Chile, Santiago, Chile,* [3] *Department of Neuroscience, Faculty of Medicine, Universidad de Chile, Santiago, Chile*

***Correspondence:**
Marco Tulio Núñez
mnunez@uchile.cl

Iron and calcium share the common feature of being essential for normal neuronal function. Iron is required for mitochondrial function, synaptic plasticity, and the development of cognitive functions whereas cellular calcium signals mediate neurotransmitter exocytosis, axonal growth and synaptic plasticity, and control the expression of genes involved in learning and memory processes. Recent studies have revealed that cellular iron stimulates calcium signaling, leading to downstream activation of kinase cascades engaged in synaptic plasticity. The relationship between calcium and iron is Janus-faced, however. While under physiological conditions iron-mediated reactive oxygen species generation boosts normal calcium-dependent signaling pathways, excessive iron levels promote oxidative stress leading to the upsurge of unrestrained calcium signals that damage mitochondrial function, among other downstream targets. Similarly, increases in mitochondrial calcium to non-physiological levels result in mitochondrial dysfunction and a predicted loss of iron homeostasis. Hence, if uncontrolled, the iron/calcium self-feeding cycle becomes deleterious to neuronal function, leading eventually to neuronal death. Here, we review the multiple cell-damaging responses generated by the unregulated iron/calcium self-feeding cycle, such as excitotoxicity, free radical-mediated lipid peroxidation, and the oxidative modification of crucial components of iron and calcium homeostasis/signaling: the iron transporter DMT1, plasma membrane, and intracellular calcium channels and pumps. We discuss also how iron-induced dysregulation of mitochondrial calcium contributes to the generation of neurodegenerative conditions, including Alzheimer's disease (AD) and Parkinson's disease (PD).

Keywords: neurodegenerative diseases, reactive oxygen species, mitochondria, HIF-1, Nrf-2, inflammation, ferroptosis

INTRODUCTION

Iron and calcium ions are both essential for maintaining normal brain function. Iron is required for oxidative phosphorylation, Krebs cycle, iron–sulfur cluster and heme synthesis, synaptic plasticity, and the development of cognitive functions (Oexle et al., 1999; Bolton et al., 2000; Hidalgo and Núñez, 2007;Tong and Rouault, 2007; Zorov et al., 2007; Huang et al., 2011; Muñoz et al., 2011; Murray-Kolb, 2013; Mena et al., 2015; Requejo-Aguilar and Bolanos, 2016), while increases in cytoplasmic calcium concentration known as calcium signals mediate the secretion of neurotransmitters, synaptic plasticity, and axonal growth (Berridge, 1998). Moreover, nuclear calcium signals command the expression of neuronal genes involved in learning and memory processes (Bading, 2013).

Recent studies have revealed that cellular iron stimulates neuronal calcium signaling, leading to downstream activation of kinase cascades engaged in synaptic plasticity, a neuronal response associated to memory and learning (Hidalgo and Núñez, 2007; Hidalgo et al., 2007; Muñoz et al., 2011). The relationship between calcium and iron is Janus-faced, however. Dysregulation of iron levels induces calcium dyshomeostasis and abnormal calcium signaling, whereas increased calcium levels enhance redox-active iron levels; neurodegenerative conditions exhibit both types of dysregulation. Thus, current evidence indicates that increased intracellular calcium and aberrant calcium signaling occur in neurodegenerative disorders that include Alzheimer's disease (AD), Parkinson's disease (PD), and amyotrophic lateral sclerosis (ALS) (reviewed in Pchitskaya et al., 2018). Similarly, disruption of neuronal iron homeostasis linked to iron accumulation is a common feature in a plethora of neurodegenerative diseases, which included and other parkinsonisms (Lee et al., 2013), AD (Bulk et al., 2018), Friedrich's ataxia, pantothenate kinase-associated neurodegeneration (Swaiman, 1991), and other neuronal pathologies that entail brain iron accumulation (Wiethoff and Houlden, 2017).

Here, we will review the evidence that points to a rarely acknowledged relationship between iron homeostasis and calcium homeostasis and signaling, in which dysregulation of one of these processes results in dysregulation of the other, generating a vicious cycle that ends up in neuronal death. The multiple cell-damaging responses generated by the unregulated iron/calcium self-feeding cycle, such as excitotoxicity, free radical-mediated lipid peroxidation, and the oxidative modification of crucial components of iron and calcium homeostasis and signaling, including the iron transporter DMT1, plasma membrane and intracellular calcium channels and pumps will be presented. This review article concludes with a discussion of how dysregulation of calcium homeostasis and signaling contributes to the generation of neurodegenerative diseases with an iron accumulation component, focusing in particular on AD and PD.

IRON HOMEOSTASIS IN NEURONAL CELLS

Through the Fenton reaction, redox-active iron is a net producer of the hydroxyl radical, the most reactive radical species in nature (Davies, 2005). In a reductive environment, such as the intracellular milieu, through redox cycling redox-active iron promotes the production of hydroxyl radicals at the expense of O_2 and GSH consumption (Núñez et al., 2012). Consequently, under physiological conditions, redox-active iron levels that conform the labile iron pool are very tightly regulated to a cytosolic concentration of 0.5–1.5 μM, which comprises <5% of total intracellular iron (Cabantchik, 2014). In mammals, cellular iron levels are maintained by transcriptional, translational, and vesicular flux mechanisms (Núñez, 2010). The iron regulatory protein (IRPs: IRP1 and IRP2)/iron-responsive element (IRE) is the best-characterized system that regulates at the translation level the expression of iron homeostasis proteins. These proteins include the transferrin receptor 1 (TfR1, involved in iron uptake), the divalent metal transporter 1 (DMT1, involved in iron uptake), ferroportin 1 (FPN1), involved in iron efflux from cells), and ferritin (involved in iron storage) (Wilkinson and Pantopoulos, 2014). The IRP/IRE is a plentiful-oriented system, since it is activated under low iron conditions to ensure an adequate supply of iron for cellular processes. Of note, the IRE–IRP regulatory system is not only regulated by cellular iron status but it is also regulated by reactive oxygen species (ROS), whereby cells elicit a defense mechanism against iron toxicity and iron-catalyzed oxidative stress (Ray et al., 2012).

The iron uptake protein DMT1 (SLC11A2) is a crucial component of cell iron homeostasis. *SLC11A2* transcription generates four alternatively spliced mRNAs that differ at their 5′-untranslated region (coding for the DMT1 isoforms 1A and 1B) and at its 3′-untranslated region (coding for isoforms +IRE and -IRE) (Garrick et al., 2006). Thus, the expression of the 1A and 1B isoforms of DMT1 is subjected to differential transcriptional regulation.

THE CRUCIAL RELATIONSHIP BETWEEN IRON AND THE HYPOXIA-INDUCIBLE TRANSCRIPTION FACTOR (HIF)

At the systemic level, the hypoxia-inducible transcription factor (HIF) transcription factor family coordinates the cellular response to low oxygen levels by regulating the expression of a large array of target genes during hypoxia, which results in adaptive changes in the hematopoietic, cardiovascular, and respiratory systems (Smith et al., 2008; Mole et al., 2009). The HIF-1 is kept at basal levels by HIF prolyl hydroxylase domain (PHD) enzymes; prolyl-hydroxylation of HIF-1 via PHD signals for its degradation via the ubiquitin-proteasome system (Bruick and McKnight, 2001; Myllyharju, 2013; Yeh et al., 2017). The PHD enzymes are both oxygen- and iron-dependent; thus, hypoxia and iron chelation results in decreased PHD activity and increased HIF-1α activity (Hewitson et al., 2003; Nandal et al., 2011; Flagg et al., 2012).

In recent years, a series of iron chelating agents that exert neuroprotective effects have been developed (Núñez and Chana-Cuevas, 2018). In particular, M30, which is an 8-hydroxyquinoline-based iron chelator developed by the group of Moussa Youdim at Technion-Israel Institute of Technology (Weinreb et al., 2016), stabilizes HIF-1α, most probably by inactivating HIF-1α PHD. In the brain, HIF-1α stabilization by M30 leads to the expression of a broad number of neuroprotective-adaptive mechanisms and pro-survival signaling pathways (Kupershmidt et al., 2011). Real-time RT-PCR revealed that M30 differentially induces the expression of a variety of cellular components, including vascular endothelial growth factor, erythropoietin, enolase-1, TfR1, heme oxygenase-1, inducible nitric oxide synthase (iNOS), glucose transporter 1, brain-derived neurotrophic factor (BDNF), glial cell-derived neurotrophic factor, and the antioxidant enzymes catalase, superoxide dismutase-1, and glutathione peroxidase (Kupershmidt et al., 2009). Further reports have supported the role of iron chelators in inducing neuronal survival pathways (Mechlovich et al., 2014; Guo et al., 2015, 2016; Xiao et al., 2015). It follows that the capacity of iron chelators to induce HIF-1α-mediated neuroprotection adds to the recognized neuroprotective effects of iron chelators, through their ability to prevent hydroxyl radical production via the Fenton reaction. A tempering note comes from the report that treatment of human skin cells with the iron chelator *N*-(2-hydroxybenzyl)-L-serine (HBSer) does not induce HIF-1α activation, as opposed to desferrioxamine (DFO) and salicylaldehyde isonicotinoyl hydrazone (SIH) used as positive controls (Creighton-Gutteridge and Tyrrell, 2002). The authors conjectured that the lack of HIF-1α activation by HBSer might be related to its lower affinity for iron as compared to DFO and SIH. Of relevance to the theme of this review, however, is the fact that the transcription factor HIF-1α activates the expression of several genes associated with iron homeostasis (Lee and Andersen, 2006), which in non-excitable cells results in an increase in cellular iron content (Qian et al., 2011).

INCREASED REACTIVE OXYGEN/NITROGEN SPECIES GENERATION INDUCES IRON DYSHOMEOSTASIS

A significant number of studies have shown that physiological levels of ROS and reactive nitrogen species (RNS) act as signaling molecules in a variety of biological responses (Sen, 2001; Ray et al., 2012; Asiimwe et al., 2016; Lourenco et al., 2017; Moldogazieva et al., 2018; Nemes et al., 2018). The brain is an organ highly susceptible to oxidative stress (Cobley et al., 2018). Hence, neuronal cells have to maintain physiological levels of ROS and RNS to avoid oxidative or nitrosative stress, which arises when excessive ROS/RNS production overcomes the cellular antioxidant systems, which by affecting the redox environment favors excitotoxicity. Henceforth, we will use the broad term oxidative stress to refer to both oxidative and nitrosative stress. Oxidative stress perturbs the function of many cellular processes; it causes glutathione deficiency (Wu et al., 2004) and promotes cell death by inducing mitochondrial depolarization, membrane lipid peroxidation, and DNA damage, among other harmful effects. To counteract the damaging effects of excess ROS/RNS (Duncan and Heales, 2005; Halliwell, 2006; Moncada and Bolaños, 2006), cells make use of enzymatic and non-enzymatic defense mechanisms, some of which engage calcium signals (Gordeeva et al., 2003). Depending on the extent and persistence of the cellular damage, oxidative stress may play a key role as a causative agent of neurodegenerative disease emergence and or progression.

Iron uptake into primary hippocampal neurons stimulates ROS generation (Muñoz et al., 2011), and decreases the redox potential established by the intracellular levels of oxidized and reduced glutathione in neuroblastoma cells (Núñez et al., 2004). The relationship between increased redox-active iron and increased oxidative stress is well accepted (Núñez et al., 2012). Similarly, in cellular models convincing evidence points to a link between increased oxidative tone and iron accumulation. Initial observations indicated that hydrogen peroxide activates IRP1 (Martins et al., 1995; Pantopoulos and Hentze, 1995; Hanson and Leibold, 1999; Caltagirone et al., 2001; Mueller et al., 2001), and that this activation results in increased cellular iron uptake mediated by increased translation of TfR1 and decreased ferritin synthesis (Caltagirone et al., 2001; Sureda et al., 2005). A subsequent study reported that, besides activation of IRP1, exposure of SH-SY5Y cells to H_2O_2 results in the degradation of the exo-transporter FPN1, which coupled to a decrease in ferritin translation leads to a time-dependent increase in the cellular labile iron pool (Dev et al., 2015), with the ensuing generation of oxidative damage through the production of hydroxyl radicals by the Fenton reaction. In animal models, evidence linking increased ROS as a cause, and iron homeostasis loss as an effect, is still lacking. An early report indicated that vitamin A deficiency results in increased hepcidin mRNA expression and increased iron spleen concentrations, accompanied by increased protein oxidation. These results suggest that vitamin A protects the liver against protein oxidation by maintaining iron homeostasis (Arruda et al., 2009). In a mouse model of experimentally induced hemolysis, excess heme increases intracellular ROS production, which signals for the induction of the unique iron exporter ferroportin, resulting in iron export from macrophages (Jeney et al., 2002; Marro et al., 2010). Of note, decreasing ROS levels by treatment with the antioxidant N-acetylcysteine prevents ferroportin induction and normalizes intracellular iron levels in a mice model of experimentally induced hemolysis (Tangudu et al., 2018). In a separate study using the APPswe/PS1ΔE9 AD mice model, administration for 3 months of antioxidants of plant origin decreased iron levels and malondialdehyde content and increased antioxidant defenses (Zhang et al., 2018). Overall, these results are consistent with the notion that oxidative stress dysregulates iron homeostasis both in cellular and animal models.

Nitric oxide also modifies IRP1 activity; it increases IRP1 binding to IRE and the increase IRE binding activity of IRP1 is coincident with inhibited ferritin synthesis and increased TfR1 mRNA levels (Phillips et al., 1996). Nitric oxide activates IRP1 directly by destabilizing the 4Fe-4S cluster of IRP1 (Drapier et al., 1993; Soum and Drapier, 2003), and may activate IRP1 indirectly by mobilizing intracellular Fe, thus decreasing the intracellular labile iron pool and activating IRP1 (Pantopoulos et al., 1996; Wardrop et al., 2000).

Altogether, these studies point to a robust association between increased ROS, nitric oxide, and increased levels of redox-active iron, which in turn mediate oxidative damage to lipids, protein, and nucleic acids. Yet, a recent study showed that in cultured macrophages, the labile iron pool apparently attenuates peroxynitrite-dependent damage (Damasceno et al., 2018). Whether this protective effect of the labile iron pool is translatable to other cell types and to neurons in particular, remains to be established.

IRON DYSHOMEOSTASIS IN NEURODEGENERATION

Increased iron levels and the associated ROS generation are important initiators and mediators of cell death (Dixon and Stockwell, 2014), whereas iron dyshomeostasis has a key role in neurodegeneration. Mutations of genes encoding proteins involved in iron homeostasis are associated with degeneration of central nervous system (CNS) cells (Ponka, 2004; Zecca et al., 2004), while oxidative stress induces cell injury by disrupting cellular iron balance (Carocci et al., 2018; Kerins and Ooi, 2018), thus leading to a vicious circle. Both AD and PD entail increased brain iron content and oxidative stress (Crichton et al., 2011; Ward et al., 2014; Tonnies and Trushina, 2017; Guo et al., 2018), with the implied threat of hydroxyl radical-induced neuronal damage. Of note, binding of Cu or Fe to Aβ peptides generates H_2O_2 (Huang et al., 1999), which may induce neuronal oxidative stress during AD progression (Cristovao et al., 2016). Moreover, iron overload increases neuronal amyloid-β production and enhances cognitive impairment in a transgenic mice model of AD (Becerril-Ortega et al., 2014) while accumulating evidence suggests that impaired iron homeostasis is an early event in AD progression (Peters et al., 2015).

Parkinson's disease is a progressive neurodegenerative disease characterized by rigidity, tremor, and slowness of movement as well as by a wide range of debilitating non-motor symptoms. A key feature of PD is the selective loss of the dopaminergic neurons of the substantia nigra; ample evidence shows iron accumulation in these neurons (Jellinger, 1999; Zecca et al., 2004; Berg and Youdim, 2006; Muñoz et al., 2016; An et al., 2018). The observation that pharmacological agents with iron chelation capacity prevent neuronal death in AD or PD experimental models (recently reviewed in Núñez and Chana-Cuevas, 2018) highlights the pivotal role of iron as a mediator of neuronal death in AD and PD.

In addition, spinal neurons from ALS patients display increased iron and calcium levels (Kasarskis et al., 1995). The success of iron chelation therapy in ALS mouse models sustains the central role of iron in ALS pathogenesis (Jeong et al., 2009; Kupershmidt et al., 2009). Alterations of proteins involved in iron metabolism, inhibition of anterograde axonal transport leading to iron accumulation in ventral motor neurons, and increased mitochondrial iron load in neurons and glia have been proposed as pathogenic mechanisms to explain the abnormal iron accumulation displayed by the neurons and glia of ALS mice (Jeong et al., 2009).

IRON DYSHOMEOSTASIS IN INFLAMMATION

Inflammation, a condition often found in neurodegenerative environments, is yet another factor that induces iron accumulation (reviewed in Urrutia et al., 2014). Both the p50 and the p65 subunits of the transcription factor NF-κB bind to a NFκB-responsive element present in the 5′ untranslated region of the DMT1-1B promoter, inducing the expression of the 1B isoforms of DMT1 (Paradkar and Roth, 2006a,b). The transcription factor NF-κB is often activated by inflammatory signals (Rothwell and Luheshi, 2000; Hanke and Kielian, 2011; Shih et al., 2015). Accordingly, the possible association between inflammation and iron accumulation has been recently explored (Pelizzoni et al., 2013; Urrutia et al., 2013, 2014; McCarthy et al., 2018). To this purpose, the effects of lipopolysaccharide (LPS) and the pro-inflammatory cytokines TNF-α and IL-6 on mRNA and protein levels of DMT1, FPN1, and hepcidin were investigated in astrocytes, microglia, and neurons isolated from rat brain. A causal association between inflammation and iron accumulation was reported, since in addition to increasing neuronal iron content, treatment with LPS, TNF-α, or IL-6 increases DMT1 expression and protein levels in neurons (Urrutia et al., 2013). Similar results were reported in studies of ventral mesencephalic neurons in primary culture, in which treatment with TNF-α or IL-1β induces an increment in DMT1 and TfR1 protein levels, together with a reduction of FPN1 levels (Wang et al., 2013). Considering that NFκB activation is downstream of the TNF-α, IL-1, and LPS signaling pathways, these results are consistent with a circuit in which inflammatory stimuli induce DMT1 expression and iron accumulation via NFκB activation and hepcidin expression.

An additional link between inflammation and increased oxidative stress resides in the observation that inflammatory stimuli activate the NADPH oxidase (NOX) enzyme, the main regulated source of cellular ROS generation (Green et al., 2001; Urrutia et al., 2014; Sorce et al., 2017). In particular, pro-inflammatory cytokines activate the phagocytic NOX2 enzyme, which is highly expressed in microglia (Sorce and Krause, 2009; Lim et al., 2013; Barrett et al., 2017). In turn, NOX2 activation generates an oxidative extracellular environment that increases ROS levels in neighboring neurons (Schiavone et al., 2009; Gao et al., 2012; Surace and Block, 2012; Zhang et al., 2014).

Of note, NOX activation has also been reported in experimental models of PD and AD. In particular treatment with MPTP (1-methyl-4-phenyl-1,2,3,6-tetrahydropyridine), a prodrug to the Parkinsonian neurotoxin 1-methyl-4-phenylpyridinium (MPP+), results in increased synthesis of the pro-inflammatory cytokine IL-1β, and increased membrane translocation of the cytosolic NOX sub-unit $p67^{phox}$, which is prevented by minocycline, a tetracycline derivative that exerts multiple anti-inflammatory effects (Wu et al., 2002). In addition, iron supplementation to midbrain neuron-glia cell cultures causes the selective death of dopaminergic neurons. This death is mediated by microglial NOX2 since cells derived from NOX2−/− mice do not present iron-induced neuronal death (Zhang et al., 2014). Similarly, brain tissue from AD patients reveals an elevation in NOX activity coupled to membrane translocation of cytosolic NOX2 subunits and increased NOX1 and NOX3 mRNA transcripts (Shimohama et al., 2000; Ansari and Scheff, 2011). Significantly, the authors found an inverse correlation between postmortem NOX activity and ante-mortem cognitive status (Ansari and Scheff, 2011). Altogether, these results indicate that inflammatory stimuli generate a neuronal phenotype of increased iron influx and increased NOX-produced ROS, with the consequent risk of oxidative damage observed in neurodegenerative diseases.

ROLE OF IRON IN EXCITOTOXICITY

Earlier reports indicate that iron plays a role in excitotoxicity, a death process mediated by high levels of intracellular calcium caused by excessive activity of excitatory neurotransmitters. Seminal observations by Cheah and colaborators described a signaling cascade in which stimulation of *N*-methyl-D-aspartate (NMDA) receptors activates the small GTPase Dexras1 via S-nitrosylation, mediated by activation of neuronal nitric oxide synthase (nNOS). Activated Dexras binds to the peripheral benzodiazepine receptor-associated protein PAP7, which in turn binds to the iron transporter DMT1 (Cheah et al., 2006). Most importantly, treatment with neurotoxic concentrations of NMDA elicits a major increase in iron uptake, resulting in three- to fivefold increase of hydroxyl radical levels and the death of more than 90% of cells, whereas co-treatment with NMDA and a cell-permeant iron chelator largely blocked NMDA-induced cell death. Overall, these results indicate that glutamate-NMDA excitotoxicity elicits DMT1 activation and iron-mediated cell death (Cheah et al., 2006). Although the role of calcium was not explored, the authors hypothesized initial calcium entrance through the NMDA receptor may activate nNOS, thus initiating this neurodegenerative process. As discussed below, crosstalk between NMDA receptor-mediated calcium influx and iron is likely to have a relevant role in neurodegenerative diseases such as AD and PD.

NEURONAL CALCIUM HOMEOSTASIS AND SIGNALING

Calcium is a universal second messenger that regulates numerous cellular processes over a wide temporal range (Berridge et al., 2003). In neurons, the free calcium concentration at rest lies in the 70–100 nM range (Clapham, 2007), whereas extracellular calcium concentration is $\sim$1.5 mM. This large concentration gradient, combined with resting potential values of 70–90 mV (negative inside), generate a significant electrochemical gradient that favors calcium entry. Calcium homeostasis and signaling are vital for cellular function and survival; thus, neuronal cells possess powerful systems to maintain calcium homeostatic and signaling systems (Berridge, 1998; Brini et al., 2014), which regulate the neuronal processes underlying synaptic plasticity and complex brain cognitive functions, such as information processing, learning, and memory. Calcium is stored also in intracellular organelles such as the endoplasmic reticulum (ER), where its free concentration lies in the 0.5 mM range. The main systems in charge of maintaining calcium homeostasis are two plasma membrane calcium (PMCA) transporters, the PMCA pump and the sodium/calcium exchanger (NCX), plus the sarco/ER Ca^{2+}-ATPase (SERCA) pump that maintains the steep concentration gradient between the ER and the cytoplasm (Brini et al., 2014). These transporters utilize different mechanisms and display a range of calcium affinities, transport rates, and capacities to ensure the proper managing of the variety of intracellular increases in free calcium concentration, known as calcium signals, generated by the diverse stimuli neuronal cells receive.

Neuronal activity generates calcium signals that via sequential activation of calcium-dependent signaling cascades and transcription factors promote the expression of genes underlying dendritic development, synaptic plasticity, and neuronal survival (Brini et al., 2014). In response to neuronal stimulation, calcium influx through plasma membrane pathways, including agonist-operated, store-operated, or voltage-gated calcium channels (VGCCs), generates neuronal calcium signals. In addition, the release of calcium from intracellular stores such as the ER also contributes to neuronal calcium signal generation (Brini et al., 2014). All neuronal compartments crucial for neurotransmission have the two types of calcium release channels: the inositol 1,4,5-trisphosphate (IP_3) receptor (IP_3R) and the ryanodine receptor (RyR) channels (Berridge, 1998). These large channels have complex gating and regulation and mediate a cellular process known as calcium-induced calcium release (CICR), whereby calcium promotes its own release from intracellular calcium stores (Berridge, 1998). This CICR mechanism likely contributes to propagate calcium signals that reach distant targets such as the nucleus (Berridge, 1998), where calcium promotes short or long-lasting changes in neuronal function and structure (Bading, 2013).

ROS LEVELS INFLUENCE CALCIUM HOMEOSTASIS AND SIGNALING

Significant evidence gathered in the last years indicates that increased cellular ROS levels modify the function of key proteins engaged in calcium homeostasis and signaling (Gordeeva et al., 2003; Hidalgo and Donoso, 2008; Gorlach et al., 2015). Redox-dependent regulation of components that maintain neuronal Ca^{2+} homeostasis may influence the direction and/or the efficiency of Ca^{2+}-signaling pathways. Interactions among ROS and calcium-dependent signaling pathways are bidirectional; while ROS regulate cellular calcium signaling, calcium signals are essential for ROS production because a number of ROS-generating and antioxidant systems of living cells are calcium-dependent (Gordeeva et al., 2003).

Reversible modifications of proteins via ROS-promoted oxidation of their amino acids modify the properties of neuronal proteins engaged in signal transduction, such as protein kinases, protein phosphatases, and transcription factors (Wang et al., 2012). An increase in cellular ROS levels results in the inhibition of NMDA receptor function and in decreased activity of both the PMCA and the SERCA calcium pumps, while it enhances the activity of IP_3R and RyR calcium channels (Hidalgo and Donoso, 2008; Joseph et al., 2018). Consequently, ROS generation in neuronal cells increases cellular calcium levels by promoting calcium release mediated by IP_3R and RyR channels and by inhibiting both the PMCA and the SERCA pumps: the ROS-mediated increase in calcium levels promotes changes in several calcium-dependent neuronal pathways (Yermolaieva et al., 2000; Riquelme et al., 2011). Depending on the magnitude of the calcium increase, activation of kinases or phosphatases implicated in synaptic plasticity process will occur (reviewed in Hidalgo and Arias-Cavieres, 2016). In addition, activation of the large-conductance Ca^{2+}-activated K^+ (BKCa) by oxidation of SH cysteine residues, by decreasing neuronal excitability reduces the vulnerability of hippocampal neurons to hypoxia (Hepp et al., 2005).

DEFECTIVE CALCIUM HOMEOSTASIS AND SIGNALING IN NEURODEGENERATION

A link between excessive intracellular calcium accumulation and neuronal death is by now firmly established (Demuro et al., 2010; Stefani et al., 2012; Fukui, 2016). Neuronal cells are particularly sensitive to calcium-mediated cytotoxic damage and the failure of neurons to maintain Ca^{2+} homeostasis is a common feature of aged-linked neurodegenerative pathologies (Berrocal et al., 2015; Brini et al., 2017; Pchitskaya et al., 2018; Strehler and Thayer, 2018). Calcium dyshomeostasis (Pchitskaya et al., 2018) and altered neuronal calcium signaling (Chan et al., 2009; Overk et al., 2015) have been reported in a number of disease conditions, including AD, PD, and ALS (for recent reviews, see Franco-Iborra et al., 2018; Popugaeva et al., 2018; Post et al., 2018; Sirabella et al., 2018). Likewise, defective calcium signaling in glia and autophagy-related pathways has been implicated in neurodegenerative disease (Mustaly-Kalimi et al., 2018). Accruing evidence implicates decreased levels and functional decline of PMCA isoforms in neurodegeneration (Hajieva et al., 2018; Strehler and Thayer, 2018). In addition, in many pathological conditions, disruptions of ER Ca^{2+} signaling disrupt neuronal function and promote neuronal cell death (Okubo et al., 2018). To date, however, the detailed mechanisms of how neuronal Ca^{2+} homeostasis and signaling are perturbed in neurodegenerative diseases are not well understood.

The most common neurodegenerative disorder and the leading cause of dementia in the elderly is AD, whereas PD is the most prevalent age-associated movement disorder that entails early and selective degeneration of dopaminergic neurons. The pathological hallmarks of AD are neuronal loss and the presence of amyloid plaques and neurofibrillary tangles in the brain of affected individuals. Yet, before the emergence of plaques and/or neurofibrillary tangles other defects, including Ca^{2+} and iron dyshomeostasis, mitochondrial dysfunction, increased contacts between the ER and the mitochondria, neuro-inflammation, and alterations in lipid metabolism have been reported (Mattson, 2010; Area-Gomez and Schon, 2017; Lane et al., 2018). How these early defects relate to the emergence and progression of AD remains to be established. Of note, a recent report by the Alzheimer's Association Calcium Hypothesis Workgroup [AACHW] (2017) analyzed how defective calcium signaling may be an early upstream event in AD progression, and how alterations of the many cellular components that control calcium hemostasis and signaling leads to the decline in the function of more vulnerable neuronal cells. In particular, these more vulnerable neuronal cells present early synaptic dysfunction, upregulation of some calcium signaling related genes and significant decreases in the expression of genes related to synaptic neurotransmission, neurotrophic factor activity, mitochondrial metabolism, and energy production, among others (Alzheimer's Association Calcium Hypothesis Workgroup [AACHW], 2017).

In PD, dopaminergic neurons of the substantia nigra are especially vulnerable to Ca^{2+} dyshomeostasis, because their autonomous pace-making activity, through which these neurons generate action potentials in the absence of synaptic input (Guzman et al., 2009). This particular property of dopaminergic neurons imposes a high pressure on adequate handling of activity-generated Ca^{2+} signals, presumably mediated by the significant calcium influx through plasma membrane L-type calcium channels that markedly surpasses the calcium influx displayed by other neurons (Surmeier et al., 2010).

Dopaminergic neurons are highly vulnerable to oxidants and mitochondrial inhibition compared to other neuronal types (Sherer et al., 2003; Halliwell, 2006; Burbulla et al., 2017). Thus, brain permeant toxins such as rotenone, an inhibitor of NADH dehydrogenase, exclusively affect dopaminergic neurons (Sherer et al., 2003; Cannon et al., 2009). This special vulnerability is likely to produce the mitochondrial Ca^{2+} imbalance that occurs in PD (Ludtmann and Abramov, 2018). As discussed below, iron-induced ROS increases result in calcium signal generation, which may contribute to the basal calcium burden of dopaminergic neurons.

Several studies have reported defective Ca^{2+} signaling in other neurodegenerative conditions such as ALS (Siklos et al., 1998; Grosskreutz et al., 2010; Jaiswal, 2013; Muhling et al., 2014) and multiple sclerosis (MS; Gonsette, 2008). The death of motor neuron is a characteristic feature of ALS. Excitotoxicity, which involves glutamate and calcium overload, or cell death caused by high levels of intracellular calcium caused by excessive activity of excitatory neurotransmitters, may contribute to ALS pathology. Calcium dysregulation is also present in MS, where the associated disability results from neuronal and axonal loss initiated by microglia activation and mediated by oxidative stress, excitotoxicity, calcium dysregulation, and mitochondrial dysfunction, leading to proteolytic enzyme production and apoptosis (Gonsette, 2008).

Additionally, calcium dysregulation has been associated with neuroinflammation, a CNS response that comprises biochemical and cellular responses to injury, infection, or neurodegenerative diseases (DiSabato et al., 2016). Neuroinflammation markers increase in some neurodegenerative conditions; microglia, the innate CNS immune cells, play key roles as mediators of these neuroinflammatory responses. Of note, Ca^{2+} and neuroinflammatory signaling mechanisms exhibit extensive crosstalk and bidirectional interactions. As an example, chronic brain inflammation leads to a feedback reduction in NMDA receptors caused by excess synaptic glutamate activity during microglial activation (Rosi et al., 2004).

Despite the abundant literature that points to defective calcium homeostasis and signaling in neurodegeneration, scarce information is available in the literature regarding the protective effects of calcium modulators in preventing these defects. Yet, all recent reports on this subject highlight the fact that this is an urgent task. The non-competitive NMDA receptor antagonist Memantine, which reduces excitoxicity by inhibiting neuronal calcium entry (Bezprozvanny and Mattson, 2008), has been the most common drug for treating moderate to severe AD; nevertheless, Memantine provides only limited benefits for AD patients. A recent report showed that immunotherapy with a murine analog of the anti-Aβ antibody Aducanumab restores calcium homeostasis in a transgenic AD mice model (Kastanenka et al., 2016), whereas a recent review addresses the evidence linking neurodegeneration to RyR dysfunction and describes novel therapeutic approaches to target abnormal RyR function (Kushnir et al., 2018). There are no reports, however, on the efficacy of these strategies for treating AD patients.

THE HIF-1–CALCIUM RELATIONSHIP

In SH-SY5Y neuroblastoma cells, chelation of calcium by 1,2-bis(2-aminophenoxy)ethane-N,N,N',N'-tetraacetic acid (BAPTA) induces HIF-1α protein accumulation and nuclear localization, whereas the cytosolic calcium elevation produced by inhibition of the SERCA pump attenuates these effects (Berchner-Pfannschmidt et al., 2004). Further experiments indicated that calcium chelation attenuates the interaction of HIF-1α with the von-Hippel-Lindau protein, thus decreasing the proteasomal degradation of HIF-1α (Berchner-Pfannschmidt et al., 2004). Control experiments indicated that BAPTA did not complex intracellular iron ions, thus the above effects were caused by calcium chelation and not by stimulation of iron-activated PHD enzymes (Berchner-Pfannschmidt et al., 2004). Subsequent studies showed that intermittent hypoxia causes HIF-1α accumulation through a mechanism that involves increased cell calcium and increased generation of ROS by NOX, which induces a complex signaling pathway that results in increased HIF-1α synthesis and decreased hydroxylase-dependent HIF-1α degradation (Yuan et al., 2008).

Although brain levels of HIF-1α are considered neuroprotective (Kietzmann et al., 2001; Siddiq et al., 2005; Guo et al., 2016; Lee et al., 2017; Merelli et al., 2018), under certain conditions, HIF-1α acts as a pro-apoptotic factor (Piret et al., 2002; Zhang et al., 2007; Merelli et al., 2018). For example, the anesthetic isoflurane induces apoptotic neurodegeneration in a process mediated by HIF-1α, since knockdown of HIF-1α expression attenuates isoflurane-induced neurotoxicity (Jiang et al., 2012). In addition, isoflurane induces a significant elevation of cytoplasmic calcium levels in cultured neurons. Based on previous observations, showing that calcium mediates HIF-1α expression (Yuan et al., 2005; Riganti et al., 2009), the authors hypothesized that the high calcium levels induced by isofluorane promote HIF-1α-mediated apoptotic neurodegeneration. Studies discerning the calcium concentrations and other cell physiological condition, which elicit each of the above responses, should shed light on these apparent contradictory responses.

Overall, the emerging picture from the above results is consistent with the idea that low calcium concentrations stabilize HIF-1α protein levels by decreasing its proteasomal degradation. The effect of calcium concentrations above homeostatic levels is not clear and may depend on cell type: high calcium levels may induce a protective response consisting in increased HIF-1α synthesis coupled to decreased degradation or may mediate HIF-1α degradation.

IRON MODIFIES NEURONAL CALCIUM HOMEOSTASIS AND CALCIUM SIGNALING PATHWAYS

Iron overload increases intracellular calcium levels, which in turn activate calcineurin (Lee et al., 2016), a calcium-dependent phosphatase which has a key role in synaptic plasticity and memory processes (Baumgartel and Mansuy, 2012). Increases in cytoplasmic calcium levels via the NMDA receptor stimulate the neuronal NOS enzyme (Ghosh and Salerno, 2003) and generate superoxide anion in hippocampal neurons (Brennan et al., 2009), while in cortical neurons, this calcium increase induces a signaling cascade that enhances superoxide generation through NOX activation (Girouard et al., 2009).

Both synaptic plasticity and memory processes require activity-dependent hippocampal ROS generation (Bindokas et al., 1996; Kahlert et al., 2005; Kishida and Klann, 2007). In primary hippocampal neurons, the ROS increase induced by iron promotes calcium release from the ER mediated by redox-sensitive RyR channels; the resulting increase in intracellular calcium levels link NMDA receptor stimulation to ERK1/2 activation and nuclear translocation (Muñoz, 2012). Since several reports indicate that CREB-dependent transcription of synaptic plasticity related genes entails ERK1/2-mediated long-term CREB phosphorylation (Wu et al., 2001; Lynch, 2004; Thomas and Huganir, 2004). Accordingly, these findings indicate that iron-induced, RyR-mediated, calcium release contributes to this activity-dependent neuronal response.

In summary, the current evidence suggests that crosstalk between ROS and calcium plays an essential role in many pathophysiological conditions including neurodegenerative diseases such as PD and AD. Here we complement this idea by adding the component of iron overload, and the ensuing oxidative stress, as a significant factor in promoting calcium dysregulation in neurodegeneration.

THE SYNERGISM BETWEEN IRON AND CALCIUM IN LIPID PEROXIDATION

A link between iron-mediated lipid peroxidation and calcium dyshomeostasis was reported more than 30 years ago. Peroxidation of rat brain synaptosomes by Fe^{2+} and

H_2O_2 generates rapid and large uptake of Ca^{2+} by isolated synaptosomes; Fe^{2+} also enhances Ca^{2+} uptake by spinal cord neurons in culture, an effect that is coupled to lipid peroxidation and the release of arachidonic acid from cells, in a process prevented by the iron chelator DFO (Braughler et al., 1985). The authors concluded that Fe^{2+} and Ca^{2+} act synergistically to produce lipid peroxidation and damage to neuronal membranes (Braughler et al., 1985). A further report proposed that this is not a direct effect of calcium but the result of independently initiated processes of lipid peroxidation and Ca^{2+} translocation, which interact subsequently in a synergistic manner (Bors et al., 1990).

The relationship between iron-induced lipid peroxidation and dysregulation of Ca^{2+}-ATPase is long-dated (Pelizzoni et al., 2008; Mata and Sepulveda, 2010; Zaidi, 2010). Plasma membrane lipid peroxidation initiated by the Fenton reaction results in increased calcium content, derived from the inhibition of the plasma membrane and ER Ca^{2+}-ATPases (Pereira et al., 1996). This inhibitory effect is shared by other radical species, in particular by peroxynitrite (Zaidi and Michaelis, 1999). Oxidants also inhibit SERCA activity while promoting calcium release from the ER (Gordeeva et al., 2003; Hidalgo and Donoso, 2008). Arguably, the observed upsurge in intracellular Ca^{+2} induced by iron-mediated lipid peroxidation could be compounded by an oxidant-induced loss of PMCA and SERCA activity, which combined with ROS-mediated activation of IP_3R/RyR channels would result in further and deleterious increases in the intracellular Ca^{2+} concentration.

IRON, CALCIUM, AND HIF-1 ACTIVITY

Considering the overlapping effects of iron and calcium on HIF-1 activity detailed above, a Fe/Ca bipartisan regulation of HIF-1 can be hypothesized (**Figure 1**). In neurodegenerative diseases with an iron accumulation component, decreased HIF-1 activity is predicted by a mechanism that involves the maintenance of maximal HIF-1 hydrolase activities and the increase of intracellular calcium mediated by dysregulation of redox-sensitive calcium homeostatic and signaling pathways. In neurons, decreased HIF-1 activity results in decreased neuroprotective, neuroregenerative, and antioxidant responses associated to HIF-1 activity (see above).

CALCIUM-INDUCED IRON DYSHOMEOSTASIS: POSSIBLE ROLE IN NEURODEGENERATION

Excessive intracellular calcium levels, such as those associated with neurodegenerative conditions, are likely to produce high H_2O_2 levels via NOX2 and to enhance mitochondrial calcium uptake and ROS production. These two ROS sources, NOX2, and mitochondria should affect jointly iron homeostasis by increasing the cellular labile iron pool, as occurs in SH-SY5Y cells exposed to H_2O_2 (Dev et al., 2015). These findings raise the possibility that conditions that increase postsynaptic calcium levels following NMDA receptor activation, which promote H_2O_2 generation in neocortical neurons via a cascade engaging the NOS and NOX2

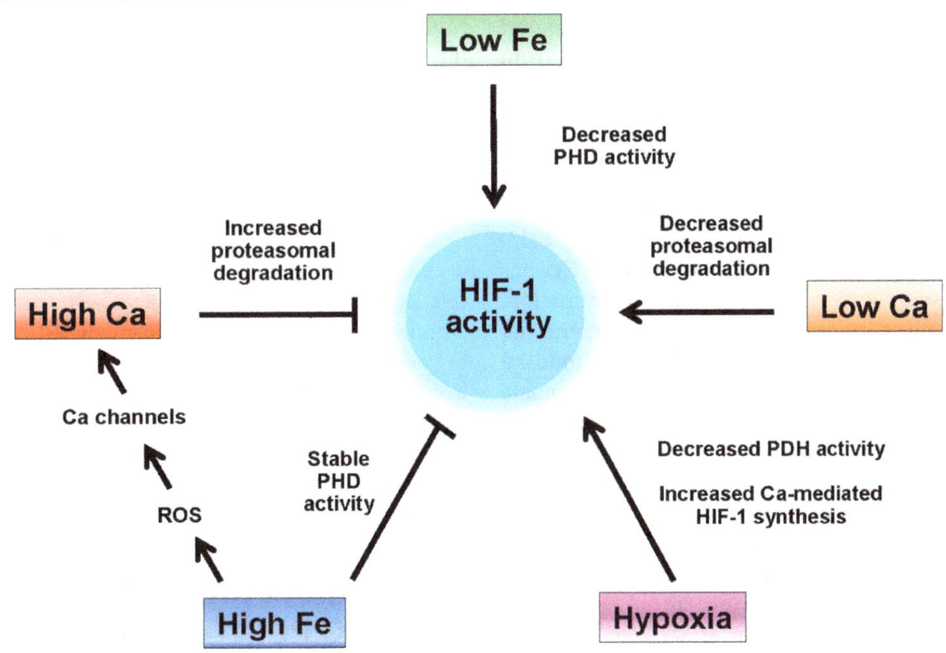

FIGURE 1 | Regulation of HIF-1 activity by iron and calcium. HIF-1 activity is induced by hypoxia, which decreases the activity of HIF-1 hydrolases (PHD), by low iron (e.g., iron chelation), which also decreases the activity of HIF-1 hydrolases, and by low intracellular calcium, which decreases the interaction of HIF-1α with the von-Hippel-Lindau protein (see text). High intracellular calcium levels increase the rate of HIF-1 proteasomal degradation while high levels of iron both maintain the activity of HIF-1 hydrolases and, through enhanced ROS production increase the cellular levels of calcium by activation of RyR, IP_3R, and L-type calcium channels.

enzymes (Girouard et al., 2009), may lead to an upsurge of the labile iron pool.

The role of voltage-gated Ca^{2+} channels as mediators of iron transport into neuronal cells is well established (Gaasch et al., 2007; Lockman et al., 2012). Another link between iron and calcium during neurodegeneration was provided by the observation that the hippocampal and nigral neuron loss induced by intra-cerebroventricular $FeCl_3$ injection in rats is largely prevented by pre-treatment with nicardipine, a blocker of L-type VGCCs (Bostanci and Bagirici, 2013). The authors concluded that these channels mediate the neurotoxic effects of extracellular iron by inducing either calcium and/or iron uptake. The question remains as to whether the protective effect of nicardipine is due to decreased iron influx, decreased calcium influx, or to a calcium-mediated process leading to neurodegeneration downstream of iron-induced oxidative stress. Other studies have also provided evidence of iron influx through NMDA receptors or voltage-operated calcium channels in primary hippocampal neurons (Pelizzoni et al., 2011) and the dopaminergic MES23.5 cell line (Wang et al., 2017).

THE MITOCHONDRION MELTING POT: CALCIUM, IRON, AND APOPTOTIC CELL DEATH

Mitochondria, by taking up and releasing calcium, act as important regulators of cellular calcium levels. The large mitochondrial membrane potential difference (negative inside) provides the driving force for calcium entry through the mitochondrial calcium uniporter (MCU), a component of the inner mitochondrial membrane; in physiological conditions, calcium antiporters rapidly extrude calcium from the mitochondria and restore the basal calcium levels (Giorgi et al., 2018). Mitochondrial calcium concentration modulates ATP production and mitochondrial metabolism, whereas mitochondrial calcium overload induced by deregulated intracellular calcium levels promotes apoptotic cell death, necrosis, and autophagy (Giorgi et al., 2012; Rimessi et al., 2013; Marchi et al., 2018). In pathological conditions, the MCU has been implicated in excitotoxicity, iron overload, inflammation, and oxidative stress-induced mitochondrial dysfunction and cell death (Liao et al., 2017). The ROS generated by mitochondrial enzymes or the electron transport chain presumably regulate diverse cellular physiological pathways, whereas dysregulated ROS generation may contribute to the development of human diseases (Angelova and Abramov, 2017).

Neurodegenerative disorders such as AD, PD, and ALS display dysregulation of calcium homeostasis and mitochondrial dysfunction; in addition, excitotoxicity leads to mitochondrial calcium overload and promotes necrotic or apoptotic-like excitotoxic cell death (Hansson Petersen et al., 2008; Rosales-Corral et al., 2012; Bose and Beal, 2016; Gibson and Thakkar, 2017; Giorgi et al., 2018). An increase in mitochondrial calcium is of particular importance in dopaminergic neurons, which are constantly exposed to calcium influx (Surmeier et al., 2011). The interaction between calcium overload and excessive ROS production (Chinopoulos and Adam-Vizi, 2006) causes further damage to the electron transport chain and promotes oxidative stress, which induces the oxidation of mitochondrial lipids, proteins, and DNA leading to cytotoxicity (Muravchick and Levy, 2006). The vicious cycle between calcium overload and oxidative stress favors the sustained opening of the mitochondrial permeability transition pore (mPTP), leading to the collapse of the mitochondrial membrane potential and mitochondrial swelling, which in turn promote the apoptotic response (Di Lisa and Bernardi, 2009). Opening of the mPTP has a central role in the pathogenesis of neurodegenerative disorders (Vila and Przedborski, 2003; Perier et al., 2005).

Excessive iron levels promote oxidative stress leading to the upsurge of unrestrained calcium signals that damage mitochondrial function. Iron accumulation in the cytoplasm induces excessive iron influx into mitochondria through mitoferrin1/2 (Paradkar et al., 2009), which causes mitochondrial dysfunction by increased ROS production leading to oxidative damage. Hence, if uncontrolled, this calcium/iron self-feeding cycle becomes deleterious to mitochondrial and neuronal function, leading eventually to neuronal death. In this regard, it is of note that, by preserving mitochondrial calcium homeostasis, the iron-binding protein lactoferrin protects vulnerable dopamine neurons from degeneration (Rousseau et al., 2013).

In primary hippocampal neurons, iron-induced stimulation of redox-sensitive RyR-mediated calcium release causes significant mitochondrial fragmentation (Sanmartin et al., 2014). Iron overload induces oxidative stress in the ER earlier than in the mitochondria, thereby increasing ER stress and calcium levels, and consequently causing mitochondrial fragmentation and neuronal cell death (Lee et al., 2016). Mitochondrial fragmentation presumably contributes to the impairment of neuronal function produced by iron overload, since inhibition of mitochondrial division protects neuronal cells from excitotoxicity (Ruiz et al., 2018). Moreover, iron overload of HT-22 hippocampal neuron cells increases intracellular calcium levels, causes mitochondrial fragmentation via dephosphorylation of Drp1, and increases apoptotic neuronal death; of note, calcium chelation and inhibition of calcineurin prevented mitochondrial fragmentation and cell death (Lee et al., 2016). Based on these findings, the authors suggested that calcium-mediated calcineurin signaling, by regulating mitochondrial dynamics, has a key role in iron-induced neurotoxicity.

In summary, mitochondrial calcium overload combined with excessive iron-mediated ROS generation and mPTP opening compose a cell death-inducing sequence implicated in neuronal dysfunction and neurodegeneration.

OXYTOSIS/FERROPTOSIS A POSSIBLE MEETING POINT FOR CALCIUM AND IRON-INDUCED CELL DEATH

Oxytosis was first described as a glutamate-induced, calcium-dependent form of cell death (Murphy et al., 1988). Initial studies on the molecular mechanisms of oxytosis pointed to a decrease in intracellular glutathione levels, enhanced mitochondrial ROS production, lipid peroxidation, and massive calcium influx as causes of death (Miyamoto et al., 1989). The mechanistic link between glutamate exposure and glutathione depletion was the inhibition of the cysteine/glutamate antiporter xc- by glutamate, which deprived cells of cystine, a precursor in glutamate synthesis (Murphy et al., 1989). As glutathione levels decrease, ROS levels increase exponentially (Tan et al., 1998), which gives rise to the activation of signaling pathways that culminate in large influx of calcium and cell death (Maher et al., 2018). Thus, the increased calcium influx is an essential mediator of the cell death program, as cells do not die in calcium-free medium.

Ferroptosis is a form of regulated cell death that occurs because of lethal lipid peroxidation. Ferroptotic cell death is blocked by iron chelators, lipophilic antioxidants, and by agents that block propagation of lipid peroxidation (Stockwell et al., 2017; Fricker et al., 2018). Ferroptosis is induced by inhibition of the cystine-glutamate antiporter xc- or by inhibition of glutathione peroxidase 4 (Gpx4). Induction of ferroptosis by erastin (an inhibitor of the antiporter xc-) results in cell death, which is morphologically characterized by mitochondrial shrinkage, with no overt signs of apoptosis or necrosis (Dixon et al., 2012). Ferroptotic death derives from depletion of cell glutathione, increased oxidative stress, and iron-mediated lipid peroxidation to lethal levels (Stockwell et al., 2017). Inhibition of Gpx4 also causes ferroptosis (Yang et al., 2014). Gpx4 is a lipid peroxidase that directly reduces phospholipid hydroperoxides at the expense of reduced glutathione. In mice, conditional deletion in forebrain neurons of Gpx4 resulted in hippocampal neurodegeneration and behavior dysfunction, associated with markers of ferroptosis such as elevated lipid peroxidation, ERK1/2 activation, and neuroinflammation (Hambright et al., 2017). Given the large similarity in their cell death mechanisms, the current view is that oxytosis and ferroptosis are similar forms of cell death (Fricker et al., 2018; Lewerenz et al., 2018; Maher et al., 2018).

Although a lethal influx of calcium is an intrinsic feature of oxytosis, the participation of calcium in ferroptosis is still poorly defined. Initial work by Dixon et al. (2012) revealed that calcium chelators do not inhibit erastin-induced HT-1080 cell death. Nevertheless, as mentioned above, an increase in cellular ROS levels enhances the activity of IP_3R and RyR calcium release channels and decreases the activity of both the PMCA and the SERCA calcium pumps. These effects increase cellular calcium levels by promoting calcium release from the ER while inhibiting its removal by the calcium pumps.

Lipid peroxidation-derived modification of some calcium channels could also be intermediates in ferroptotic death (Maher et al., 2018). In particular, 4-hydroxynonenal, a product of hydroxyl radical-mediated lipid peroxidation, induces the opening of NMDA receptor and VGCCs (Lu et al., 2002). Indeed,

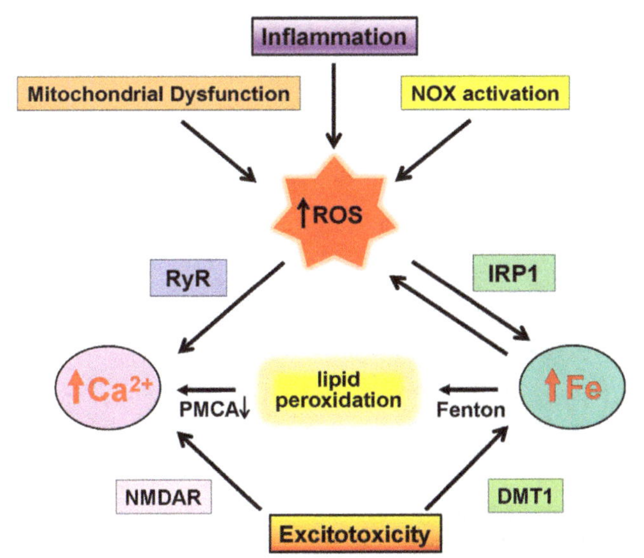

FIGURE 2 | Neuronal pathways that increase calcium and iron levels. Increases in ROS due to mitochondrial dysfunction, inflammation, and NOX activation promote excessive ROS generation that promotes calcium release via RyR channels and increases redox-active iron by IRP1 activation. Through the Fenton reaction, iron induces lipid peroxidation that inhibits the PMCA calcium pump. In addition, excitotoxic conditions over-activate NMDA receptors (NMDAR), which results in increased cytoplasmic calcium levels and increases iron levels via DMT1 activation.

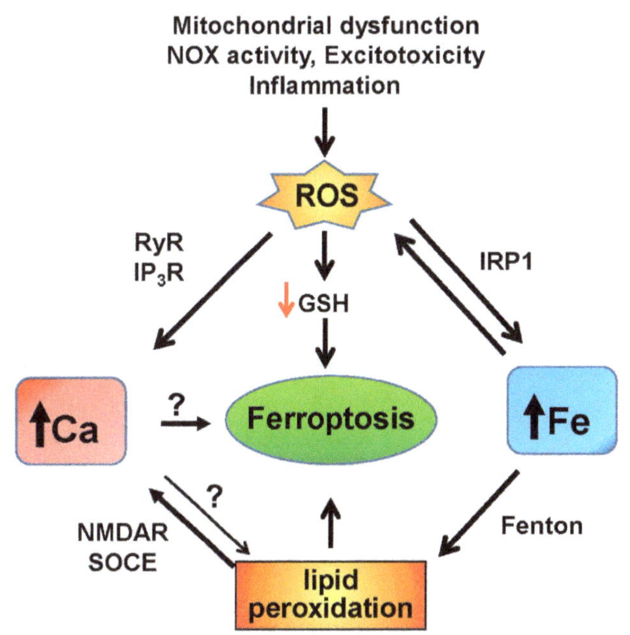

FIGURE 3 | Iron and calcium-mediated cell death by ferroptosis. Increases in ROS due to mitochondrial dysfunction, non-physiological activation of NOX, excitotoxicity, inflammation, or other factors result in the increase of redox-active iron mediated by activation of IRP1. Through the Fenton reaction, iron induces lipid peroxidation that activates NMDAR and the SOCE system, which results in increased cytoplasmic calcium. Increased iron levels and lipid peroxidation mediate ferroptotic cell death, which may also be induced by unregulated calcium levels. Increased ROS levels decrease the intracellular GSH content, leading to ferroptosis, and activate the intracellular calcium channels RyR and IP3R, which adds to the increase in cytoplasmic calcium caused by iron-induced lipid peroxidation.

the store-operated calcium entry (SOCE) system, which activates calcium influx channels in the plasma membrane upon the release of intracellular calcium from the ER participates in the neuronal death induced by MPP+, a Parkinsonian toxin that inhibits mitochondria electron transport chain complex I. Inhibition of the SOCE response decreased apoptotic cell death, reduced ROS production, and decreased lipid peroxidation induced by MPP+ (Li et al., 2013). In the same vein, a recent report shows that the pharmacological or transcriptional inhibition of SOCE proteins protects against oxidative glutamate toxicity and against MPP+ injury (Maher et al., 2018).

Overall, these results point to a possible participation of calcium in ferroptosis, a participation driven by raises in cytoplasmic calcium because of oxidative- and lipid peroxidation-derived modifications of the calcium homeostasis machinery (**Figure 3**). This participation may be specific to cells with weak antioxidant defenses, which could allow for the oxidative activation of calcium channels.

PROTECTION OF IRON OVERLOAD BY NRF2; THE CALCIUM CONNECTION

Under oxidative stress conditions, the transcription factor known as nuclear factor (erythroid-derived 2)-like 2 (Nrf2) directs the expression of a large array of cytoprotective genes (Tonelli et al., 2018). In particular, Nrf2 protects cells from the injurious effects of iron overload by regulating the expression of genes involved in iron storage and iron export (Chorley et al., 2012; Kerins and Ooi, 2018). These findings raise the possibility that Nrf2 may counteract the oxidative stress induced in neuronal cells by iron overload. Thus, Nrf2 may restore the intracellular labile iron pool by inducing the expression of the iron exporter FPN1 and ferritin, which oxidizes Fe^{2+} to Fe^{3+} and stores it within its structure making it unavailable for the Fenton reaction (Orino et al., 2001). In addition, intracellular iron levels act as a link between HIF-1α and Nrf2: Nrf2-induced ferritin upregulation activates HIF-1α by making iron unavailable to HIF prolyl-hydroxylase (Siegert et al., 2015), whereas Nrf2 inhibition results in decreased activation of HIF-1α by hypoxia (Kim et al., 2011; Ji et al., 2014).

Recent studies point to a connection between ROS, cellular calcium signals, and Nrf2. The neurotrophin BDNF, besides inducing complex neuronal signaling cascades underlying synaptic plasticity (Bolton et al., 2000), also induces neuronal antioxidant responses through BDNF-induced Nrf2 nuclear translocation (Bouvier et al., 2017; Bruna et al., 2018). In this regard, a recent study showed that BDNF-mediated activation of Nrf2 in astrocytes, which is under circadian control, protects dopaminergic neurons from ferroptosis (Ishii et al., 2018). Of note, in primary hippocampal neurons, ROS and RyR-mediated calcium signals are required for BDNF-induced nuclear translocation of Nrf2 (Bruna et al., 2018). It remains to be established if iron overload in hippocampal neurons engages BDNF and RyR-mediated calcium signals to promote Nrf2-induced expression of protective genes.

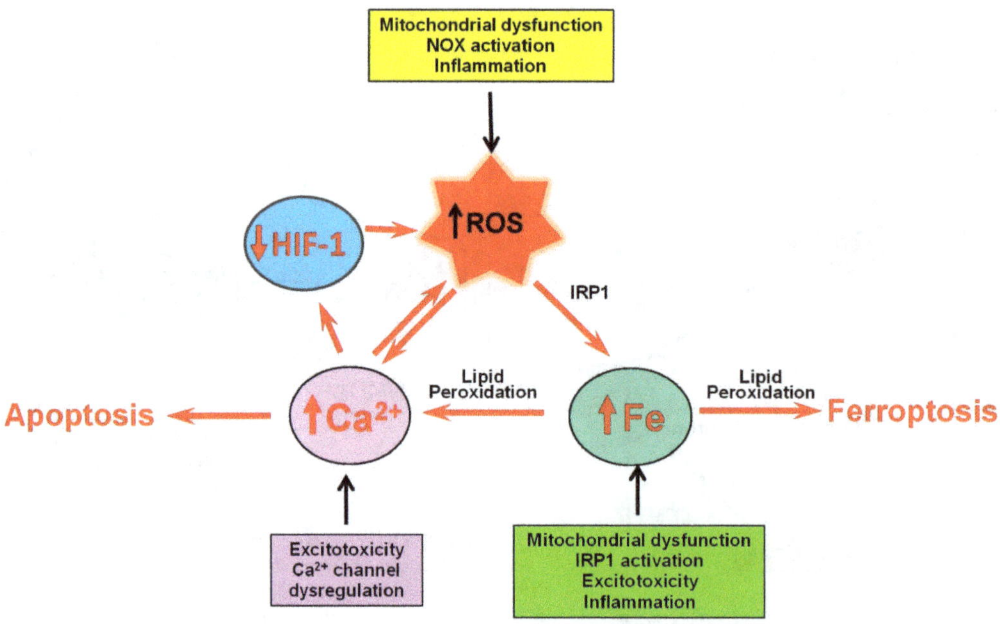

FIGURE 4 | The self-feeding cycle ROS–Fe–Ca. Mitochondrial dysfunction promotes in increased ROS and activation IRP1, which results in increased iron accumulation. Excess iron promotes lipid peroxidation by hydroxyl radicals derived from the Fenton reaction. Lipid peroxidation modifies the activity of a variety of proteins involved in calcium homeostasis that results in massive calcium influx. Increased cytoplasmic calcium levels result in increased mitochondrial calcium and accentuated mitochondrial dysfunction, oxidative stress, and damage. If uncontrolled, this ROS–iron–calcium self-feeding cycle becomes deleterious to mitochondrial and neuronal function, leading eventually to apoptotic or ferroptotic cell death. In yet another aspect of this cycle, high intracellular calcium levels increase the rate of HIF-1 proteasome degradation, which results in increased ROS levels, product of decreased expression of antioxidant proteins.

CONCLUSION

This article reviews the little acknowledged relationship between iron and calcium in neurodegeneration. The main premise of this article is that increased ROS production generated by iron accumulation profoundly influences calcium homeostasis and signaling (**Figure 4**).

The influence of increased ROS is clearly shown in the process of oxytosis, in which lipid peroxidation initiated by Fenton-derived hydroxyl radicals results in the modification of a variety of proteins involved in calcium homeostasis that brings to calcium upsurges and cell death. Increased cytoplasmic calcium levels caused by iron dysregulation result in increased mitochondrial calcium and accentuated oxidative stress and damage. If uncontrolled, this calcium/iron self-feeding cycle becomes deleterious to mitochondrial and neuronal function, leading eventually to neuronal death. In yet another aspect of neurodegeneration, high intracellular calcium levels increase the rate of HIF-1 proteasomal degradation while high levels of iron both maintain the activity of HIF-1 hydrolases and, through oxidative stress increase the cellular levels of calcium by activation of ER and PMCA channels. The main conclusion we draw from this review is that dysregulated iron or calcium levels promote deleterious crosstalk between iron and calcium that can result in neuronal dysfunction and death. To our knowledge, this is the first attempt in literature to systemize this important relationship.

AUTHOR CONTRIBUTIONS

MN and CH wrote this article.

FUNDING

This work was supported by FONDEF project 17I10095 from the National Commission of Science and Technology (CONICYT) of Chile; Fondo Nacional de Desarrollo Científico y Tecnológico (FONDECYT; Grants Nos. 1170053 and 11140580), and by Biomedical Neuroscience Institute (Grant No. BNI P09-015-F).

REFERENCES

Alzheimer's Association Calcium Hypothesis Workgroup [AACHW] (2017). Calcium hypothesis of Alzheimer's disease and brain aging: a framework for integrating new evidence into a comprehensive theory of pathogenesis. *Alzheimers Dement.* 13, 178.e17–182.e17. doi: 10.1016/j.jalz.2016.12.006

An, H., Zeng, X., Niu, T., Li, G., Yang, J., Zheng, L., et al. (2018). Quantifying iron deposition within the substantia nigra of Parkinson's disease by quantitative susceptibility mapping. *J. Neurol. Sci.* 386, 46–52. doi: 10.1016/j.jns.2018.01.008

Angelova, P. R., and Abramov, A. Y. (2017). Alpha-synuclein and beta-amyloid - different targets, same players: calcium, free radicals and mitochondria in the mechanism of neurodegeneration. *Biochem. Biophys. Res. Commun.* 483, 1110–1115. doi: 10.1016/j.bbrc.2016.07.103

Ansari, M. A., and Scheff, S. W. (2011). NADPH-oxidase activation and cognition in Alzheimer disease progression. *Free Radic. Biol. Med.* 51, 171–178. doi: 10.1016/j.freeradbiomed.2011.03.025

Area-Gomez, E., and Schon, E. A. (2017). On the pathogenesis of Alzheimer's Disease: the MAM hypothesis. *FASEB J.* 31, 864–867. doi: 10.1096/fj.201601309

Arruda, S. F., Siqueira, E. M., and De Valencia, F. F. (2009). Vitamin A deficiency increases hepcidin expression and oxidative stress in rat. *Nutrition* 25, 472–478. doi: 10.1016/j.nut.2008.11.030

Asiimwe, N., Yeo, S. G., Kim, M. S., Jung, J., and Jeong, N. Y. (2016). Nitric oxide: exploring the contextual link with alzheimer's disease. *Oxid. Med. Cell. Longev.* 2016:7205747. doi: 10.1155/2016/7205747

Bading, H. (2013). Nuclear calcium signalling in the regulation of brain function. *Nat. Rev. Neurosci.* 14, 593–608. doi: 10.1038/nrn3531

Barrett, J. P., Henry, R. J., Villapol, S., Stoica, B. A., Kumar, A., Burns, M. P., et al. (2017). NOX2 deficiency alters macrophage phenotype through an IL-10/STAT3 dependent mechanism: implications for traumatic brain injury. *J. Neuroinflammation* 14:65. doi: 10.1186/s12974-017-0843-4

Baumgartel, K., and Mansuy, I. M. (2012). Neural functions of calcineurin in synaptic plasticity and memory. *Learn. Mem.* 19, 375–384. doi: 10.1101/lm.027201.112

Becerril-Ortega, J., Bordji, K., Freret, T., Rush, T., and Buisson, A. (2014). Iron overload accelerates neuronal amyloid-beta production and cognitive impairment in transgenic mice model of Alzheimer's disease. *Neurobiol. Aging* 35, 2288–2301. doi: 10.1016/j.neurobiolaging.2014.04.019

Berchner-Pfannschmidt, U., Petrat, F., Doege, K., Trinidad, B., Freitag, P., Metzen, E., et al. (2004). Chelation of cellular calcium modulates hypoxia-inducible gene expression through activation of hypoxia-inducible factor-1alpha. *J. Biol. Chem.* 279, 44976–44986. doi: 10.1074/jbc.M313995200

Berg, D., and Youdim, M. B. (2006). Role of iron in neurodegenerative disorders. *Top. Magn. Reson. Imaging* 17, 5–17. doi: 10.1097/01.rmr.0000245461.90406.ad

Berridge, M. J. (1998). Neuronal calcium signaling. *Neuron* 21, 13–26. doi: 10.1016/S0896-6273(00)80510-3

Berridge, M. J., Bootman, M. D. and Roderick, H. L. (2003). Calcium signalling: dynamics, homeostasis and remodelling. *Nat. Rev. Mol. Cell Biol.* 4, 517–529. doi: 10.1038/nrm1155

Berrocal, M., Corbacho, I., Vazquez-Hernandez, M., Avila, J., Sepulveda, M. R., and Mata, A. M. (2015). Inhibition of PMCA activity by tau as a function of aging and Alzheimer's neuropathology. *Biochim. Biophys. Acta* 1852, 1465–1476. doi: 10.1016/j.bbadis.2015.04.007

Bezprozvanny, I., and Mattson, M. P. (2008). Neuronal calcium mishandling and the pathogenesis of Alzheimer's disease. *Trends Neurosci.* 31, 454–463. doi: 10.1016/j.tins.2008.06.005

Bindokas, V. P., Jordan, J., Lee, C. C., and Miller, R. J. (1996). Superoxide production in rat hippocampal neurons: selective imaging with hydroethidine. *J. Neurosci.* 16, 1324–1336. doi: 10.1523/JNEUROSCI.16-04-01324.1996

Bolton, M. M., Pittman, A. J., and Lo, D. C. (2000). Brain-derived neurotrophic factor differentially regulates excitatory and inhibitory synaptic transmission in hippocampal cultures. *J. Neurosci.* 20, 3221–3232. doi: 10.1523/JNEUROSCI.20-09-03221.2000

Bors, W., Buettner, G. R., Michel, C., and Saran, M. (1990). Calcium in lipid peroxidation: does calcium interact with superoxide? *Arch. Biochem. Biophys.* 278, 269–272. doi: 10.1016/0003-9861(90)90258-Z

Bose, A., and Beal, M. F. (2016). Mitochondrial dysfunction in Parkinson's disease. *J. Neurochem.* 139(Suppl. 1), 216–231. doi: 10.1111/jnc.13731

Bostanci, M. O., and Bagirici, F. (2013). Blocking of L-type calcium channels protects hippocampal and nigral neurons against iron neurotoxicity. The role of L-type calcium channels in iron-induced neurotoxicity. *Int. J. Neurosci.* 123, 876–882. doi: 10.3109/00207454.2013.813510

Bouvier, E., Brouillard, F., Molet, J., Claverie, D., Cabungcal, J. H., Cresto, N., et al. (2017). Nrf2-dependent persistent oxidative stress results in stress-induced vulnerability to depression. *Mol. Psychiatry* 22, 1701–1713. doi: 10.1038/mp.2016.211

Braughler, J. M., Duncan, L. A., and Chase, R. L. (1985). Interaction of lipid peroxidation and calcium in the pathogenesis of neuronal injury. *Cent. Nerv. Syst. Trauma* 2, 269–283. doi: 10.1089/cns.1985.2.269

Brennan, A. M., Suh, S. W., Won, S. J., Narasimhan, P., Kauppinen, T. M., Lee, H., et al. (2009). NADPH oxidase is the primary source of superoxide induced by NMDA receptor activation. *Nat. Neurosci.* 12, 857–863. doi: 10.1038/nn.2334

Brini, M., Cali, T., Ottolini, D., and Carafoli, E. (2014). Neuronal calcium signaling: function and dysfunction. *Cell. Mol. Life Sci.* 71, 2787–2814. doi: 10.1007/s00018-013-1550-7

Brini, M., Leanza, L., and Szabo, I. (2017). Lipid-mediated modulation of intracellular ion channels and redox state: physiopathological implications. *Antioxid. Redox Signal.* doi: 10.1089/ars.2017.7215 [Epub ahead of print].

Bruick, R. K., and McKnight, S. L. (2001). A conserved family of prolyl-4-hydroxylases that modify HIF. *Science* 294, 1337–1340. doi: 10.1126/science.1066373

Bruna, B., Lobos, P., Herrera-Molina, R., Hidalgo, C., Paula-Lima, A., and Adasme, T. (2018). The signaling pathways underlying BDNF-induced Nrf2 hippocampal nuclear translocation involve ROS, RyR-Mediated Ca(2+) signals, ERK and PI3K. *Biochem. Biophys. Res. Commun.* 505, 201–207. doi: 10.1016/j.bbrc.2018.09.080

Bulk, M., Van Der Weerd, L., Breimer, W., Lebedev, N., Webb, A., Goeman, J. J., et al. (2018). Quantitative comparison of different iron forms in the temporal cortex of Alzheimer patients and control subjects. *Sci. Rep.* 8:6898. doi: 10.1038/s41598-018-25021-7

Burbulla, L. F., Song, P., Mazzulli, J. R., Zampese, E., Wong, Y. C., Jeon, S., et al. (2017). Dopamine oxidation mediates mitochondrial and lysosomal dysfunction in Parkinson's disease. *Science* 357, 1255–1261. doi: 10.1126/science.aam9080

Cabantchik, Z. I. (2014). Labile iron in cells and body fluids: physiology, pathology, and pharmacology. *Front. Pharmacol.* 5:45. doi: 10.3389/fphar.2014.00045

Caltagirone, A., Weiss, G., and Pantopoulos, K. (2001). Modulation of cellular iron metabolism by hydrogen peroxide. Effects of H2O2 on the expression and function of iron-responsive element-containing mRNAs in B6 fibroblasts. *J. Biol. Chem.* 276, 19738–19745. doi: 10.1074/jbc.M100245200

Cannon, J. R., Tapias, V., Na, H. M., Honick, A. S., Drolet, R. E., and Greenamyre, J. T. (2009). A highly reproducible rotenone model of Parkinson's disease. *Neurobiol. Dis.* 34, 279–290. doi: 10.1016/j.nbd.2009.01.016

Carocci, A., Catalano, A., Sinicropi, M. S., and Genchi, G. (2018). Oxidative stress and neurodegeneration: the involvement of iron. *Biometals* 31, 715–735. doi: 10.1007/s10534-018-0126-2

Chan, C. S., Gertler, T. S., and Surmeier, D. J. (2009). Calcium homeostasis, selective vulnerability and Parkinson's disease. *Trends Neurosci.* 32, 249–256. doi: 10.1016/j.tins.2009.01.006

Cheah, J. H., Kim, S. F., Hester, L. D., Clancy, K. W., Patterson, S. E. III, Papadopoulos, V., et al. (2006). NMDA receptor-nitric oxide transmission mediates neuronal iron homeostasis via the GTPase Dexras1. *Neuron* 51, 431–440. doi: 10.1016/j.neuron.2006.07.011

Chinopoulos, C., and Adam-Vizi, V. (2006). Calcium, mitochondria and oxidative stress in neuronal pathology. Novel aspects of an enduring theme. *FEBS J.* 273, 433–450. doi: 10.1111/j.1742-4658.2005.05103.x

Chorley, B. N., Campbell, M. R., Wang, X., Karaca, M., Sambandan, D., Bangura, F., et al. (2012). Identification of novel NRF2-regulated genes by ChIP-Seq: influence on retinoid X receptor alpha. *Nucleic Acids Res.* 40, 7416–7429. doi: 10.1093/nar/gks409

Clapham, D. E. (2007). Calcium signaling. *Cell* 131, 1047–1058. doi: 10.1016/j.cell.2007.11.028

Cobley, J. N., Fiorello, M. L., and Bailey, D. M. (2018). 13 reasons why the brain is susceptible to oxidative stress. *Redox Biol.* 15, 490–503. doi: 10.1016/j.redox.2018.01.008

Creighton-Gutteridge, M., and Tyrrell, R. M. (2002). A novel iron chelator that does not induce HIF-1 activity. *Free Radic. Biol. Med.* 33, 356–363. doi: 10.1016/S0891-5849(02)00884-5

Crichton, R. R., Dexter, D. T., and Ward, R. J. (2011). Brain iron metabolism and its perturbation in neurological diseases. *J. Neural Transm.* 118, 301–314. doi: 10.1007/s00702-010-0470-z

Cristovao, J. S., Santos, R., and Gomes, C. M. (2016). Metals and neuronal metal binding proteins implicated in Alzheimer's Disease. *Oxid. Med. Cell. Longev.* 2016:9812178. doi: 10.1155/2016/9812178

Damasceno, F. C., Condeles, A. L., Lopes, A. K. B., Facci, R. R., Linares, E., Truzzi, D. R., et al. (2018). The labile iron pool attenuates peroxynitrite-dependent damage and can no longer be considered solely a pro-oxidative cellular iron source. *J. Biol. Chem.* 293, 8530–8542. doi: 10.1074/jbc.RA117.000883

Davies, M. J. (2005). The oxidative environment and protein damage. *Biochim. Biophys. Acta* 1703, 93–109. doi: 10.1016/j.bbapap.2004.08.007

Demuro, A., Parker, I., and Stutzmann, G. E. (2010). Calcium signaling and amyloid toxicity in Alzheimer disease. *J. Biol. Chem.* 285, 12463–12468. doi: 10.1074/jbc.R109.080895

Dev, S., Kumari, S., Singh, N., Kumar Bal, S., Seth, P., and Mukhopadhyay, C. K. (2015). Role of extracellular hydrogen peroxide in regulation of iron homeostasis genes in neuronal cells: implication in iron accumulation. *Free Radic. Biol. Med.* 86, 78–89. doi: 10.1016/j.freeradbiomed.2015.05.025

Di Lisa, F., and Bernardi, P. (2009). A CaPful of mechanisms regulating the mitochondrial permeability transition. *J. Mol. Cell Cardiol.* 46, 775–780. doi: 10.1016/j.yjmcc.2009.03.006

DiSabato, D. J., Quan, N., and Godbout, J. P. (2016). Neuroinflammation: the devil is in the details. *J. Neurochem.* 139(Suppl. 2), 136–153. doi: 10.1111/jnc.13607

Dixon, S. J., Lemberg, K. M., Lamprecht, M. R., Skouta, R., Zaitsev, E. M., Gleason, C. E., et al. (2012). Ferroptosis: an iron-dependent form of nonapoptotic cell death. *Cell* 149, 1060–1072. doi: 10.1016/j.cell.2012.03.042

Dixon, S. J., and Stockwell, B. R. (2014). The role of iron and reactive oxygen species in cell death. *Nat. Chem. Biol.* 10, 9–17. doi: 10.1038/nchembio.1416

Drapier, J. C., Hirling, H., Wietzerbin, J., Kaldy, P., and Kuhn, L. C. (1993). Biosynthesis of nitric oxide activates iron regulatory factor in macrophages. *EMBO J.* 12, 3643–3649. doi: 10.1002/j.1460-2075.1993.tb06038.x

Duncan, A. J., and Heales, S. J. (2005). Nitric oxide and neurological disorders. *Mol. Aspects Med.* 26, 67–96. doi: 10.1016/j.mam.2004.09.004

Flagg, S. C., Martin, C. B., Taabazuing, C. Y., Holmes, B. E., and Knapp, M. J. (2012). Screening chelating inhibitors of HIF-prolyl hydroxylase domain 2 (PHD2) and factor inhibiting HIF (FIH). *J. Inorg. Biochem.* 113, 25–30. doi: 10.1016/j.jinorgbio.2012.03.002

Franco-Iborra, S., Vila, M., and Perier, C. (2018). Mitochondrial quality control in neurodegenerative diseases: focus on parkinson's disease and huntington's disease. *Front. Neurosci.* 12:342. doi: 10.3389/fnins.2018.00342

Fricker, M., Tolkovsky, A. M., Borutaite, V., Coleman, M., and Brown, G. C. (2018). Neuronal cell death. *Physiol. Rev.* 98, 813–880. doi: 10.1152/physrev.00011.2017

Fukui, K. (2016). Reactive oxygen species induce neurite degeneration before induction of cell death. *J. Clin. Biochem. Nutr.* 59, 155–159. doi: 10.3164/jcbn.16-34

Gaasch, J. A., Geldenhuys, W. J., Lockman, P. R., Allen, D. D., and Van Der Schyf, C. J. (2007). Voltage-gated calcium channels provide an alternate route for iron uptake in neuronal cell cultures. *Neurochem. Res.* 32, 1686–1693. doi: 10.1007/s11064-007-9313-1

Gao, H. M., Zhou, H., and Hong, J. S. (2012). NADPH oxidases: novel therapeutic targets for neurodegenerative diseases. *Trends Pharmacol. Sci.* 33, 295–303. doi: 10.1016/j.tips.2012.03.008

Garrick, M. D., Singleton, S. T., Vargas, F., Kuo, H. C., Zhao, L., Knopfel, M., et al. (2006). DMT1: which metals does it transport? *Biol. Res.* 39, 79–85. doi: 10.4067/S0716-97602006000100009

Ghosh, D. K., and Salerno, J. C. (2003). Nitric oxide synthases: domain structure and alignment in enzyme function and control. *Front. Biosci.* 8, D193–D209. doi: 10.2741/959

Gibson, G. E., and Thakkar, A. (2017). Interactions of mitochondria/metabolism and calcium regulation in alzheimer's disease: a calcinist point of view. *Neurochem. Res.* 42, 1636–1648. doi: 10.1007/s11064-017-2182-3

Giorgi, C., Baldassari, F., Bononi, A., Bonora, M., De Marchi, E., Marchi, S., et al. (2012). Mitochondrial Ca(2+) and apoptosis. *Cell Calcium* 52, 36–43. doi: 10.1016/j.ceca.2012.02.008

Giorgi, C., Marchi, S., and Pinton, P. (2018). The machineries, regulation and cellular functions of mitochondrial calcium. *Nat. Rev. Mol. Cell Biol.* 19, 713–730. doi: 10.1038/s41580-018-0052-8

Girouard, H., Wang, G., Gallo, E. F., Anrather, J., Zhou, P., Pickel, V. M., et al. (2009). NMDA receptor activation increases free radical production through nitric oxide and NOX2. *J. Neurosci.* 29, 2545–2552. doi: 10.1523/JNEUROSCI.0133-09.2009

Gonsette, R. E. (2008). Neurodegeneration in multiple sclerosis: the role of oxidative stress and excitotoxicity. *J. Neurol. Sci.* 274, 48–53. doi: 10.1016/j.jns.2008.06.029

Gordeeva, A. V., Zvyagilskaya, R. A., and Labas, Y. A. (2003). Cross-talk between reactive oxygen species and calcium in living cells. *Biochemistry* 68, 1077–1080.

Gorlach, A., Bertram, K., Hudecova, S., and Krizanova, O. (2015). Calcium and ROS: a mutual interplay. *Redox Biol.* 6, 260–271. doi: 10.1016/j.redox.2015.08.010

Green, S. P., Cairns, B., Rae, J., Errett-Baroncini, C., Hongo, J. A., Erickson, R. W., et al. (2001). Induction of gp91-phox, a component of the phagocyte NADPH oxidase, in microglial cells during central nervous system inflammation. *J. Cereb. Blood Flow Metab.* 21, 374–384. doi: 10.1097/00004647-200104000-00006

Grosskreutz, J., Van Den Bosch, L., and Keller, B. U. (2010). Calcium dysregulation in amyotrophic lateral sclerosis. *Cell Calcium* 47, 165–174. doi: 10.1016/j.ceca.2009.12.002

Guo, C., Hao, L. J., Yang, Z. H., Chai, R., Zhang, S., Gu, Y., et al. (2016). Deferoxamine-mediated up-regulation of HIF-1alpha prevents dopaminergic neuronal death via the activation of MAPK family proteins in MPTP-treated mice. *Exp. Neurol.* 280, 13–23. doi: 10.1016/j.expneurol.2016.03.016

Guo, C., Zhang, Y. X., Wang, T., Zhong, M. L., Yang, Z. H., Hao, L. J., et al. (2015). Intranasal deferoxamine attenuates synapse loss via up-regulating the P38/HIF-1alpha pathway on the brain of APP/PS1 transgenic mice. *Front. Aging Neurosci.* 7:104. doi: 10.3389/fnagi.2015.00104

Guo, J. D., Zhao, X., Li, Y., Li, G. R., and Liu, X. L. (2018). Damage to dopaminergic neurons by oxidative stress in Parkinson's disease (Review). *Int. J. Mol. Med.* 41, 1817–1825. doi: 10.3892/ijmm.2018.3406

Guzman, J. N., Sanchez-Padilla, J., Chan, C. S., and Surmeier, D. J. (2009). Robust pacemaking in substantia nigra dopaminergic neurons. *J. Neurosci.* 29, 11011–11019. doi: 10.1523/JNEUROSCI.2519-09.2009

Hajieva, P., Baeken, M. W., and Moosmann, B. (2018). The role of plasma membrane calcium atpases (PMCAS) in neurodegenerative disorders. *Neurosci. Lett.* 663, 29–38. doi: 10.1016/j.neulet.2017.09.033

Halliwell, B. (2006). Oxidative stress and neurodegeneration: where are we now? *J. Neurochem.* 97, 1634–1658. doi: 10.1111/j.1471-4159.2006.03907.x

Hambright, W. S., Fonseca, R. S., Chen, L., Na, R., and Ran, Q. (2017). Ablation of ferroptosis regulator glutathione peroxidase 4 in forebrain neurons promotes cognitive impairment and neurodegeneration. *Redox Biol.* 12, 8–17. doi: 10.1016/j.redox.2017.01.021

Hanke, M. L., and Kielian, T. (2011). Toll-like receptors in health and disease in the brain: mechanisms and therapeutic potential. *Clin. Sci.* 121, 367–387. doi: 10.1042/CS20110164

Hanson, E. S., and Leibold, E. A. (1999). Regulation of the iron regulatory proteins by reactive nitrogen and oxygen species. *Gene Expr.* 7, 367–376.

Hansson Petersen, C. A., Alikhani, N., Behbahani, H., Wiehager, B., Pavlov, P. F., Alafuzoff, I., et al. (2008). The amyloid beta-peptide is imported into mitochondria via the TOM import machinery and localized to mitochondrial cristae. *Proc. Natl. Acad. Sci. U.S.A.* 105, 13145–13150. doi: 10.1073/pnas.0806192105

Hepp, S., Gerich, F. J., and Muller, M. (2005). Sulfhydryl oxidation reduces hippocampal susceptibility to hypoxia-induced spreading depression by activating BK channels. *J. Neurophysiol.* 94, 1091–1103. doi: 10.1152/jn.00291.2005

Hewitson, K. S., Mcneill, L. A., Elkins, J. M., and Schofield, C. J. (2003). The role of iron and 2-oxoglutarate oxygenases in signalling. *Biochem. Soc. Trans.* 31, 510–515. doi: 10.1042/bst0310510

Hidalgo, C., and Arias-Cavieres, A. (2016). Calcium, reactive oxygen species, and synaptic plasticity. *Physiology* 31, 201–215. doi: 10.1152/physiol.00038.2015

Hidalgo, C., Carrasco, M. A., Muñoz, P., and Núñez, M. T. (2007). A role for reactive oxygen/nitrogen species and iron on neuronal synaptic plasticity. *Antioxid. Redox. Signal.* 9, 245–255. doi: 10.1089/ars.2007.9.245

Hidalgo, C., and Donoso, P. (2008). Crosstalk between calcium and redox signaling: from molecular mechanisms to health implications. *Antioxid. Redox Signal.* 10, 1275–1312. doi: 10.1089/ars.2007.1886

Hidalgo, C., and Núñez, M. T. (2007). Calcium, iron and neuronal function. *IUBMB Life* 59, 280–285. doi: 10.1080/15216540701222906

Huang, M. L., Lane, D. J., and Richardson, D. R. (2011). Mitochondrial mayhem: the mitochondrion as a modulator of iron metabolism and its role in disease. *Antioxid. Redox Signal.* 15, 3003–3019. doi: 10.1089/ars.2011.3921

Huang, X., Atwood, C. S., Hartshorn, M. A., Multhaup, G., Goldstein, L. E., Scarpa, R. C., et al. (1999). The A beta peptide of Alzheimer's disease directly produces hydrogen peroxide through metal ion reduction. *Biochemistry* 38, 7609–7616. doi: 10.1021/bi990438f

Ishii, T., Warabi, E., and Mann, G. E. (2018). Circadian control of BDNF-mediated Nrf2 activation in astrocytes protects dopaminergic neurons from ferroptosis. *Free Radic. Biol. Med.* doi: 10.1016/j.freeradbiomed.2018.09.002 [Epub ahead of print].

Jaiswal, M. K. (2013). Calcium, mitochondria, and the pathogenesis of ALS: the good, the bad, and the ugly. *Front. Cell. Neurosci.* 7:199. doi: 10.3389/fncel.2013.00199

Jellinger, K. A. (1999). The role of iron in neurodegeneration: prospects for pharmacotherapy of Parkinson's disease. *Drugs Aging* 14, 115–140. doi: 10.2165/00002512-199914020-00004

Jeney, V., Balla, J., Yachie, A., Varga, Z., Vercellotti, G. M., Eaton, J. W., et al. (2002). Pro-oxidant and cytotoxic effects of circulating heme. *Blood* 100, 879–887. doi: 10.1182/blood.V100.3.879

Jeong, S. Y., Rathore, K. I., Schulz, K., Ponka, P., Arosio, P., and David, S. (2009). Dysregulation of iron homeostasis in the CNS contributes to disease progression in a mouse model of amyotrophic lateral sclerosis. *J. Neurosci.* 29, 610–619. doi: 10.1523/JNEUROSCI.5443-08.2009

Ji, X., Wang, H., Zhu, J., Zhu, L., Pan, H., Li, W., et al. (2014). Knockdown of Nrf2 suppresses glioblastoma angiogenesis by inhibiting hypoxia-induced activation of HIF-1alpha. *Int. J. Cancer* 135, 574–584. doi: 10.1002/ijc.28699

Jiang, L., Bechtel, M. D., Galeva, N. A., Williams, T. D., Michaelis, E. K., and Michaelis, M. L. (2012). Decreases in plasma membrane Ca(2)(+)-ATPase in brain synaptic membrane rafts from aged rats. *J. Neurochem.* 123, 689–699. doi: 10.1111/j.1471-4159.2012.07918.x

Joseph, S. K., Young, M. P., Alzayady, K., Yule, D. I., Ali, M., Booth, D. M., et al. (2018). Redox regulation of type-I inositol trisphosphate receptors in intact mammalian cells. *J. Biol. Chem.* 293, 17464–17476. doi: 10.1074/jbc.RA118.005624

Kahlert, S., Zundorf, G., and Reiser, G. (2005). Glutamate-mediated influx of extracellular Ca2+ is coupled with reactive oxygen species generation in cultured hippocampal neurons but not in astrocytes. *J. Neurosci. Res.* 79, 262–271. doi: 10.1002/jnr.20322

Kasarskis, E. J., Tandon, L., Lovell, M. A., and Ehmann, W. D. (1995). Aluminum, calcium, and iron in the spinal cord of patients with sporadic amyotrophic lateral sclerosis using laser microprobe mass spectroscopy: a preliminary study. *J. Neurol. Sci.* 130, 203–208. doi: 10.1016/0022-510X(95)00037-3

Kastanenka, K. V., Bussiere, T., Shakerdge, N., Qian, F., Weinreb, P. H., Rhodes, K., et al. (2016). Immunotherapy with aducanumab restores calcium homeostasis in Tg2576 Mice. *J. Neurosci.* 36, 12549–12558. doi: 10.1523/JNEUROSCI.2080-16.2016

Kerins, M. J., and Ooi, A. (2018). The roles of NRF2 in modulating cellular iron homeostasis. *Antioxid. Redox Signal.* 29, 1756–1773. doi: 10.1089/ars.2017.7176

Kietzmann, T., Knabe, W., and Schmidt-Kastner, R. (2001). Hypoxia and hypoxia-inducible factor modulated gene expression in brain: involvement in neuroprotection and cell death. *Eur. Arch. Psychiatry Clin. Neurosci.* 251, 170–178. doi: 10.1007/s004060170037

Kim, T. H., Hur, E. G., Kang, S. J., Kim, J. A., Thapa, D., Lee, Y. M., et al. (2011). NRF2 blockade suppresses colon tumor angiogenesis by inhibiting hypoxia-induced activation of HIF-1alpha. *Cancer Res.* 71, 2260–2275. doi: 10.1158/0008-5472.CAN-10-3007

Kishida, K. T., and Klann, E. (2007). Sources and targets of reactive oxygen species in synaptic plasticity and memory. *Antioxid. Redox Signal.* 9, 233–244. doi: 10.1089/ars.2007.9.233

Kupershmidt, L., Weinreb, O., Amit, T., Mandel, S., Bar-Am, O., and Youdim, M. B. (2011). Novel molecular targets of the neuroprotective/neurorescue multimodal iron chelating drug M30 in the mouse brain. *Neuroscience* 189, 345–358. doi: 10.1016/j.neuroscience.2011.03.040

Kupershmidt, L., Weinreb, O., Amit, T., Mandel, S., Carri, M. T., and Youdim, M. B. (2009). Neuroprotective and neuritogenic activities of novel multimodal iron-chelating drugs in motor-neuron-like NSC-34 cells and transgenic mouse model of amyotrophic lateral sclerosis. *FASEB J.* 23, 3766–3779. doi: 10.1096/fj.09-130047

Kushnir, A., Wajsberg, B., and Marks, A. R. (2018). Ryanodine receptor dysfunction in human disorders. *Biochim. Biophys. Acta Mol. Cell. Res.* doi: 10.1016/j.bbamcr.2018.07.011 [Epub ahead of print].

Lane, D. J. R., Ayton, S., and Bush, A. I. (2018). Iron and Alzheimer's disease: an update on emerging mechanisms. *J. Alzheimers Dis.* 64, S379–S395. doi: 10.3233/JAD-179944

Lee, D. G., Park, J., Lee, H. S., Lee, S. R., and Lee, D. S. (2016). Iron overload-induced calcium signals modulate mitochondrial fragmentation in HT-22 hippocampal neuron cells. *Toxicology* 365, 17–24. doi: 10.1016/j.tox.2016.07.022

Lee, D. W., and Andersen, J. K. (2006). Role of HIF-1 in iron regulation: potential therapeutic strategy for neurodegenerative disorders. *Curr. Mol. Med.* 6, 883–893. doi: 10.2174/156652406779010849

Lee, J. C., Tae, H. J., Kim, I. H., Cho, J. H., Lee, T. K., Park, J. H., et al. (2017). Roles of HIF-1alpha, VEGF, and NF-kappaB in ischemic preconditioning-mediated neuroprotection of hippocampal CA1 pyramidal neurons against a subsequent transient cerebral ischemia. *Mol. Neurobiol.* 54, 6984–6998. doi: 10.1007/s12035-016-0219-2

Lee, J. H., Han, Y. H., Kang, B. M., Mun, C. W., Lee, S. J., and Baik, S. K. (2013). Quantitative assessment of subcortical atrophy and iron content in progressive supranuclear palsy and parkinsonian variant of multiple system atrophy. *J. Neurol.* 260, 2094–2101. doi: 10.1007/s00415-013-6951-x

Lewerenz, J., Ates, G., Methner, A., Conrad, M., and Maher, P. (2018). Oxytosis/ferroptosis-(Re-) emerging roles for oxidative stress-dependent non-apoptotic cell death in diseases of the central nervous system. *Front. Neurosci.* 12:214. doi: 10.3389/fnins.2018.00214

Li, X., Chen, W., Zhang, L., Liu, W. B., and Fei, Z. (2013). Inhibition of store-operated calcium entry attenuates MPP(+)-induced oxidative stress via preservation of mitochondrial function in PC12 cells: involvement of Homer1a. *PLoS One* 8:e83638. doi: 10.1371/journal.pone.0083638

Liao, Y., Dong, Y., and Cheng, J. (2017). The function of the mitochondrial calcium uniporter in neurodegenerative disorders. *Int. J. Mol. Sci.* 18:E248. doi: 10.3390/ijms18020248

Lim, H., Kim, D., and Lee, S. J. (2013). Toll-like receptor 2 mediates peripheral nerve injury-induced NADPH oxidase 2 expression in spinal cord microglia. *J. Biol. Chem.* 288, 7572–7579. doi: 10.1074/jbc.M112.414904

Lockman, J. A., Geldenhuys, W. J., Bohn, K. A., Desilva, S. F., Allen, D. D., and Van Der Schyf, C. J. (2012). Differential effect of nimodipine in attenuating iron-induced toxicity in brain- and blood-brain barrier-associated cell types. *Neurochem. Res.* 37, 134–142. doi: 10.1007/s11064-011-0591-2

Lourenco, C. F., Ledo, A., Barbosa, R. M., and Laranjinha, J. (2017). Neurovascular-neuroenergetic coupling axis in the brain: master regulation by nitric oxide and consequences in aging and neurodegeneration. *Free Radic. Biol. Med.* 108, 668–682. doi: 10.1016/j.freeradbiomed.2017.04.026

Lu, C., Chan, S. L., Fu, W., and Mattson, M. P. (2002). The lipid peroxidation product 4-hydroxynonenal facilitates opening of voltage-dependent Ca2+ channels in neurons by increasing protein tyrosine phosphorylation. *J. Biol. Chem.* 277, 24368–24375. doi: 10.1074/jbc.M201924200

Ludtmann, M. H. R., and Abramov, A. Y. (2018). Mitochondrial calcium imbalance in Parkinson's disease. *Neurosci. Lett.* 663, 86–90. doi: 10.1016/j.neulet.2017.08.044

Lynch, M. A. (2004). Long-term potentiation and memory. *Physiol. Rev.* 84, 87–136. doi: 10.1152/physrev.00014.2003

Maher, P., Van Leyen, K., Dey, P. N., Honrath, B., Dolga, A., and Methner, A. (2018). The role of Ca(2+) in cell death caused by oxidative glutamate toxicity and ferroptosis. *Cell Calcium* 70, 47–55. doi: 10.1016/j.ceca.2017.05.007

Marchi, S., Patergnani, S., Missiroli, S., Morciano, G., Rimessi, A., Wieckowski, M. R., et al. (2018). Mitochondrial and endoplasmic reticulum calcium homeostasis and cell death. *Cell Calcium* 69, 62–72. doi: 10.1016/j.ceca.2017.05.003

Marro, S., Chiabrando, D., Messana, E., Stolte, J., Turco, E., Tolosano, E., et al. (2010). Heme controls ferroportin1 (FPN1) transcription involving Bach1, Nrf2 and a MARE/ARE sequence motif at position -7007 of the FPN1 promoter. *Haematologica* 95, 1261–1268. doi: 10.3324/haematol.2009.020123

Martins, E. A., Robalinho, R. L., and Meneghini, R. (1995). Oxidative stress induces activation of a cytosolic protein responsible for control of iron uptake. *Arch. Biochem. Biophys.* 316, 128–134. doi: 10.1006/abbi.1995.1019

Mata, A. M., and Sepulveda, M. R. (2010). Plasma membrane Ca-ATPases in the nervous system during development and ageing. *World J. Biol. Chem.* 1, 229–234. doi: 10.4331/wjbc.v1.i7.229

Mattson, M. P. (2010). ER calcium and Alzheimer's disease: in a state of flux. *Sci. Signal.* 3:e10. doi: 10.1126/scisignal.3114pe10

McCarthy, R. C., Sosa, J. C., Gardeck, A. M., Baez, A. S., Lee, C. H., and Wessling-Resnick, M. (2018). Inflammation-induced iron transport and metabolism by brain microglia. *J. Biol. Chem.* 293, 7853–7863. doi: 10.1074/jbc.RA118.001949

Mechlovich, D., Amit, T., Bar-Am, O., Mandel, S., Youdim, M. B., and Weinreb, O. (2014). The novel multi-target iron chelator, M30 modulates HIF-1alpha-related glycolytic genes and insulin signaling pathway in the frontal cortex of APP/PS1 Alzheimer's disease mice. *Curr. Alzheimer Res.* 11, 119–127. doi: 10.2174/1567205010666131212112529

Mena, N. P., Urrutia, P. J., Lourido, F., Carrasco, C. M., and Núñez, M. T. (2015). Mitochondrial iron homeostasis and its dysfunctions in neurodegenerative disorders. *Mitochondrion* 21, 92–105. doi: 10.1016/j.mito.2015.02.001

Merelli, A., Rodriguez, J. C. G., Folch, J., Regueiro, M. R., Camins, A., and Lazarowski, A. (2018). Understanding the role of hypoxia inducible factor during neurodegeneration for new therapeutics opportunities. *Curr. Neuropharmacol.* 16, 1484–1498. doi: 10.2174/1570159X16666180110130253

Miyamoto, M., Murphy, T. H., Schnaar, R. L., and Coyle, J. T. (1989). Antioxidants protect against glutamate-induced cytotoxicity in a neuronal cell line. *J. Pharmacol. Exp. Ther.* 250, 1132–1140.

Moldogazieva, N. T., Lutsenko, S. V., and Terentiev, A. A. (2018). Reactive oxygen and nitrogen species-induced protein modifications: implication in carcinogenesis and anticancer therapy. *Cancer Res.* 78, 6040–6047. doi: 10.1158/0008-5472.CAN-18-0980

Mole, D. R., Blancher, C., Copley, R. R., Pollard, P. J., Gleadle, J. M., Ragoussis, J., et al. (2009). Genome-wide association of hypoxia-inducible factor (HIF)-1alpha and HIF-2alpha DNA binding with expression profiling of hypoxia-inducible transcripts. *J. Biol. Chem.* 284, 16767–16775. doi: 10.1074/jbc.M901790200

Moncada, S., and Bolaños, J. P. (2006). Nitric oxide, cell bioenergetics and neurodegeneration. *J. Neurochem.* 97, 1676–1689. doi: 10.1111/j.1471-4159.2006.03988.x

Mueller, S., Pantopoulos, K., Hubner, C. A., Stremmel, W., and Hentze, M. W. (2001). IRP1 activation by extracellular oxidative stress in the perfused rat liver. *J. Biol. Chem.* 276, 23192–23196. doi: 10.1074/jbc.M100654200

Muhling, T., Duda, J., Weishaupt, J. H., Ludolph, A. C., and Liss, B. (2014). Elevated mRNA-levels of distinct mitochondrial and plasma membrane Ca(2+) transporters in individual hypoglossal motor neurons of endstage SOD1 transgenic mice. *Front. Cell. Neurosci.* 8:353. doi: 10.3389/fncel.2014.00353

Muñoz, P. (2012). Iron-mediated redox modulation in neural plasticity. *Commun. Integr. Biol.* 5, 166–168. doi: 10.4161/cib.18710

Muñoz, P., Humeres, A., Elgueta, C., Kirkwood, A., Hidalgo, C., and Núñez, M. T. (2011). Iron mediates N-methyl-D-aspartate receptor-dependent stimulation of calcium-induced pathways and hippocampal synaptic plasticity. *J. Biol. Chem.* 286, 13382–13392. doi: 10.1074/jbc.M110.213785

Muñoz, Y., Carrasco, C. M., Campos, J. D., Aguirre, P., and Núñez, M. T. (2016). Parkinson's Disease: the mitochondria-iron link. *Parkinsons Dis.* 2016:7049108. doi: 10.1155/2016/7049108

Muravchick, S., and Levy, R. J. (2006). Clinical implications of mitochondrial dysfunction. *Anesthesiology* 105, 819–837. doi: 10.1097/00000542-200610000-00029

Murphy, T. H., Malouf, A. T., Sastre, A., Schnaar, R. L., and Coyle, J. T. (1988). Calcium-dependent glutamate cytotoxicity in a neuronal cell line. *Brain Res.* 444, 325–332. doi: 10.1016/0006-8993(88)90941-9

Murphy, T. H., Miyamoto, M., Sastre, A., Schnaar, R. L., and Coyle, J. T. (1989). Glutamate toxicity in a neuronal cell line involves inhibition of cystine transport leading to oxidative stress. *Neuron* 2, 1547–1558. doi: 10.1016/0896-6273(89)90043-3

Murray-Kolb, L. E. (2013). Iron and brain functions. *Curr. Opin. Clin. Nutr. Metab. Care* 16, 703–707. doi: 10.1097/MCO.0b013e3283653ef8

Mustaly-Kalimi, S., Littlefield, A. M., and Stutzmann, G. E. (2018). Calcium signaling deficits in glia and autophagic pathways contributing to neurodegenerative disease. *Antioxid. Redox Signal.* 29, 1158–1175. doi: 10.1089/ars.2017.7266

Myllyharju, J. (2013). Prolyl 4-hydroxylases, master regulators of the hypoxia response. *Acta Physiol.* 208, 148–165. doi: 10.1111/apha.12096

Nandal, A., Ruiz, J. C., Subramanian, P., Ghimire-Rijal, S., Sinnamon, R. A., Stemmler, T. L., et al. (2011). Activation of the HIF prolyl hydroxylase by the iron chaperones PCBP1 and PCBP2. *Cell Metab.* 14, 647–657. doi: 10.1016/j.cmet.2011.08.015

Nemes, R., Koltai, E., Taylor, A. W., Suzuki, K., Gyori, F., and Radak, Z. (2018). Reactive oxygen and nitrogen species regulate key metabolic, anabolic, and catabolic pathways in skeletal muscle. *Antioxidants* 7:E85. doi: 10.3390/antiox7070085

Núñez, M. T. (2010). Regulatory mechanisms of intestinal iron absorption-uncovering of a fast-response mechanism based on DMT1 and ferroportin endocytosis. *Biofactors* 36, 88–97. doi: 10.1002/biof.84

Núñez, M. T., and Chana-Cuevas, P. (2018). New perspectives in iron chelation therapy for the treatment of neurodegenerative diseases. *Pharmaceuticals* 11:E109. doi: 10.3390/ph11040109

Núñez, M. T., Gallardo, V., Muñoz, P., Tapia, V., Esparza, A., Salazar, J., et al. (2004). Progressive iron accumulation induces a biphasic change in the glutathione content of neuroblastoma cells. *Free Radic. Biol. Med.* 37, 953–960. doi: 10.1016/j.freeradbiomed.2004.06.005

Núñez, M. T., Urrutia, P., Mena, N., Aguirre, P., Tapia, V., and Salazar, J. (2012). Iron toxicity in neurodegeneration. *Biometals* 25, 761–776. doi: 10.1007/s10534-012-9523-0

Oexle, H., Gnaiger, E., and Weiss, G. (1999). Iron-dependent changes in cellular energy metabolism: influence on citric acid cycle and oxidative phosphorylation. *Biochim. Biophys. Acta* 1413, 99–107. doi: 10.1016/S0005-2728(99)00088-2

Okubo, Y., Mikami, Y., Kanemaru, K., and Iino, M. (2018). Role of endoplasmic reticulum-mediated Ca(2+) signaling in neuronal cell death. *Antioxid. Redox Signal.* 29, 1147–1157. doi: 10.1089/ars.2018.7498

Orino, K., Lehman, L., Tsuji, Y., Ayaki, H., Torti, S. V., and Torti, F. M. (2001). Ferritin and the response to oxidative stress. *Biochem. J.* 357, 241–247. doi: 10.1042/bj3570241

Overk, C. R., Rockenstein, E., Florio, J., Cheng, Q., and Masliah, E. (2015). Differential calcium alterations in animal models of neurodegenerative disease: reversal by FK506. *Neuroscience* 310, 549–560. doi: 10.1016/j.neuroscience.2015.08.068

Pantopoulos, K., and Hentze, M. W. (1995). Rapid responses to oxidative stress mediated by iron regulatory protein. *EMBO J.* 14, 2917–2924. doi: 10.1002/j.1460-2075.1995.tb07291.x

Pantopoulos, K., Weiss, G., and Hentze, M. W. (1996). Nitric oxide and oxidative stress (H2O2) control mammalian iron metabolism by different pathways. *Mol. Cell. Biol.* 16, 3781–3788. doi: 10.1128/MCB.16.7.3781

Paradkar, P. N., and Roth, J. A. (2006a). Nitric oxide transcriptionally down-regulates specific isoforms of divalent metal transporter (DMT1) via NF-kappaB. *J. Neurochem.* 96, 1768–1777.

Paradkar, P. N., and Roth, J. A. (2006b). Post-translational and transcriptional regulation of DMT1 during P19 embryonic carcinoma cell differentiation by retinoic acid. *Biochem. J.* 394, 173–183.

Paradkar, P. N., Zumbrennen, K. B., Paw, B. H., Ward, D. M., and Kaplan, J. (2009). Regulation of mitochondrial iron import through differential turnover of mitoferrin 1 and mitoferrin 2. *Mol. Cell. Biol.* 29, 1007–1016. doi: 10.1128/MCB.01685-08

Pchitskaya, E., Popugaeva, E., and Bezprozvanny, I. (2018). Calcium signaling and molecular mechanisms underlying neurodegenerative diseases. *Cell Calcium* 70, 87–94. doi: 10.1016/j.ceca.2017.06.008

Pelizzoni, I., Macco, R., Morini, M. F., Zacchetti, D., Grohovaz, F., and Codazzi, F. (2011). Iron handling in hippocampal neurons: activity-dependent iron entry and mitochondria-mediated neurotoxicity. *Aging Cell* 10, 172–183. doi: 10.1111/j.1474-9726.2010.00652.x

Pelizzoni, I., Macco, R., Zacchetti, D., Grohovaz, F., and Codazzi, F. (2008). Iron and calcium in the central nervous system: a close relationship in health and sickness. *Biochem. Soc. Trans.* 36, 1309–1312. doi: 10.1042/BST0361309

Pelizzoni, I., Zacchetti, D., Campanella, A., Grohovaz, F., and Codazzi, F. (2013). Iron uptake in quiescent and inflammation-activated astrocytes: a potentially neuroprotective control of iron burden. *Biochim. Biophys. Acta* 1832, 1326–1333. doi: 10.1016/j.bbadis.2013.04.007

Pereira, C., Ferreira, C., Carvalho, C., and Oliveira, C. (1996). Contribution of plasma membrane and endoplasmic reticulum Ca(2+)-ATPases to the synaptosomal [Ca2+]i increase during oxidative stress. *Brain Res.* 713, 269–277. doi: 10.1016/0006-8993(95)01554-X

Perier, C., Tieu, K., Guegan, C., Caspersen, C., Jackson-Lewis, V., Carelli, V., et al. (2005). Complex I deficiency primes Bax-dependent neuronal apoptosis through mitochondrial oxidative damage. *Proc. Natl. Acad. Sci. U.S.A.* 102, 19126–19131. doi: 10.1073/pnas.0508215102

Peters, D. G., Connor, J. R., and Meadowcroft, M. D. (2015). The relationship between iron dyshomeostasis and amyloidogenesis in Alzheimer's disease: two sides of the same coin. *Neurobiol. Dis.* 81, 49–65. doi: 10.1016/j.nbd.2015.08.007

Phillips, J. D., Kinikini, D. V., Yu, Y., Guo, B., and Leibold, E. A. (1996). Differential regulation of IRP1 and IRP2 by nitric oxide in rat hepatoma cells. *Blood* 87, 2983–2992.

Piret, J. P., Mottet, D., Raes, M., and Michiels, C. (2002). Is HIF-1alpha a pro- or an anti-apoptotic protein? *Biochem. Pharmacol.* 64, 889–892.

Ponka, P. (2004). Hereditary causes of disturbed iron homeostasis in the central nervous system. *Ann. N. Y. Acad. Sci.* 1012, 267–281. doi: 10.1196/annals.1306.022

Popugaeva, E., Pchitskaya, E., and Bezprozvanny, I. (2018). Dysregulation of intracellular calcium signaling in alzheimer's disease. *Antioxid. Redox Signal.* 29, 1176–1188. doi: 10.1089/ars.2018.7506

Post, M. R., Lieberman, O. J., and Mosharov, E. V. (2018). Can interactions between alpha-synuclein, dopamine and calcium explain selective neurodegeneration in Parkinson's disease? *Front. Neurosci.* 12:161. doi: 10.3389/fnins.2018.00161

Qian, Z. M., Wu, X. M., Fan, M., Yang, L., Du, F., Yung, W. H., et al. (2011). Divalent metal transporter 1 is a hypoxia-inducible gene. *J. Cell Physiol.* 226, 1596–1603. doi: 10.1002/jcp.22485.

Ray, P. D., Huang, B. W., and Tsuji, Y. (2012). Reactive oxygen species (ROS) homeostasis and redox regulation in cellular signaling. *Cell. Signal.* 24, 981–990. doi: 10.1016/j.cellsig.2012.01.008

Requejo-Aguilar, R., and Bolanos, J. P. (2016). Mitochondrial control of cell bioenergetics in Parkinson's disease. *Free Radic. Biol. Med.* 100, 123–137. doi: 10.1016/j.freeradbiomed.2016.04.012

Riganti, C., Doublier, S., Viarisio, D., Miraglia, E., Pescarmona, G., Ghigo, D., et al. (2009). Artemisinin induces doxorubicin resistance in human colon cancer cells via calcium-dependent activation of HIF-1alpha and P-glycoprotein overexpression. *Br. J. Pharmacol.* 156, 1054–1066. doi: 10.1111/j.1476-5381.2009.00117.x

Rimessi, A., Bonora, M., Marchi, S., Patergnani, S., Marobbio, C. M., Lasorsa, F. M., et al. (2013). Perturbed mitochondrial Ca2+ signals as causes or consequences of mitophagy induction. *Autophagy* 9, 1677–1686. doi: 10.4161/auto.24795

Riquelme, D., Alvarez, A., Leal, N., Adasme, T., Espinoza, I., Valdes, J. A., et al. (2011). High-frequency field stimulation of primary neurons enhances ryanodine receptor-mediated Ca2+ release and generates hydrogen peroxide, which jointly stimulate NF-kappaB activity. *Antioxid. Redox Signal.* 14, 1245–1259. doi: 10.1089/ars.2010.3238

Rosales-Corral, S., Acuna-Castroviejo, D., Tan, D. X., Lopez-Armas, G., Cruz-Ramos, J., Muñoz, R., et al. (2012). Accumulation of exogenous amyloid-beta peptide in hippocampal mitochondria causes their dysfunction: a protective role for melatonin. *Oxid. Med. Cell. Longev.* 2012:843649. doi: 10.1155/2012/843649

Rosi, S., Ramirez-Amaya, V., Hauss-Wegrzyniak, B., and Wenk, G. L. (2004). Chronic brain inflammation leads to a decline in hippocampal NMDA-R1 receptors. *J Neuroinflammation* 1:12. doi: 10.1186/1742-2094-1-12

Rothwell, N. J., and Luheshi, G. N. (2000). Interleukin 1 in the brain: biology, pathology and therapeutic target. *Trends Neurosci.* 23, 618–625. doi: 10.1016/S0166-2236(00)01661-1

Rousseau, E., Michel, P. P., and Hirsch, E. C. (2013). The iron-binding protein lactoferrin protects vulnerable dopamine neurons from degeneration by preserving mitochondrial calcium homeostasis. *Mol. Pharmacol.* 84, 888–898. doi: 10.1124/mol.113.087965

Ruiz, A., Alberdi, E., and Matute, C. (2018). Mitochondrial division inhibitor 1 (mdivi-1) protects neurons against excitotoxicity through the modulation of mitochondrial function and intracellular Ca(2+) signaling. *Front. Mol. Neurosci.* 11:3. doi: 10.3389/fnmol.2018.00003

Sanmartin, C. D., Paula-Lima, A. C., Garcia, A., Barattini, P., Hartel, S., Núñez, M. T., et al. (2014). Ryanodine receptor-mediated Ca(2+) release underlies iron-induced mitochondrial fission and stimulates mitochondrial Ca(2+)

uptake in primary hippocampal neurons. *Front. Mol. Neurosci.* 7:13. doi: 10.3389/fnmol.2014.00013

Schiavone, S., Sorce, S., Dubois-Dauphin, M., Jaquet, V., Colaianna, M., Zotti, M., et al. (2009). Involvement of NOX2 in the development of behavioral and pathologic alterations in isolated rats. *Biol. Psychiatry* 66, 384–392. doi: 10.1016/j.biopsych.2009.04.033

Sen, C. K. (2001). Antioxidants in exercise nutrition. *Sports Med.* 31, 891–908. doi: 10.2165/00007256-200131130-00001

Sherer, T. B., Betarbet, R., Testa, C. M., Seo, B. B., Richardson, J. R., Kim, J. H., et al. (2003). Mechanism of toxicity in rotenone models of Parkinson's disease. *J. Neurosci.* 23, 10756–10764. doi: 10.1523/JNEUROSCI.23-34-10756.2003

Shih, R. H., Wang, C. Y., and Yang, C. M. (2015). NF-kappaB signaling pathways in neurological inflammation: a mini review. *Front. Mol. Neurosci.* 8:77. doi: 10.3389/fnmol.2015.00077

Shimohama, S., Tanino, H., Kawakami, N., Okamura, N., Kodama, H., Yamaguchi, T., et al. (2000). Activation of NADPH oxidase in Alzheimer's disease brains. *Biochem. Biophys. Res. Commun.* 273, 5–9. doi: 10.1006/bbrc.2000.2897

Siddiq, A., Ayoub, I. A., Chavez, J. C., Aminova, L., Shah, S., Lamanna, J. C., et al. (2005). Hypoxia-inducible factor prolyl 4-hydroxylase inhibition. A target for neuroprotection in the central nervous system. *J. Biol. Chem.* 280, 41732–41743. doi: 10.1074/jbc.M504963200

Siegert, I., Schodel, J., Nairz, M., Schatz, V., Dettmer, K., Dick, C., et al. (2015). Ferritin-Mediated iron sequestration stabilizes hypoxia-inducible factor-1alpha upon LPS activation in the presence of ample oxygen. *Cell Rep.* 13, 2048–2055. doi: 10.1016/j.celrep.2015.11.005

Siklos, L., Engelhardt, J. I., Alexianu, M. E., Gurney, M. E., Siddique, T., and Appel, S. H. (1998). Intracellular calcium parallels motoneuron degeneration in SOD-1 mutant mice. *J. Neuropathol. Exp. Neurol.* 57, 571–587. doi: 10.1097/00005072-199806000-00005

Sirabella, R., Valsecchi, V., Anzilotti, S., Cuomo, O., Vinciguerra, A., Cepparulo, P., et al. (2018). Ionic homeostasis maintenance in ALS: focus on new therapeutic targets. *Front. Neurosci.* 12:510. doi: 10.3389/fnins.2018.00510

Smith, T. G., Robbins, P. A., and Ratcliffe, P. J. (2008). The human side of hypoxia-inducible factor. *Br. J. Haematol.* 141, 325–334. doi: 10.1111/j.1365-2141.2008.07029.x

Sorce, S., and Krause, K. H. (2009). NOX enzymes in the central nervous system: from signaling to disease. *Antioxid. Redox Signal.* 11, 2481–2504. doi: 10.1089/ARS.2009.2578

Sorce, S., Stocker, R., Seredenina, T., Holmdahl, R., Aguzzi, A., Chio, A., et al. (2017). NADPH oxidases as drug targets and biomarkers in neurodegenerative diseases: what is the evidence? *Free Radic. Biol. Med.* 112, 387–396. doi: 10.1016/j.freeradbiomed.2017.08.006

Soum, E., and Drapier, J. C. (2003). Nitric oxide and peroxynitrite promote complete disruption of the [4Fe-4S] cluster of recombinant human iron regulatory protein 1. *J. Biol. Inorg. Chem.* 8, 226–232. doi: 10.1007/s00775-002-0412-9

Stefani, I. C., Wright, D., Polizzi, K. M., and Kontoravdi, C. (2012). The role of ER stress-induced apoptosis in neurodegeneration. *Curr. Alzheimers Res.* 9, 373–387. doi: 10.2174/156720512800107618

Stockwell, B. R., Friedmann Angeli, J. P., Bayir, H., Bush, A. I., Conrad, M., Dixon, S. J., et al. (2017). Ferroptosis: a regulated cell death nexus linking metabolism, redox biology, and disease. *Cell* 171, 273–285. doi: 10.1016/j.cell.2017.09.021

Strehler, E. E., and Thayer, S. A. (2018). Evidence for a role of plasma membrane calcium pumps in neurodegenerative disease: recent developments. *Neurosci. Lett.* 663, 39–47. doi: 10.1016/j.neulet.2017.08.035

Surace, M. J., and Block, M. L. (2012). Targeting microglia-mediated neurotoxicity: the potential of NOX2 inhibitors. *Cell. Mol. Life Sci.* 69, 2409–2427. doi: 10.1007/s00018-012-1015-4

Sureda, A., Hebling, U., Pons, A., and Mueller, S. (2005). Extracellular H2O2 and not superoxide determines the compartment-specific activation of transferrin receptor by iron regulatory protein 1. *Free Radic. Res.* 39, 817–824. doi: 10.1080/10715760500164045

Surmeier, D. J., Guzman, J. N., and Sanchez-Padilla, J. (2010). Calcium, cellular aging, and selective neuronal vulnerability in Parkinson's disease. *Cell. Calcium* 47, 175–182. doi: 10.1016/j.ceca.2009.12.003

Surmeier, D. J., Guzman, J. N., Sanchez-Padilla, J., and Goldberg, J. A. (2011). The origins of oxidant stress in Parkinson's disease and therapeutic strategies. *Antioxid. Redox Signal.* 14, 1289–1301. doi: 10.1089/ars.2010.3521

Swaiman, K. F. (1991). Hallervorden-Spatz syndrome and brain iron metabolism. *Arch. Neurol.* 48, 1285–1293. doi: 10.1001/archneur.1991.00530240091029

Tan, S., Sagara, Y., Liu, Y., Maher, P., and Schubert, D. (1998). The regulation of reactive oxygen species production during programmed cell death. *J. Cell. Biol.* 141, 1423–1432. doi: 10.1083/jcb.141.6.1423

Tangudu, N. K., Alan, B., Vinchi, F., Worle, K., Lai, D., Vettorazzi, S., et al. (2018). Scavenging reactive oxygen species production normalizes ferroportin expression and ameliorates cellular and systemic iron disbalances in hemolytic mouse model. *Antioxid. Redox Signal.* 29, 484–499. doi: 10.1089/ars.2017.7089

Thomas, G. M., and Huganir, R. L. (2004). MAPK cascade signalling and synaptic plasticity. *Nat. Rev. Neurosci.* 5, 173–183. doi: 10.1038/nrn1346

Tonelli, C., Chio, I. I. C., and Tuveson, D. A. (2018). Transcriptional regulation by Nrf2. *Antioxid. Redox Signal.* 29, 1727–1745. doi: 10.1089/ars.2017.7342

Tong, W. H., and Rouault, T. A. (2007). Metabolic regulation of citrate and iron by aconitases: role of iron-sulfur cluster biogenesis. *Biometals* 20, 549–564. doi: 10.1007/s10534-006-9047-6

Tonnies, E., and Trushina, E. (2017). Oxidative stress, synaptic dysfunction, and Alzheimer's Disease. *J. Alzheimers Dis.* 57, 1105–1121. doi: 10.3233/JAD-161088

Urrutia, P., Aguirre, P., Esparza, A., Tapia, V., Mena, N. P., Arredondo, M., et al. (2013). Inflammation alters the expression of DMT1, FPN1 and hepcidin, and it causes iron accumulation in central nervous system cells. *J. Neurochem.* 126, 541–549. doi: 10.1111/jnc.12244

Urrutia, P. J., Mena, N. P., and Núñez, M. T. (2014). The interplay between iron accumulation, mitochondrial dysfunction, and inflammation during the execution step of neurodegenerative disorders. *Front. Pharmacol.* 5:38. doi: 10.3389/fphar.2014.00038

Vila, M., and Przedborski, S. (2003). Targeting programmed cell death in neurodegenerative diseases. *Nat. Rev. Neurosci.* 4, 365–375. doi: 10.1038/nrn1100

Wang, J., Song, N., Jiang, H., Wang, J., and Xie, J. (2013). Pro-inflammatory cytokines modulate iron regulatory protein 1 expression and iron transportation through reactive oxygen/nitrogen species production in ventral mesencephalic neurons. *Biochim. Biophys. Acta* 1832, 618–625. doi: 10.1016/j.bbadis.2013.01.021

Wang, Q. M., Xu, Y. Y., Liu, S., and Ma, Z. G. (2017). Isradipine attenuates MPTP-induced dopamine neuron degeneration by inhibiting up-regulation of L-type calcium channels and iron accumulation in the substantia nigra of mice. *Oncotarget* 8, 47284–47295. doi: 10.18632/oncotarget.17618

Wang, Y., Yang, J., and Yi, J. (2012). Redox sensing by proteins: oxidative modifications on cysteines and the consequent events. *Antioxid. Redox Signal.* 16, 649–657. doi: 10.1089/ars.2011.4313

Ward, R. J., Zucca, F. A., Duyn, J. H., Crichton, R. R., and Zecca, L. (2014). The role of iron in brain ageing and neurodegenerative disorders. *Lancet Neurol.* 13, 1045–1060. doi: 10.1016/S1474-4422(14)70117-6

Wardrop, S. L., Watts, R. N., and Richardson, D. R. (2000). Nitrogen monoxide activates iron regulatory protein 1 RNA-binding activity by two possible mechanisms: effect on the [4Fe-4S] cluster and iron mobilization from cells. *Biochemistry* 39, 2748–2758. doi: 10.1021/bi991099t

Weinreb, O., Amit, T., Bar-Am, O., and Youdim, M. B. (2016). Neuroprotective effects of multifaceted hybrid agents targeting MAO, cholinesterase, iron and beta-amyloid in ageing and Alzheimer's disease. *Br. J. Pharmacol.* 173, 2080–2094. doi: 10.1111/bph.13318

Wiethoff, S., and Houlden, H. (2017). Neurodegeneration with brain iron accumulation. *Handb. Clin. Neurol.* 145, 157–166. doi: 10.1016/B978-0-12-802395-2.00011-0

Wilkinson, N., and Pantopoulos, K. (2014). The IRP/IRE system in vivo: insights from mouse models. *Front. Pharmacol.* 5:176. doi: 10.3389/fphar.2014.00176

Wu, D. C., Jackson-Lewis, V., Vila, M., Tieu, K., Teismann, P., Vadseth, C., et al. (2002). Blockade of microglial activation is neuroprotective in the 1-methyl-4-phenyl-1,2,3,6-tetrahydropyridine mouse model of Parkinson disease. *J. Neurosci.* 22, 1763–1771. doi: 10.1523/JNEUROSCI.22-05-01763.2002

Wu, G., Fang, Y. Z., Yang, S., Lupton, J. R., and Turner, N. D. (2004). Glutathione metabolism and its implications for health. *J. Nutr.* 134, 489–492. doi: 10.1093/jn/134.3.489

Wu, G. Y., Deisseroth, K., and Tsien, R. W. (2001). Activity-dependent CREB phosphorylation: convergence of a fast, sensitive calmodulin kinase pathway and a slow, less sensitive mitogen-activated protein kinase pathway. *Proc. Natl. Acad. Sci. U.S.A.* 98, 2808–2813. doi: 10.1073/pnas.051634198

Xiao, J., Lv, Y., Lin, B., Tipoe, G. L., Youdim, M. B., Xing, F., et al. (2015). A novel antioxidant multitarget iron chelator M30 protects hepatocytes against ethanol-induced injury. *Oxid. Med. Cell. Longev.* 2015:607271. doi: 10.1155/2015/607271

Yang, W. S., Sriramaratnam, R., Welsch, M. E., Shimada, K., Skouta, R., Viswanathan, V. S., et al. (2014). Regulation of ferroptotic cancer cell death by GPX4. *Cell* 156, 317–331. doi: 10.1016/j.cell.2013.12.010

Yeh, T. L., Leissing, T. M., Abboud, M. I., Thinnes, C. C., Atasoylu, O., Holt-Martyn, J. P., et al. (2017). Molecular and cellular mechanisms of HIF prolyl hydroxylase inhibitors in clinical trials. *Chem. Sci.* 8, 7651–7668. doi: 10.1039/c7sc02103h

Yermolaieva, O., Brot, N., Weissbach, H., Heinemann, S. H., and Hoshi, T. (2000). Reactive oxygen species and nitric oxide mediate plasticity of neuronal calcium signaling. *Proc. Natl. Acad. Sci. U.S.A.* 97, 448–453. doi: 10.1073/pnas.97.1.448

Yuan, G., Nanduri, J., Bhasker, C. R., Semenza, G. L., and Prabhakar, N. R. (2005). Ca2+/calmodulin kinase-dependent activation of hypoxia inducible factor 1 transcriptional activity in cells subjected to intermittent hypoxia. *J. Biol. Chem.* 280, 4321–4328. doi: 10.1074/jbc.M407706200

Yuan, G., Nanduri, J., Khan, S., Semenza, G. L., and Prabhakar, N. R. (2008). Induction of HIF-1alpha expression by intermittent hypoxia: involvement of NADPH oxidase, Ca2+ signaling, prolyl hydroxylases, and mTOR. *J. Cell. Physiol.* 217, 674–685. doi: 10.1002/jcp.21537

Zaidi, A. (2010). Plasma membrane Ca-ATPases: targets of oxidative stress in brain aging and neurodegeneration. *World J. Biol. Chem.* 1, 271–280. doi: 10.4331/wjbc.v1.i9.271

Zaidi, A., and Michaelis, M. L. (1999). Effects of reactive oxygen species on brain synaptic plasma membrane Ca(2+)-ATPase. *Free Radic. Biol. Med.* 27, 810–821. doi: 10.1016/S0891-5849(99)00128-8

Zecca, L., Youdim, M. B., Riederer, P., Connor, J. R., and Crichton, R. R. (2004). Iron, brain ageing and neurodegenerative disorders. *Nat. Rev. Neurosci.* 5, 863–873. doi: 10.1038/nrn1537

Zhang, W., Yan, Z. F., Gao, J. H., Sun, L., Huang, X. Y., Liu, Z., et al. (2014). Role and mechanism of microglial activation in iron-induced selective and progressive dopaminergic neurodegeneration. *Mol. Neurobiol.* 49, 1153–1165. doi: 10.1007/s12035-013-8586-4

Zhang, X., Zhou, K., Wang, R., Cui, J., Lipton, S. A., Liao, F. F., et al. (2007). Hypoxia-inducible factor 1alpha (HIF-1alpha)-mediated hypoxia increases BACE1 expression and beta-amyloid generation. *J. Biol. Chem.* 282, 10873–10880. doi: 10.1074/jbc.M608856200

Zhang, Y., Kong, W. N., and Chai, X. Q. (2018). Compound of icariin, astragalus, and puerarin mitigates iron overload in the cerebral cortex of Alzheimer's disease mice. *Neural Regen. Res.* 13, 731–736. doi: 10.4103/1673-5374.230302

Zorov, D. B., Isaev, N. K., Plotnikov, E. Y., Zorova, L. D., Stelmashook, E. V., Vasileva, A. K., et al. (2007). The mitochondrion as janus bifrons. *Biochemistry* 72, 1115–1126.

7

The Dual Role of Hepcidin in Brain Iron Load and Inflammation

*Driton Vela**

Department of Physiology, Faculty of Medicine, University of Pristina, Pristina, Kosovo

Correspondence:
Driton Vela
driton.vela@uni-pr.edu

Hepcidin is the major regulator of systemic iron metabolism, while the role of this peptide in the brain has just recently been elucidated. Studies suggest a dual role of hepcidin in neuronal iron load and inflammation. This is important since neuronal iron load and inflammation are pathophysiological processes frequently associated with neurodegeneration. Furthermore, manipulation of hepcidin activity has recently been used to recover neuronal damage due to brain inflammation in animal models and cultured cells. Therefore, understanding the mechanistic insights of hepcidin action in the brain is important to uncover its role in treating neuronal damage in neurodegenerative diseases.

Keywords: hepcidin, brain, neurodegenerative diseases, glial cells, inflammation, iron load

INTRODUCTION

Iron is a crucial element for maintaining brain homeostasis. It is used by brain cells to synthesize myelin, produce neurotransmitters, and realize a wide range of important cellular biochemical reactions (Ward et al., 2014). But, iron excess is toxic for brain cells. This is observed during brain hemorrhage, where inflammatory signaling is responsible for the increase in brain iron load, which is associated with oxidative damage and cognitive decline (Wu et al., 2003; Ward et al., 2014; Garton et al., 2016). Furthermore, iron dysregulation has been proposed as a pathogenic factor in neurodegenerative diseases as well (Ward et al., 2014). Recent research suggests that brain iron dysmetabolism can be tackled via hepcidin manipulation, since local hepcidin production in the brain has been shown to affect cellular iron transport (Urrutia et al., 2013; Du et al., 2015; Gong et al., 2016; Xiong et al., 2016; Zhou et al., 2017). But, it seems that the presence or absence of inflammation dictates the deleterious vs. beneficial effects of hepcidin in the brain. Therefore, unraveling mechanistic aspects of the dual nature of hepcidin in the brain is important to understand its therapeutic potential.

REGULATION OF SYSTEMIC HEPCIDIN AND ITS ACTIONS

Most of systemic hepcidin is produced in hepatocytes via paracrine signaling from liver sinusoidal endothelial cells (LSECs) (Canali et al., 2017). LSECs respond to iron-mediated pathways by producing bone morphogenetic protein 6 (BMP6), which then activates BMP receptor (BMPR) in hepatocytes (Steinbicker et al., 2011). Activated BMPR induces s-mothers against decapentaplegic (SMAD) protein phosphorylation. Phosphorylated SMADs migrate to nucleus where they cause hepcidin upregulation (Casanovas et al., 2009). Although iron-mediated signals act mainly through BMP/SMAD pathway, other pathways are also involved, like mediation through transferrin receptor 2 (TFR2) and hemochromatosis protein (HFE) (Fleming, 2009). The second most studied stimulator of hepcidin expression is inflammation. It induces hepcidin expression via interleukin-6/janus kinase 2/signal transducer and activator of transcription 3 (IL-6/JAK2/STAT3) pathway (Pietrangelo et al., 2007). This pathway does not dominate hepcidin expression in basal conditions, but during high levels of inflammation it can override hepcidin regulation by iron signaling. In addition to these pathways, hepcidin is controlled by negative regulation, which includes signaling via erythroferrone (ERFE), heparin, vitamin D (Poli et al., 2011; Bacchetta et al., 2014; Kautz et al., 2014). Tight regulation of hepcidin production ensures a direct control of iron metabolism. This is attributed to the ability of hepcidin to induce ferroportin (FPN) degradation in target cells (Ramey et al., 2010; Zhang et al., 2011). FPN is known as the major cellular iron exporter, which is the main target protein of hepcidin.

REGULATION OF BRAIN IRON METABOLISM

Iron homeostasis in the brain must be finely regulated to serve the purposes of brain cells without damaging cell structures. There are different mechanisms that allow for this to occur; first, blood brain barrier (BBB) is a natural barrier that does not allow passing of iron with ease, which means that iron has to be transported transcellularly via TFR (Bien-Ly et al., 2014; McCarthy and Kosman, 2015a). The iron-TFR complex undergoes endocytosis, while iron gets released intracellularly through divalent metal transporter 1 (DMT1) (Ward et al., 2014). Iron exits from brain cells via FPN (Ward et al., 2014). Higher density of FPN in neurons compared to other brain cells shows why FPN downregulation causes more marked cellular iron load in neurons (Moos and Rosengren Nielsen, 2006; Boserup et al., 2011; Urrutia et al., 2013). Studies suggest that astrocytes encircling brain microvascular endothelial cells (BMVECs) influence their FPN activity by releasing local hepcidin, but also by secreting ferroxidases [including amyloid-β precursor protein (APP)] to stabilize FPN (McCarthy and Kosman, 2014, 2015a,b). In any case, iron released into brain parenchyma enters neuronal cells via TFR1, transient receptor potential canonical (TRPC) channel, DMT1 and newly discovered players, such as Zip8 and Steap2, with DMT1 role being more prominent during pathophysiological processes (Ji and Kosman, 2015; Skjørringe et al., 2015).

ROLE OF SYSTEMIC HEPCIDIN IN BRAIN HOMEOSTASIS

It is believed that systemic hepcidin can cross blood barriers such as BBB (Xiong et al., 2016). Hepcidin is a member of the big family of antimicrobial peptides (AMPs), which have been shown to cross BBB via different pathways (Welling et al., 2015). This argument is further enforced by the ability of a specific group of AMPs named defensins (which includes hepcidin) to cross intact BBB rather easily (Schluesener and Meyermann, 1995). On the other hand, the idea that hepcidin passes intact BBB has been proposed by Raha-Chowdhury et al. (2015). Authors base their conclusion on their observation that hepcidin expression was seen in nearly all cellular layers of BBB, and also due to the fact that protein expression of hepcidin is higher and more robust than its mRNA expression, which has also been corroborated by other studies (Zechel et al., 2006). The idea that hepcidin could pass through intact BBB has been shared by other authors as well (Myhre et al., 2013; Hofer and Perry, 2016). It seems that the amphipathic and cationic chemical structure of defensins in general and hepcidin in particular, might make them potential candidates for BBB pass via transcytosis (Kumagai et al., 1987; Rousselle et al., 2000; Hunter et al., 2002), though this property of hepcidin has still not been conclusively shown in intact BBB. Still, hepcidin passage through BBB is significantly increased with its disruption, and it is observed even with larger peptides than hepcidin (Ostergaard et al., 2009).

It has to be mentioned that models with liver hepcidin knockout do not result in significant brain iron dysmetabolism (Xiong et al., 2016). This would be the reason why we do not observe significant brain iron overload in hemochromatosis (Rutgers et al., 2007). This means that autonomous mechanisms in the brain are responsible for keeping iron metabolism in check. These mechanisms are mostly realized through the activity of glial cells, which are capable of buffering excess iron (Pelizzoni et al., 2013; Codazzi et al., 2015; McCarthy et al., 2018). Astrocytes are especially active during iron transport through BBB (McCarthy and Kosman, 2015b), while microglia are responsible for the control of parenchymal brain iron transport (McCarthy et al., 2018). Microglia are important "managers" of the response to brain damage due to their first-time reaction and commanding role in this respect (Shinozaki et al., 2017). On the other hand, astrocytes are able to transport the much needed iron for neuronal needs as well, which is why conditional deletion of FPN in astrocytes damages the process of myelination (Schulz et al., 2012). FPN is also important for the iron transport through BMVEC, which is why specific BMVEC FPN mutations cause transient brain iron deficiency. This process is reversible due to upregulation of iron import proteins in BMVEC (Iacovelli et al., 2009). This means that significant injury to brain cells from iron overload will occur if both, cellular iron import and export proteins are affected. Cellular iron overload seems to be more detrimental to neurons due to their lower iron buffering capacity (Bishop et al., 2011). But, studies suggest that glial cell beneficial phenotype can also be dysregulated in the presence of high ironload (Song et al., 2018).

Animal models suggest that liver hepcidin has important consequences in brain pathologies, such as brain hemorrhage/ischemia. During brain hemorrhage/ischemia liver hepcidin is upregulated, which is accompanied with increased global brain iron content after peak levels of hepcidin (Xiong et al., 2016). Importantly, hepcidin knockout decreases brain iron content in models with brain hemorrhage, but not in physiological conditions (Tan et al., 2016; Xiong et al., 2016). Xiong et al. (2016) study found a significantly lower brain iron content in hepcidin knockout rodents compared to normal rodents during intracerebral hemorrhage (ICH). In addition, brain markers of oxidative stress and brain water content were lower in hepcidin knockout rodents compared to the brain of normal rodents during ICH. Finally, hepcidin knockout rodents performed better than their normal counterparts during cognitive tests. Together these data suggest that the presence of hepcidin impacts brain iron content and function during ICH. Data from human studies seem to complement findings from animal studies because they suggest that systemic hepcidin could contribute to increased brain damage during ICH. This observation is based on the existence of the correlation between serum levels of hepcidin and clinical scores that predict poor outcome in these patients (Xiong et al., 2015). This is the reason why Xiong et al. (2016) conclude that hepcidin affects brain iron efflux during ICH, but how could this action occur is unknown. It is interesting to notice that hepcidin has opposite effects on brain iron content during brain iron-overload that occurs without inflammation (Du et al., 2015; Gong et al., 2016). Du et al. (2015) study showed that the use ad-hepcidin after injection of holotransferrin into left carotid artery results in reduced brain iron content compared to rodents not treated with ad-hepcidin (Du et al., 2015). *In vitro* results from this study showed that ad-hepcidin and hepcidin peptide reduced brain iron uptake by decreasing TFR1, DMT1, and FPN expression in brain endothelial cells. So, how could hepcidin presence during ICH cause opposite results? During ICH brain iron is increased even many weeks after the insult (Dietrich and Bradley, 1988; Wu et al., 2003; Hua et al., 2006; Liu et al., 2016). The increase in brain iron content in this setting might occur because during BBB disruption iron leakage to brain parenchyma cannot be accompanied with reactive iron efflux since hepcidin blocks excess iron from getting out of brain cells. In this respect, hepcidin further enhances the effect of inflammatory signals on cellular iron accumulation (Sansing et al., 2011; Urrutia et al., 2013; Zhou et al., 2014; Xiong et al., 2016; Goldstein et al., 2017). This occurs because during brain inflammation, cytokines, and hepcidin have agonistic effects in suppressing cellular iron efflux (Urrutia et al., 2013; Xiong et al., 2016; Zhao Y. et al., 2018). In addition, inflammatory signaling overrides the blocking effect of hepcidin on cellular iron uptake which creates an ideal environment that promotes brain iron overload by both, inflammatory signals and hepcidin (Urrutia et al., 2013; Du et al., 2015; Gong et al., 2016; Xiong et al., 2016; Zhou et al., 2017; Zhao Y. et al., 2018).

BRAIN HEPCIDIN EXPRESSION AND MECHANISMS OF REGULATION

Local hepcidin expression in the brain has been an object of investigation of different studies. In physiological conditions hepcidin expression in brain structures and cells (neurons, glial cells, endothelial cells, epithelial cells of choroid plexus) has been consistently observed by *in vivo* studies in humans and rodents, albeit in low levels (Krause et al., 2000; Pigeon et al., 2001; Zechel et al., 2006; Wang et al., 2008, 2010; Hänninen et al., 2009; Raha et al., 2013; Wei et al., 2014; Farajdokht et al., 2015; Raha-Chowdhury et al., 2015; Graf et al., 2016; Li Y. et al., 2016; Pan et al., 2016; Tan et al., 2016; Lu et al., 2017; You et al., 2017; Zhang et al., 2017). Data from human and animal studies suggest that local hepcidin is more robustly expressed in pathophysiological states (Sun et al., 2012; Urrutia et al., 2013; Tan et al., 2016; Xiong et al., 2016; You et al., 2017; Zhang et al., 2017). Similar to other cells, hepcidin main target protein in brain cells is FPN, but also iron import proteins (Sun et al., 2012; Urrutia et al., 2013; Tan et al., 2016; Xiong et al., 2016; You et al., 2017; Zhang et al., 2017).

Hepcidin upregulation can be elicited by acute iron load in astrocytes and microglia, while in neurons this response seems to become more evident with higher doses of iron supplementation (Sun et al., 2012; Urrutia et al., 2013; Simpson et al., 2015). On the other hand, according to Burkhart et al. (2016) hepcidin expression in the brain stem is scarce and probably has no effect during physiological conditions. It has to be mentioned that Burkhart et al. (2016) model of study has many differences compared to other authors. Burkhart et al. (2016) study did not include a bichamber model of BBB as compared to others, which imitates the cellular environment of brain endothelial cells and adjacent astrocytes (McCarthy and Kosman, 2014; Simpson et al., 2015). Still, even authors of this study acknowledge that hepcidin has an important role in brain iron homeostasis during iron-overload and conditions associated with BBB disruption (Burkhart et al., 2016). Unfortunately, compared to liver hepcidin, we still do not know the detailed mechanistic aspects of iron-induced regulation of hepcidin expression in brain cells. It is interesting to notice that results from studies with BMP6 pretreatment experiments are similar to those that have used pretreatment with hepcidin in terms of protection of brain cells from oxidative stress. But, whether BMP6 can control hepcidin expression in response to ironload in brain cells is still not known (Wang et al., 2001; Urrutia et al., 2017).

On the other hand, there is quite robust data concerning hepcidin regulation in the brain via an inflammatory cascade which involves lipopolysaccharide (LPS), toll-like receptor 4 (TLR4), IL-6, STAT3 molecules (**Figure 1**). The magnitude of cell-specific response to LPS is highest in glial cells and lowest in neurons (Urrutia et al., 2013; You et al., 2017). Furthermore, TLR4 as the main membrane receptor for LPS is more consistently present in microglia (Trotta et al., 2014). In addition, studies suggest that IL-6 (which is a downstream molecule induced by LPS activity) is the mediator of hepcidin upregulation in the brain during inflammation (Zhang et al., 2017). Knockdown of IL-6 during brain inflammation reduces significantly the extent of STAT3 phosphorylation and resultant hepcidin upregulation and FPN downregulation (Zhang et al., 2017). Furthermore, IL-6 activity is associated with overexpression of DMT1, though this effect is not as robust as the consequences in reduction of iron export through FPN (Zhang et al., 2017). Urrutia et al. (2013) and Zhang et al. (2017) have revealed that although the effect of IL-6 in brain hepcidin expression is robust, it is not the only cytokine through which LPS regulates hepcidin. Intriguingly, FPN downregulation during inflammation is not related only to STAT3 or hepcidin levels, but due to an unknown IL-6 dependent pathway (Zhang et al., 2017). This finding is in-line with the suggestion that inflammatory signaling independent of hepcidin expression is the main culprit

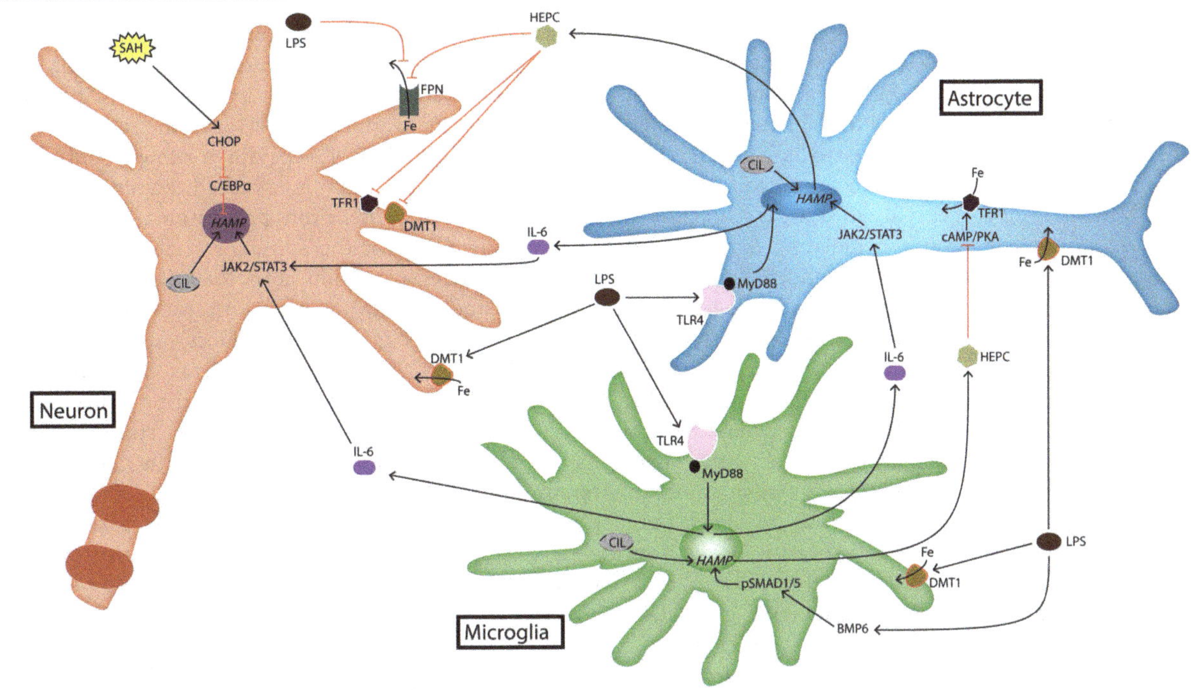

FIGURE 1 | Expression and regulation of hepcidin in brain cells. Brain hepcidin expression is upregulated during inflammation. LPS is a product of inflammation that activates TLR4 receptor. Activated TLR4 induces the production of cytokines such as IL-6, which then goes on to upregulate hepcidin expression via JAK2/STAT3 pathway. Recently, it has been shown that LPS can induce hepcidin expression in microglia through BMP/SMAD pathway as well. LPS is a strong stimulus for iron import, because it induces upregulation of DMT1. Another pathway that can induce hepcidin expression in neurons is realized through CHOP and C/EBPα molecules. This occurs during SAH. In any case, most of hepcidin is produced by glial cells during inflammatory conditions. It acts on target cells by degrading FPN, which reduces iron export out of brain cells. Hepcidin also downregulates iron import proteins, DMT1 and TFR1. In astrocytes this action is realized through cAMP/PKA pathway. BMP6, bone morphogenetic protein 6; cAMP, cyclic adenosine monophosphate; C/EBPα, CCAAT/enhancer-binding protein α; CHOP, C/EBP homologous protein; CIL, cellular iron load; DMT1, divalent metal transporter 1; Fe, iron; FPN, ferroportin; *HAMP*, hepcidin antimicrobial peptide gene; HEPC, hepcidin; IL-6, interleukin-6; JAK2, janus kinase 2; LPS, lipopolysaccharide; MyD88, myeloid differentiation primary response 88; PKA, protein kinase A; SAH, subarachnoid hemorrhage; SMAD1/5, s-mothers against decapentaplegic 1/5; STAT3, signal transducer and activator of transcription 3; TFR1, transferrin receptor 1; TLR4, toll-like receptor 4.

behind downregulation of FPN in brain cells. Cellular analysis shows that in an inflammatory setting the most evident changes in cellular iron load are observed in neurons and microglia, but less in astrocytes (Urrutia et al., 2013). This is probably due to the ability of astrocytes to facilitate iron transport in and out of their cellular environment (Xu H. et al., 2017). This would make sense if we take into account the general role of astrocytes as supporting cells that mediate transport and metabolism of different molecules.

Recently, two other pathways have been observed as inducers of brain hepcidin expression. This includes the canonical BMP/SMAD pathway, which is the classical pathway of hepcidin regulation in liver, and CCAAT/enhancer-binding protein (C/EBP) homologous protein (CHOP), which has also been involved in regulating liver hepcidin expression during endoplasmic reticulum (ER) stress (Oliveira et al., 2009). BMP/SMAD pathway has been shown to be involved in hepcidin expression in activated microglia in response to LPS, albeit in a reduced manner compared to IL-6/STAT3 pathway (Qian et al., 2014; Shin et al., 2018). On the other hand, CHOP pathway is involved in hepcidin expression in neurons, especially during brain hemorrhage. Similarly to liver, data suggest that CHOP regulates hepcidin expression in neurons via C/EBPα (Zhao J. et al., 2018). In this way, the picture of hepcidin regulation in the brain is unfolding, which will help in choosing the appropriate therapeutic strategies in different brain pathologies. Indeed, experiments with brain hepcidin knockout have resulted in decreased brain iron content in models with brain hemorrhage, while BMP/SMAD pathway suppression has recently been used in animal models to treat iron overload caused by hepcidin upregulation during brain ischemia (Ding et al., 2011; Tan et al., 2016; Shin et al., 2018). Similarly, CHOP silencing with siRNA reduces brain edema and improves neuronal function (Zhao J. et al., 2018). Also, TLR4 knockdown prevents brain iron accumulation during inflammation (Xiong et al., 2016).

DUAL ROLE OF HEPCIDIN IN BRAIN PATHOLOGIES; IMPLICATIONS FOR ITS THERAPEUTIC POTENTIAL

It is evident that local and/or systemic hepcidin is induced during brain inflammation and iron load (Urrutia et al., 2013; Xiong et al., 2016). *In vivo* experiments during brain inflammation show that the use of iron chelation protects from brain iron overload, reduces microglial activation and improves cognitive functions in rodents by reducing levels of hepcidin and increasing levels of FPN in hippocampus (Li Y. et al., 2016; Pan et al., 2016). In addition, maternal diet and calorie restriction have been proposed as factors that offer neuroprotection by reducing brain iron load through suppression of brain hepcidin (Wei et al., 2014; Graf et al., 2016). But, it is interesting to notice that accumulating data suggest that hepcidin role in neuronal iron load and inflammation is ambiguous; hepcidin can protect from iron load, but also can cause iron load during inflammation. The reason for this duality seems to occur due to the timing of hepcidin action; studies show that pretreatment with hepcidin protects brain cells from iron load, while hepcidin induction during inflammation aggravates iron load (Xiong et al., 2016; Urrutia et al., 2017; Zhao Y. et al., 2018). Inflammation in the brain is a strong stimulus for the increase in iron import, which increases iron load. But, inflammation has a double effect on iron export; it blocks iron export via FPN inhibition through hepcidin-independent and hepcidin-dependent mechanisms in neurons and glial cells (Urrutia et al., 2013; Zhang et al., 2017). The double effect of inflammation in blocking iron export enhances the cellular iron load in the brain even further. Previous studies have indicated that LPS can indeed affect FPN expression independently of cytokines, though cellular specific differences do exist (Liu et al., 2005; Deschemin and Vaulont, 2013). Cellular specific reactions to inflammatory stimuli have revealed that astrocytes and microglia (compared to neurons) react more strongly to LPS by increasing their hepcidin expression and decreasing FPN expression (Urrutia et al., 2013; Ma et al., 2018). Isolated neurons do not show signs of robust increase in hepcidin levels and FPN downregulation in reaction to inflammatory stimuli (Ma et al., 2018; Puy et al., 2018). But, when neurons are stimulated with high dose of inflammatory cytokines their hepcidin expression is increased significantly (Urrutia et al., 2013). This environment is created when neurons are co-cultured with microglia and astrocytes (You et al., 2017). In this scenario, prime responders to LPS are microglia, which through IL-6 act on astrocytes to increase hepcidin expression. Then, hepcidin acts on neurons in a paracrine manner to reduce FPN expression (You et al., 2017). It has to be mentioned that microglia can also affect neuronal hepcidin expression via LPS (Qian et al., 2014; Li Y. et al., 2016). So, the present picture suggests that during inflammation astrocytes are responsible for directing iron influx from plasma into the brain, where this iron is deposited in neurons via microglial and astrocyte activity, which can increase neuronal oxidative damage and even cause neurodegeneration.

On the other hand, hepcidin pretreatment has the potential to relieve the damage caused by inflammatory signaling. This happens because hepcidin pretreatment downregulates IL-6 and tumor necrosis α (TNFα) expression in astrocytes and microglia (Urrutia et al., 2017) (**Figure 2**). Treatment with hepcidin in these conditions protects neurons from oxidative stress (Urrutia et al., 2017). In addition, treatment with ad-hepcidin in non-inflammatory conditions protects neurons from iron load (Du et al., 2015; Gong et al., 2016; Zhou et al., 2017). The protective role of hepcidin occurs due to its effect in inhibiting iron transport through BMVEC and through its effects in reducing iron import in neuronal cells (Du et al., 2015; Gong et al., 2016; Zhou et al., 2017). These data show that timing of hepcidin treatment and presence of inflammation dramatically influences hepcidin actions in brain cells. It seems that hepcidin pretreatment primes the brain cellular milieu against the stimulative effects of inflammatory signals in increasing brain iron load (Urrutia et al., 2017). Previous studies with cultured macrophages have revealed that hepcidin-FPN interaction induces suppressor of cytokine signaling 3 (SOCS3) activity, which as its name suggest, is a suppressor of cytokine signaling during inflammation (De Domenico et al., 2010). Also, human studies have shown that levels of hepcidin are related with the inflammatory response (Burté et al., 2013). It would be interesting for future studies to reveal if beneficial effects of pretreatment with hepcidin can be sustained with increasing levels of inflammation.

ROLE OF INFLAMMATION AND IRON LOAD IN NEURODEGENERATIVE DISEASES

Pathogenesis of neurodegenerative diseases is complex and still not entirely understood. But, in recent years accumulating evidence are linking neurodegenerative processes with iron metabolism and neuroinflammation. Iron dysmetabolism is an early feature of Alzheimer's disease (AD) and in isolated nuclei in Parkinson's disease (PD) (Nunomura et al., 2001; Smith et al., 2010; Guan et al., 2017). In AD, levels of ferritin in cerebrospinal fluid (CSF) are predictors of worsening cognitive performance and are also correlated with apolipoprotein E (ApoE) CSF levels and AD risk allele ε4 (Ayton et al., 2015). Similarly, higher iron deposition in substantia nigra (SN) of AD patients makes them more prone to develop PD (Brar et al., 2009). Use of compounds with moderate iron-binding potency reduces levels of α-synclein and protects neurons from oxidative damage in PD (Finkelstein et al., 2017). This effect is realized by restoring the function of FPN as a cellular iron exporter (Finkelstein et al., 2017). Iron load as a risk factor in PD has been further confirmed in a meta-analysis, which has identified the presence of iron overload in SN of PD patients (Wang et al., 2016). It seems that in PD iron overload is generally more present in advanced stages of the disease compared to AD (Wang et al., 2016; Guan et al., 2017). In patients with mild and moderate PD there is also evidence of systemic perturbations of iron metabolism, with ferritin and malondialdehyde (MDA) serum levels (marker of oxidative damage) serving as significant biomarkers of PD (De Farias et al., 2017). On the other hand, it has to be mentioned that the most affected brain structure in PD, that is SN, is characterized with iron overload and significant damage in early stages of the disease (Ziegler et al., 2013; Guan et al., 2017). This would imply that iron dysmetabolism in SN in PD could occur due to a similar pathogenic mechanism observed in AD.

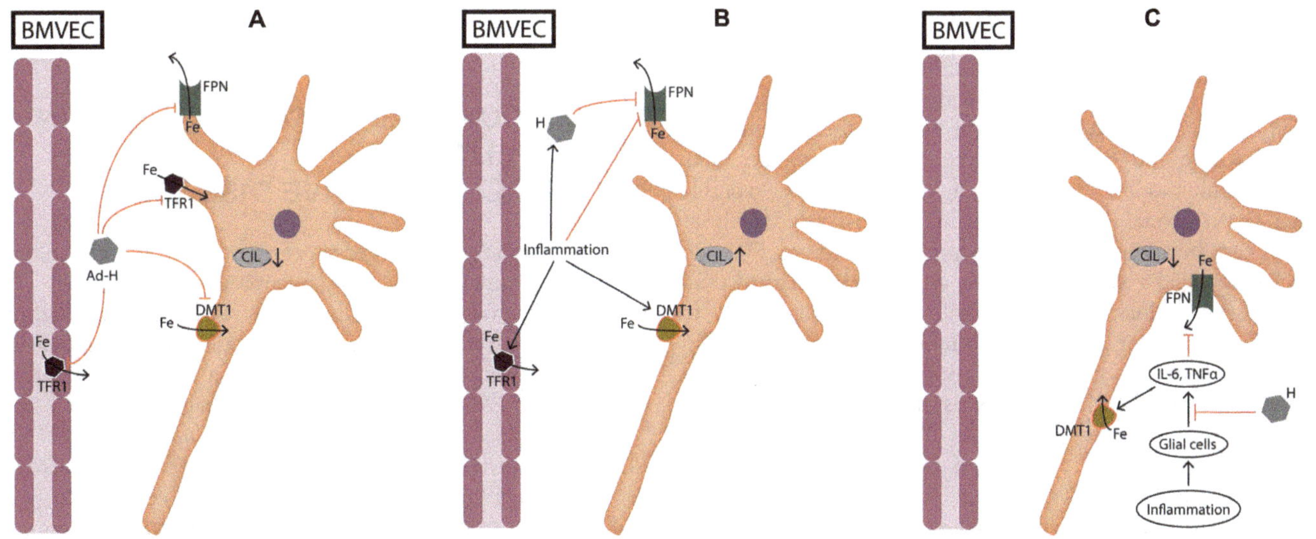

FIGURE 2 | Dual role of hepcidin during neuronal cellular iron load and inflammation. **(A)** During cellular iron load not caused by inflammation hepcidin protects neurons by reducing iron transport through BMVEC and by reducing iron import into neurons. **(B)** During inflammation hepcidin production induced by cytokines is deleterious for neurons because it increases iron load by inhibiting iron export through FPN. On the other hand, inflammation increases iron import into cells which further aggravates cellular iron load. **(C)** When glial cells are pretreated with hepcidin, cellular iron load is decreased because hepcidin suppresses the release of cytokines from glial cells. Ad-H, ad-hepcidin; BMVEC, brain microvascular endothelial cells; CIL, cellular iron load; DMT1, divalent metal transporter 1; Fe, iron; FPN, ferroportin; IL-6, interleukin-6; TFR1, transferrin receptor 1; TNFα, tumor necrosis factor α.

It is interesting to notice that APP dysfunction (which is a hallmark of AD) induces dementia-like symptoms in PD (Lei et al., 2012). Importantly, APP dysfunction in AD results in its inability to stabilize the function of FPN as a cellular iron exporter, which would affect intracellular iron load (Duce et al., 2010).

Similar to iron load, inflammation is also being recognized as an important pathogenic marker of neurodegenerative diseases. It is observed early in AD and PD, often bearing evidence of peripheral (intestinal) aberrant response to different stimuli (Qin et al., 2016; Houser and Tansey, 2017; Raj et al., 2017; Gelders et al., 2018; Gurel et al., 2018; King et al., 2018; Steeland et al., 2018). This means that in AD and PD the pathogenic process is initiated and "fueled" by immunologic disturbances occurring in the gastrointestinal tract. In relation to this scenario are data coming from studies with the TNF receptor (TNFR), which have caught attention for their importance in neurodegenerative diseases. TNF and Aβ-induced inflammation is significantly reduced via TNFR1 loss (Steeland et al., 2018). It seems that TNF and Aβ oligomers act as agonists on TNFR1 to activate microglial cells. In addition, TNFR1 loss protects brain cells from propagation of peripheral inflammatory reaction by restoring blood-CSF barrier functionality (Steeland et al., 2018). In addition, direct evidence from human studies with inflammatory bowel disease (IBD) suggests that early TNF inhibition dramatically reduces the incidence of PD (Peter et al., 2018). TNF involvement in PD is further strengthened by the increased risk of early onset of PD in patients with higher expression of TNF (Lindenau et al., 2017). On the other hand, role of inflammation in AD and PD is characterized with subtle but important differences between these conditions; *in vivo* models with mice have shown that Aβ oligomer accumulation in AD is related to TLR4 activity, which is in contrast with α-synuclein accumulation in PD, where the role of TLR4 is low or inexistent (Noelker et al., 2013; Forloni et al., 2016; Calvo-Rodríguez et al., 2017). Also, microglial activation is somewhat more prominent with AD related oligomers than with PD related oligomers (Forloni et al., 2016). Furthermore, in PD, microglial activity is accompanied with increased number of lymphocytes in damaged brain nuclei (Wang et al., 2015). These data suggest distinct inflammatory routes of activation by pathogenic oligomers in AD and PD.

Alzheimer's disease and PD are diseases that increase in prevalence with age. It is believed that the ability of microglia and astrocytes to secure the homeostatic equilibrium for neurons is reduced with aging. The homeostatic disequilibrium might be a result of the genetic factors that are related with increased activity of inflammatory signals, decreased ability of microglia to clear oligomer accumulation and other factors (Heppner et al., 2015; Lindenau et al., 2017; Hansen et al., 2018). "Pathogenic" microglia release cytokines which are responsible for neuronal damage, partly by inducing iron load. In experiments with cultured neurons, accumulation of pathological Aβ oligomers produces significant neurotoxic effects when neurons are co-cultured with glial cells (Urrutia et al., 2017). This shows that glial cell activity is an important factor in potentiating the toxic effect of Aβ oligomers. In order to protect themselves from cellular damage neurons increase ferritin depots, but the accumulating iron is very reactive and once it accumulates in sufficient amount it will cause oxidative damage. Iron load initiates a vicious cycle of neuronal damage, caused by the ability of excess iron to accelerate oligomer toxicity (Rottkamp et al., 2001; Wan et al., 2017).

Although evidence for the role of inflammation and resultant iron load in neurodegenerative diseases is accumulating, it is of therapeutic importance to explain how do these pathogenic factors change the dynamic of cellular biochemistry. Data from animal models show that aging creates a favorable milieu for neuronal damage via iron load. In rats, levels of DMT1 and hepcidin are increased, while levels of FPN do not change (Wang et al., 2010; Lu et al., 2017). This would indicate that cellular iron load with aging occurs due to increased iron import. Increased cellular iron stimulates hepcidin expression, which is not able to control FPN expression. It is interesting to notice that FPN is downregulated in aged rats with APP knockout (Belaidi et al., 2018). Furthermore, APP knockout increases the rate of brain iron accumulation that occurs with aging. This means that the preservation of cellular iron efflux is important for slowing age-related brain iron overload. In brains of AD patients and mice hepcidin expression is located in damaged neurons and blood vessels of amyloid plaques (Raha et al., 2013). On the other hand, similar to changes occurring with age, we observe increased DMT1 expression, but also co-localization of DMT1 with amyloid plaques in AD patients and in animal models with AD (Zheng et al., 2009). Animal models suggest that DMT1 expression is directly linked with the metabolism of pathogenic peptides that accumulate during AD (Zheng et al., 2009). Furthermore, DMT1 silencing increases cell viability in AD (Zheng et al., 2009). Similarly, in human patients, animal models and cell cultures with PD, DMT1 is also upregulated and related to oxidative stress (Salazar et al., 2008; Chen et al., 2015). Consequently, blocking DMT1 and hepcidin improves cell viability, while FPN upregulation rescues neuronal function in cultured cells and mice brain with PD (Chen et al., 2015; Xu et al., 2016; Xu Q. et al., 2017). So, at least in animal models with neurodegenerative disease, suppression of iron import and stimulation of iron export (via hepcidin manipulation) ameliorates neuronal degeneration.

In other diseases accompanied with neurodegeneration (Huntington disease, amyotrophic lateral sclerosis) iron deposition is also increased in different brain structures (Chen et al., 2013; Muller and Leavitt, 2014; Szeliga et al., 2016; Moreau et al., 2018). Changes in expression of iron protein carriers and the therapeutic potential of iron chelation evoke striking similarities with AD and PD (Salazar et al., 2008; Zheng et al., 2009; Chen et al., 2013; Belaidi and Bush, 2016; Szeliga et al., 2016; Moreau et al., 2018). It is speculative to suggest that the role of hepcidin in neurodegenerative diseases might be of primary importance, due to the dominating role of innate immune system in the pathophysiology of these diseases. Hepcidin has been evidenced quite robustly as part of our innate immune response, which is helpful in acute situations, because it controls iron availability to pathogens, but also it can regulate actions of inflammatory cytokines (De Domenico et al., 2010; Armitage et al., 2011; Burté et al., 2013). But, during chronic innate immune activity the negative feedback control between hepcidin and inflammation observed in acute situations turns into an agonistic relationship which will eventually deteriorate brain cell damage.

THE RATIONALE FOR USING HEPCIDIN THERAPEUTICS IN NEURODEGENERATIVE DISEASES

Stimulation and inhibition of hepcidin has been used in cultured cells and animal models to ameliorate brain damage. The rationale is evident; hepcidin affects FPN and iron import proteins, which means its manipulation can control cellular iron load. Furthermore, it has been shown that decreased activity or expression of FPN promotes neuronal damage (Song et al., 2010; Yang et al., 2011; Crespo et al., 2014). In animal models with PD neurodegeneration is associated with increased microglial activity and FPN downregulation (Zhang et al., 2014). In addition, human trials with iron chelators have shown promise in retarding the progress of neuronal damage (Crapper McLachlan et al., 1991; Martin-Bastida et al., 2017; Moreau et al., 2018). But, long-term results of this therapy are still unknown and pending future trials (Adlard and Bush, 2018).

In animal models with brain inflammation and increased oxidative stress, direct and indirect suppression of local and systemic hepcidin offers neuroprotection (Chen et al., 2015; Li W.-Y. et al., 2016; Pan et al., 2016; Xiong et al., 2016). But, in conditions with lack of inflammation, the use of ad-hepcidin has also beneficial effects in neuronal function, probably due to hepcidin ability to protect neurons during iron overload via suppression of cellular iron import proteins. Still, there exist practical issues concerning the use of delivery methods for hepcidin in these scenarios. In animal models this has been done via intracerebroventricular injections, but the feasibility of this method in humans is unknown (Gong et al., 2016; Urrutia et al., 2017). Recent advances suggest that nanotechnology could make an important breakthrough in treating brain diseases with targeted delivery of peptides (Goldsmith et al., 2014; Silva Adaya et al., 2017).

Based on the accumulating evidence about the role of inflammation on cellular iron content, it is reasonable to assume that neuroprotection can be achieved by blocking the inflammatory pathways through already established drugs. One such drug is acetylsalicylic acid, which has already been used in cultured cells to protect neuronal cells and microglia from inflammation-induced damage (Li W.-Y. et al., 2016; Huang et al., 2018) (**Table 1**). The protective effect of acetylsalicylic acid is realized through increase in iron export in neuronal cells (Huang et al., 2018), while in microglia it reduces iron import and increases iron export (Xu et al., 2015).

As it was previously mentioned heparins can affect liver hepcidin expression. One such heparin, called dalteparin, has been administered via intraperitoneal injections in mice to suppress brain hepcidin expression during inflammatory conditions (Farajdokht et al., 2015). Dalteparin can also suppress serum IL-6 levels in these conditions, which means that its beneficial properties in reducing increased brain iron during inflammation could be due to suppression if

TABLE 1 | Therapeutic potential of the manipulation of hepcidin and its target proteins in neurodegeneration.

Condition	Method of study	Main results	Reference
Brain inflammation	Effects of hepcidin suppression in brains of mice with intracerebral hemorrhage and in cultured cells	Liver hepcidin knockout reduces brain damage Treatment with hepcidin aggravates brain damage Suppression of brain hepcidin by blocking inflammatory stimuli reduces brain damage	Xiong et al., 2016
Brain inflammation	Effects of hepcidin suppression in rat brains with brain ischemia	Knockdown of brain hepcidin reduces iron load by increasing FPN expression	Ding et al., 2011
Brain inflammation	Effects of hepcidin suppression in rat brains with subarachnoid hemorrhage	Hepcidin injections increase cellular apoptosis Knockdown of brain hepcidin ameliorates brain damage	Tan et al., 2016
Brain inflammation	Effects of aspirin on cytokine actions in cultured microglial cells	Aspirin protects cultured microglial cells from LPS-induced damage Aspirin induces FPN upregulation and reduces ferritin levels in microglial cells treated with LPS Aspirin suppresses IL-6, TNFα and hepcidin expression in microglial cells treated with LPS	Xu et al., 2015
Brain inflammation	Effects of aspirin on cytokine actions in cultured microglial cells	Aspirin protects cultured microglial cells from LPS-induced damage Aspirin suppresses hepcidin expression in microglial cells treated with LPS Aspirin suppresses IL-6 expression in microglial cells treated with or without LPS	Li W.-Y. et al., 2016
Brain inflammation	Effects of aspirin on cytokine actions in cultured neuronal cells	Aspirin protects neuronal cells from inflammation-induced signaling Aspirin increases FPN expression and decreases hepcidin and ferritin levels in neuronal cells treated with IL-6	Huang et al., 2018
Brain ischemia/inflammation	Effects of L-LYC on cytokine actions in rat brains with ischemia/inflammation	L-LYC protects brain cells during brain ischemia/inflammation L-LYC reduces hepcidin expression and increases FPN expression in neuronal cells L-LYC reduces IL-6 expression and hepcidin expression in rat brains	Zhao Y. et al., 2018
Brain inflammation	Effects of dalteparin on IL-6 and hepcidin in mouse model with chronic mild stress	Dalteparin protects from brain iron load Dalteparin reduces brain hepcidin expression Dalteparin reduces serum IL-6	Farajdokht et al., 2015
Brain inflammation/ischemia	Effects of tanshinone IIA on iron-related proteins in rat brains and cultured neurons	Tanshinone IIA has neuroprotective properties during brain ischemia Tanshinone IIA downregulates TFR1, DMT1, while it upregulates FPN expression in rat brains Tanshinone IIA downregulates TFR1, DMT1, while it upregulates FPN expression in cultured neurons	Yang et al., 2011
Brain amyloid-β toxicity	Effects of hepcidin pretreatment in mice brain and cultured mice brain cells	Hepcidin pretreatment reduces IL-6 and TNFα expression in astrocytes and microglia treated with amyloid-β aggregates Hepcidin pretreatment reduces astrocyte and microglia activation in mice brain Hepcidin pretreatment protects from amyloid-β induced oxidative damage in mice brain Hepcidin pretreatment suppresses the ability of microglia and astrocytes treated with amyloid-β to induce oxidative damage in neurons	Urrutia et al., 2017
Alzheimer's disease	Effects of DMT1 silencing in neuronal cell cultures	DMT1 silencing reduces cellular iron load DMT1 silencing reduces the expression of APP and Aβ peptide DMT1 silencing increases cell viability	Zheng et al., 2009
Parkinson's disease	Effects of EGCG on neuronal cultured cells with Parkinson's disease model induced by 6-OHDA	EGCG protects neurons from cellular death and increases cell viability EGCG decreases DMT1, hepcidin, ferritin expression, while it increases FPN expression	Chen et al., 2015
Parkinson's disease	Effect of hepcidin on neuronal cultured cells with Parkinson's disease model induced by 6-OHDA	Hepcidin knockdown with siRNA protects neurons from cytotoxic effects of 6-OHDA	Xu et al., 2016
Brain iron-overload without inflammation	Effects of ad-hepcidin in rat brains and cultured cells with iron overload	Ad-hepcidin reduces brain iron overload Ad-hepcidin reduces iron uptake proteins (DMT1, TFR1) and iron release protein (FPN) in cultured BMVEC Ad-hepcidin reduces iron uptake proteins (DMT1, TFR1) and iron release protein (FPN) in cultured neurons	Du et al., 2015
Brain iron-overload without inflammation	Effects of ad-hepcidin in rat brains with iron overload	Ad-hepcidin reduces iron load in iron overload brains	Gong et al., 2016
Brain iron-overload without inflammation	Effects of ad-hepcidin in cultured neurons during hemin-induced injury	Ad-hepcidin reduces cellular iron content in cultured neurons treated with hemin Hepcidin downregulates the levels of DMT1, TFR1, and FPN in cultured neurons treated with hemin	Zhou et al., 2017

6-OHDA, 6-hydroxydopamine; APP, amyloid precursor protein; BMVEC, brain microvascular endothelial cells; DMT1, divalent metal transporter 1; EGCG, epigallocatechin-3-gallate; FPN, ferroportin; IL-6, interleukin-6; L-LYC, liposomal lycopene; LPS, lipopolysaccharide; siRNA, small interfering RNA; TFR1, transferrin receptor 1; TNFα, tumor necrosis factor α.

systemic inflammation and brain hepcidin. Still the cause/effect relationship of dalteparin in the brain has not been studied thoroughly in terms of its impact on brain iron metabolism via hepcidin regulation. Future studies should also explain whether dalteparin-induced brain hepcidin suppression is dose-dependent, because of the side effects of this drug on brain homeostasis (Perry et al., 2010).

Another therapeutic option that has been used is based on methods of delivery that increase the efficiency of neuroprotective substances. One example is the use of liposomes, which serve as particles that deliver drugs to target cells, whilst keeping intact the stability of the substance that is being used for therapeutic purposes. Liposomal lycopene has been delivered in rat brains to reduce oxidative stress and ameliorate apoptosis caused by ischemia. This effect is at least partly attributed to the ability of lycopene to reduce hepcidin expression in astrocytes via its suppressive effect on IL-6 signaling (Zhao Y. et al., 2018).

CONCLUSION

Hepcidin is emerging as an important peptide for brain (patho)physiology. The source of hepcidin in the brain is local and probably systemic. It is believed that systemic hepcidin can pass through BBB, especially during BBB leakage (for example during inflammation). Neurons, glial cells, endothelial cells, and other brain cells may express hepcidin, although basal levels of brain hepcidin are low. They increase significantly during inflammation and most likely during brain iron load. The local molecular regulation of brain hepcidin expression is unfolding, while studies suggest that it bears resemblance with liver hepcidin regulation. Still, the details of this regulation await further clarification from future studies. Hepcidin produced by the brain cells in pathological conditions may limit iron transport through BMVEC, and thereby also limit neuronal iron load. High iron load is detrimental for neuronal function. In addition, high iron load can also affect glial cell activity by turning them into cells that promote neuronal damage. The observation of robust production of hepcidin by glial cells compared to neurons during changes in brain homeostasis is in-line with the already established role of glia as supportive, regulatory and protective cells in the brain milieu. During inflammatory conditions hepcidin promotes neuronal iron load, while the opposite occurs in non-inflammatory conditions. This observation is based on studies that have revealed the neuroprotective nature of hepcidin suppression during inflammation. This occurs due to the increase in iron import caused by inflammation, which is further exacerbated by FPN downregulation caused by hepcidin-dependent and hepcidin-independent mechanisms. On the other hand, use of ad-hepcidin during neuronal iron load (not caused by inflammation) protects these cells from oxidative stress. Intriguingly, hepcidin pretreatment also protects neurons from the deleterious effects of inflammation. It seems that pretreatment with hepcidin blocks the initiation of inflammation-induced biochemical cascade inside brain cells. This effect of hepcidin is not without precedent, because it has been observed in mice and human studies. Unfortunately, therapeutic implications of this physiological effect of hepcidin have not been studied in details, despite its potential crucial importance in brain and other pathologies. Still, pharmacologic manipulation of hepcidin is emerging as e new therapeutic territory in neurodegenerative diseases. Animal models have shown that the use of ad-hepcidin and suppression of hepcidin protects brain cells in models of neurodegenerative diseases. This has been further confirmed with the use of standard anti-inflammatory drugs such as acetylsalicylic acid or lycopene.

Finally, considering the ever increasing importance of hepcidin for brain physiology, it is paramount for future studies to examine models with different cell specific hepcidin knockout in AD and PD that will reveal the temporal changes of hepcidin, but that will also define whether hepcidin is of primary importance for the pathophysiology of neurodegenerative diseases.

AUTHOR CONTRIBUTIONS

The author confirms being the sole contributor of this work and has approved it for publication.

REFERENCES

Adlard, P. A., and Bush, A. I. (2018). Metals and Alzheimer's disease: how far have we come in the clinic? *J. Alzheimers Dis.* 62, 1369–1379. doi: 10.3233/JAD-170662

Armitage, A. E., Eddowes, L. A., Gileadi, U., Cole, S., Spottiswoode, N., Selvakumar, T. A., et al. (2011). Hepcidin regulation by innate immune and infectious stimuli. *Blood* 118, 4129–4139. doi: 10.1182/blood-2011-04-351957

Ayton, S., Faux, N. G., Bush, A. I., Initiative, A. D. N., Weiner, M. W., Aisen, P., et al. (2015). Ferritin levels in the cerebrospinal fluid predict Alzheimer's disease outcomes and are regulated by APOE. *Nat. Commun.* 6:6760. doi: 10.1038/ncomms7760

Bacchetta, J., Zaritsky, J. J., Sea, J. L., Chun, R. F., Lisse, T. S., Zavala, K., et al. (2014). Suppression of iron-regulatory hepcidin by vitamin D. *J. Am. Soc. Nephrol.* 25, 564–572. doi: 10.1681/ASN.2013040355

Belaidi, A. A., and Bush, A. I. (2016). Iron neurochemistry in Alzheimer's disease and Parkinson's disease: targets for therapeutics. *J. Neurochem.* 139, 179–197. doi: 10.1111/jnc.13425

Belaidi, A. A., Gunn, A. P., Wong, B. X., Ayton, S., Appukuttan, A. T., Roberts, B. R., et al. (2018). Marked age-related changes in brain iron homeostasis in amyloid protein precursor knockout mice. *Neurotherapeutics* doi: 10.1007/s13311-018-0656-x

Bien-Ly, N., Yu, Y. J., Bumbaca, D., Elstrott, J., Boswell, C. A., Zhang, Y., et al. (2014). Transferrin receptor (TfR) trafficking determines brain uptake of TfR antibody affinity variants. *J. Exp. Med.* 211, 233–244. doi: 10.1084/jem.20131660

Bishop, G. M., Dang, T. N., Dringen, R., and Robinson, S. R. (2011). Accumulation of non-transferrin-bound iron by neurons, astrocytes, and microglia. *Neurotox. Res.* 19, 443–451. doi: 10.1007/s12640-010-9195-x

Boserup, M. W., Lichota, J., Haile, D., and Moos, T. (2011). Heterogenous distribution of ferroportin-containing neurons in mouse brain. *Biometals* 24, 357–375. doi: 10.1007/s10534-010-9405-2

Brar, S., Henderson, D., Schenck, J., and Zimmerman, E. A. (2009). Iron accumulation in the substantia nigra of patients with Alzheimer disease and parkinsonism. *Arch. Neurol.* 66, 371–374. doi: 10.1001/archneurol.2008.586

Burkhart, A., Skjørringe, T., Johnsen, K. B., Siupka, P., Thomsen, L. B., Nielsen, M. S., et al. (2016). Expression of iron-related proteins at the neurovascular unit supports reduction and reoxidation of iron for transport through the blood-brain barrier. *Mol. Neurobiol.* 53, 7237–7253. doi: 10.1007/s12035-015-9582-7

Burté, F., Brown, B. J., Orimadegun, A. E., Ajetunmobi, W. A., Afolabi, N. K., Akinkunmi, F., et al. (2013). Circulatory hepcidin is associated with the anti-inflammatory response but not with iron or anemic status in childhood malaria. *Blood* 121, 3016–3022. doi: 10.1182/blood-2012-10-461418

Calvo-Rodríguez, M., de la Fuente, C., García-Durillo, M., García-Rodríguez, C., Villalobos, C., and Núñez, L. (2017). Aging and amyloid β oligomers enhance TLR4 expression, LPS-induced Ca^{2+} responses, and neuron cell death in cultured rat hippocampal neurons. *J. Neuroinflamm.* 14:24. doi: 10.1186/s12974-017-0802-0

Canali, S., Zumbrennen-Bullough, K. B., Core, A. B., Wang, C.-Y., Nairz, M., Bouley, R., et al. (2017). Endothelial cells produce bone morphogenetic protein 6 required for iron homeostasis in mice. *Blood* 129, 405–414. doi: 10.1182/blood-2016-06-721571

Casanovas, G., Mleczko-Sanecka, K., Altamura, S., Hentze, M. W., and Muckenthaler, M. U. (2009). Bone morphogenetic protein (BMP)-responsive elements located in the proximal and distal hepcidin promoter are critical for its response to HJV/BMP/SMAD. *J. Mol. Med.* 87, 471–480. doi: 10.1007/s00109-009-0447-2

Chen, D., Kanthasamy, A. G., and Reddy, M. B. (2015). EGCG protects against 6-OHDA-induced neurotoxicity in a cell culture model. *Parkinsons. Dis.* 2015:843906. doi: 10.1155/2015/843906

Chen, J., Marks, E., Lai, B., Zhang, Z., Duce, J. A., Lam, L. Q., et al. (2013). Iron accumulates in Huntington's disease neurons: protection by deferoxamine. *PLoS One* 8:e77023. doi: 10.1371/journal.pone.0077023

Codazzi, F., Pelizzoni, I., Zacchetti, D., and Grohovaz, F. (2015). Iron entry in neurons and astrocytes: a link with synaptic activity. *Front. Mol. Neurosci.* 8:18. doi: 10.3389/fnmol.2015.00018

Crapper, McLachlan, D. R., Dalton, A. J., Kruck, T. P., Bell, M. Y., Smith, W. L., et al. (1991). Intramuscular desferrioxamine in patients with Alzheimer's disease. *Lancet* 337, 1304–1308.

Crespo, Â. C., Silva, B., Marques, L., Marcelino, E., Maruta, C., Costa, S., et al. (2014). Genetic and biochemical markers in patients with Alzheimer's disease support a concerted systemic iron homeostasis dysregulation. *Neurobiol. Aging* 35, 777–785. doi: 10.1016/j.neurobiolaging.2013.10.078

De Domenico, I., Zhang, T. Y., Koening, C. L., Branch, R. W., London, N., Lo, E., et al. (2010). Hepcidin mediates transcriptional changes that modulate acute cytokine-induced inflammatory responses in mice. *J. Clin. Invest.* 120, 2395–2405. doi: 10.1172/JCI42011

De Farias, C. C., Maes, M., Bonifacio, K. L., Matsumoto, A. K., Bortolasci, C. C., Nogueira, A. S., et al. (2017). Parkinson's disease is accompanied by intertwined alterations in iron metabolism and activated immune-inflammatory and oxidative stress pathways. *CNS Neurol. Disord. – Drug Targets* 16, 484–491. doi: 10.2174/1871527316666170223161004

Deschemin, J.-C., and Vaulont, S. (2013). Role of hepcidin in the setting of hypoferremia during acute inflammation. *PLoS One* 8:e61050. doi: 10.1371/journal.pone.0061050

Dietrich, R. B., and Bradley, W. G. (1988). Iron accumulation in the basal ganglia following severe ischemic-anoxic insults in children. *Radiology* 168, 203–206. doi: 10.1148/radiology.168.1.3380958

Ding, H., Yan, C.-Z., Shi, H., Zhao, Y.-S., Chang, S.-Y., Yu, P., et al. (2011). Hepcidin is involved in iron regulation in the ischemic brain. *PLoS One* 6:e25324. doi: 10.1371/journal.pone.0025324

Du, F., Qian, Z.-M., Luo, Q., Yung, W.-H., and Ke, Y. (2015). Hepcidin suppresses brain iron accumulation by downregulating iron transport proteins in iron-overloaded rats. *Mol. Neurobiol.* 52, 101–114. doi: 10.1007/s12035-014-8847-x

Duce, J. A., Tsatsanis, A., Cater, M. A., James, S. A., Robb, E., Wikhe, K., et al. (2010). Iron-export ferroxidase activity of β-amyloid precursor protein is inhibited by zinc in Alzheimer's disease. *Cell* 142, 857–867. doi: 10.1016/j.cell.2010.08.014

Farajdokht, F., Soleimani, M., Mehrpouya, S., Barati, M., and Nahavandi, A. (2015). The role of hepcidin in chronic mild stress-induced depression. *Neurosci. Lett.* 588, 120–124. doi: 10.1016/j.neulet.2015.01.008

Finkelstein, D. I., Billings, J. L., Adlard, P. A., Ayton, S., Sedjahtera, A., Masters, C. L., et al. (2017). The novel compound PBT434 prevents iron mediated neurodegeneration and alpha-synuclein toxicity in multiple models of Parkinson's disease. *Acta Neuropathol. Commun.* 5:53. doi: 10.1186/s40478-017-0456-2

Fleming, R. E. (2009). Iron sensing as a partnership: HFE and transferrin receptor 2. *Cell Metab.* 9, 211–212. doi: 10.1016/J.CMET.2009.02.004

Forloni, G., Artuso, V., La Vitola, P., and Balducci, C. (2016). Oligomeropathies and pathogenesis of Alzheimer and Parkinson's diseases. *Mov. Disord.* 31, 771–781. doi: 10.1002/mds.26624

Garton, T., Keep, R. F., Hua, Y., and Xi, G. (2016). Brain iron overload following intracranial haemorrhage. *Stroke Vasc. Neurol.* 1, 172–184. doi: 10.1136/svn-2016-000042

Gelders, G., Baekelandt, V., and Van der Perren, A. (2018). Linking neuroinflammation and neurodegeneration in Parkinson's disease. *J. Immunol. Res.* 2018, 1–12. doi: 10.1155/2018/4784268

Goldsmith, M., Abramovitz, L., and Peer, D. (2014). Precision nanomedicine in neurodegenerative diseases. *ACS Nano* 8, 1958–1965. doi: 10.1021/nn501292z

Goldstein, E. Z., Church, J. S., Pukos, N., Gottipati, M. K., Popovich, P. G., and McTigue, D. M. (2017). Intraspinal TLR4 activation promotes iron storage but does not protect neurons or oligodendrocytes from progressive iron-mediated damage. *Exp. Neurol.* 298, 42–56. doi: 10.1016/j.expneurol.2017.08.015

Gong, J., Du, F., Qian, Z. M., Luo, Q. Q., Sheng, Y., Yung, W., et al. (2016). Pre-treatment of rats with ad-hepcidin prevents iron-induced oxidative stress in the brain. *Free Radic. Biol. Med.* 90, 126–132. doi: 10.1016/j.freeradbiomed.2015.11.016

Graf, A. E., Lallier, S. W., Waidyaratne, G., Thompson, M. D., Tipple, T. E., Hester, M. E., et al. (2016). Maternal high fat diet exposure is associated with increased hepcidin levels, decreased myelination, and neurobehavioral changes in male offspring. *Brain. Behav. Immun.* 58, 369–378. doi: 10.1016/j.bbi.2016.08.005

Guan, X., Xuan, M., Gu, Q., Huang, P., Liu, C., Wang, N., et al. (2017). Regionally progressive accumulation of iron in Parkinson's disease as measured by quantitative susceptibility mapping. *NMR Biomed.* 30:e3489. doi: 10.1002/nbm.3489

Gurel, B., Cansev, M., Sevinc, C., Kelestemur, S., Ocalan, B., Cakir, A., et al. (2018). Early stage alterations in CA1 extracellular region proteins indicate dysregulation of IL6 and iron homeostasis in the 5XFAD Alzheimer's disease mouse model. *J. Alzheimer's Dis.* 61, 1399–1410. doi: 10.3233/JAD-170329

Hänninen, M. M., Haapasalo, J., Haapasalo, H., Fleming, R. E., Britton, R. S., Bacon, B. R., et al. (2009). Expression of iron-related genes in human brain and brain tumors. *BMC Neurosci.* 10:36. doi: 10.1186/1471-2202-10-36

Hansen, D. V., Hanson, J. E., and Sheng, M. (2018). Microglia in Alzheimer's disease. *J. Cell Biol.* 217, 459–472. doi: 10.1083/jcb.201709069

Heppner, F. L., Ransohoff, R. M., and Becher, B. (2015). Immune attack: the role of inflammation in Alzheimer disease. *Nat. Rev. Neurosci.* 16, 358–372. doi: 10.1038/nrn3880

Hofer, T., and Perry, G. (2016). Nucleic acid oxidative damage in Alzheimer's disease-explained by the hepcidin-ferroportin neuronal iron overload hypothesis? *J. Trace Elem. Med. Biol.* 38, 1–9. doi: 10.1016/j.jtemb.2016.06.005

Houser, M. C., and Tansey, M. G. (2017). The gut-brain axis: is intestinal inflammation a silent driver of Parkinson's disease pathogenesis? *NPJ Parkinsons Dis.* 3:3. doi: 10.1038/s41531-016-0002-0

Hua, Y., Nakamura, T., Keep, R. F., Wu, J., Schallert, T., Hoff, J. T., et al. (2006). Long-term effects of experimental intracerebral hemorrhage: the role of iron. *J. Neurosurg.* 104, 305–312. doi: 10.3171/jns.2006.104.2.305

Huang, S.-N., Ruan, H.-Z., Chen, M. Y.-J., Zhou, G., and Qian, Z. M. (2018). Aspirin increases ferroportin 1 expression by inhibiting hepcidin via the JAK/STAT3 pathway in interleukin 6-treated PC-12 cells. *Neurosci. Lett.* 662, 1–5. doi: 10.1016/j.neulet.2017.10.001

Hunter, H. N., Fulton, D. B., Ganz, T., and Vogel, H. J. (2002). The solution structure of human hepcidin, a peptide hormone with antimicrobial activity that is involved in iron uptake and hereditary hemochromatosis. *J. Biol. Chem.* 277, 37597–37603. doi: 10.1074/jbc.M205305200

Iacovelli, J., Mlodnicka, A. E., Veldman, P., Ying, G.-S., Dunaief, J. L., and Schumacher, A. (2009). Brain and retinal ferroportin 1 dysregulation in polycythaemia mice. *Brain Res.* 1289, 85–95. doi: 10.1016/j.brainres.2009.06.098

Ji, C., and Kosman, D. J. (2015). Molecular mechanisms of non-transferrin-bound and transferring-bound iron uptake in primary hippocampal neurons. *J. Neurochem.* 133, 668–683. doi: 10.1111/jnc.13040

Kautz, L., Jung, G., Valore, E. V., Rivella, S., Nemeth, E., and Ganz, T. (2014). Identification of erythroferrone as an erythroid regulator of iron metabolism. *Nat. Genet.* 46, 678–684. doi: 10.1038/ng.2996

King, E., O'Brien, J. T., Donaghy, P., Morris, C., Barnett, N., Olsen, K., et al. (2018). Peripheral inflammation in prodromal Alzheimer's and Lewy body dementias. *J. Neurol. Neurosurg. Psychiatry* 89, 339–345. doi: 10.1136/jnnp-2017-317134

Krause, A., Neitz, S., Mägert, H.-J., Schulz, A., Forssmann, W.-G., Schulz-Knappe, P., et al. (2000). LEAP-1, a novel highly disulfide-bonded human peptide, exhibits antimicrobial activity. *FEBS Lett.* 480, 147–150. doi: 10.1016/S0014-5793(00)01920-7

Kumagai, A. K., Eisenberg, J. B., and Pardridge, W. M. (1987). Absorptive-mediated endocytosis of cationized albumin and a beta-endorphin-cationized albumin chimeric peptide by isolated brain capillaries. Model system of blood-brain barrier transport. *J. Biol. Chem.* 262, 15214–15219.

Lei, P., Ayton, S., Finkelstein, D. I., Spoerri, L., Ciccotosto, G. D., Wright, D. K., et al. (2012). Tau deficiency induces parkinsonism with dementia by impairing APP-mediated iron export. *Nat. Med.* 18, 291–295. doi: 10.1038/nm.2613

Li, W.-Y., Li, F.-M., Zhou, Y.-F., Wen, Z.-M., Ma, J., Ya, K., et al. (2016). Aspirin down regulates hepcidin by inhibiting NF-κB and IL6/JAK2/STAT3 pathways in BV-2 microglial cells treated with lipopolysaccharide. *Int. J. Mol. Sci.* 17:1921. doi: 10.3390/ijms17121921

Li, Y., Pan, K., Chen, L., Ning, J.-L., Li, X., Yang, T., et al. (2016). Deferoxamine regulates neuroinflammation and iron homeostasis in a mouse model of postoperative cognitive dysfunction. *J. Neuroinflamm.* 13, 268. doi: 10.1186/s12974-016-0740-2

Lindenau, J. D., Altmann, V., Schumacher-Schuh, A. F., Rieder, C. R., and Hutz, M. H. (2017). Tumor necrosis factor alpha polymorphisms are associated with Parkinson's disease age at onset. *Neurosci. Lett.* 658, 133–136. doi: 10.1016/j.neulet.2017.08.049

Liu, X.-B., Nguyen, N.-B. H., Marquess, K. D., Yang, F., and Haile, D. J. (2005). Regulation of hepcidin and ferroportin expression by lipopolysaccharide in splenic macrophages. *Blood Cells Mol. Dis.* 35, 47–56. doi: 10.1016/j.bcmd.2005.04.006

Liu, Y., Liu, J., Liu, H., Liao, Y., Cao, L., Ye, B., et al. (2016). Investigation of cerebral iron deposition in aged patients with ischemic cerebrovascular disease using susceptibility-weighted imaging. *Ther. Clin. Risk Manage.* 12, 1239–1247. doi: 10.2147/TCRM.S107783

Lu, L.-N., Qian, Z.-M., Wu, K.-C., Yung, W.-H., and Ke, Y. (2017). Expression of iron transporters and pathological hallmarks of Parkinson's and Alzheimer's diseases in the brain of young, adult, and aged rats. *Mol. Neurobiol.* 54, 5213–5224. doi: 10.1007/s12035-016-0067-0

Ma, J., Zhang, F.-L., Zhou, G., Bao, Y.-X., Shen, Y., and Qian, Z.-M. (2018). Different characteristics of hepcidin expression in IL-6 + / + and IL-6-/- neurons and astrocytes treated with lipopolysaccharides. *Neurochem. Res.* 43, 1624–1630. doi: 10.1007/s11064-018-2577-9

Martin-Bastida, A., Ward, R. J., Newbould, R., Piccini, P., Sharp, D., Kabba, C., et al. (2017). Brain iron chelation by deferiprone in a phase 2 randomised double-blinded placebo controlled clinical trial in Parkinson's disease. *Sci. Rep.* 7:1398. doi: 10.1038/s41598-017-01402-2

McCarthy, R. C., and Kosman, D. J. (2014). Glial cell ceruloplasmin and hepcidin differentially regulate iron efflux from brain microvascular endothelial cells. *PLoS One* 9:e89003. doi: 10.1371/journal.pone.0089003

McCarthy, R. C., and Kosman, D. J. (2015a). Iron transport across the blood-brain barrier: development, neurovascular regulation and cerebral amyloid angiopathy. *Cell. Mol. Life Sci.* 72, 709–727. doi: 10.1007/s00018-014-1771-4

McCarthy, R. C., and Kosman, D. J. (2015b). Mechanisms and regulation of iron trafficking across the capillary endothelial cells of the blood-brain barrier. *Front. Mol. Neurosci.* 8:31. doi: 10.3389/fnmol.2015.00031

McCarthy, R. C., Sosa, J. C., Gardeck, A. M., Baez, A. S., Lee, C.-H., and Wessling-Resnick, M. (2018). Inflammation-induced iron transport and metabolism by brain microglia. *J. Biol. Chem.* 293, 7853–7863. doi: 10.1074/jbc.RA118.001949

Moos, T., and Rosengren Nielsen, T. (2006). Ferroportin in the postnatal rat brain: implications for axonal transport and neuronal export of iron. *Semin. Pediatr. Neurol.* 13, 149–157. doi: 10.1016/j.spen.2006.08.003

Moreau, C., Danel, V., Devedjian, J. C., Grolez, G., Timmerman, K., Laloux, C., et al. (2018). Could conservative iron chelation lead to neuroprotection in amyotrophic lateral sclerosis? *Antioxid. Redox Signal.* 29, 742–748. doi: 10.1089/ars.2017.7493

Muller, M., and Leavitt, B. R. (2014). Iron dysregulation in Huntington's disease. *J. Neurochem.* 130, 328–350. doi: 10.1111/jnc.12739

Myhre, O., Utkilen, H., Duale, N., Brunborg, G., and Hofer, T. (2013). Metal dyshomeostasis and inflammation in Alzheimer's and Parkinson's diseases: possible impact of environmental exposures. *Oxid. Med. Cell. Longev.* 2013:726954. doi: 10.1155/2013/726954

Noelker, C., Morel, L., Lescot, T., Osterloh, A., Alvarez-Fischer, D., Breloer, M., et al. (2013). Toll like receptor 4 mediates cell death in a mouse MPTP model of Parkinson disease. *Sci. Rep.* 3:1393. doi: 10.1038/srep01393

Nunomura, A., Perry, G., Aliev, G., Hirai, K., Takeda, A., Balraj, E. K., et al. (2001). Oxidative damage is the earliest event in Alzheimer disease. *J. Neuropathol. Exp. Neurol.* 60, 759–767.

Oliveira, S. J., Pinto, J. P., Picarote, G., Costa, V. M., Carvalho, F., Rangel, M., et al. (2009). ER stress-inducible factor CHOP affects the expression of hepcidin by modulating C/EBPalpha activity. *PLoS One* 4:e6618. doi: 10.1371/journal.pone.0006618

Ostergaard, C., Sandvang, D., Frimodt-Møller, N., and Kristensen, H.-H. (2009). High cerebrospinal fluid (CSF) penetration and potent bactericidal activity in CSF of NZ2114, a novel plectasin variant, during experimental pneumococcal meningitis. *Antimicrob. Agents Chemother.* 53, 1581–1585. doi: 10.1128/AAC.01202-08

Pan, K., Li, X., Chen, Y., Zhu, D., Li, Y., Tao, G., et al. (2016). Deferoxamine pre-treatment protects against postoperative cognitive dysfunction of aged rats by depressing microglial activation via ameliorating iron accumulation in hippocampus. *Neuropharmacology* 111, 180–194. doi: 10.1016/j.neuropharm.2016.09.004

Pelizzoni, I., Zacchetti, D., Campanella, A., Grohovaz, F., and Codazzi, F. (2013). Iron uptake in quiescent and inflammation-activated astrocytes: a potentially neuroprotective control of iron burden. *Biochim. Biophys. Acta – Mol. Basis Dis.* 1832, 1326–1333. doi: 10.1016/J.BBADIS.2013.04.007

Perry, J. R., Julian, J. A., Laperriere, N. J., Geerts, W., Agnelli, G., Rogers, L. R., et al. (2010). PRODIGE: a randomized placebo-controlled trial of dalteparin low-molecular-weight heparin thromboprophylaxis in patients with newly diagnosed malignant glioma. *J. Thromb. Haemost.* 8, 1959–1965. doi: 10.1111/j.1538-7836.2010.03973.x

Peter, I., Dubinsky, M., Bressman, S., Park, A., Lu, C., Chen, N., et al. (2018). Anti-tumor necrosis factor therapy and incidence of parkinson disease among patients with inflammatory bowel disease. *JAMA Neurol.* 75, 939–946. doi: 10.1001/jamaneurol.2018.0605

Pietrangelo, A., Dierssen, U., Valli, L., Garuti, C., Rump, A., Corradini, E., et al. (2007). STAT3 is required for IL-6-gp130–dependent activation of hepcidin in vivo. *Gastroenterology* 132, 294–300. doi: 10.1053/j.gastro.2006.10.018

Pigeon, C., Ilyin, G., Courselaud, B., Leroyer, P., Turlin, B., Brissot, P., et al. (2001). A new mouse liver-specific gene, encoding a protein homologous to human antimicrobial peptide hepcidin, is overexpressed during iron overload. *J. Biol. Chem.* 276, 7811–7819. doi: 10.1074/jbc.M008923200

Poli, M., Girelli, D., Campostrini, N., Maccarinelli, F., Finazzi, D., Luscieti, S., et al. (2011). Heparin: a potent inhibitor of hepcidin expression in vitro and in vivo. *Blood* 117, 997–1004. doi: 10.1182/blood-2010-06-289082

Puy, V., Darwiche, W., Trudel, S., Gomila, C., Lony, C., Puy, L., et al. (2018). Predominant role of microglia in brain iron retention in sanfilippo syndrome, a pediatric neurodegenerative disease. *Glia* 66, 1709–1723. doi: 10.1002/glia.23335

Qian, Z.-M., He, X., Liang, T., Wu, K.-C., Yan, Y.-C., Lu, L.-N., et al. (2014). Lipopolysaccharides upregulate hepcidin in neuron via microglia and the IL-6/STAT3 signaling pathway. *Mol. Neurobiol.* 50, 811–820. doi: 10.1007/s12035-014-8671-3

Qin, X.-Y., Zhang, S.-P., Cao, C., Loh, Y. P., and Cheng, Y. (2016). Aberrations in peripheral inflammatory cytokine levels in parkinson disease. *JAMA Neurol.* 73, 1316. doi: 10.1001/jamaneurol.2016.2742

Raha, A. A., Vaishnav, R. A., Friedland, R. P., Bomford, A., and Raha-Chowdhury, R. (2013). The systemic iron-regulatory proteins hepcidin and ferroportin are reduced in the brain in Alzheimer's disease. *Acta Neuropathol. Commun.* 1:55. doi: 10.1186/2051-5960-1-55

Raha-Chowdhury, R., Raha, A. A., Forostyak, S., Zhao, J.-W., Stott, S. R. W., and Bomford, A. (2015). Expression and cellular localization of hepcidin mRNA and protein in normal rat brain. *BMC Neurosci.* 16:24. doi: 10.1186/s12868-015-0161-7

Raj, D., Yin, Z., Breur, M., Doorduin, J., Holtman, I. R., Olah, M., et al. (2017). Increased white matter inflammation in aging- and Alzheimer's disease brain. *Front. Mol. Neurosci.* 10:206. doi: 10.3389/fnmol.2017.00206

Ramey, G., Deschemin, J.-C., Durel, B., Canonne-Hergaux, F., Nicolas, G., and Vaulont, S. (2010). Hepcidin targets ferroportin for degradation in hepatocytes. *Haematologica* 95, 501–504. doi: 10.3324/haematol.2009.014399

Rottkamp, C. A., Raina, A. K., Zhu, X., Gaier, E., Bush, A. I., Atwood, C. S., et al. (2001). Redox-active iron mediates amyloid-beta toxicity. *Free Radic. Biol. Med.* 30, 447–450.

Rousselle, C., Clair, P., Lefauconnier, J. M., Kaczorek, M., Scherrmann, J. M., and Temsamani, J. (2000). New advances in the transport of doxorubicin through the blood-brain barrier by a peptide vector-mediated strategy. *Mol. Pharmacol.* 57, 679–686. doi: 10.1124/mol.57.4.679

Rutgers, M. P., Pielen, A., and Gille, M. (2007). Chronic cerebellar ataxia and hereditary hemochromatosis: causal or coincidental association? *J. Neurol.* 254, 1296–1297. doi: 10.1007/s00415-006-0507-2

Salazar, J., Mena, N., Hunot, S., Prigent, A., Alvarez-Fischer, D., Arredondo, M., et al. (2008). Divalent metal transporter 1 (DMT1) contributes to neurodegeneration in animal models of Parkinson's disease. *Proc. Natl. Acad. Sci. U.S.A.* 105, 18578–18583. doi: 10.1073/pnas.0804373105

Sansing, L. H., Harris, T. H., Welsh, F. A., Kasner, S. E., Hunter, C. A., and Kariko, K. (2011). Toll-like receptor 4 contributes to poor outcome after intracerebral hemorrhage. *Ann. Neurol.* 70, 646–656. doi: 10.1002/ana.22528

Schluesener, H., and Meyermann, R. (1995). Neutrophilic defensins penetrate the blood-brain barrier. *J. Neurosci. Res.* 42, 718–723. doi: 10.1002/jnr.490420515

Schulz, K., Kroner, A., and David, S. (2012). Iron efflux from astrocytes plays a role in remyelination. *J. Neurosci.* 32, 4841–4847. doi: 10.1523/JNEUROSCI.5328-11.2012

Shin, J. A., Kim, Y. A., Kim, H. W., Kim, H.-S., Lee, K.-E., Kang, J. L., et al. (2018). Iron released from reactive microglia by noggin improves myelin repair in the ischemic brain. *Neuropharmacology* 133, 202–215. doi: 10.1016/j.neuropharm.2018.01.038

Shinozaki, Y., Shibata, K., Yoshida, K., Shigetomi, E., Gachet, C., Ikenaka, K., et al. (2017). Transformation of astrocytes to a neuroprotective phenotype by microglia via $P2Y_1$ receptor downregulation. *Cell Rep.* 19, 1151–1164. doi: 10.1016/j.celrep.2017.04.047

Silva Adaya, D., Aguirre-Cruz, L., Guevara, J., and Ortiz-Islas, E. (2017). Nanobiomaterials' applications in neurodegenerative diseases. *J. Biomater. Appl.* 31, 953–984. doi: 10.1177/0885328216659032

Simpson, I. A., Ponnuru, P., Klinger, M. E., Myers, R. L., Devraj, K., Coe, C. L., et al. (2015). A novel model for brain iron uptake: introducing the concept of regulation. *J. Cereb. Blood Flow Metab.* 35, 48–57. doi: 10.1038/jcbfm.2014.168

Skjørringe, T., Burkhart, A., Johnsen, K. B., and Moos, T. (2015). Divalent metal transporter 1 (DMT1) in the brain: implications for a role in iron transport at the blood-brain barrier, and neuronal and glial pathology. *Front. Mol. Neurosci.* 8:19. doi: 10.3389/fnmol.2015.00019

Smith, M. A., Zhu, X., Tabaton, M., Liu, G., McKeel, D. W., Cohen, M. L., et al. (2010). Increased iron and free radical generation in preclinical Alzheimer disease and mild cognitive impairment. *J. Alzheimer's Dis.* 19, 363–372. doi: 10.3233/JAD-2010-1239

Song, N., Wang, J., Jiang, H., and Xie, J. (2010). Ferroportin 1 but not hephaestin contributes to iron accumulation in a cell model of Parkinson's disease. *Free Radic. Biol. Med.* 48, 332–341. doi: 10.1016/j.freeradbiomed.2009.11.004

Song, N., Wang, J., Jiang, H., and Xie, J. (2018). Astroglial and microglial contributions to iron metabolism disturbance in Parkinson's disease. *Biochim. Biophys. Acta – Mol. Basis Dis.* 1864, 967–973. doi: 10.1016/j.bbadis.2018.01.008

Steeland, S., Gorlé, N., Vandendriessche, C., Balusu, S., Brkic, M., Van Cauwenberghe, C., et al. (2018). Counteracting the effects of TNF receptor-1 has therapeutic potential in Alzheimer's disease. *EMBO Mol. Med.* 10:e8300. doi: 10.15252/emmm.201708300

Steinbicker, A. U., Bartnikas, T. B., Lohmeyer, L. K., Leyton, P., Mayeur, C., Kao, S. M., et al. (2011). Perturbation of hepcidin expression by BMP type I receptor deletion induces iron overload in mice. *Blood* 118, 4224–4230. doi: 10.1182/blood-2011-03-339952

Sun, C., Song, N., Xie, A., Xie, J., and Jiang, H. (2012). High hepcidin level accounts for the nigral iron accumulation in acute peripheral iron intoxication rats. *Toxicol. Lett.* 212, 276–281. doi: 10.1016/J.TOXLET.2012.05.022

Szeliga, M., Róñycka, A., Jędrak, P., Barańska, S., Janik, P., Jamrozik, Z., et al. (2016). Expression of RNAs coding for metal transporters in blood of patients with Huntington's disease. *Neurochem. Res.* 41, 101–106. doi: 10.1007/s11064-015-1737-4

Tan, G., Liu, L., He, Z., Sun, J., Xing, W., and Sun, X. (2016). Role of hepcidin and its downstream proteins in early brain injury after experimental subarachnoid hemorrhage in rats. *Mol. Cell. Biochem.* 418, 31–38. doi: 10.1007/s11010-016-2730-1

Trotta, T., Porro, C., Calvello, R., and Panaro, M. A. (2014). Biological role of Toll-like receptor-4 in the brain. *J. Neuroimmunol.* 268, 1–12. doi: 10.1016/j.jneuroim.2014.01.014

Urrutia, P., Aguirre, P., Esparza, A., Tapia, V., Mena, N. P., Arredondo, M., et al. (2013). Inflammation alters the expression of DMT1, FPN1 and hepcidin, and it causes iron accumulation in central nervous system cells. *J. Neurochem.* 126, 541–549. doi: 10.1111/jnc.12244

Urrutia, P. J., Hirsch, E. C., González-Billault, C., and Núñez, M. T. (2017). Hepcidin attenuates amyloid beta-induced inflammatory and pro-oxidant responses in astrocytes and microglia. *J. Neurochem.* 142, 140–152. doi: 10.1111/jnc.14005

Wan, W., Jin, L., Wang, Z., Wang, L., Fei, G., Ye, F., et al. (2017). Iron deposition leads to neuronal α-synuclein pathology by inducing autophagy dysfunction. *Front. Neurol.* 8:1. doi: 10.3389/fneur.2017.00001

Wang, J.-Y., Zhuang, Q.-Q., Zhu, L.-B., Zhu, H., Li, T., Li, R., et al. (2016). Meta-analysis of brain iron levels of Parkinson's disease patients determined by postmortem and MRI measurements. *Sci. Rep.* 6:36669. doi: 10.1038/srep36669

Wang, Q., Du, F., Qian, Z.-M., Ge, X. H., Zhu, L., Yung, W. H., et al. (2008). Lipopolysaccharide induces a significant increase in expression of iron regulatory hormone hepcidin in the cortex and substantia nigra in rat brain. *Endocrinology* 149, 3920–3925. doi: 10.1210/en.2007-1626

Wang, Q., Liu, Y., and Zhou, J. (2015). Neuroinflammation in Parkinson's disease and its potential as therapeutic target. *Transl. Neurodegener.* 4:19. doi: 10.1186/s40035-015-0042-0

Wang, S.-M., Fu, L.-J., Duan, X.-L., Crooks, D. R., Yu, P., Qian, Z.-M., et al. (2010). Role of hepcidin in murine brain iron metabolism. *Cell. Mol. Life Sci.* 67, 123–133. doi: 10.1007/s00018-009-0167-3

Wang, Y., Chang, C. F., Morales, M., Chou, J., Chen, H. L., Chiang, Y. H., et al. (2001). Bone morphogenetic protein-6 reduces ischemia-induced brain damage in rats. *Stroke* 32, 2170–2178.

Ward, R. J., Zucca, F. A., Duyn, J. H., Crichton, R. R., and Zecca, L. (2014). The role of iron in brain ageing and neurodegenerative disorders. *Lancet Neurol.* 13, 1045–1060. doi: 10.1016/S1474-4422(14)70117-6

Wei, S., Shi, W., Li, M., and Gao, Q. (2014). Calorie restriction down-regulates expression of the iron regulatory hormone hepcidin in normal and d -galactose-induced aging mouse brain. *Rejuvenation Res.* 17, 19–26. doi: 10.1089/rej.2013.1450

Welling, M. M., Nabuurs, R. J. A., and van der Weerd, L. (2015). Potential role of antimicrobial peptides in the early onset of Alzheimer's disease. *Alzheimer's Dement.* 11, 51–57. doi: 10.1016/j.jalz.2013.12.020

Wu, J., Hua, Y., Keep, R. F., Nakamura, T., Hoff, J. T., and Xi, G. (2003). Iron and iron-handling proteins in the brain after intracerebral hemorrhage. *Stroke* 34, 2964–2969. doi: 10.1161/01.STR.0000103140.52838.45

Xiong, X.-Y., Chen, J., Zhu, W.-Y., Zhao, T., Zhong, Q., Zhou, K., et al. (2015). Serum hepcidin concentrations correlate with serum iron level and outcome in patients with intracerebral hemorrhage. *Neurol. Sci.* 36, 1843–1849. doi: 10.1007/s10072-015-2266-2

Xiong, X.-Y., Liu, L., Wang, F.-X., Yang, Y.-R., Hao, J.-W., Wang, P.-F., et al. (2016). Toll-like receptor 4/MyD88–mediated signaling of hepcidin expression causing brain iron accumulation, oxidative injury, and cognitive impairment after intracerebral hemorrhage. *Circulation* 134, 1025–1038. doi: 10.1161/CIRCULATIONAHA.116.021881

Xu, H., Wang, Y., Song, N., Wang, J., Jiang, H., and Xie, J. (2017). New progress on the role of glia in iron metabolism and iron-induced degeneration of dopamine neurons in Parkinson's disease. *Front. Mol. Neurosci.* 10:455. doi: 10.3389/fnmol.2017.00455

Xu, Q., Langley, M., Kanthasamy, A. G., and Reddy, M. B. (2017). Epigallocatechin gallate has a neurorescue effect in a mouse model of parkinson disease. *J. Nutr.* 147, 1926–1931. doi: 10.3945/jn.117.255034

Xu, Q., Kanthasamy, A. G., Jin, H., and Reddy, M. B. (2016). Hepcidin plays a key role in 6-OHDA induced iron overload and apoptotic cell death in a cell culture model of parkinson's disease. *Parkinsons Dis.* 2016:8684130. doi: 10.1155/2016/8684130

Xu, Y. X., Du, F., Jiang, L. R., Gong, J., Zhou, Y.-F., Luo, Q. Q., et al. (2015). Effects of aspirin on expression of iron transport and storage proteins in BV-2 microglial cells. *Neurochem. Int.* 91, 72–77. doi: 10.1016/j.neuint.2015.10.014

Yang, L., Zhang, B., Yin, L., Cai, B., Shan, H., Zhang, L., et al. (2011). Tanshinone IIA prevented brain iron dyshomeostasis in cerebral ischemic rats. *Cell. Physiol. Biochem.* 27, 23–30. doi: 10.1159/000325202

You, L.-H., Yan, C.-Z., Zheng, B.-J., Ci, Y.-Z., Chang, S.-Y., Yu, P., et al. (2017). Astrocyte hepcidin is a key factor in LPS-induced neuronal apoptosis. *Cell Death Dis.* 8:e2676. doi: 10.1038/cddis.2017.93

Zechel, S., Huber-Wittmer, K., and von Bohlen und Halbach, O. (2006). Distribution of the iron-regulating protein hepcidin in the murine central nervous system. *J. Neurosci. Res.* 84, 790–800. doi: 10.1002/jnr.20991

Zhang, D.-L., Senecal, T., Ghosh, M. C., Ollivierre-Wilson, H., Tu, T., and Rouault, T. A. (2011). Hepcidin regulates ferroportin expression and intracellular iron homeostasis of erythroblasts. *Blood* 118, 2868–2877. doi: 10.1182/blood-2011-01-330241

Zhang, F.-L., Hou, H.-M., Yin, Z.-N., Chang, L., Li, F.-M., Chen, Y.-J., et al. (2017). Impairment of hepcidin upregulation by lipopolysaccharide in the interleukin-6 knockout mouse brain. *Front. Mol. Neurosci.* 10:367. doi: 10.3389/fnmol.2017.00367

Zhang, Z., Hou, L., Song, J.-L., Song, N., Sun, Y.-J., Lin, X., et al. (2014). Pro-inflammatory cytokine-mediated ferroportin down-regulation contributes to the nigral iron accumulation in lipopolysaccharide-induced Parkinsonian models. *Neuroscience* 257, 20–30. doi: 10.1016/J.NEUROSCIENCE.2013.09.037

Zhao, J., Xiang, X., Zhang, H., Jiang, D., Liang, Y., Qing, W., et al. (2018). CHOP induces apoptosis by affecting brain iron metabolism in rats with subarachnoid hemorrhage. *Exp. Neurol.* 302, 22–33. doi: 10.1016/j.expneurol.2017.12.015

Zhao, Y., Xin, Z., Li, N., Chang, S., Chen, Y., Geng, L., et al. (2018). Nano-liposomes of lycopene reduces ischemic brain damage in rodents by regulating iron metabolism. *Free Radic. Biol. Med.* 124, 1–11. doi: 10.1016/j.freeradbiomed.2018.05.082

Zheng, W., Xin, N., Chi, Z.-H., Zhao, B.-L., Zhang, J., Li, J.-Y., et al. (2009). Divalent metal transporter 1 is involved in amyloid precursor protein processing and Aβ generation. *FASEB J.* 23, 4207–4217. doi: 10.1096/fj.09-135749

Zhou, Y., Wang, Y., Wang, J., Anne Stetler, R., and Yang, Q.-W. (2014). Inflammation in intracerebral hemorrhage: from mechanisms to clinical translation. *Prog. Neurobiol.* 115, 25–44. doi: 10.1016/j.pneurobio.2013.11.003

Zhou, Y.-F., Zhang, C., Yang, G., Qian, Z.-M., Zhang, M.-W., Ma, J., et al. (2017). Hepcidin protects neuron from hemin-mediated injury by reducing iron. *Front. Physiol.* 8:332. doi: 10.3389/fphys.2017.00332

Ziegler, D. A., Wonderlick, J. S., Ashourian, P., Hansen, L. A., Young, J. C., Murphy, A. J., et al. (2013). Substantia nigra volume loss before basal forebrain degeneration in early parkinson disease. *JAMA Neurol.* 70:241. doi: 10.1001/jamaneurol.2013.597

8

The Relevancy of Data Regarding the Metabolism of Iron to Our Understanding of Deregulated Mechanisms in ALS: Hypotheses and Pitfalls

*Camille Petillon[1], Rudolf Hergesheimer[2], Hervé Puy[3], Philippe Corcia[2,4], Patrick Vourc'h[1,2], Christian Andres[1,2], Zoubida Karim[3] and Hélène Blasco[1,2]**

[1] Laboratoire de Biochimie, CHRU de Tours, Tours, France, [2] INSERM, U1253, Université de Tours, Tours, France, [3] Centre de Recherches sur l'Inflammation, Equipe "Hème, Fer et Maladies Inflammatoires", UMR 1149/ERL CNRS 8252, Université Paris Diderot Paris 7, UFR de Médecine Site Bichat, Paris, France, [4] Centre SLA, Service de Neurologie, CHRU de Tours, Tours, France

***Correspondence:**
Hélène Blasco
helene.blasco@univ-tours.fr

Amyotrophic lateral sclerosis (ALS) is a neurodegenerative disease caused by the loss of motor neurons. Its etiology remains unknown, but several pathophysiological mechanisms are beginning to explain motor neuronal death, as well as oxidative stress. Iron accumulation has been observed in both sporadic and familial forms of ALS, including mouse models. Therefore, the dysregulation of iron metabolism could play a role in the pathological oxidative stress in ALS. Several studies have been undertaken to describe iron-related metabolic markers, in most cases focusing on metabolites in the bloodstream due to few available data in the central nervous system. Reports of accumulation of iron, high serum ferritin, and low serum transferrin levels in ALS patients have encouraged researchers to consider dysregulated iron metabolism as an integral part of ALS pathophysiology. However, it appears complicated to suggest a general mechanism due to the diversity of models and iron markers studied, including the lack of consensus among all of the studies. Regarding clinical study reports, most of them do not take into account confusion biases such as inflammation, renal dysfunction, and nutritional status. Furthermore, the iron regulatory pathways, particularly involving hepcidin, have not been thoroughly explored yet within the pathogenesis of iron overload in ALS. In this sense, it is also essential to explore the relation between iron overload and other ALS-related events, such as neuro-inflammation, protein aggregation, and iron-driven cell death, termed ferroptosis. In this review, we point out limits of the designs of certain studies that may prevent the understanding of the role of iron in ALS and discuss the relevance of the published data regarding the pathogenic impact of iron metabolism deregulation in this disease and the therapeutics targeting this pathway.

Keywords: iron metabolism, amyotrophic lateral sclerosis, ferritin, biomarkers, ALS

INTRODUCTION

Amyotrophic lateral sclerosis (ALS) is a fatal, neurodegenerative disorder characterized by the selective loss of motor neurons (MN) in the spinal cord, brainstem, and cerebral cortex. This leads to progressive paralysis and death by respiratory failure (Hadzhieva et al., 2013). The median survival is three to five years from onset, and the only drug approved for treatment in Europe is riluzole that extends the average patient's lifespan for only a few more months. ALS is either familial (5–10% of cases) or sporadic (90–95% of cases). Genetic factors including mutations in the *C9orf72*, *SOD1* (Superoxide Dismutase 1), *TARDBP* (Transactive Response DNA-Binding Protein 43), and *FUS* (Fused in Sarcoma) genes could explain nearly 50% of familial cases (van Blitterswijk et al., 2012). Although the specific etiology of sporadic ALS remains unknown, several pathophysiological mechanisms have been described, such as oxidative stress, glutamate-mediated excitotoxicity, impaired axonal transport, mitochondrial dysfunction, and protein aggregation (Shaw, 2005).

Oxidative stress, characterized by reactive oxygen species (ROS), has been suggested to play a major role in the disease, because it has been described in all cases (D'Amico et al., 2013), even in those independent of mutations in SOD1 (corresponding to 80% of familial ALS patients, and most of the cases of sporadic forms). One of the crucial factors associated with the production and presence of ROS is iron, especially via the Fenton reaction, producing highly reactive hydroxyl radicals (Hadzhieva et al., 2013). Furthermore, an iron-dependent mechanism of cell death has recently been described, termed ferroptosis (Dixon et al., 2012). Various reports have suggested a neurodegenerative role of ferroptosis in which the affected neurons exhibit an accumulation of iron and lowered glutathione levels in rodent models (Wu et al., 2018).

Interestingly, perturbed iron regulation has notably been observed in many pre-clinical and clinical studies of ALS (Kwan et al., 2012; Golko-Perez et al., 2017). Determining the etiology of this deregulation, the specific role of iron, whether or not iron is only linked to oxidative stress and, finally, its potential as a diagnostic tool, prognostic marker, or therapeutic target all remain challenges. Studies evaluating iron metabolism in ALS, yet rarely included confusion biases or related these mechanisms to other pathophysiological pathways. In addition, many studies have focused on metabolic markers in the bloodstream, but ALS is mainly a disease of the central nervous system (CNS) and iron metabolism is different in the brain.

Accordingly, we question whether the quantity and the quality of the published data enable us to propose one or several mechanisms linking iron to ALS and to justify their relevance in clinical practice.

We focus this review on the publications concerning the metabolism of iron in the brain, the methods applied to explore iron metabolism in ALS, and on the published data on ALS patients and mutant SOD1 mice. We discuss the role of each marker of iron metabolism evaluated in this pathological context. We also highlight limits of the designs of certain studies that may prevent the understanding of the role of iron in ALS. Lastly, we offer suggestions regarding pitfalls to avoid when determining the role of iron metabolism in this disease's pathogenesis and discuss the associated therapeutic perspectives.

BODY IRON METABOLISM

Body iron metabolism relies on the coordination of several proteins having crucial roles in iron maintenance. Ferritin and transferrin (Tf) are the main carriers of iron in the blood, while proteins such as intracellular iron regulatory proteins (IRPs) and systemic hepcidin are key factors of iron metabolism regulation. Other proteins, including divalent metal transporter-1 (DMT1) and ferroportin (FPN1) in association with ferroxidases such as duodenal cytochrome B (DcytB), hephastin (Hp) and ceruloplasmin (Cp), are involved in the cellular membrane trafficking of iron. Finally, the production of hemoglobin (Hb), myoglobin, and various enzymes (cytochromes, aconitases, etc.) that require iron to function, are the final actors of iron metabolism.

Iron storage and recycling are directed by the liver and the spleen's macrophages that store excess iron with ferritin. They recycle iron following phagocytosis of senescent red blood cells and degradation of hemoglobin. Released iron is exported by FPN1 then oxidized by Cp to be re-bound to serum Tf for reuse. Iron absorption is mediated by the duodenal epithelial cells, which absorb both heme and non-heme iron from the diet according to the body's needs. Heme is taken up by specific carrier proteins and is catabolized by heme-oxygenase-1 to release ferrous iron (Fe^{2+}). Non-heme ferric iron (Fe^{3+}), is reduced to $Fe2^{+}$ by the duodenal Dcytb before uptake by the apically expressed DMT1. Ferrous iron is delivered to the circulation via the basolateral exporter FPN1 in association with the ferroxidase Hp. The complex (Fe^{3+}-Tf) is delivered to cells by binding to its receptor, transferrin receptor 1 (TfR1), then the complex is taken up by the cell through the invagination of the membrane, initiating endocytosis. Finally, iron is released from transferrin and is transported out of the endosome by DMT1. In all cells of the body, excess Fe^{2+} is converted to Fe^{3+} by the ferroxidase activity of ferritin H-chain (Ft-H) before storage in the ferritin mineral core (Ft-H and Ft-L) (Hentze et al., 2010).

Hepcidin is a central player in iron homeostasis, acting as a 25 amino-acid mature peptide predominantly expressed in the liver (Nicolas et al., 2001). Hepcidin acts by triggering FPN1 activity and/or protein level and degradation of duodenal DMT1 protein (Nemeth et al., 2004; Brasse-Lagnel et al., 2011; Aschemeyer et al., 2018). Therefore, hepcidin is a hyposideremic factor that reduces both the intestinal absorption of iron and its release by macrophages, hepatocytes, and other cell types. Hepcidin is eliminated in the urine, and small fragments from degradation of 20–25 aa have been found (Park et al., 2001). Hepcidin is expressed by the *HAMP* gene located on chromosome 19 (19q13.1). This gene is upregulated by iron overload, infection, and inflammation. It is downregulated by iron deficiency, hypoxia, anemia, and stimulated erythropoiesis (Hentze et al., 2010).

BRAIN IRON METABOLISM

Iron is a vital cofactor in many metabolic processes of the CNS, including oxidative phosphorylation, myelin synthesis, neurotransmitter production, and oxygen transport (Crichton et al., 2011). The presence of the blood–brain barrier (BBB) protects the brain from the daily fluctuations of systemic iron and also from iron disorders that affect all peripheral tissues. The precise mechanism by which the BBB mediates iron influx from the blood to the parenchyma of the brain still remains to be uncovered (**Figure 1**). One hypothesis currently accepted for the transfer of iron across the blood capillary endothelial cells (BCECs) states that Tf-TfR1 transcytosis creates a passive conduit without intracellular processing. However, a new model based on the classical process of iron and experimental data has been recently proposed (Simpson et al., 2015). In this model, iron that enters the CNS is delivered to BCECs by the Tf-TfR complex. Upon internalization into the endosome, iron is released from Tf, exported to the cytosol by DMT1, then exported out of the cell by FPN with the help of Cp ferroxidase expressed at the external cell surface of astrocytes (Jeong and David, 2003; Wu et al., 2004). The *bioGPS* database also shows Cp and FPN transcripts evenly distributed throughout the CNS (BioGPS - your Gene Portal System [Internet], 2018).

Released iron is most likely captured by brain Tf that is synthesized and secreted by oligodendrocytes and the choroid plexus into the brain interstitium. Intriguingly, in this proposed model, evidence of the presence of DMT1 in BCECs is yet to be demonstrated since, not until recently, there are conflicting studies indicating both the presence and absence of DMT1 transcripts and protein (Gunshin et al., 1997; Moos et al., 2006; Skjørringe et al., 2015). However, several arguments promote that in BCECs, the expression level of DMT1 is probably low but that its amount is sufficient to ensure the iron export from the endosome (Skjørringe et al., 2015). A third, alternative explanation of iron delivery involving the uptake of ferritin across the BBB has been proposed, but further support is still necessary to confirm this mechanism (Fisher et al., 2007; Todorich et al., 2011).

The acquisition of iron by brain cells is mediated by different pathways. Neurons express abundant TfR1 and acquire most of their iron via transferrin. Astrocytes do not appear to express TfR1 (Dringen et al., 2007), although this is controversial (Qian et al., 1999). However, they express DMT1 and FPN at the plasma membrane (Wu et al., 2004; Lane et al., 2010). Oligodendrocytes accumulate the most amount of brain iron and are the predominant producers of Tf in the brain (Burdo and Connor, 2003). Transferrin is widely distributed in the CNS but is preferentially expressed in the spinal cord, pre-frontal cortex, and hypothalamus (Mackenzie et al., 2007). Oligodendrocytes also express the ferritin receptor Tim-2, suggestive of an ability to acquire iron from ferritin (Hulet et al., 1999). Most brain cells express cytosolic ferritin for storing excess iron, and relatively high transcript levels are found in the spinal cord, hypothalamus, and pre-frontal cortex; neurons contain the least, while microglia contain the most (Mackenzie et al., 2007; Crichton et al., 2011; Singh et al., 2014).

Despite the high concentration of hepcidin in the liver, recent studies have also revealed the widespread expression of hepcidin in the brain, specifically in the spinal cord, hippocampus, and olfactory bulb (Zechel et al., 2006; Mackenzie et al., 2007; Wang et al., 2008). These findings imply that hepcidin might also

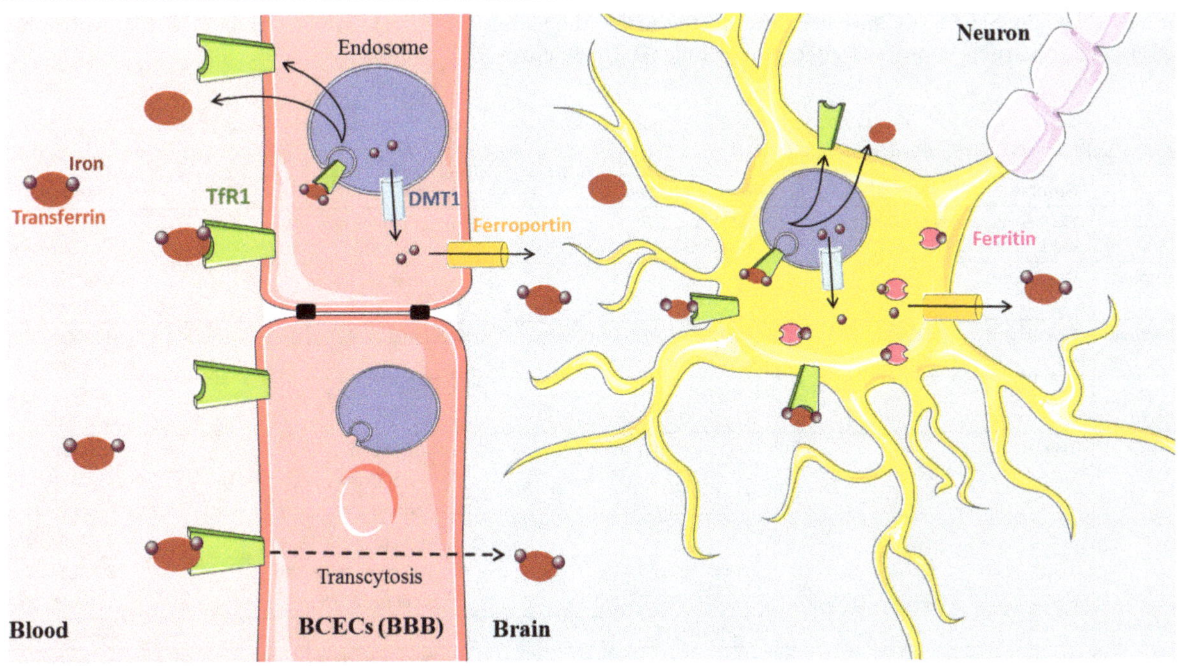

FIGURE 1 | Brain iron metabolism (Medical images: https://smart.servier.com).

be a key regulator in brain iron homeostasis. Hepcidin, similar to its action in the intestine, may regulate the expression of iron transport proteins DMT1 and ferroportin (Puy et al., 2018). This could explain the maintenance of iron balance in neurons and glial cells through the control of their iron uptake and release (Du et al., 2015).

One regulatory protein of brain iron that is currently receiving increased attention is the HFE protein. Mutations in the *HFE* gene are commonly associated with hereditary hemochromatosis in which an iron overload is the consequence of hepcidin deficiency. HFE transcripts in the CNS are relatively concentrated in the spinal cord, temporal and occipital lobes, and the cortex (Mackenzie et al., 2007). The presence of the HFE protein at the interface between the brain and endothelial cells of the microvasculature, and in the cerebrospinal fluid (CSF), may also affect iron content and contribute to iron overload in neurodegenerative disorders. Indeed, HFE mutations have been investigated as risk factors for neurodegenerative disorders (Nandar and Connor, 2011).

METHODS TO STUDY IRON METABOLISM

Imaging and biological methods have been utilized on cohorts of patients as tools to study the dysregulation of iron metabolism. In SOD1 transgenic mice and cell models, several approaches, such as concentration measurements, protein expression followed by Western blotting and/or immunofluorescence, and measuring mRNA expression have been employed. **Table 1** summarizes the different studies performed to explore iron metabolism in ALS. It is important to notice the significant diversity among models, tissues, and markers studied. For example, cell lines, especially neurons or MN (NSC-34, SH-SY5Y), have been transfected with mutant SOD1 gene constructs in order to attempt to mimic ALS in humans (Schlachetzki et al., 2013). Glial cells are also used in co-culture with neurons, given the hypothesis that ALS is a non-cell-autonomous disease, meaning that multiple cell types can play into the disease's pathogenesis (Smethurst et al., 2016; Zeineddine et al., 2017). Astrocytes expressing WT or mutant SOD1 have been co-cultured with primary cortical neurons (Kunze et al., 2013). Microglia expressing mutant SOD1 have been co-cultured, as well, with iPSC-derived MN (Frakes et al., 2014). Another example is the co-culture of human adult primary sALS astrocytes and human embryonic stem cell-derived MN (Re et al., 2014).

Nevertheless, transgenic mice and rats represent the gold standard of preclinical ALS modeling. Rodent models exist for the genetic mutations in *SOD1, TARDBP,* and *FUS* and mouse models for *C9orf72* repeat expansions have also been developed (Chew et al., 2015; Jiang et al., 2016; Liu et al., 2016). In particular, the models in which human genomic mutant SOD1 is overexpressed have been used extensively with the following most studied mutations: SOD1 G93A, SOD1 G37R, and SOD1 G85R (Shaw, 2005). Clinical studies of cohorts of ALS patients also add to the knowledge of iron metabolism.

MARKERS OF DEREGULATED IRON METABOLISM IN ALS

We searched the *Pubmed* database to identify potentially relevant studies on the association between iron metabolism and ALS. We used free text and the medical subject heading (MeSH) terms "amyotrophic lateral sclerosis," "ALS," "iron," "iron metabolism," "iron accumulation," "biomarker," and "iron chelation." Then, we searched for each marker of iron metabolism (DMT1, TfR1, ferritin, ferroportin, hepcidin, *HFE*,...) AND ALS (OR "amyotrophic lateral sclerosis").

TABLE 1 | Models and iron metabolism markers studied.

Model	Sample	Marker studied	Studies	Workforce
G93A-SOD1 cells	SH-Y5Y human NeurobLastoma cells	DMT1 and TfRI	Hadzhieva et al., 2013	–
SOD1 G93A mouse	Spinal cord	Iron	Lee et al., 2015	4 SOD1 G93A/4 wild-type
SOD1 G37R mouse	Spinal cord	Iron DMT1, TfR1 ferroportin, ceruloplasmin	Jeong et al., 2009	4 SOD1 G37R/ 3 wild-type
SOD 1G93A rats	Serum	Hepcidin	Halon et al., 2014	15 SOD1 G93A/15 wild-type
ALS patients	Serum	Iron, transferrin, ferritin, TSC	Nadjar et al., 2012	629 ALS/297 controls
			Veyrat-Durebex et al., 2014	104 ALS/145 controls
			Goodall et al., 2008	60 ALS/ 44 controls
			Ikeda et al., 2012	92 ALS/ 92 controls
		Ferritin	Qureshi et al., 2008	30 ALS/ 30 controls
			Su et al., 2015	138 ALS/152 controls
		Pro-hepcidin	Mitchell et al., 2010	30 ALS/ 36 controls
	Cerebral cortex	Iron	Oba et al., 1993	15 ALS/49 controls
			Ignjatovic et al., 2013	46 ALS/ 26 controls

BCECs, blood capillary endothelial cells; BBB, blood–brain barrier; TfR1, receptor transferrin 1; DMT1, divalent metal ion transporter 1.

Iron Accumulation

Increased iron levels were reported in spinal cord MN in two ALS SOD1-mouse models, SOD1 G93A (Lee et al., 2015) and SOD1 G37R (Jeong et al., 2009), by staining ventral MN with Perl's (Fe^{3+}) and Turnbull's (Fe^{2+}) reactants.

Iron accumulation was also observed in the CNS of ALS patients by magnetic resonance imaging (MRI) (Oba et al., 1993; Ignjatovic et al., 2013). T2-weighted MRI scans were used to detect areas of hypo-intensity (iron deposits) in the cerebral cortex of ALS patients. Likewise, they used Perl's-reactant for the analyses of postmortem brains and revealed a large amount of ferric iron in the pre-central cortices (Oba et al., 1993). More recently, accumulated iron was detected in multiple brain regions, including the motor cortex, substantia nigra, globus pallidus, red nucleus, and the putamen in ALS patients by quantitative susceptibility mapping (Acosta-Cabronero et al., 2018).

The Alteration of Iron Transport

A study reported the upregulation of DMT1 and TfR1 mRNAs in G93A-SOD1 cells (SH-SY5Y) (Hadzhieva et al., 2013). In another study, the expression of various proteins involved in iron transport, such as DMT1, TfR1, ferroportin, and ceruloplasmin was evaluated in the spinal cord of SOD1 G37R mice (Jeong et al., 2009). Data at 12 months of age (end stage) showed an increase in the mRNA and protein expression of DMT1, ferroportin, and ceruloplasmin in the cervical spinal cord. Furthermore, double immunofluorescence labeling revealed that in 12-month-old SOD1 G37R transgenic mice the expression of DMT1 was augmented in MN in the ventral horn of the spinal cord. It was also shown that these iron transport markers were more abundant in SOD1 G37R mice at 4 months of age, and mRNA levels were higher in the lumbar region of the spinal cord in the early stages of the disease.

Two independent clinical studies have shown increased values of transferrin saturation (TS) in a cohort of ALS patients and controls (Nadjar et al., 2012; Veyrat-Durebex et al., 2014). However, only the study by Nadjar et al. (2012), performed on a large ALS population (694 patients), thus presenting higher statistical power (Veyrat-Durebex et al., 2014), showed a significant decrease in serum transferrin levels in ALS subjects. Interestingly, it was also demonstrated that low serum transferrin concentrations were associated with a higher loss in body weight at diagnosis in ALS patients (Veyrat-Durebex et al., 2014), which could link iron metabolism to nutritional status – largely associated with energetic metabolism in ALS.

Increased Serum Ferritin

Serum ferritin is also increased in ALS patients (Goodall et al., 2008; Qureshi et al., 2008; Su et al., 2015). Six case-control studies published between 2008 and 2015 investigating the possible relationship between ALS patients and their susceptibility to elevated serum ferritin levels were included in a meta-analysis (Hu et al., 2016), including 1053 cases of ALS and 760 healthy control cases from the United Kingdom, United States, France, and Japan. The serum ferritin concentrations in ALS were statistically higher compared to healthy controls ($p < 0.00001$). The limitations revealed by this meta-analysis were a high heterogeneity ($p = 0.03$; $I^2 = 50\%$) and a publisher bias.

Alteration of *HFE* Gene and Hepcidin Alteration

A meta-analysis assessing the roles of the H63D and C282Y variants of the *HFE* gene in ALS from 14 observational studies illustrated a significant association of the C282Y variant to the disease, meaning a decreased risk for ALS, while confirming that the H63D variant showed no relevant association (Li et al., 2014). In fact, hemochromatosis linked to mutations in the *HFE* gene has been attributed solely to the homozygous C282Y variant. The results of this meta-analysis imply that the C282Y *HFE* variant could be a protective factor against ALS, which is *a priori* surprising given the physiopathology of ALS, in which iron is expected to play a toxic role.

In one report, hepcidin plasma concentrations were measured in SOD1 transgenic rats (G93A) at 12 weeks (asymptomatic, ALS stage I), 21 weeks (disease onset, ALS stage II) and 24 weeks (end-stage disease, ALS stage III) of age, and were significantly increased in the blood of ALS II and III animals (Halon et al., 2014). On the other hand, the plasma concentrations of pro-hepcidin, the precursor to hepcidin, were not significantly altered in a cohort of 29 ALS patients (from nine to 28 months post-diagnosis) compared to control group. Nevertheless, there was a positive correlation between pro-hepcidin and IL-6 levels in ALS patients compared to controls, suggesting exacerbated iron release by macrophages and inflammation in ALS patients (Mitchell et al., 2010).

CAN WE INTEGRATE PUBLISHED DATA TO SUGGEST A ROLE OF IRON DEREGULATION IN ALS?

Regarding the diversity of models and the methodology used, as well as the studied markers, the findings with respect to iron metabolism seem heterogeneous. It appears complicated to suggest a global mechanism of dysregulation. Accumulation of iron, higher serum ferritin, and lower serum transferrin levels in ALS patients have clearly encouraged researchers to consider iron deregulation as an essential mechanism in ALS. The critical review of the literature led us to identify the limits preventing the understanding of iron metabolism disturbance in ALS, and more specific findings in the context of ALS must be provided.

PITFALLS TO AVOID WHEN STUDYING IRON METABOLISM IN ALS

Types of Models

The lack of the complex interplay between MN and their surrounding environment is the precise problem that we face with the published data on cellular models, encouraging us to turn to other models. Although SOD1 mutations are rare in sALS, there are phenotypic similarities with fALS, and it has been assumed that studying the familial form could provide insight into the sporadic form. However, the validity of these assumptions has been questioned (Clerc et al., 2016) and, even if clinical manifestations are not so different, the pathophysiological mechanisms are obviously distinct. For instance, TDP-43 aggregates were not observed in patients suffering from ALS forms associated with SOD1 mutations (Mackenzie et al., 2007), whereas they were in a $SOD1^{G93A}$ mouse model (Jeon et al., 2018). Due to this discrepancy between postmortem patient and mouse tissues, one should consider the TDP-43 aggregation to be unrelated to the SOD1 ALS pathology if this artifactual aggregation is unavoidable in SOD1 mouse models. Moreover, exploring iron metabolism closely linked with the consequence of SOD1 activity, i.e., production of ROS, seems biased. So, this model that is subjected to oxidative stress may not fit with the investigation of iron metabolism. In addition, the relatively rapid neurodegeneration that occurs in these mice can reduce the quantity of iron in the affected neurons, potentially confounding the interpretation of the corresponding results. Altogether, we are aware that SOD1 mouse models remain valid for the study of certain aspects of ALS pathogenesis, but the scope of the conclusions must be limited in relation to the restraints of this model, especially in the exploration of iron metabolism.

Localization of Iron Metabolism Exploration

Data reporting the main genetic loci involved in iron accumulation would be the first step to the understanding of the role of iron in ALS. Another study, in fact, showed that inducing inflammation with intravenous injections of lipopolysaccharide (LPS) in mice led to hepcidin expression in the cortex, hippocampus, and striatum (Wang et al., 2008). In fact, hepcidin along with the other iron regulators are shown to be expressed in the spinal cord and cortex, the two main areas affected by ALS. Therefore, investigating their behavior in these tissues in ALS models could yield insight regarding iron accumulation hot spots. Published data on mouse models have revealed that the spinal cord is especially affected with increased expression of iron transporters (DMT1, ferroportin, and TfR1). Much attention has been turned toward ALS patients' brains, but incomplete data prevent us from drawing conclusions in humans. Although there is limited data for factors of iron metabolism in the CSF of ALS patients, data from MRI and postmortem brain exploration have presented interesting information to locate the main regions of accumulation.

In addition, the identification of cells types is also essential to integrate all of these findings. Some researchers have highlighted the role of glia (Jeong et al., 2009) by observing an increased cytosolic ferritin expression not identified in MN, suggesting that neurons and glia accumulate iron via different mechanisms.

Finally, it is necessary to be aware of the differences in the expression levels between mice and humans, since murine models are the "gold standard" in studying ALS. Indeed, the differences in distribution and expression levels pose limitations on the conclusions inferred from these models (**Supplementary Table S1**). Even though certain regulators exhibit differential distributions and expression levels in the mouse CNS compared to that of humans, mouse microglia consistently show expression for most, if not all, the regulators mentioned here. Because cells other than neurons can also become affected in ALS and that microglia have quite an unequivocal relationship with iron-driven inflammation, paying attention to the levels of these iron regulators in the microglia of murine ALS models could increase the relevancy and decrease the limitations of murine models.

Extrapolation From Liver to the Brain

The interaction between the liver and the brain regarding iron metabolism must be taken into account, but it is difficult to extrapolate from the published data. Indeed, most of the factors of iron metabolism have not yet been studied in the brain, and we cannot deduce a mechanism from their activity in other organs. For example, it was suggested that the HFE C282Y variant could be a potentially protective factor for ALS. But, it is difficult to extrapolate the role of HFE from the liver to the brain, given that ALS is not a disease primarily affecting the liverapart from the manifestation of a fatty liver (Dupuis et al., 2008). Similarly, it could be misleading to compare the levels of metabolic regulators of iron in the serum and the brain, since the main carriers and regulatory processes are not fully understood in healthy persons and even less so in ALS patients.

RELEVANT PARAMETERS TO INCLUDE IN IRON METABOLISM EXPLORATION IN ALS PATIENTS

Dynamic Variation of Iron Metabolism

Importantly, a multi-factorial disease, such as ALS, is characterized by regulation and counter-regulation, which is dependent on the progress of the disease and on other pathophysiological mechanisms. Information regarding the relation between iron metabolism and disease progression would help the integration of iron's role in the pathogenesis. One does, therefore, wonder if iron accumulation in the CNS of ALS patients is a factor for poor prognosis and if increasing concentrations of iron might cause the disease to progress more quickly over time. However, very few data on iron concentrations in the brain of ALS patients are available, and even fewer about variations in these concentrations throughout the progression of the disease. Nadjar et al. (2012) showed that high levels of serum ferritin (>156 μg/L), were significantly associated with a reduced survival time. ALS patients with low levels of ferritin lived around 300 days longer than patients with high levels ($p < 0{,}04$). But, serum ferritin does not necessarily reflect the iron accumulation in the CNS.

The pathophysiological mechanisms that could explain why ALS patients have increased iron body storage and how that is responsible for a decreased survival is, at present, unknown.

With respect to the largely unknown mechanism of regulation and/or rebound effect, very little can be concluded for a general mechanism of iron metabolism in ALS, such as with data concerning hepcidin that has been clearly understudied and whose studies yield contradictory outcomes.

Confounding Factors for the Interpretation of Iron Metabolism Status

Regarding clinical studies, the first issue is the heterogeneity among ALS patients, since the site of onset, the form of ALS, the evolution, and genetic mutations add and multiply the diversity among patients. To add to this expected and known limit of all cohort studies of ALS, some biological concerns are often overlooked. Several parameters that can disrupt iron metabolism are not taken into account. For example, inflammation, renal dysfunction, and nutritional status are commonly overlooked. Since serum ferritin is an acute-phase reactive protein whose concentration can rise in the presence of acute or chronic inflammation, it might fluctuate depending on the inflammatory status of ALS patients (Hu et al., 2016). Also, CRP concentrations were not measured in all the clinical studies (Qureshi et al., 2008; Ikeda et al., 2012; Nadjar et al., 2012). This was taken into account in the study by Veyrat-Durebex et al. (2014), and CRP values were not significantly different between patients and controls. In Goodall et al. (2008), CRP and ceruloplasmin levels were both negatively correlated with iron and iron saturation in ALS patients showing that iron metabolism disturbance was not due to inflammation.

Kidney dysfunction may alter some parameters of iron metabolism (Maras et al., 2015). The age at onset of ALS [between 50 and 60 years (Shaw, 2005)] could suggest that kidney function starts to be altered, but this data has not been directly reported; no ideal marker has been identified or used in these cases, and clinicians are hesitant to insist on kidney function exploration. Unfortunately, creatinine is not a very reliable marker of kidney function in the context of ALS due to muscular atrophy (Corbett et al., 1982), leading to the mis-evaluation of the glomerular filtration rate (eGF). Veyrat-Durebex et al. (2014) reported a creatinine value, used in the MDRD (modified diet in renal disease) equation, to estimate the glomerular filtration rate. The estimated eGFR was higher ($p < 0.0001$) in ALS patients than in controls, showing not that renal function was better but that creatinine levels were low probably due to muscular atrophy and that the role of potential defective renal elimination on differences in iron metabolism cannot be explored by this approach (Veyrat-Durebex et al., 2014). The evaluation of creatinine values after taking into account body composition (impedancemetry) or using other markers of renal function (cystatin C, iohexol, etc.) may help with the interpretation of iron metabolism, independent of muscle atrophy and renal elimination. Similarly, nutritional factors essential to ALS have to be included in iron metabolism interpretation, as it may completely influence the results, either due to disease or management. For example, it has been illustrated that low serum transferrin concentrations are associated with a higher body weight loss at the time of diagnosis in ALS patients (Veyrat-Durebex et al., 2014). Further investigations on nutritional care in ALS patients will be necessary.

We expect promising and complementary findings from CSF studies, but few data has been published to date (Goodall et al., 2008).

THERAPEUTIC PROSPECTS

The pathogenic impact of iron metabolism deregulation in ALS has been further supported by the partially protective effects of iron chelators in ALS mouse models (Hadzhieva et al., 2014). In recent years, various iron chelators have demonstrated a prolonged survival of SOD1 transgenic mice. A classic iron chelator, desferrioxamine, previously studied in models of neurodegenerative diseases, such as Huntington's disease or Parkinson's disease (Hilditch-Maguire et al., 2000; Zhang et al., 2005), as well as the new iron chelators 5-[4-(2-hydroxyethyl) piperazine-1-ylmethyl]-8- hydroxyquinoline (VK-28) and 5-(*N*-methyl-*N*-propargylaminomethyl)-8-hydroxyquinoline (M30), have also been studied in models of ALS disease (Wang et al., 2011).

Iron chelators significantly delay disease onset (6–12 days on average, $p < 0.05$), extend the lifespan (8–13 days on average, $p < 0.05$), and reduce spinal cord motor neuron loss in ALS SOD1 transgenic mice. These chelators are able to prevent ferroptosis, as well (Masaldan et al., 2018). In support of this, a mouse model of aggravated ferroptosis displayed ALS features, such as intense muscular atrophy, rapid paralysis, and ferroptotic neurodegeneration of the motor neurons of the spinal cord (Chen et al., 2015; Masaldan et al., 2018). Thus, the therapeutic effects of iron chelation in SOD1 mice seem to partly stem from the suppression of ferroptosis, which could result from iron accumulation. Besides these findings, VK-28 and M30 reduced ROS generation and inhibited activation of glial cells in the spinal cord (Wang et al., 2011).

In both a SOD1 murine model of fALS and sALS, a low dose of deferiprone, another classic iron chelator, was associated with a decrease in pathological iron accumulation in the central motor pathways (Moreau et al., 2018).

In ALS patients, iron chelation could reduce iron accumulation and the related excess of oxidative stress in the motor pathways. Classical iron chelation could induce systemic iron depletion. For this reason, the safety and efficacy of conservative iron chelation (chelation with a low risk of iron depletion) was assessed in a single-center, single-arm, 12-month-long pilot clinical trial (NCT02164253). After 12 months of treatment with deferiprone, none of the 23 ALS patients enrolled in the trial displayed signs of anemia. The decreases in the ALS Functional Rating Scale (ALSFRS-R) and in the body mass index were significantly smaller in the first 3 months of deferiprone treatment than in the parallel 3-month treatment-free period (Moreau et al., 2018). A significant decrease in iron concentration, shown by MRI, was observed in the cervical spinal cord and the motor cortex while not in areas outside the motor system (the cerebellum and the occipital cortex) (Moreau et al., 2018).

Currently, the efficacy of deferiprone in ALS patients is being evaluated in a randomized, double-blind, placebo-controlled, multi-center French study (FAIR-ALS II) with an estimated enrollment of 210 participants and a 12-month period (NCT03293069).

Evidence has revealed that the neuroprotection of iron chelation may result from the attenuation of iron-related oxidative stress, iron accumulation, and ferroptosis. However, we have little perspective on the long term regarding the effects of these iron chelators, and we are not yet certain about their precise mechanism of action. It could very well be that the chelation treatment brings about a long-term effect; it could also simply be temporarily effective, requiring life-long treatment. Moreover, to our knowledge no study has determined the exact specificity of these chelators for iron. We question to which extent one can attribute the therapeutic effect of iron chelators in animal models to the interaction with iron. Therefore, future studies should pay attention to the concentrations of other heavy metals besides iron in order to better assess the overall effect of the chelator on the cell.

CONCLUSION

Since iron heavily participates in ROS production and has been seen to accumulate in the context of ALS, we have focused this review on the published findings concerning iron metabolism in this disease. Future studies will need to address the experimental limitations that we have acknowledged in this review. The limitations in the murine models originate from the experimental bias projected from the use of pathogenic SOD1. Because this condition primarily generates ROS, the conclusions relating iron metabolic regulators drawn from these studies are confined to the ALS cases in which SOD1 is mutated, which is only a minute proportion of both familial and sporadic cases. Therefore, it would be of particular interest to compare the effects on iron regulation between the SOD1 models and another type, such as TDP-43 models.

Other limitations in clinical studies analyzing the metabolic alterations of iron stem from the fact that many overlook the roles of the inflammatory status, renal function, and nutritional status. These factors become very important when considering therapeutic strategies relying on iron chelation. The clinical trials attempt to employ chelators as an early form of treatment but, even though patients show a considerable retention in body mass and a decrease in iron levels in the spinal cord (Wang et al., 2011), this seems only temporary. Furthermore, studies on patients do not necessarily contain a homogeneous cohort of people affected by SOD1-driven ALS, unlike SOD1 murine models. This confounds the interpretations of iron metabolism, since the sub-type of ALS is not controlled. However, these clinical limitations might be nearly impossible to avoid. Therefore, while complementing treatment with nutritional maintenance and keeping track of kidney and inflammatory status, the chelation-guided therapy could be prolonged and possibly more applicable to the general population of ALS patients. Indeed, there appears to be a global dysregulation of iron in ALS cases, and we must gain a more complete understanding of the causes and consequences.

AUTHOR CONTRIBUTIONS

CP and RH wrote most of the sections of the manuscript. CP did the bibliography and the literature review on iron in ALS. ZK wrote Section "Body Iron Metabolism" and completed Section "Brain Iron Metabolism". RH did the article proofreading (English). All authors contributed to manuscript revision, read and approved the submitted version.

REFERENCES

Acosta-Cabronero, J., Machts, J., Schreiber, S., Abdulla, S., Kollewe, K., Petri, S., et al. (2018). Quantitative susceptibility MRI to detect brain iron in amyotrophic lateral sclerosis. *Radiology* 289, 195–203. doi: 10.1148/radiol.2018180112

Aschemeyer, S., Qiao, B., Stefanova, D., Valore, E. V., Sek, A. C., Ruwe, T. A., et al. (2018). Structure-function analysis of ferroportin defines the binding site and an alternative mechanism of action of hepcidin. *Blood* 131, 899–910. doi: 10.1182/blood-2017-05-786590

BioGPS – your Gene Portal System [Internet] (2018). *[cité 10 déc]: Disponible sur.* Available at: http://biogps.org/#goto=welcome

Brasse-Lagnel, C., Karim, Z., Letteron, P., Bekri, S., Bado, A., and Beaumont, C. (2011). Intestinal DMT1 cotransporter is down-regulated by hepcidin via proteasome internalization and degradation. *Gastroenterology* 140, 1261–1271.e1. doi: 10.1053/j.gastro.2010.12.037

Burdo, J. R., and Connor, J. R. (2003). Brain iron uptake and homeostatic mechanisms: an overview. *Biometals* 16, 63–75. doi: 10.1023/A:1020718718550

Chen, L., Hambright, W. S., Na, R., and Ran, Q. (2015). Ablation of the ferroptosis inhibitor glutathione peroxidase 4 in neurons results in rapid motor neuron degeneration and paralysis. *J. Biol. Chem.* 290, 28097–28106. doi: 10.1074/jbc.M115.680090

Chew, J., Gendron, T. F., Prudencio, M., Sasaguri, H., Zhang, Y.-J., Castanedes-Casey, M., et al. (2015). Neurodegeneration. C9ORF72 repeat expansions in mice cause TDP-43 pathology, neuronal loss, and behavioral deficits. *Science* 348, 1151–1154. doi: 10.1126/science.aaa9344

Clerc, P., Lipnick, S., and Willett, C. (2016). A look into the future of ALS research. *Drug Discov. Today* 21, 939–949. doi: 10.1016/j.drudis.2016.02.002

Corbett, A. J., Griggs, R. C., and Moxley, R. T. (1982). Skeletal muscle catabolism in amyotrophic lateral sclerosis and chronic spinal muscular atrophy. *Neurology* 32, 550–552. doi: 10.1212/WNL.32.5.550

Crichton, R. R., Dexter, D. T., and Ward, R. J. (2011). Brain iron metabolism and its perturbation in neurological diseases. *J. Neural Transm.* 118, 301–314. doi: 10.1007/s00702-010-0470-z

D'Amico, E., Factor-Litvak, P., Santella, R. M., and Mitsumoto, H. (2013). Clinical perspective on oxidative stress in sporadic amyotrophic lateral sclerosis. *Free Radic. Biol. Med.* 65, 509–527. doi: 10.1016/j.freeradbiomed.2013.06.029

Dixon, S. J., Lemberg, K. M., Lamprecht, M. R., Skouta, R., Zaitsev, E. M., Gleason, C. E., et al. (2012). Ferroptosis: an iron-dependent form of nonapoptotic cell death. *Cell* 149, 1060–1072. doi: 10.1016/j.cell.2012.03.042

Dringen, R., Bishop, G. M., Koeppe, M., Dang, T. N., and Robinson, S. R. (2007). The pivotal role of astrocytes in the metabolism of iron in the brain. *Neurochem. Res.* 32, 1884–1890. doi: 10.1007/s11064-007-9375-0

Du, F., Qian, Z.-M., Luo, Q., Yung, W.-H., and Ke, Y. (2015). Hepcidin suppresses brain iron accumulation by downregulating iron transport proteins in iron-overloaded rats. *Mol. Neurobiol.* 52, 101–114. doi: 10.1007/s12035-014-8847-x

Dupuis, L., Corcia, P., Fergani, A., Gonzalez De Aguilar, J.-L., Bonnefont-Rousselot, D., Bittar, R., et al. (2008). Dyslipidemia is a protective factor in amyotrophic lateral sclerosis. *Neurology* 70, 1004–1009. doi: 10.1212/01.wnl.0000285080.70324.27

Fisher, J., Devraj, K., Ingram, J., Slagle-Webb, B., Madhankumar, A. B., Liu, X., et al. (2007). Ferritin: a novel mechanism for delivery of iron to the brain and other organs. *Am. J. Physiol. Cell Physiol.* 293, C641–C649. doi: 10.1152/ajpcell.00599.2006

Frakes, A. E., Ferraiuolo, L., Haidet-Phillips, A. M., Schmelzer, L., Braun, L., Miranda, C. J., et al. (2014). Microglia induce motor neuron death via the classical NF-κB pathway in amyotrophic lateral sclerosis. *Neuron* 81, 1009–1023. doi: 10.1016/j.neuron.2014.01.013

Golko-Perez, S., Amit, T., Bar-Am, O., Youdim, M. B. H., and Weinreb, O. (2017). A novel iron chelator-radical scavenger ameliorates motor dysfunction and improves life span and mitochondrial biogenesis in SOD1^{G93A} ALS mice. *Neurotox. Res.* 31, 230–244. doi: 10.1007/s12640-016-9677-6

Goodall, E. F., Haque, M. S., and Morrison, K. E. (2008). Increased serum ferritin levels in amyotrophic lateral sclerosis (ALS) patients. *J. Neurol.* 255, 1652–1656. doi: 10.1007/s00415-008-0945-0

Gunshin, H., Mackenzie, B., Berger, U. V., Gunshin, Y., Romero, M. F., Boron, W. F., et al. (1997). Cloning and characterization of a mammalian proton-coupled metal-ion transporter. *Nature* 388, 482–488. doi: 10.1038/41343

Hadzhieva, M., Kirches, E., and Mawrin, C. (2014). Review: iron metabolism and the role of iron in neurodegenerative disorders. *Neuropathol. Appl. Neurobiol.* 40, 240–257. doi: 10.1111/nan.12096

Hadzhieva, M., Kirches, E., Wilisch-Neumann, A., Pachow, D., Wallesch, M., Schoenfeld, P., et al. (2013). Dysregulation of iron protein expression in the G93A model of amyotrophic lateral sclerosis. *Neuroscience* 230, 94–101. doi: 10.1016/j.neuroscience.2012.11.021

Halon, M., Kaczor, J. J., Ziolkowski, W., Flis, D. J., Borkowska, A., Popowska, U., et al. (2014). Changes in skeletal muscle iron metabolism outpace amyotrophic lateral sclerosis onset in transgenic rats bearing the G93A hmSOD1 gene mutation. *Free Radic. Res.* 48, 1363–1370. doi: 10.3109/10715762.2014.955484

Hentze, M. W., Muckenthaler, M. U., Galy, B., and Camaschella, C. (2010). Two to tango: regulation of Mammalian iron metabolism. *Cell* 142, 24–38. doi: 10.1016/j.cell.2010.06.028

Hilditch-Maguire, P., Trettel, F., Passani, L. A., Auerbach, A., Persichetti, F., and MacDonald, M. E. (2000). Huntingtin: an iron-regulated protein essential for normal nuclear and perinuclear organelles. *Hum. Mol. Genet.* 9, 2789–2797. doi: 10.1093/hmg/9.19.2789

Hu, X., Yang, Y., Su, J., and Yao, C. (2016). Meta-analysis of the relationship between amyotrophic lateral sclerosis and susceptibility to serum ferritin level elevation. *Neurosciences* 21, 120–125. doi: 10.17712/nsj.2016.2.20150482

Hulet, S. W., Hess, E. J., Debinski, W., Arosio, P., Bruce, K., Powers, S., et al. (1999). Characterization and distribution of ferritin binding sites in the adult mouse brain. *J. Neurochem.* 72, 868–874. doi: 10.1046/j.1471-4159.1999.720868.x

Ignjatovic, A., Steviæ, Z., Lavrniæ, S., Dakoviæ, M., and Baèiæ, G. (2013). Brain iron MRI: a biomarker for amyotrophic lateral sclerosis. *J. Magn. Reson. Imaging* 38, 1472–1479. doi: 10.1002/jmri.24121

Ikeda, K., Hirayama, T., Takazawa, T., Kawabe, K., and Iwasaki, Y. (2012). Relationships between disease progression and serum levels of lipid, urate, creatinine and ferritin in Japanese patients with amyotrophic lateral sclerosis: a cross-sectional study. *Intern. Med.* 51, 1501–1508. doi: 10.2169/internalmedicine.51.7465

Jeon, G. S., Shim, Y.-M., Lee, D.-Y., Kim, J.-S., Kang, M., Ahn, S. H., et al. (2018). Pathological modification of TDP-43 in amyotrophic lateral sclerosis with SOD1 mutations. *Mol. Neurobiol.* doi: 10.1007/s12035-018-1218-2 [Epub ahead of print].

Jeong, S. Y., and David, S. (2003). Glycosylphosphatidylinositol-anchored ceruloplasmin is required for iron efflux from cells in the central nervous system. *J. Biol. Chem.* 278, 27144–27148. doi: 10.1074/jbc.M301988200

Jeong, S. Y., Rathore, K. I., Schulz, K., Ponka, P., Arosio, P., and David, S. (2009). Dysregulation of iron homeostasis in the CNS contributes to disease progression in a mouse model of amyotrophic lateral sclerosis. *J. Neurosci.* 29, 610–619. doi: 10.1523/JNEUROSCI.5443-08.2009

Jiang, J., Zhu, Q., Gendron, T. F., Saberi, S., McAlonis-Downes, M., Seelman, A., et al. (2016). Gain of toxicity from ALS/FTD-linked repeat expansions in C9ORF72 is alleviated by antisense oligonucleotides targeting GGGGCC-containing RNAs. *Neuron* 90, 535–550. doi: 10.1016/j.neuron.2016.04.006

Kunze, A., Lengacher, S., Dirren, E., Aebischer, P., Magistretti, P. J., and Renaud, P. (2013). Astrocyte-neuron co-culture on microchips based on the model of SOD mutation to mimic ALS. *Integr. Biol.* 5, 964–975. doi: 10.1039/c3ib40022k

Kwan, J. Y., Jeong, S. Y., Van Gelderen, P., Deng, H.-X., Quezado, M. M., Danielian, L. E., et al. (2012). Iron accumulation in deep cortical layers accounts for MRI signal abnormalities in ALS: correlating 7 tesla MRI and pathology. *PLoS One* 7:e35241. doi: 10.1371/journal.pone.0035241

Lane, D. J. R., Robinson, S. R., Czerwinska, H., Bishop, G. M., and Lawen, A. (2010). Two routes of iron accumulation in astrocytes: ascorbate-dependent ferrous iron uptake via the divalent metal transporter (DMT1) plus an independent route for ferric iron. *Biochem. J.* 432, 123–132. doi: 10.1042/BJ20101317

Lee, J. K., Shin, J. H., Gwag, B. J., and Choi, E.-J. (2015). Iron accumulation promotes TACE-mediated TNF-α secretion and neurodegeneration in a mouse model of ALS. *Neurobiol. Dis.* 80, 63–69. doi: 10.1016/j.nbd.2015.05.009

Li, M., Wang, L., Wang, W., Qi, X. L., and Tang, Z. Y. (2014). Mutations in the HFE gene and sporadic amyotrophic lateral sclerosis risk: a meta-analysis of observational studies. *Braz. J. Med. Biol. Res.* 47, 215–222. doi: 10.1590/1414-431X20133296

Liu, Y., Pattamatta, A., Zu, T., Reid, T., Bardhi, O., Borchelt, D. R., et al. (2016). C9orf72 BAC mouse model with motor deficits and neurodegenerative features of ALS/FTD. *Neuron* 90, 521–534. doi: 10.1016/j.neuron.2016.04.005

Mackenzie, I. R. A., Bigio, E. H., Ince, P. G., Geser, F., Neumann, M., Cairns, N. J., et al. (2007). Pathological TDP-43 distinguishes sporadic amyotrophic lateral sclerosis from amyotrophic lateral sclerosis with SOD1 mutations. *Ann. Neurol.* 61, 427–434. doi: 10.1002/ana.21147

Maras, J. S., Maiwall, R., Harsha, H. C., Das, S., Hussain, M. S., Kumar, C., et al. (2015). Dysregulated iron homeostasis is strongly associated with multiorgan failure and early mortality in acute-on-chronic liver failure. *Hepatology* 61, 1306–1320. doi: 10.1002/hep.27636

Masaldan, S., Bush, A. I., Devos, D., Rolland, A. S., and Moreau, C. (2018). Striking while the iron is hot: iron metabolism and ferroptosis in neurodegeneration. *Free Radic. Biol. Med.* doi: 10.1016/j.freeradbiomed.2018.09.033 [Epub ahead of print].

Mitchell, R. M., Simmons, Z., Beard, J. L., Stephens, H. E., and Connor, J. R. (2010). Plasma biomarkers associated with ALS and their relationship to iron homeostasis. *Muscle Nerve* 42, 95–103. doi: 10.1002/mus.21625

Moos, T., Skjoerringe, T., Gosk, S., and Morgan, E. H. (2006). Brain capillary endothelial cells mediate iron transport into the brain by segregating iron from transferrin without the involvement of divalent metal transporter 1. *J. Neurochem.* 98, 1946–1958. doi: 10.1111/j.1471-4159.2006.04023.x

Moreau, C., Danel, V., Devedjian, J. C., Grolez, G., Timmerman, K., Laloux, C., et al. (2018). Could conservative iron chelation lead to neuroprotection in amyotrophic lateral sclerosis? *Antioxid. Redox Signal.* 29, 742–748. doi: 10.1089/ars.2017.7493

Nadjar, Y., Gordon, P., Corcia, P., Bensimon, G., Pieroni, L., Meininger, V., et al. (2012). Elevated serum ferritin is associated with reduced survival in amyotrophic lateral sclerosis. *PLoS One* 7:e45034. doi: 10.1371/journal.pone.0045034

Nandar, W., and Connor, J. R. (2011). HFE gene variants affect iron in the brain. *J. Nutr.* 141, 729S–739S. doi: 10.3945/jn.110.130351

Nemeth, E., Tuttle, M. S., Powelson, J., Vaughn, M. B., Donovan, A., Ward, D. M., et al. (2004). Hepcidin regulates cellular iron efflux by binding to ferroportin and inducing its internalization. *Science* 306, 2090–2093. doi: 10.1126/science.1104742

Nicolas, G., Bennoun, M., Devaux, I., Beaumont, C., Grandchamp, B., Kahn, A., et al. (2001). Lack of hepcidin gene expression and severe tissue iron overload in upstream stimulatory factor 2 (USF2) knockout mice. *Proc. Natl. Acad. Sci. U.S.A.* 98, 8780–8785. doi: 10.1073/pnas.151179498

Oba, H., Araki, T., Ohtomo, K., Monzawa, S., Uchiyama, G., Koizumi, K., et al. (1993). Amyotrophic lateral sclerosis: T2 shortening in motor cortex at MR imaging. *Radiology* 189, 843–846. doi: 10.1148/radiology.189.3.8234713

Park, C. H., Valore, E. V., Waring, A. J., and Ganz, T. (2001). Hepcidin, a urinary antimicrobial peptide synthesized in the liver. *J. Biol. Chem.* 276, 7806–7810. doi: 10.1074/jbc.M008922200

Puy, V., Darwiche, W., Trudel, S., Gomila, C., Lony, C., Puy, L., et al. (2018). Predominant role of microglia in brain iron retention in Sanfilippo syndrome, a pediatric neurodegenerative disease. *Glia* doi: 10.1002/glia.23335 [Epub ahead of print].

Qian, Z. M., To, Y., Tang, P. L., and Feng, Y. M. (1999). Transferrin receptors on the plasma membrane of cultured rat astrocytes. *Exp. Brain Res.* 129, 473–476. doi: 10.1007/s002210050916

Qureshi, M., Brown, R. H., Rogers, J. T., and Cudkowicz, M. E. (2008). Serum ferritin and metal levels as risk factors for amyotrophic lateral sclerosis. *Open Neurol. J.* 2, 51–54. doi: 10.2174/1874205X00802010051

Re, D. B., Le Verche, V., Yu, C., Amoroso, M. W., Politi, K. A., Phani, S., et al. (2014). Necroptosis drives motor neuron death in models of both sporadic and familial ALS. *Neuron* 81, 1001–1008. doi: 10.1016/j.neuron.2014.01.011

Schlachetzki, J. C. M., Saliba, S. W., and de Oliveira, A. C. P. (2013). Studying neurodegenerative diseases in culture models. *Braz. J. Psychiatry* 35, S92–S100. doi: 10.1590/1516-4446-2013-1159

Shaw, P. J. (2005). Molecular and cellular pathways of neurodegeneration in motor neurone disease. *J. Neurol. Neurosurg. Psychiatry* 76, 1046–1057. doi: 10.1136/jnnp.2004.048652

Simpson, I. A., Ponnuru, P., Klinger, M. E., Myers, R. L., Devraj, K., Coe, C. L., et al. (2015). A novel model for brain iron uptake: introducing the concept of regulation. *J. Cereb. Blood Flow Metab.* 35, 48–57. doi: 10.1038/jcbfm.2014.168

Singh, N., Haldar, S., Tripathi, A. K., Horback, K., Wong, J., Sharma, D., et al. (2014). Brain iron homeostasis: from molecular mechanisms to clinical significance and therapeutic opportunities. *Antioxid. Redox Signal.* 20, 1324–1363. doi: 10.1089/ars.2012.4931

Skjørringe, T., Burkhart, A., Johnsen, K. B., and Moos, T. (2015). Divalent metal transporter 1 (DMT1) in the brain: implications for a role in iron transport at the blood-brain barrier, and neuronal and glial pathology. *Front. Mol. Neurosci.* 8:19. doi: 10.3389/fnmol.2015.00019

Smethurst, P., Newcombe, J., Troakes, C., Simone, R., Chen, Y.-R., Patani, R., et al. (2016). In vitro prion-like behaviour of TDP-43 in ALS. *Neurobiol. Dis.* 96, 236–247. doi: 10.1016/j.nbd.2016.08.007

Su, X. W., Clardy, S. L., Stephens, H. E., Simmons, Z., and Connor, J. R. (2015). Serum ferritin is elevated in amyotrophic lateral sclerosis patients. *Amyotroph. Lateral Scler. Frontotemporal Degener.* 16, 102–107. doi: 10.3109/21678421.2014.984723

Todorich, B., Zhang, X., and Connor, J. R. (2011). H-ferritin is the major source of iron for oligodendrocytes. *Glia* 59, 927–935. doi: 10.1002/glia.21164

van Blitterswijk, M., van Es, M. A., Hennekam, E. A. M., Dooijes, D., van Rheenen, W., Medic, J., et al. (2012). Evidence for an oligogenic basis of amyotrophic lateral sclerosis. *Hum. Mol. Genet.* 21, 3776–3784. doi: 10.1093/hmg/dds199

Veyrat-Durebex, C., Corcia, P., Mucha, A., Benzimra, S., Mallet, C., Gendrot, C., et al. (2014). Iron metabolism disturbance in a French cohort of ALS patients. *Biomed Res. Int.* 2014:485723. doi: 10.1155/2014/485723

Wang, Q., Du, F., Qian, Z.-M., Ge, X. H., Zhu, L., Yung, W. H., et al. (2008). Lipopolysaccharide induces a significant increase in expression of iron regulatory hormone hepcidin in the cortex and *Substantia nigra* in rat brain. *Endocrinology* 149, 3920–3925. doi: 10.1210/en.2007-1626

Wang, Q., Zhang, X., Chen, S., Zhang, X., Zhang, S., Youdium, M., et al. (2011). Prevention of motor neuron degeneration by novel iron chelators in SOD1(G93A) transgenic mice of amyotrophic lateral sclerosis. *Neurodegener. Dis.* 8, 310–321. doi: 10.1159/000323469

Wu, J.-R., Tuo, Q.-Z., and Lei, P. (2018). Ferroptosis, a recent defined form of critical cell death in neurological disorders. *J. Mol. Neurosci.* 66, 197–206. doi: 10.1007/s12031-018-1155-6

Wu, L. J., Leenders, A. G. M., Cooperman, S., Meyron-Holtz, E., Smith, S., Land, W., et al. (2004). Expression of the iron transporter ferroportin in synaptic vesicles and the blood-brain barrier. *Brain Res.* 1001, 108–117. doi: 10.1016/j.brainres.2003.10.066

Zechel, S., Huber-Wittmer, K., and von Bohlen und Halbach, O. (2006). Distribution of the iron-regulating protein hepcidin in the murine central nervous system. *J. Neurosci. Res.* 84, 790–800. doi: 10.1002/jnr.20991

Zeineddine, R., Whiten, D. R., Farrawell, N. E., McAlary, L., Hanspal, M. A., Kumita, J. R., et al. (2017). Flow cytometric measurement of the cellular propagation of TDP-43 aggregation. *Prion* 11, 195–204. doi: 10.1080/19336896.2017.1314426

Zhang, X., Xie, W., Qu, S., Pan, T., Wang, X., and Le, W. (2005). Neuroprotection by iron chelator against proteasome inhibitor-induced nigral degeneration. *Biochem. Biophys. Res. Commun.* 333, 544–549. doi: 10.1016/j.bbrc.2005.05.150

9

Unraveling the Role of Heme in Neurodegeneration

Deborah Chiabrando*†, Veronica Fiorito†, Sara Petrillo and Emanuela Tolosano

Molecular Biotechnology Center, Department of Molecular Biotechnology and Health Sciences, University of Torino, Turin, Italy

***Correspondence:**
Deborah Chiabrando
deborah.chiabrando@unito.it

†These authors have contributed equally to this work

Heme (iron-protoporphyrin IX) is an essential co-factor involved in several biological processes, including neuronal survival and differentiation. Nevertheless, an excess of free-heme promotes oxidative stress and lipid peroxidation, thus leading to cell death. The toxic properties of heme in the brain have been extensively studied during intracerebral or subarachnoid hemorrhages. Recently, a growing number of neurodegenerative disorders have been associated to alterations of heme metabolism. Hence, the etiology of such diseases remains undefined. The aim of this review is to highlight the neuropathological role of heme and to discuss the major heme-regulated pathways that might be crucial for the survival of neuronal cells. The understanding of the molecular mechanisms linking heme to neurodegeneration will be important for therapeutic purposes.

Keywords: heme, neurodegeneration, FLVCR, FLVCR1, FLVCR1a, neuropathy

INTRODUCTION

Neurodegeneration is a complex process leading to the progressive and selective loss of neurons. Mitochondrial dysfunction, oxidative stress, protein aggregation and endoplasmic reticulum stress are well established pathways driving the neurodegenerative process (Lansbury and Lashuel, 2006; Lin and Beal, 2006; Xiang et al., 2017; Morris et al., 2018). Recent data suggest that iron and heme metabolism dysfunction may also play a crucial role. The involvement of iron in neurodegeneration has been well documented (Levi and Finazzi, 2014; Mena et al., 2015; Stockwell et al., 2017) and iron chelation has been proposed as a therapeutic option (Ward et al., 2015; Ashraf et al., 2018). Moreover, several neurodegenerative disorders have been associated to dysfunction of heme metabolism, thus supporting a crucial role for heme in the pathogenesis of such diseases.

The neurotoxicity of heme is evident during intracerebral or subarachnoid hemorrhages. In these pathological conditions, large amount of hemoglobin and heme are released in the brain promoting oxidative stress, lipid peroxidation, inflammatory response and finally cell death (Righy et al., 2016). To counteract the toxic effects exerted by hemoglobin and heme, human cells have evolved several detoxification mechanisms. During brain injury, the plasma proteins Haptoglobin and Hemopexin have proved to be protective against free hemoglobin and heme as primary scavenger systems (Hahl et al., 2013; Ma et al., 2016). Moreover, the induction of the heme-degrading enzyme heme oygenase-1 (HMOX1) in the brain has been reported in intracerebral and subarachnoid hemorrhage, and other neurodegenerative conditions (Panahian et al., 1999; Wang and Doré, 2007; Guan et al., 2009; Gozzelino, 2016).

Hemoglobin-derived heme is not the only form of heme that the nervous system can handle. Endogenously synthesized heme is also deleterious if not properly managed. Heme synthesis is an endogenous and essential process occurring in almost all tissues, including the nervous system (Smith et al., 2011; Gozzelino, 2016). Heme is endogenously synthesized to regulate a plethora of biological processes that may be particularly relevant in the nervous system. Among them, heme regulates energy production, ion channels, gene expression and microRNA processing (Smith et al., 2011). For these reasons, heme is essential for neuronal survival and differentiation. Recent data clearly indicate that the amount of intracellular heme available for regulatory functions (the so called "Heme Regulatory Pool" or "Labile Heme") is determined by the balance between heme synthesis, catabolism, import and export (Chiabrando et al., 2014b; Reddi and Hamza, 2016). The identification of a growing number of neurodegenerative disorders due to mutations in genes involved in heme metabolism strongly support the idea that the control of labile heme is crucial to avoid neurodegeneration. How heme drives the neurodegenerative process is still incompletely understood. However, it is becoming clear that heme neurotoxicity could be only partially explained by the release of toxic iron.

Here, we provide an overview of heme-related neurodegenerative disorders. Moreover, we discuss the potential mechanisms leading to heme neurotoxicity. We believe that the understanding of these mechanisms will be essential in the future to identify novel therapeutic targets.

NEURODEGENERATIVE DISORDERS CAUSED BY HEME METABOLISM DYSFUNCTIONS

The physiological relevance to control labile heme in the nervous system is highlighted by the identification of neurodegenerative disease-causing mutations in genes involved in heme metabolism. Indeed, mutations in genes involved in heme biosynthesis are responsible for neuropathic Porphyrias and Friederich Ataxia; mutations in the heme importer FLVCR2 have been found in Fowler Syndrome; mutations in the heme exporter FLVCR1 cause Posterior Column Ataxia and Retinitis Pigmentosa, non-syndromic Retinitis Pigmentosa and Hereditary Sensory and Autonomic Neuropathies (**Figure 1**). However, the molecular mechanisms underlying heme neurotoxicity are still unclear. Below, we summarize the major clinical features and the molecular genetics of these rare disorders.

Neurodegenerative Disorders Due to Defects in Heme Synthesis

Heme synthesis is a well characterized and ubiquitous process that involves eight enzymatic steps. Briefly, ALAS1 (δ-aminolevulinic acid synthase 1) catalyzes the condensation of succynil-CoA and glycine in the mitochondrial matrix, to form δ-aminolevulinic acid (ALA). ALA is transported into the cytosol where it is converted to coproporphyrinogen III through a series of enzymatic reactions. Then, coproporphyrinogen III is translocated back into mitochondria for the final steps of heme synthesis (Chiabrando et al., 2014a). Mutations in each gene involved in the heme biosynthetic pathway are responsible for a group of rare disorders collectively named porphyrias (Besur et al., 2014; Ramanujam and Anderson, 2015). The partial deficiency of these enzymes results in reduced heme synthesis and accumulation of toxic porphyrin precursors in multiple organ systems, including the skin, liver and nervous system. Here we focus on neuropathic porphyrias which are associated with neurologic manifestations. Furthermore, defects in the last steps of heme synthesis have been reported in Friederic Ataxia (Schoenfeld et al., 2005; Huang et al., 2009).

Neuropathic Porphyrias

The most common neurologic manifestations in neuropathic Porphyrias are a combination of autonomic and peripheral neuropathy. The autonomic neuropathy is characterized by abdominal pain, tachycardia, hypertension, constipation and nausea. The peripheral neuropathy is predominantly a motor axonal neuropathy leading to muscle pain and weakness. Sensory neuropathy is manifested as neuropathic pain and distal paraesthesiaes. The central nervous system (CNS) may also be affected, leading to psychosis, anxiety, depression and seizures. Porphyric neuropathies are characterized by relative quiescent phases followed by acute neurovisceral attacks involving severe abdominal pain, peripheral neuropathies and psychiatric disturbances. Such attacks are often exacerbated by external stimuli (drugs and hormones) that induce endogenous heme synthesis thus leading to an increase of toxic heme precursors (Albers and Fink, 2004; Simon and Herkes, 2011; Tracy and Dyck, 2014). Neuropathic Porphyrias include delta-aminolevulinate dehydratase deficiency, acute intermittent porphyria, hereditary coproporphyria and variegate porphyria.

Delta-aminolevulinate dehydratase deficiency (ALAD deficiency; OMIM: #612740) is the only type of neuropathic porphyria with an autosomal recessive mode of inheritance. ALAD deficiency is an extremely rare disorder with childhood onset and severe neurologic implications. ALAD deficiency is caused by mutations in the gene encoding the second enzyme in the heme biosynthetic pathway. These mutations cause almost complete lack of ALAD activity and patients excrete a large amount of ALA into urine (Ramanujam and Anderson, 2015).

Acute intermittent porphyria (AIP; OMIM: #176000) is an autosomal dominant disorder with incomplete penetrance. It is the most common type of neuropathic porphyria. AIP is caused by mutations in the hydroxymethylbilane synthase (*HMBS*) gene, resulting in the partial deficiency of porphobilinogen deaminase (PBGD). PBGD is the third enzyme in the heme biosynthetic pathway and its reduced activity leads to the accumulation and urine excretion of ALA and porphobilinogen (PBG) (Pischik and Kauppinen, 2015; Ramanujam and Anderson, 2015).

Hereditary coproporphyria (HCP; OMIM: #121300) is an autosomal dominant disorder with incomplete penetrance. HCP results from mutations in the gene encoding coproporphyrinogen oxidase (*CPOX*). CPOX represents the sixth enzyme in the heme biosynthetic pathway. Its partial deficiency

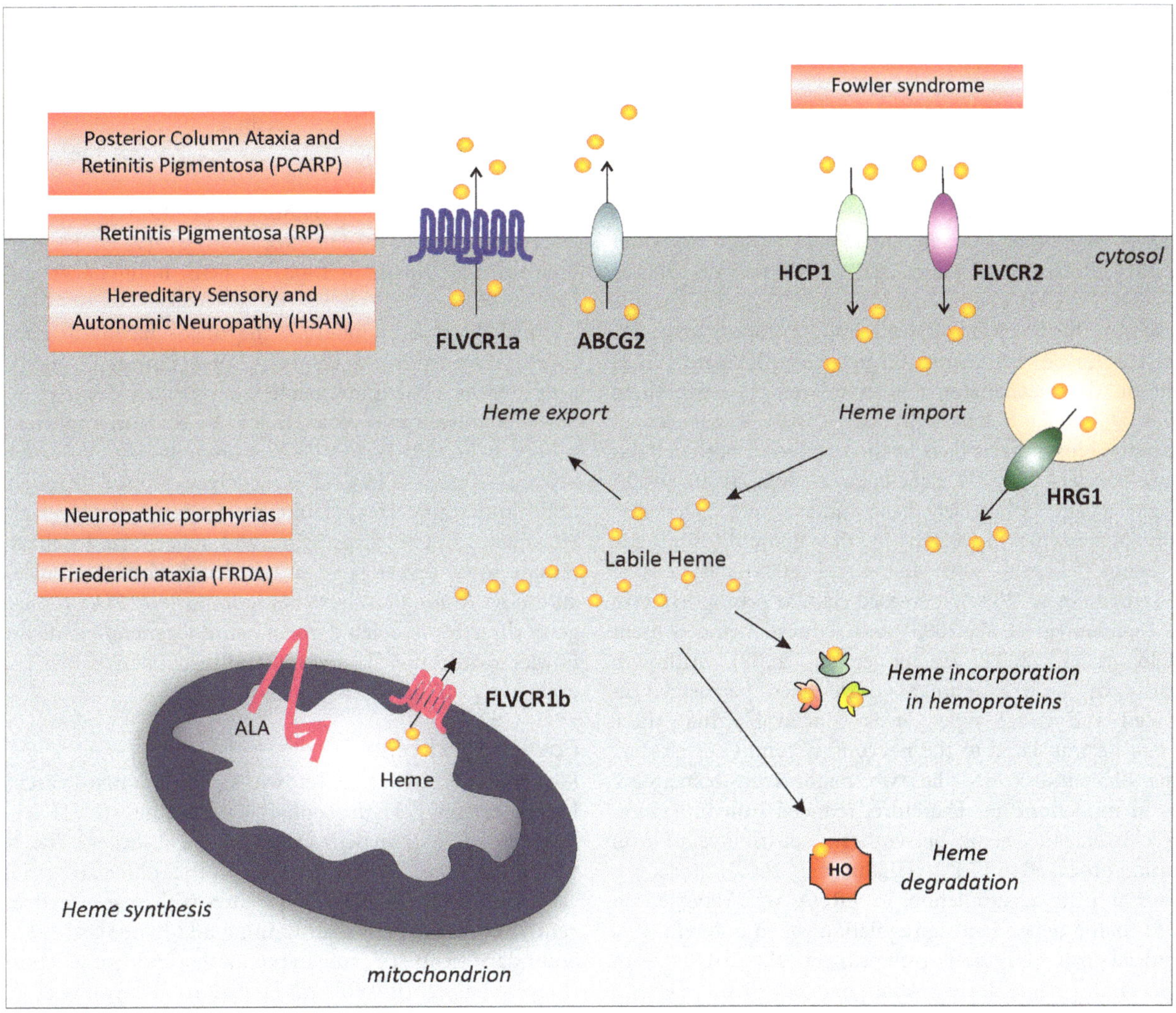

FIGURE 1 | Neurodegenerative disorders associated to heme metabolism dysfunction. Schematic representation of the main pathways involved in the regulation of intracellular labile heme: heme synthesis, heme incorporation into hemoproteins, heme degradation, heme export and import. The picture highlights rare neurodegenerative disorders directly associated to heme metabolism dysfunction: defective heme biosynthesis causes neuropathic porphyria and is observed in FRDA; defective heme export (*FLVCR1* mutations) is responsible for PCARP, RP and HSAN. For simplicity, these disorders have been depicted near FLVCR1a; however, the specific contribution of FLVCR1a and FLVCR1b to these disorders still remains to be addressed. Finally, defective heme import (*FLVCR2* mutations) leads to the Fowler syndrome. Alteration of heme incorporation into hemoproteins and heme degradation have not been directly associated to a specific neurodegenerative disorder. However, we cannot exclude a role for these pathways in neurodegeneration.

causes the accumulation of ALA, PBG and coproporphyrin III (Horner et al., 2013; Ramanujam and Anderson, 2015).

Variegate porphyria (VP; OMIM: #176200) is an autosomal dominant disorder with incomplete penetrance. VP is due to mutations in the gene encoding protoporphyrinogen oxidase (*PPOX*). PPOX catalyzes the oxidation of protoporphyrinogen IX to form protoporphyrin IX and its partial deficiency causes the elevation of plasma porphyrins (Horner et al., 2013; Ramanujam and Anderson, 2015).

The clinical presentation is generally milder in HCP and VP compared to AIP and ALAD deficiency.

The etiology of the neurological manifestations in neuropathic porphyrias remained undefined for long time. Nowadays, two major mechanisms have been proposed to contribute to the nerve failure: direct neurotoxicity of the porphyrin precursors and mitochondrial dysfunction (Lin et al., 2011).

Friederich Ataxia

Friederich Ataxia (FRDA; OMIM #229300) is a progressive neurodegenerative disease usually associated with cardiomyopathy and diabetes. Although a rare disorder, FRDA represents the most frequent type of inherited ataxia. FRDA is characterized by progressive gait and limb ataxia, dysarthria, areflexia, loss of vibratory and position sense, and a progressive motor weakness of central origin. Neurodegeneration first affects the dorsal root ganglia (DRG) but then involves spinal cord, peripheral nerves and cerebellum (Marmolino, 2011; Bürk, 2017).

FRDA is an autosomal recessive disorder caused by the abnormal expansion of the GAA triplet in the first intron of *FRATAXIN* (*FXN*) gene (Campuzano et al., 1996). FXN function remained elusive for long time. FXN is a mitochondrial iron chaperone involved in iron–sulfur (Fe–S) clusters and heme biosynthesis. Here we focus on the role of FXN on heme biosynthesis and readers are referred to more comprehensive reviews on the role of FXN in Fe–S clusters biosynthesis (Stemmler et al., 2010; Martelli and Puccio, 2014; Braymer and Lill, 2017; Rouault and Maio, 2017). FXN delivers iron to Ferrochelatase (FECH) (Yoon and Cowan, 2004), the enzyme responsible for the insertion of iron into protoporphyrin IX. Structural studies on the interaction between FXN and FECH shed light on the mechanism of iron delivery between them (Bencze et al., 2007; Söderberg et al., 2016). Evidences of defective heme biosynthesis have been reported in both cellular and mouse models of FXN deficiency as well as in FRDA patient-derived cells. Collectively these studies showed decreased expression of enzymes involved in the heme biosynthetic pathway (Schoenfeld et al., 2005; Huang et al., 2009), induction of HMOX1 (Huang et al., 2009), increased cellular protoporphyrin IX levels (Schoenfeld et al., 2005) and reduced heme content (Schoenfeld et al., 2005; Huang et al., 2009). Although the majority of these experiments have been performed in different cell and tissue types, it is conceivable that these findings can be translated to the nervous system. Fe-S clusters and heme biosynthesis are the two major iron consuming processes in mitochondria. Therefore, reduced iron utilization for Fe–S clusters and heme biosynthesis contributes to iron accumulation observed in FRDA (Huang et al., 2009). Moreover, mitochondrial iron accumulation in FRDA was reported to be due to heme-dependent upregulation of mitoferrin-2, a mitochondrial iron importer (Martelli et al., 2015). Both Fe–S clusters and heme are essential cofactors of the electron transport chain required for energy production. Indeed, FXN deficiency finally causes mitochondrial dysfunction, that actively contributes to the disease pathogenesis (Lodi et al., 1999; Martelli et al., 2015; Chiang et al., 2018).

Several yeast and mouse models of FXN deficiency have been generated (Perdomini et al., 2013). These models have been extremely useful to understand the molecular mechanisms of neurodegeneration associated to FXN loss and to test therapeutic approaches for the disorder.

Neurodegenerative Disorders Due to Defects in Heme Import

The import of heme inside the cell is achieved through multiple transporters: the heme responsive gene 1 (HRG1), the Heme carrier protein 1/Proton-coupled folate transporter (HCP1/PCFT) and the Feline leukemia virus subgroup C receptor 2 (FLVCR2).

The role of HRG1 in the import of heme is well established (Rajagopal et al., 2008; White et al., 2013). HRG1 is highly expressed in the brain and its transient downregulation in zebrafish leads to hydrocephalus and yolk tube malformations suggesting an important role for HRG1 in neurodevelopment (Rajagopal et al., 2008). Conversely, the substrate-specificity of HCP1 and FLVCR2 have been debated. HCP1 was initially identified as a heme importer (Shayeghi et al., 2005). Nevertheless, Qiu A. et al. reported that HCP1 is a folate transporter implicated in hereditary folate malabsorption (Qiu et al., 2006). However, evidences suggest that the heme import function of HCP1 could be relevant in some cell types or in particular physiologic or pathologic situations (Chiabrando et al., 2014b). Because of the low expression level of HCP1 in the brain, the role of HCP1 in the import of heme in the nervous system is likely marginal.

FLVCR2 is a member of the major facilitator superfamily (MFS) of transporters (Pao et al., 1998; Law et al., 2008) initially proposed as a calcium-chelate transporter (Meyer et al., 2010). Subsequent studies revealed that FLVCR2 is an importer of heme (Duffy et al., 2010). FLVCR2 is ubiquitously expressed. In the nervous system, FLVCR2 is widely expressed throughout the brain and spinal cord (Duffy et al., 2010; Meyer et al., 2010). However, FLVCR2 expression and subcellular localization still remain to be investigated in detail due to the lack of a specific antibody. Among all these heme importers, *FLVCR2* is the only gene directly associated to a neurodegenerative disorder, the Fowler Syndrome. Therefore, the discussion below is focused exclusively on this disease.

Fowler Syndrome

Fowler syndrome, also known as Proliferative Vasculopathy, Hydrancephaly Hydrocephaly syndrome (PVHH; OMIM #225790), is a rare neurodegenerative disorder. The hallmark of the disease is the presence of proliferative glomerular vasculopathy in the CNS associated with severe hydrocephaly, ventriculomegaly, cortical thinning and hypoplastic cerebellum. Secondary features are hypokinesia and joint contractures (Meyer et al., 2010; Williams et al., 2010; Kvarnung et al., 2016). It is still unclear whether the proliferative vasculopathy is the primary or secondary event in the disease pathogenesis. Massive endothelial cells proliferation might be the first event leading to adjacent tissue damage, calcification and neuronal cells loss. Otherwise, proliferative vasculopathy might be a consequence of neurodegeneration (Meyer et al., 2010). The Fowler syndrome is characterized by early prenatal onset and is incompatible with life in most cases (Lalonde et al., 2010; Meyer et al., 2010; Thomas et al., 2010; Williams et al., 2010). Recently, two cases of survival beyond infancy have been reported. These patients were characterized by severe intellectual and neurologic disability (Kvarnung et al., 2016).

The Fowler syndrome is an autosomal recessive disorder caused by mutations in the *FLVCR2* gene (Meyer et al., 2010). Different kinds of mutations in the *FLVCR2* gene have been reported (Lalonde et al., 2010; Meyer et al., 2010; Thomas et al., 2010; Kvarnung et al., 2016), including missense and nonsense mutations, deletions and insertions. Homology modeling of FLVCR2 structure suggests that the missense mutations related with Fowler syndrome affect transmembrane domains that may modify the channel proper function or folding (Radio et al., 2018). It has been proposed that the mutations might lead to alteration of heme-iron metabolism. However, this is merely an hypothesis since *in vitro* or *in vivo* evidences are still lacking. The generation of appropriate *in vitro* and *in vivo* model systems will be important to investigate the molecular mechanisms underlying Fowler syndrome.

Neurodegenerative Disorders Due to Defects in Heme Export

The export of heme is mediated by two widely expressed proteins: the ATP binding cassette subfamily G member 2 (ABCG2) and the Feline Leukemia Virus Subgroup C Receptor 1 (FLVCR1).

Besides heme, ABCG2 is involved in the transport of a variety of substrates: urate, chemotherapeutics, antibiotics, xenobiotics and food metabolites (Krishnamurthy and Schuetz, 2006). In the nervous system, ABCG2 is mainly located on the luminal side of endothelial cells (ECs) (Krishnamurthy and Schuetz, 2006), suggesting an important role for ABCG2 in the blood-brain-barrier to protect brain from drugs. Furthermore, ABCG2 has been implicated in brain protection following ischemic reperfusion injury (Shin et al., 2018) and in Alzheimer's disease (Xiong et al., 2009; Zeng et al., 2012; Shen et al., 2010). However, the relevance of ABCG2-mediated heme efflux to neurodegeneration still remains to be elucidated.

Feline Leukemia Virus Subgroup C Receptor 1 (FLVCR1) is a member of the MFS of transporters (Pao et al., 1998; Law et al., 2008), implicated in the transport of heme and other planar porphyrins (Yang et al., 2010). *FLVCR1* gene encodes for two isoforms: FLVCR1a expressed at the plasma membrane and FLVCR1b in mitochondria (Chiabrando et al., 2012). FLVCR1 is ubiquitously expressed (Quigley et al., 2004; Keel et al., 2008; Chiabrando et al., 2012; Fiorito et al., 2014, 2015; Vinchi et al., 2014; Mercurio et al., 2015; Petrillo et al., 2017). In the nervous system, Flvcr1 mRNA has been detected in the mouse brain (neocortex, striatum, hippocampus, and cerebellum), posterior column of the spinal cord, retina and retinal pigment epithelium. The highest Flvcr1 mRNA levels have been found in the retina and spinal cord (Rajadhyaksha et al., 2010; Gnana-Prakasam et al., 2011). Unfortunately, no information is available concerning FLVCR1 protein expression levels and localization in neurons and glia, due to the lack of a reliable antibody against FLVCR1. Mutations in *FLVCR1* gene have been reported in distinct disorders affecting the sensory nervous system: Posterior Column Ataxia and Retinitis Pigmentosa, Retinitis Pigmentosa and Hereditary Sensory and Autonomic Neuropathy, as reviewed below.

Posterior Column Ataxia and Retinitis Pigmentosa (PCARP)

PCARP (OMIM: #609033) is a rare neurodegenerative syndrome characterized by sensory ataxia and retinitis pigmentosa. Sensory ataxia is a consequence of the degeneration of the posterior columns of the spinal cord, resulting in loss of proprioception. Retinitis pigmentosa is due to the progressive degeneration of photoreceptors in the retina, leading to night blindness and progressive restriction of the visual field (Higgins et al., 1997; Rajadhyaksha et al., 2010). PCARP has been described for the first time in Higgins et al. (1997) as an autosomal recessive disorder associated with the AXPC1 locus (Higgins et al., 1999). In 2010, the analysis of three inbreed families of different ethnic origins revealed that mutations in the *FLVCR1* gene were responsible for the disorder (Rajadhyaksha et al., 2010). In the majority of cases, PCARP is caused by homozygous mutations in the *FLVCR1* gene (c.361A > G – c.721G > A – c.574T > C – c.1477G < C) (Rajadhyaksha et al., 2010; Ishiura et al., 2011). The identified mutations are missense mutations that affect highly conserved residues in potential transmembrane domains of the heme exporter. *In vitro* studies suggest that these mutations result in the mislocalization of FLVCR1 protein and in the loss of its heme export function. Compound heterozygous mutations in the *FLVCR1* gene have been also reported in three siblings (c.1547G > A and c.1593 + 5_ + 8delGTAA) (Shaibani et al., 2015).

Retinitis Pigmentosa (RP)

Non-syndromic retinitis pigmentosa (RP; OMIM: #268000) encompasses a group of genetically heterogeneous disorders characterized by the progressive neurodegeneration of photoreceptors. RP-associated genes are involved in different processes: phototransduction, retinal metabolism, tissue development and maintenance, cellular structure and splicing (Hartong et al., 2006). Recently, *FLVCR1* mutations have been reported in some patients with retinitis pigmentosa (RP) without evidences of posterior column degeneration or cerebellar degeneration (Tiwari et al., 2016; Yusuf et al., 2018). Interestingly, all the patients carry a specific splice-site variant in *FLVCR1* (c.1092 + 5G > A) in homozygosity or as compound heterozygosity. Functional studies showed that the c.1092 + 5G > A mutation interferes with the correct splicing of *FLVCR1* resulting in the skipping of exon 4, the frame-shift deletion of 68bp and a premature stop codon (Tiwari et al., 2016; Yusuf et al., 2018).

Hereditary Sensory and Autonomic Neuropathy (HSAN)

HSANs are a group of neurodegenerative disorders of the peripheral nervous system mainly characterized by impaired nociception and autonomic dysfunction. The hallmark of the disease is the degeneration of sensory neurons, which transmit information about sensations such as pain, temperature and touch. The inability to experience pain causes unintentional self-injuries and chronic ulcerations. Soft tissue infections and osteomyelitis, often requiring amputations, are common. The disease is also associated to mild abnormalities of the autonomic nervous system: swallowing and feeding problems, apnea, gastro-esophageal reflux and delayed development are variable features of the disorder (Verpoorten et al., 2006; Rotthier et al., 2012; Auer-Grumbach, 2013).

HSANs arise from mutations in genes that are crucial for distinct molecular pathways: sphingolipid-metabolism, membrane-shaping of organelles, neurotrophin action, DNA methylation, regulation of ion channels, endoplasmic reticulum turnover and axonal trafficking and heme metabolism (Rotthier et al., 2012; Khaminets et al., 2015; Chiabrando et al., 2016; Tanaka et al., 2016). Recently, mutations in the *FLVCR1* gene have been reported in a subset of HSAN patients. Compound heterozygous mutations in *FLVCR1* (c.574T > C and c.610del – c.661C > T and c.1324dup) have been reported (Chiabrando et al., 2016). Functional studies in patient-derived cells showed that these mutations reduce heme export activity, enhance oxidative stress and increase the sensitivity to programmed cell death (Chiabrando et al., 2016). Finally, Castori et al. (2017) reported the homozygosity for a previously identified pc.661C > T variation in a sporadic case with a mixed phenotype of HSAN, PCARP and acute lymphocytic leukemia.

Due to the limited number of cases described to date, it is very difficult to understand whether FLVCR1-related PCARP, RP and HSAN are distinct disorders or rather a single clinical spectrum.

The finding of *FLVCR1* mutations in PCARP, RP and HSAN indicates that heme is particularly required for the survival of specific subpopulation of neurons. However, the elucidation of the role of heme in these subpopulations is far to be clearly understood.

The available mouse models of FLVCR1 deficiency did not recapitulate the major disease features of HSAN, PCARP or RP. The targeted disruption of *Flvcr1* gene causes embryonic lethality in two different mouse models. Mice lacking both Flvcr1a and Flvcr1b die *in utero* because of a block of erythropoiesis (Keel et al., 2008). Mice lacking only Flvcr1a die during embryonic development due to severe hemorrhages, edema and skeletal malformations (Chiabrando et al., 2012). The downregulation of FLVCR1 isoforms in zebrafish confirm the essential role of FLVCR1 isoforms in erythropoiesis and ECs maintenance (Mercurio et al., 2015).

The discrepancy between the phenotype of these animal models and the human diseases is likely due to different degree of Flvcr1a downregulation. Indeed, HSAN patients-derived cells still expressed FLVCR1a but are characterized by reduced heme export activity (Chiabrando et al., 2016). Moreover, treatment of patient-derived cells with Hemopexin, that facilitates heme export through FLVCR1a (Chiabrando et al., 2016), improved cell survival. These data clearly indicate that *FLVCR1* mutations do not completely abrogate FLVCR1a function (Chiabrando et al., 2016). Reasonably, embryonic lethality is expected for patients carrying null mutations in the *FLVCR1* gene.

The reason why the loss of an ubiquitously expressed heme exporter affects specific sensory modalities (vision, proprioception and/or nociception) is still unknown. The development of appropriate cellular and mouse models will help dissecting the role of FLVCR1 in these disorders.

HEME-REGULATED PROCESSES CRUCIAL FOR NEUROURODEGENERATION

In the paragraphs above, we summarized the most relevant neurodegenerative disorders associated to alterations in heme metabolism. However, the etiology of such diseases remains mostly undefined. Heme bears toxic properties due to its ability to promote iron mediated Fenton's reaction. This awareness contributed over the years to underestimate the importance of iron-independent mechanisms of heme toxicity in neuronal diseases. The misconception that heme neurotoxicity is due to iron release from protoporphyrin IX mainly contributed to the lack of interest in the topic. To stimulate research in the field, we will discuss the major heme-regulated pathways that might be relevant during neurodegeneration (**Figure 2**).

Heme and Oxidative Stress: Implications for Neurodegenerative Disorders

Oxidative stress is a condition occurring when the production of reactive oxygen species (ROS) overcomes the endogenous antioxidant defenses. Accumulation of ROS causes the oxidative damage of cellular components, included lipids, proteins and nucleic acids. As a pro-oxidant molecule, heme can itself promote oxidative stress, eventually leading to cell death. In particular, due to its hydrophobic nature, free heme tends to aggregate and bind to cell membranes. Oxidation of membrane components leads to increased permeability and altered lipid organization, in turn promoting cell lysis and death (Schmitt et al., 1993). The redox activity of heme-derived iron also contributes to the cytotoxic effects of heme. Indeed, in aqueous phase heme becomes unstable and releases free iron, responsible for the formation of ROS via the Fenton's reaction (Kumar and Bandyopadhyay, 2005). The CNS is particularly susceptible to oxidative stress due to its high oxygen consumption rates and weak antioxidant systems. Consistently, oxidative stress is involved in the pathogenesis of several neurodegenerative disorders as Parkinson's disease, Alzheimer's disease, Huntington's disease and FRDA (Schulz et al., 2000; Calabrese et al., 2005; de Vries et al., 2008; Li et al., 2013; Puspita et al., 2017). Increased ROS levels have been observed also in HSAN patient-derived cells (Chiabrando et al., 2016; Castori et al., 2017). To counteract the toxic effects exerted by ROS accumulation, human cells have evolved several detoxification mechanisms. In particular, the primary defense systems against ROS consists of oxidant-inactivating enzymes, such as superoxide dismutase or HMOX1, and endogenous antioxidants, including glutathione and thioredoxin (Li et al., 2013). The transcriptional response to oxidative stress is mediated by a *cis*-regulatory element known as ARE (antioxidant response element) found in the promoters of genes codifying for antioxidant proteins. Nuclear factor E2-related factor 2 (Nrf2) is the major trans-acting factor responsible for the activation of gene transcription through its binding to the AREs (Nguyen et al., 2009). Notably, alterations in Nrf2 signaling pathway have been found in Parkinson's disease, Alzheimer's disease, and Huntington's disease (PMID: 18824091) as well as in a cardiac mouse model of FRDA (Anzovino et al., 2017). Several proteins and kinases modulate the Nrf2 pathway at various levels to ensure a tight control of its activity. Among these regulators, BTB domain and CNC homolog 1 (Bach1) acts as a repressor of Nrf2 activity by competing with Nrf2 for ARE binding sites. Notably, the activity and localization of Bach1 is regulated by heme (Sun et al., 2004; Suzuki et al., 2004; Marro et al., 2010), thus suggesting that alterations in heme homeostasis might affect the Nrf2-Bach1 axis and the cell ability to respond to the oxidative insult. This mechanism could be particularly relevant in the progression

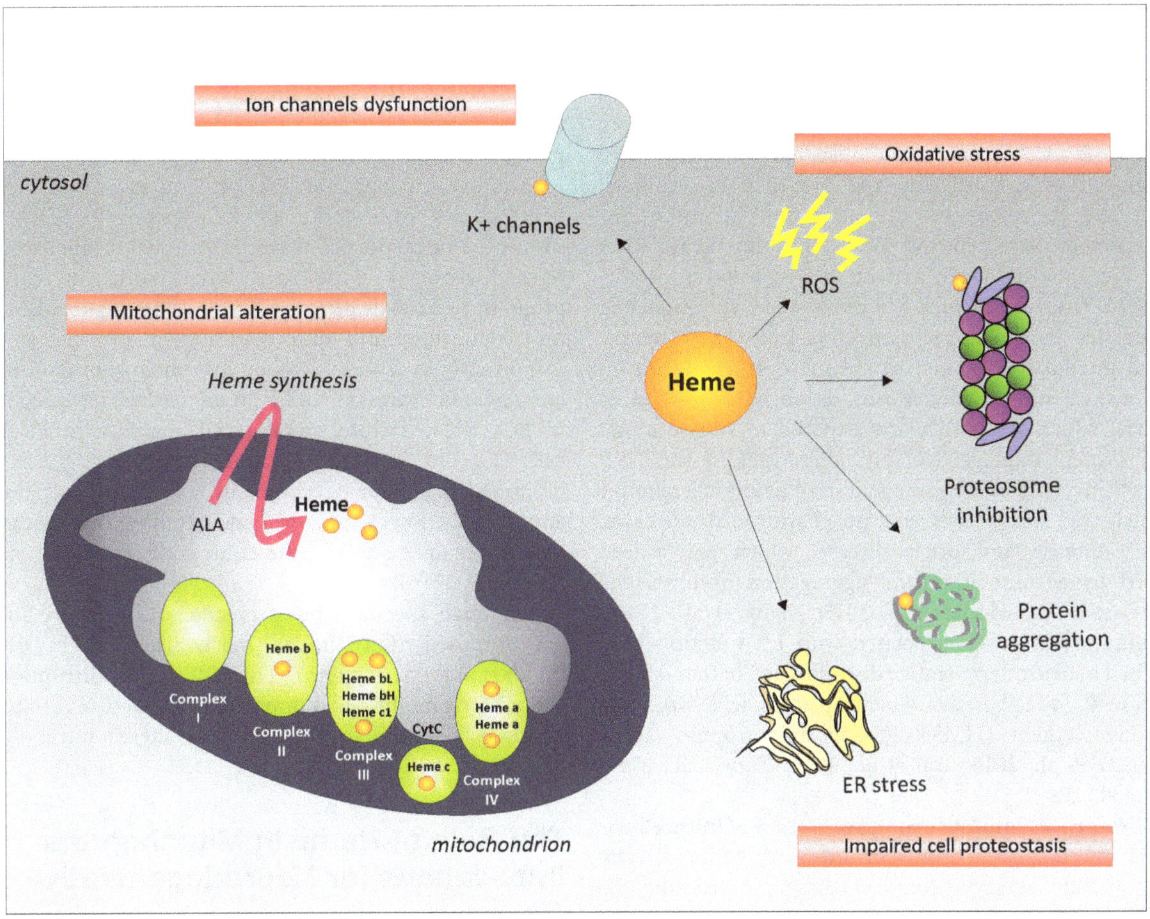

FIGURE 2 | Potential mechanisms leading to neurodegeneration. The picture summarizes the major heme-regulated processes that might be relevant during neurodegeneration. The alteration of intracellular labile heme may affect cell proteostasis, oxidative phosphorylation, ion channels function and/or induce oxidative stress, leading to neurodegeneration.

of neurodegenerative diseases, which is indeed exacerbated by oxidative stress. Hence, oxidative stress might exert neurotoxicity also by impairing the ubiquitin-proteasome system, as found in Parkinson's disease (PD) where a decreased protein clearance rate due to elevated ROS results in the accumulation of alpha-synuclein (Hashimoto et al., 1999; McNaught and Jenner, 2001).

The Role of Heme in Cellular Proteostasis: Implications for Neurodegenerative Disorders

The maintenance of protein homeostasis, also called proteostasis, is essential for cell function and survival (Hartl et al., 2011; Morimoto and Cuervo, 2014; Kaushik and Cuervo, 2015). The constant control of cellular proteostasis requires the proper activity of two main cellular components (Kaushik and Cuervo, 2015). On one hand, the activity of chaperones is fundamental to correct protein misfolding eventually occurring during protein synthesis, assembly in three-dimensional and functional structures and trafficking. On the other hand, protein clearance mechanisms mediate the removal of irreversibly misfolded proteins. In particular, this second purpose is achieved most prominently through two molecular systems: the ubiquitin-proteasome system (UPS) and the autophagy system. These systems are able to sense disturbances in the proteome and to be rapidly activated, thus exerting a constant protein quality control. In this way, the proteostasis network ensures the cell the ability to adapt to environmental changes and transitory stress. Reduced proteostasis capacity may lead to the accumulation of misfolded proteins, which form cytotoxic aggregates (Morimoto and Cuervo, 2014). Deficiencies in the machinery of protein homeostasis promote the onset and progression of several human pathologies, including neurodegenerative diseases (Hartl et al., 2011). For instance, deposits of aberrant proteins such as tau and α-synuclein, have been associated with dementia and Parkinson's disease. The use of proteasome inhibitors as Bortezomib in cancer therapy has been shown to induce peripheral neuropathy as a prominent side effect (Alé et al., 2014; Kaplan et al., 2017). Moreover, an impairment of mitochondrial turnover via selective autophagy has been found in Parkinson's disease (Andreux et al., 2013) and in sensory neuropathy (Khaminets et al., 2015). In addition to the above described classical proteostasis network, which assures the quality control of *de novo* synthetized cytosolic proteins, organelle-specific systems can be activated in response to proteotoxic stress occurring in specific subcellular compartments (Kaushik and Cuervo, 2015). These signaling pathways include the unfolded protein response (UPR) of the endoplasmic reticulum (ER) and mitochondria. In particular, the presence of unfolded proteins in the ER promotes the activation of three ER-resident transmembrane proteins: PERK (protein kinase RNA (PKR)-like ER kinase), ATF6 (activating transcription factor-6) and IRE1α (inositol-requiring enzyme-1α). The signaling cascade mediated by downstream effectors leads to an overall translational attenuation as well as enhanced transcription of ER chaperons. A similar mechanism has been described in mitochondria, which are particularly exposed to stressors that can trigger protein damage. Notably, alterations in the UPR machinery are involved in the pathogenesis of neurodegenerative diseases such as Alzheimer's disease, Parkinson's diseases, Huntington's disease and prion disease, which are indeed characterized by accumulation and aggregation of misfolded proteins (Scheper and Hoozemans, 2015; Xiang et al., 2017). Finally, mutations in genes associated with ER function have been described in neurodegenerative disorders as Charcot-Marie-Tooth disease (CMT), hereditary neuropathies with proximal dominant involvement (HMSN-P) and amyotrophic lateral sclerosis (Beetz et al., 2013; Tsai et al., 2014; Yagi et al., 2016; Murakami et al., 2017).

Growing evidences indicate that the alteration of intracellular heme levels affects proteostasis. For instance, heme directly binds and inhibits the proteasome machinery promoting the formation of perinuclear "aggresomes" of ubiquitinated proteins (Vallelian et al., 2015). In particular, Vallelian et al. (2015) analyzed changes in protein expression upon heme treatment in mouse embryo fibroblasts (MEF) isolated from wild type and mice lacking HMOX1 (*Hmox1*-null mice). The study of the proteome in *Hmox1*-null MEF by mass spectrometry revealed a specific signature characterized by a strong upregulation of networks related to the response to unfolded proteins. These data suggest that excessive intracellular heme can trigger proteostasis disruption. In particular, heme overload correlates with accumulation of ubiquitinated proteins, thus indicating a reduced protein degradation capacity in heme-stressed cells (Vallelian et al., 2015). Consistent with these previous observations, the formation of protein aggregates has been described in macrophages during heme stress (Vasconcellos et al., 2016). In particular, cell treatment with increasing concentration of heme leads to the formation of aggresome-like induced structures (ALIS), which are characterized by the presence of p62/SQSTM1 (sequestosome-1) and ubiquitinated proteins. Importantly, the pre-treatment with ROS scavengers completely abolishes heme-induced ALIS formation in bone marrow-derived macrophages, thus indicating that ROS generation has a key role in this process (Vasconcellos et al., 2016). In addition, p62 is an inhibitor of the Nrf2 repressor Keap1 (Kelch-like ECH-associated protein 1). Therefore, the heme-induced sequestration of p62 in ALIS might affect the Nrf2-Keap1 axis (PMID: 24011591), interfering with the antioxidant response mediated by Nrf2-regulated genes. Enhanced ROS production and proteasome inhibition thus represent two different activities of heme, which turned out to be extremely cytotoxic in conditions of heme excess. These findings, taken together, point out a novel model of heme toxicity mediated by accumulation of damaged proteins and disruption of cellular proteostasis.

Another evidence of the proteotoxic effect mediated by heme comes from studies on ECs lacking FLVCR1a. The loss of the heme export way in ECs leads to the accumulation of endogenously synthetized heme, which in turn triggers programmed cell death via paraptosis and impairs the angiogenic process during embryonic development (Petrillo et al., 2017). Importantly, an altered swollen morphology of the ER as well as an increased expression of ER stress markers have been described in ECs isolated from embryos lacking *Flvcr1a* in endothelial cells (Petrillo et al., 2017). Interestingly, paraptosis has been described in neural development and neurodegeneration (e.g., amyotrophic lateral sclerosis and Huntington's disease), in the ischemic damage and in the context of retina pathophysiology (Lee et al., 2016).

Although specific studies in neuronal cells are still lacking, we proposed that similar mechanisms might be relevant in the nervous system. Therefore, the disruption of cell proteostasis might be an important mechanisms contributing to neurodegeneration in conditions of altered intracellular heme levels.

The Role of Heme in Mitochondria: Implications for Neurodegenerative Disorders

An additional mechanism through which heme could potentially participate to neurodegeneration is through the control of mitochondrial function. Mitochondrial dysfunction is a common pathogenetic mechanism of several neurodegenerative disorders. Particularly, the alteration of mitochondria by different mechanisms has been proposed as one of the underlying cause of Parkinson's disease, Alzheimer's disease, Huntington's disease and amyotrophic lateral sclerosis (Shi et al., 2010; Costa and Scorrano, 2012; Bennett et al., 2014; Cabezas-Opazo et al., 2015; Arun et al., 2016; Bose and Beal, 2016).

Heme is a crucial cofactor for cytochromes *c* and cytochromes in complexes II, III and IV of the mitochondrial electron transport chain (ETC) (Kim et al., 2012), thus modulation of heme metabolism could interfere with oxidative phosphorylation. Moreover, some of the steps of heme synthesis occur in mitochondria and initiate by the condensation of succynil-CoA with glycine. Succynil-CoA is an intermediate of the TCA cycle, so heme production belongs to the group of TCA cycle cataplerotic pathways (Frezza et al., 2011; Fukuda et al., 2017), a set of processes whose function is to avoid the accumulation of TCA cycle metabolites. Alterations in heme biosynthesis, consequently, could impair this system thus altering mitochondrial function. In addition, heme has been reported to directly or indirectly influence adenosine triphosphate (ATP) translocation among mitochondria and cytosol (Sabová et al., 1993; Giraud et al., 1998; Azuma et al.,

2008) and, therefore, modulation of heme homeostasis could profoundly affect the mitochondrial contribution to cell energy supply.

Supporting the role of heme in mitochondrial function, analyses on ECs demonstrated that alterations in heme metabolism, in addition to promote lipid peroxidation and activation of autophagy, induce mitophagy and apoptosis, indicating mitochondrial dysfunction (Higdon et al., 2012). Furthermore, we previously reported that loss of FLVCR1 impairs mitochondrial function in HeLa cells (Chiabrando et al., 2012) and mitochondrial morphology in human microvascular ECs (Petrillo et al., 2017).

Considering the role of heme in mitochondria, it is tempting to speculate that, by affecting mitochondrial function, the impairment of heme metabolism in neuronal cells could potentially initiate or sustain processes responsible for neuronal cells defects and death. Supporting this hypothesis, studies in the brain of HMBS−/− mice, a model of AIP, showed alterations in the activity of ETC complexes likely related to the compromised heme biosynthesis (Homedan et al., 2014). Moreover, it has been suggested that an energy failure may lead to a defective activity of the Na/K+ ATPase in the axon, leading to its degeneration (Lin et al., 2011). Since heme is required for ATP synthesis, we cannot exclude that heme metabolism could have a role in this context. Furthermore, defects in mitochondrial iron content, in the activity of the respiratory chain complexes and in ATP production have been observed in FRDA (Lodi et al., 1999). Although these defects in FRDA can be ascribed to alterations in Fe–S clusters trafficking, the contribution of heme to these processes cannot be excluded. Finally, in three cases of Fowler syndrome it was suggested the presence of a defect in complex III and IV of the ETC (Castro-Gago et al., 1999, 2001), directly indicating that mitochondrial defects due to alterations in heme trafficking could be the underlying cause of the neurological outcomes of this syndrome.

The contribution of mitochondrial dysfunction to PCARP, HSAN and RP has not been investigated. However, the implication of heme in these pathologies suggests the possibility that mitochondrial function could contribute to them. Notably, in sensory neurons the importance of heme in mitochondria could be related not only to the production of ATP, but also to mitochondrial dynamics (fusion, fission, motility). Mitochondrial dynamics are crucial for neurotransmission, synaptic maintenance and neuronal survival. Proper mitochondrial trafficking is particularly important in neurons as compared to other cell types due to their exceptional cellular morphology. Indeed, neurons extend their axons and dendrites for very long distances. Therefore, the neurons represent an extreme case of mitochondrial distribution: dysfunctions in mitochondrial distribution that are not dangerous for other cells, could be fatal for neuronal survival (Schwarz, 2013). Supporting this concept, compromised mitochondrial motility has been reported in Alzheimer's disease (Cabezas-Opazo et al., 2015), Parkinson's disease (Yang et al., 2008; Carelli et al., 2015), Huntington's disease (Shirendeb et al., 2011) and in amyotrophic lateral sclerosis (De Vos et al., 2007; Shi et al., 2010).

In the case of human peripheral nerves or corticospinal tracts, axons can extend up to a meter, so the population of sensory neurons could be highly sensitive to defects in mitochondrial dynamics. Modulation of the cellular labile iron pool and mitochondrial iron content have been observed in FXN deficiency in association to alterations in both heme biosynthesis and OPA1 (mitochondrial dynamin like GTPase)-mediated mitochondrial fusion (Martelli et al., 2015). Although a causative link among these phenomena has not been proposed in FRDA, it is tempting to speculate that the modulation of iron and heme homeostasis could promote alterations in mitochondrial dynamics, with deleterious consequences in this pathology and, more likely, in neurological disorders affecting sensory neurons.

Heme Regulates Ion Channels: Implications for Neurodegenerative Disorders

Emerging evidences suggest that labile heme is a signaling molecule that impact on the function of various ion channels involved in neuron excitability. Among them, *voltage-gated K+ channels* are a large family of K+ channels that open on membrane depolarization and contribute to maintain the resting potential and to determine the shape and frequency of action potentials in excitable cells (Sahoo et al., 2014). Heme directly binds to the *large-conductance calcium-dependent Slo1 BK channels* and *Kv1.4 A-type K+ channels*. The high affinity binding of heme to Slo1 BK channels decreases the frequency of channel opening leading to an inhibition of transmembrane K+ currents (Tang et al., 2003). Its binding to the N-terminal domain of the Kv1.4 channels inhibits the fast inactivation of the channel, thus reducing cellular excitability (Sahoo et al., 2013).

The activity of several K+ channels is modulated by carbon monoxide (CO) (Tang et al., 2004) and ROS (Sahoo et al., 2014; Peers and Boyle, 2015). Heme may also indirectly regulate the activity of several K+ channels through the generation of CO and ROS. Indeed, the degradation of heme by HO1 produces iron, biliverdin and CO. Moreover, the released iron is responsible for the formation of ROS via the Fenton's reaction.

An alteration of the activity, function or expression of diverse K+ channels have been reported in Alzheimer's disease, Parkinson's disease, Huntington's disease and ataxias (Peers and Boyle, 2015). As mentioned before, increased ROS is common to all these neurodegenerative diseases. Oxidative modulation of diverse K+ channels has been proposed as a pathogenetic mechansim leading to neurodegeneration. Finally, several studies highlight a crucial role of K+ channels in nociception (Busserolles et al., 2016). The identification of *FLVCR1* mutations in patients affected by HSAN (Chiabrando et al., 2016; Castori et al., 2017) suggests that the alteration of K+ channels activity may explain sensory defects in these patients. Considering all these data, it is possible to speculate that the alteration of labile heme may affect the activity of K+ channels, thus contributing to the neurodegenerative process.

CONCLUDING REMARKS

The recent identification of several neurodegenerative disorders due to mutations in genes involved in heme metabolism highlights a previously unappreciated role for heme in neurodegeneration. Here, we discussed the potential mechanisms leading to heme neurotoxicity, thus suggesting future directions for investigation. The understanding of such mechanisms might be relevant for several neurodegenerative disorders. Indeed, alteration of heme metabolism have been observed also in Alzheimer's disease, Parkinson's disease and other aging-related neurodegenerative disorders (Atamna and Frey, 2004; Atamna, 2006; Scherzer et al., 2008; Dwyer et al., 2009; Smith et al., 2011; Hayden et al., 2015; Sampaio et al., 2017; Santiago and Potashkin, 2017; Fiorito et al., 2018). In the future, the comprehensive understanding of the molecular mechanisms linking heme to neurodegeneration will be potentially important for therapeutic purposes.

AUTHOR CONTRIBUTIONS

DC and VF conceptualized the study and wrote the manuscript. SP wrote the manuscript. ET wrote and reviewed the manuscript.

FUNDING

This research was funded by University of Torino (Bando Ricerca Locale ex-60%).

REFERENCES

Albers, J. W., and Fink, J. K. (2004). Porphyric neuropathy. *Muscle Nerve* 30, 410–422. doi: 10.1002/mus.20137 doi: 10.1002/mus.20137

Alé, A., Bruna, J., Navarro, X., and Udina, E. (2014). Neurotoxicity induced by antineoplastic proteasome inhibitors. *Neurotoxicology* 43, 28–35. doi: 10.1016/j.neuro.2014.02.001

Andreux, P. A., Houtkooper, R. H., and Auwerx, J. (2013). Pharmacological approaches to restore mitochondrial function. *Nat. Rev. Drug Discov.* 12, 465–483. doi: 10.1038/nrd4023

Anzovino, A., Chiang, S., Brown, B. E., Hawkins, C. L., Richardson, D. R., and Huang, M. L. (2017). Molecular alterations in a mouse cardiac model of friedreich ataxia: an impaired nrf2 response mediated via upregulation of keap1 and activation of the Gsk3β Axis. *Am. J. Pathol.* 187, 2858–2875. doi: 10.1016/j.ajpath.2017.08.021

Arun, S., Liu, L., and Donmez, G. (2016). Mitochondrial biology and neurological diseases. *Curr. Neuropharmacol.* 14, 143–154. doi: 10.2174/1570159X13666150703154541

Ashraf, A., Clark, M., and So, P. W. (2018). The aging of iron man. *Front. Aging Neurosci.* 10:65. doi: 10.3389/fnagi.2018.00065

Atamna, H. (2006). Heme binding to amyloid-beta peptide: mechanistic role in Alzheimer's disease. *J. Alzheimers Dis.* 10, 255–266. doi: 10.3233/JAD-2006-102-310

Atamna, H., and Frey, W. H. (2004). A role for heme in Alzheimer's disease: heme binds amyloid beta and has altered metabolism. *Proc. Natl. Acad. Sci. U.S.A.* 101, 11153–11158. doi: 10.1073/pnas.0404349101

Auer-Grumbach, M. (2013). Hereditary sensory and autonomic neuropathies. *Handb. Clin. Neurol.* 115, 893–906. doi: 10.1016/B978-0-444-52902-2.00050-3

Azuma, M., Kabe, Y., Kuramori, C., Kondo, M., Yamaguchi, Y., and Handa, H. (2008). Adenine nucleotide translocator transports haem precursors into mitochondria. *PLoS One* 3:e3070. doi: 10.1371/journal.pone.0003070

Beetz, C., Johnson, A., Schuh, A. L., Thakur, S., Varga, R. E., Fothergill, T., et al. (2013). Inhibition of TFG function causes hereditary axon degeneration by impairing endoplasmic reticulum structure. *Proc. Natl. Acad. Sci. U.S.A.* 110, 5091–5096. doi: 10.1073/pnas.1217197110

Bencze, K. Z., Yoon, T., Millán-Pacheco, C., Bradley, P. B., Pastor, N., Cowan, J. A., et al. (2007). Human frataxin: iron and ferrochelatase binding surface. *Chem. Commun. (Camb.)* 18, 1798–1800. doi: 10.1039/b703195e

Bennett, G. J., Doyle, T., and Salvemini, D. (2014). Mitotoxicity in distal symmetrical sensory peripheral neuropathies. *Nat. Rev. Neurol.* 10, 326–336. doi: 10.1038/nrneurol.2014.77

Besur, S., Hou, W., Schmeltzer, P., and Bonkovsky, H. L. (2014). Clinically important features of porphyrin and heme metabolism and the porphyrias. *Metabolites* 4, 977–1006. doi: 10.3390/metabo4040977

Bose, A., and Beal, M. F. (2016). Mitochondrial dysfunction in Parkinson's disease. *J. Neurochem.* 139(Suppl. 1), 216–231. doi: 10.1111/jnc.13731

Braymer, J. J., and Lill, R. (2017). Iron-sulfur cluster biogenesis and trafficking in mitochondria. *J. Biol. Chem.* 292, 12754–12763. doi: 10.1074/jbc.R117.787101

Bürk, K. (2017). Friedreich ataxia: current status and future prospects. *Cereb. Ataxias* 4:4. doi: 10.1186/s40673-017-0062-x

Busserolles, J., Tsantoulas, C., Eschalier, A., and López García, J. A. (2016). Potassium channels in neuropathic pain: advances, challenges, and emerging ideas. *Pain* 157(Suppl. 1), S7–S14. doi: 10.1097/j.pain.0000000000000368

Cabezas-Opazo, F. A., Vergara-Pulgar, K., Pérez, M. J., Jara, C., Osorio-Fuentealba, C., and Quintanilla, R. A. (2015). Mitochondrial dysfunction contributes to the pathogenesis of Alzheimer's disease. *Oxid. Med. Cell. Longev.* 2015:509654. doi: 10.1155/2015/509654

Castro-Gago, M., Alonso, A., Pintos-Martínez, E., Beiras-Iglesias, A., Campos, Y., Arenas, J. (1999). Congenital hydranencephalic-hydrocephalic syndrome associated with mitochondrial dysfunction. *J. Child Neurol.* 14, 131–135 doi: 10.1177/088307389901400213

Calabrese, V., Lodi, R., Tonon, C., D'Agata, V., Sapienza, M., Scapagnini, G., et al. (2005). Oxidative stress, mitochondrial dysfunction and cellular stress response in Friedreich's ataxia. *J. Neurol. Sci.* 233, 145–162. doi: 10.1016/j.jns.2005.03.012

Campuzano, V., Montermini, L., Moltò, M. D., Pianese, L., Cossée, M., Cavalcanti, F., et al. (1996). Friedreich's ataxia: autosomal recessive disease caused by an intronic GAA triplet repeat expansion. *Science* 271, 1423–1427. doi: 10.1126/science.271.5254.1423

Carelli, V., Musumeci, O., Caporali, L., Zanna, C., La Morgia, C., Del Dotto, V., et al. (2015). Syndromic parkinsonism and dementia associated with OPA1 missense mutations. *Ann. Neurol.* 78, 21–38. doi: 10.1002/ana.24410

Castori, M., Morlino, S., Ungelenk, M., Pareyson, D., Salsano, E., Grammatico, P., et al. (2017). Posterior column ataxia with retinitis pigmentosa coexisting with sensory-autonomic neuropathy and leukemia due to the homozygous p.Pro221Ser FLVCR1 mutation. *Am. J. Med. Genet. B Neuropsychiatr. Genet.* 174, 732–739. doi: 10.1002/ajmg.b.32570

Castro-Gago, M., Pintos-Martínez, E., Forteza-Vila, J., Iglesias-Diz, M., Ucieda-Somoza, R., Silva-Villar, I., et al. (2001). Congenital hydranencephalic-hydrocephalic syndrome with proliferative vasculopathy: a possible relation with mitochondrial dysfunction. *J. Child Neurol.* 16, 858–862. doi: 10.1177/08830738010160111401

Chiabrando, D., Castori, M., di Rocco, M., Ungelenk, M., Gießelmann, S., Di Capua, M., et al. (2016). Mutations in the heme exporter FLVCR1 cause sensory neurodegeneration with loss of pain perception. *PLoS Genet.* 12:e1006461. doi: 10.1371/journal.pgen.1006461

Chiabrando, D., Marro, S., Mercurio, S., Giorgi, C., Petrillo, S., Vinchi, F., et al. (2012). The mitochondrial heme exporter FLVCR1b mediates erythroid differentiation. *J. Clin. Invest.* 122, 4569–4579. doi: 10.1172/JCI62422

Chiabrando, D., Mercurio, S., and Tolosano, E. (2014a). Heme and erythropoieis: more than a structural role. *Haematologica* 99, 973–983. doi: 10.3324/haematol.2013.091991

Chiabrando, D., Vinchi, F., Fiorito, V., Mercurio, S., and Tolosano, E. (2014b). Heme in pathophysiology: a matter of scavenging, metabolism and trafficking across cell membranes. *Front. Pharmacol.* 5:61. doi: 10.3389/fphar.2014.00061

Chiang, S., Kalinowski, D. S., Jansson, P. J., Richardson, D. R., and Huang, M. L. (2018). Mitochondrial dysfunction in the neuro-degenerative and cardio-degenerative disease, Friedreich's ataxia. *Neurochem. Int.* 117, 35–48. doi: 10.1016/j.neuint.2017.08.002

Costa, V., and Scorrano, L. (2012). Shaping the role of mitochondria in the pathogenesis of Huntington's disease. *EMBO J.* 31, 1853–1864. doi: 10.1038/emboj.2012.65

De Vos, K. J., Chapman, A. L., Tennant, M. E., Manser, C., Tudor, E. L., Lau, K. F., et al. (2007). Familial amyotrophic lateral sclerosis-linked SOD1 mutants perturb fast axonal transport to reduce axonal mitochondria content. *Hum. Mol. Genet.* 16, 2720–2728. doi: 10.1093/hmg/ddm226

de Vries, H. E., Witte, M., Hondius, D., Rozemuller, A. J., Drukarch, B., Hoozemans, J., et al. (2008). Nrf2-induced antioxidant protection: a promising target to counteract ROS-mediated damage in neurodegenerative disease? *Free Radic. Biol. Med.* 45, 1375–1383. doi: 10.1016/j.freeradbiomed.2008.09.001

Duffy, S. P., Shing, J., Saraon, P., Berger, L. C., Eiden, M. V., Wilde, A., et al. (2010). The fowler syndrome-associated protein FLVCR2 is an importer of heme. *Mol. Cell. Biol.* 30, 5318–5324. doi: 10.1128/MCB.00690-10

Dwyer, B. E., Smith, M. A., Richardson, S. L., Perry, G., and Zhu, X. (2009). Down-regulation of aminolevulinate synthase, the rate-limiting enzyme for heme biosynthesis in Alzheimer's disease. *Neurosci. Lett.* 460, 180–184. doi: 10.1016/j.neulet.2009.05.058

Fiorito, V., Chiabrando, D., and Tolosano, E. (2018). Mitochondrial targeting in neurodegeneration: a heme perspective. *Pharmaceuticals* 11, 87. doi: 10.3390/ph11030087

Fiorito, V., Forni, M., Silengo, L., Altruda, F., and Tolosano, E. (2015). Crucial role of flvcr1a in the maintenance of intestinal heme homeostasis. *Antioxid Redox Signal.* 23, 1410–1423. doi: 10.1089/ars.2014.6216

Fiorito, V., Neri, F., Pala, V., Silengo, L., Oliviero, S., Altruda, F., et al. (2014). Hypoxia controls Flvcr1 gene expression in Caco2 cells through HIF2α and ETS1. *Biochim. Biophys. Acta* 1839, 259–264. doi: 10.1016/j.bbagrm.2014.02.010

Frezza, C., Zheng, L., Folger, O., Rajagopalan, K. N., MacKenzie, E. D., Jerby, L., et al. (2011). Haem oxygenase is synthetically lethal with the tumour suppressor fumarate hydratase. *Nature* 477, 225–228. doi: 10.1038/nature10363

Fukuda, Y., Wang, Y., Lian, S., Lynch, J., Nagai, S., Fanshawe, B., et al. (2017). Upregulated heme biosynthesis, an exploitable vulnerability in MYCN-driven leukemogenesis. *JCI Insight* 2:92409. doi: 10.1172/jci.insight.92409

Giraud, S., Bonod-Bidaud, C., Wesolowski-Louvel, M., and Stepien, G. (1998). Expression of human ANT2 gene in highly proliferative cells: GRBOX, a new transcriptional element, is involved in the regulation of glycolytic ATP import into mitochondria. *J. Mol. Biol.* 281, 409–418. doi: 10.1006/jmbi.1998.1955

Gnana-Prakasam, J. P., Reddy, S. K., Veeranan-Karmegam, R., Smith, S. B., Martin, P. M., and Ganapathy, V. (2011). Polarized distribution of heme transporters in retinal pigment epithelium and their regulation in the iron-overload disease hemochromatosis. *Invest. Ophthalmol. Vis. Sci.* 52, 9279–9286. doi: 10.1167/iovs.11-8264

Gozzelino, R. (2016). The pathophysiology of heme in the Brain. *Curr. Alzheimer Res.* 13, 174–184. doi: 10.2174/15672050126661509211033304

Guan, L., Wen, T., Zhang, Y., Wang, X., and Zhao, J. (2009). Induction of heme oxygenase-1 with hemin attenuates hippocampal injury in rats after acute carbon monoxide poisoning. *Toxicology* 262, 146–152. doi: 10.1016/j.tox.2009.06.001

Hahl, P., Davis, T., Washburn, C., Rogers, J. T., and Smith, A. (2013). Mechanisms of neuroprotection by hemopexin: modeling the control of heme and iron homeostasis in brain neurons in inflammatory states. *J. Neurochem.* 125, 89–101. doi: 10.1111/jnc.12165

Hartl, F. U., Bracher, A., and Hayer-Hartl, M. (2011). Molecular chaperones in protein folding and proteostasis. *Nature* 475, 324–332. doi: 10.1038/nature10317

Hartong, D. T., Berson, E. L., and Dryja, T. P. (2006). Retinitis pigmentosa. *Lancet* 368, 1795–1809. doi: 10.1016/S0140-6736(06)69740-7

Hashimoto, M., Hsu, L. J., Xia, Y., Takeda, A., Sisk, A., Sundsmo, M., et al. (1999). Oxidative stress induces amyloid-like aggregate formation of NACP/alpha-synuclein in vitro. *Neuroreport* 10, 717–721. doi: 10.1097/00001756-199903170-00011

Hayden, E. Y., Kaur, P., Williams, T. L., Matsui, H., Yeh, S. R., and Rousseau, D. L. (2015). Heme stabilization of α-synuclein oligomers during amyloid fibril formation. *Biochemistry* 54, 4599–4610. doi: 10.1021/acs.biochem.5b00280

Higdon, A. N., Benavides, G. A., Chacko, B. K., Ouyang, X., Johnson, M. S., Landar, A., et al. (2012). Causes mitochondrial dysfunction in endothelial cells through promoting lipid peroxidation: the protective role of autophagy. *Am. J. Physiol. Heart Circ. Physiol.* 302, H1394–H1409. doi: 10.1152/ajpheart.00584.2011

Higgins, J. J., Morton, D. H., and Loveless, J. M. (1999). Posterior column ataxia with retinitis pigmentosa (AXPC1) maps to chromosome 1q31-q32. *Neurology* 52, 146–150. doi: 10.1212/WNL.52.1.146

Higgins, J. J., Morton, D. H., Patronas, N., and Nee, L. E. (1997). An autosomal recessive disorder with posterior column ataxia and retinitis pigmentosa. *Neurology* 49, 1717–1720. doi: 10.1212/WNL.49.6.1717

Homedan, C., Laafi, J., Schmitt, C., Gueguen, N., Lefebvre, T., Karim, Z., et al. (2014). Acute intermittent porphyria causes hepatic mitochondrial energetic failure in a mouse model. *Int. J. Biochem. Cell Biol.* 51, 93–101 doi: 10.1016/j.biocel.2014.03.032

Horner, M. E., Alikhan, A., Tintle, S., Tortorelli, S., Davis, D. M., and Hand, J. L. (2013). Cutaneous porphyrias part I: epidemiology, pathogenesis, presentation, diagnosis, and histopathology. *Int. J. Dermatol.* 52, 1464–1480. doi: 10.1111/ijd.12305

Huang, M. L., Becker, E. M., Whitnall, M., Suryo Rahmanto, Y., Ponka, P., and Richardson, D. R. (2009). Elucidation of the mechanism of mitochondrial iron loading in Friedreich's ataxia by analysis of a mouse mutant. *Proc. Natl. Acad. Sci. U.S.A.* 106, 16381–16386. doi: 10.1073/pnas.0906784106

Ishiura, H., Fukuda, Y., Mitsui, J., Nakahara, Y., Ahsan, B., Takahashi, Y., et al. (2011). Posterior column ataxia with retinitis pigmentosa in a Japanese family with a novel mutation in FLVCR1. *Neurogenetics* 12, 117–121. doi: 10.1007/s10048-010-0271-4

Kaplan, G. S., Torcun, C. C., Grune, T., Ozer, N. K., and Karademir, B. (2017). Proteasome inhibitors in cancer therapy: treatment regimen and peripheral neuropathy as a side effect. *Free Radic. Biol. Med.* 103, 1–13. doi: 10.1016/j.freeradbiomed.2016.12.007

Kaushik, S., and Cuervo, A. M. (2015). Proteostasis and aging. *Nat. Med.* 21, 1406–1415. doi: 10.1038/nm.4001

Keel, S. B., Doty, R. T., Yang, Z., Quigley, J. G., Chen, J., Knoblaugh, S., et al. (2008). A heme export protein is required for red blood cell differentiation and iron homeostasis. *Science* 319, 825–828. doi: 10.1126/science.1151133

Khaminets, A., Heinrich, T., Mari, M., Grumati, P., Huebner, A. K., Akutsu, M., et al. (2015). Regulation of endoplasmic reticulum turnover by selective autophagy. *Nature* 522, 354–358. doi: 10.1038/nature14498

Kim, H. J., Khalimonchuk, O., Smith, P. M., and Winge, D. R. (2012). Structure, function, and assembly of heme centers in mitochondrial respiratory complexes. *Biochim. Biophys. Acta* 1823, 1604–1616. doi: 10.1016/j.bbamcr.2012.04.008

Krishnamurthy, P., and Schuetz, J. D. (2006). Role of ABCG2/BCRP in biology and medicine. *Annu. Rev. Pharmacol. Toxicol.* 46, 381–410. doi: 10.1146/annurev.pharmtox.46.120604.141238

Kumar, S., and Bandyopadhyay, U. (2005). Free heme toxicity and its detoxification systems in human. *Toxicol. Lett.* 157, 175–188. doi: 10.1016/j.toxlet.2005.03.004

Kvarnung, M., Taylan, F., Nilsson, D., Albåge, M., Nordenskjöld, M., Anderlid, B. M., et al. (2016). Mutations in FLVCR2 associated with Fowler syndrome and survival beyond infancy. *Clin. Genet.* 89, 99–103. doi: 10.1111/cge.12565

Lalonde, E., Albrecht, S., Ha, K. C., Jacob, K., Bolduc, N., Polychronakos, C., et al. (2010). Unexpected allelic heterogeneity and spectrum of mutations in Fowler syndrome revealed by next-generation exome sequencing. *Hum. Mutat.* 31, 918–923. doi: 10.1002/humu.21293

Lansbury, P. T., and Lashuel, H. A. (2006). A century-old debate on protein aggregation and neurodegeneration enters the clinic. *Nature* 443, 774–779. doi: 10.1038/nature05290

Law, C. J., Maloney, P. C., and Wang, D. N. (2008). Ins and outs of major facilitator superfamily antiporters. *Annu. Rev. Microbiol.* 62, 289–305. doi: 10.1146/annurev.micro.61.080706.093329

Lee, D., Kim, I. Y., Saha, S., and Choi, K. S. (2016). Paraptosis in the anti-cancer arsenal of natural products. *Pharmacol. Ther.* 162, 120–133. doi: 10.1016/j.pharmthera.2016.01.003

Levi, S., and Finazzi, D. (2014). Neurodegeneration with brain iron accumulation: update on pathogenic mechanisms. *Front. Pharmacol.* 5:99. doi: 10.3389/fphar.2014.00099

Li, J., Wuliji, O., Li, W., Jiang, Z. G., and Ghanbari, H. A. (2013). Oxidative stress and neurodegenerative disorders. *Int. J. Mol. Sci.* 14, 24438–24475. doi: 10.3390/ijms141224438

Lin, C. S., Lee, M. J., Park, S. B., and Kiernan, M. C. (2011). Purple pigments: the pathophysiology of acute porphyric neuropathy. *Clin. Neurophysiol.* 122, 2336–2344. doi: 10.1016/j.clinph.2011.07.036

Lin, M. T., and Beal, M. F. (2006). Mitochondrial dysfunction and oxidative stress in neurodegenerative diseases. *Nature* 443, 787–795. doi: 10.1038/nature05292

Lodi, R., Cooper, J. M., Bradley, J. L., Manners, D., Styles, P., Taylor, D. J., et al. (1999). Deficit of in vivo mitochondrial ATP production in patients with Friedreich ataxia. *Proc. Natl. Acad. Sci. U.S.A.* 96, 11492–11495. doi: 10.1073/pnas.96.20.11492

Ma, B., Day, J. P., Phillips, H., Slootsky, B., Tolosano, E., and Doré, S. (2016). Deletion of the hemopexin or heme oxygenase-2 gene aggravates brain injury following stroma-free hemoglobin-induced intracerebral hemorrhage. *J. Neuroinflamm.* 13:26. doi: 10.1186/s12974-016-0490-1

Marmolino, D. (2011). Friedreich's ataxia: past, present and future. *Brain Res. Rev.* 67, 311–330. doi: 10.1016/j.brainresrev.2011.04.001

Marro, S., Chiabrando, D., Messana, E., Stolte, J., Turco, E., Tolosano, E., et al. (2010). Heme controls ferroportin1 (FPN1) transcription involving Bach1, Nrf2 and a MARE/ARE sequence motif at position -7007 of the FPN1 promoter. *Haematologica* 95, 1261–1268. doi: 10.3324/haematol.2009.020123

Martelli, A., and Puccio, H. (2014). Dysregulation of cellular iron metabolism in Friedreich ataxia: from primary iron-sulfur cluster deficit to mitochondrial iron accumulation. *Front. Pharmacol.* 5:130. doi: 10.3389/fphar.2014.00130

Martelli, A., Schmucker, S., Reutenauer, L., Mathieu, J. R. R., Peyssonnaux, C., Karim, Z., et al. (2015). Iron regulatory protein 1 sustains mitochondrial iron loading and function in frataxin deficiency. *Cell Metab.* 21, 311–323. doi: 10.1016/j.cmet.2015.01.010

McNaught, K. S., and Jenner, P. (2001). Proteasomal function is impaired in substantia nigra in Parkinson's disease. *Neurosci. Lett.* 297, 191–194. doi: 10.1016/S0304-3940(00)01701-8

Mena, N. P., Urrutia, P. J., Lourido, F., Carrasco, C. M., and Núñez, M. T. (2015). Mitochondrial iron homeostasis and its dysfunctions in neurodegenerative disorders. *Mitochondrion* 21, 92–105. doi: 10.1016/j.mito.2015.02.001

Mercurio, S., Petrillo, S., Chiabrando, D., Bassi, Z. I., Gays, D., Camporeale, A., et al. (2015). Heme exporter Flvcr1 regulates expansion and differentiation of committed erythroid progenitors by controlling intracellular heme accumulation. *Haematologica* 100, 720–729. doi: 10.3324/haematol.2014.114488

Meyer, E., Ricketts, C., Morgan, N. V., Morris, M. R., Pasha, S., Tee, L. J., et al. (2010). Mutations in FLVCR2 are associated with proliferative vasculopathy and hydranencephaly-hydrocephaly syndrome (Fowler syndrome). *Am. J. Hum. Genet.* 86, 471–478. doi: 10.1016/j.ajhg.2010.02.004

Morimoto, R. I., and Cuervo, A. M. (2014). Proteostasis and the aging proteome in health and disease. *J. Gerontol. A Biol. Sci. Med. Sci.* 69(Suppl. 1), S33–S38. doi: 10.1093/gerona/glu049

Morris, G., Puri, B. K., Walder, K., Berk, M., Stubbs, B., Maes, M., et al. (2018). The Endoplasmic reticulum stress response in neuroprogressive diseases: emerging pathophysiological role and translational implications. *Mol. Neurobiol.* doi: 10.1007/s12035-018-1028-6 [Epub ahead of print].

Murakami, N., Imamura, K., Izumi, Y., Egawa, N., Tsukita, K., Enami, T., et al. (2017). Proteasome impairment in neural cells derived from HMSN-P patient iPSCs. *Mol. Brain* 10:7. doi: 10.1186/s13041-017-0286-y

Nguyen, T., Nioi, P., and Pickett, C. B. (2009). The Nrf2-antioxidant response element signaling pathway and its activation by oxidative stress. *J. Biol. Chem.* 284, 13291–13295. doi: 10.1074/jbc.R900010200

Panahian, N., Yoshiura, M., and Maines, M. D. (1999). Overexpression of heme oxygenase-1 is neuroprotective in a model of permanent middle cerebral artery occlusion in transgenic mice. *J. Neurochem.* 72, 1187–1203. doi: 10.1111/j.1471-4159.1999.721187.x

Pao, S. S., Paulsen, I. T., and Saier, M. H. (1998). Major facilitator superfamily. *Microbiol. Mol. Biol. Rev.* 62, 1–34.

Peers, C., and Boyle, J. P. (2015). Oxidative modulation of K + channels in the central nervous system in neurodegenerative diseases and aging. *Antioxid. Redox. Signal.* 22, 505–521. doi: 10.1089/ars.2014.6007

Perdomini, M., Hick, A., Puccio, H., and Pook, M. A. (2013). Animal and cellular models of Friedreich ataxia. *J. Neurochem.* 126(Suppl. 1), 65–79. doi: 10.1111/jnc.12219

Petrillo, S., Chiabrando, D., Genova, T., Fiorito, V., Ingoglia, G., Vinchi, F., et al. (2017). Heme accumulation in endothelial cells impairs angiogenesis by triggering paraptosis. *Cell Death Differ.* 25, 573–588. doi: 10.1038/s41418-017-0001-7

Pischik, E., and Kauppinen, R. (2015). An update of clinical management of acute intermittent porphyria. *Appl. Clin. Genet.* 8, 201–214. doi: 10.2147/TACG.S48605

Puspita, L., Chung, S. Y., and Shim, J. W. (2017). Oxidative stress and cellular pathologies in Parkinson's disease. *Mol. Brain* 10:53. doi: 10.1186/s13041-017-0340-9

Qiu, A., Jansen, M., Sakaris, A., Min, S. H., Chattopadhyay, S., Tsai, E., et al. (2006). Identification of an intestinal folate transporter and the molecular basis for hereditary folate malabsorption. *Cell* 127, 917–928. doi: 10.1016/j.cell.2006.09.041

Quigley, J. G., Yang, Z., Worthington, M. T., Phillips, J. D., Sabo, K. M., Sabath, D. E., et al. (2004). Identification of a human heme exporter that is essential for erythropoiesis. *Cell* 118, 757–766. doi: 10.1016/j.cell.2004.08.014

Radio, F. C., Di Meglio, L., Agolini, E., Bellacchio, E., Rinelli, M., Toscano, P., et al. (2018). Proliferative vasculopathy and hydranencephaly-hydrocephaly syndrome or Fowler syndrome: report of a family and insight into the disease's mechanism. *Mol. Genet. Genomic Med.* 6, 446–451. doi: 10.1002/mgg3.376

Rajadhyaksha, A. M., Elemento, O., Puffenberger, E. G., Schierberl, K. C., Xiang, J. Z., Putorti, M. L., et al. (2010). Mutations in FLVCR1 cause posterior column ataxia and retinitis pigmentosa. *Am. J. Hum. Genet.* 87, 643–654. doi: 10.1016/j.ajhg.2010.10.013

Rajagopal, A., Rao, A. U., Amigo, J., Tian, M., Upadhyay, S. K., Hall, C., et al. (2008). Haem homeostasis is regulated by the conserved and concerted functions of HRG-1 proteins. *Nature* 453, 1127–1131. doi: 10.1038/nature06934

Ramanujam, V. M., and Anderson, K. E. (2015). Porphyria diagnostics-part 1: a brief overview of the porphyrias. *Curr. Protoc. Hum. Genet.* 86, 17.20.1–17.20.26. doi: 10.1002/0471142905.hg1720s86 17.20.1-26, doi: 10.1002/0471142905.hg1720s86

Reddi, A. R., and Hamza, I. (2016). Heme mobilization in animals: a metallolipid's journey. *ACC Chem. Res.* 49, 1104–1110. doi: 10.1021/acs.accounts.5b00553

Righy, C., Bozza, M. T., Oliveira, M. F., and Bozza, F. A. (2016). Molecular, cellular and clinical aspects of intracerebral hemorrhage: are the enemies within? *Curr. Neuropharmacol.* 14, 392–402. doi: 10.2174/1570159X14666151230110058

Rotthier, A., Baets, J., Timmerman, V., and Janssens, K. (2012). Mechanisms of disease in hereditary sensory and autonomic neuropathies. *Nat. Rev. Neurol.* 8, 73–85. doi: 10.1038/nrneurol.2011.227

Rouault, T. A., and Maio, N. (2017). Biogenesis and functions of mammalian iron-sulfur proteins in the regulation of iron homeostasis and pivotal metabolic pathways. *J. Biol. Chem.* 292, 12744–12753. doi: 10.1074/jbc.R117.789537

Sabová, L., Zeman, I., Supek, F., and Kolarov, J. (1993). Transcriptional control of AAC3 gene encoding mitochondrial ADP/ATP translocator in *Saccharomyces cerevisiae* by oxygen, heme and ROX1 factor. *Eur. J. Biochem.* 213, 547–553. doi: 10.1111/j.1432-1033.1993.tb17793.x

Sahoo, N., Goradia, N., Ohlenschläger, O., Schönherr, R., Friedrich, M., Plass, W., et al. (2013). Heme impairs the ball-and-chain inactivation of potassium channels. *Proc. Natl. Acad. Sci. U.S.A.* 110, E4036–E4044. doi: 10.1073/pnas.1313247110

Sahoo, N., Hoshi, T., and Heinemann, S. H. (2014). Oxidative modulation of voltage-gated potassium channels. *Antioxid. Redox. Signal.* 21, 933–952. doi: 10.1089/ars.2013.5614

Sampaio, T. B., Marcondes, M. H., Sari Pesarico, A. P., and Nogueira, C. W. (2017). δ-Aminolevulinate dehydratase activity is stimulated in a mptp mouse model of Parkinson's disease: correlation with myeloperoxidase activity. *Cell Mol. Neurobiol.* 37, 911–917. doi: 10.1007/s10571-016-0428-2

Santiago, J. A., and Potashkin, J. A. (2017). Blood transcriptomic meta-analysis identifies dysregulation of hemoglobin and iron metabolism in Parkinson', disease. *Front. Aging Neurosci.* 9:73. doi: 10.3389/fnagi.2017.00073

Scheper, W., and Hoozemans, J. J. (2015). The unfolded protein response in neurodegenerative diseases: a neuropathological perspective. *Acta Neuropathol.* 130, 315–331. doi: 10.1007/s00401-015-1462-8

Scherzer, C. R., Grass, J. A., Liao, Z., Pepivani, I., Zheng, B., Eklund, A. C., et al. (2008). GATA transcription factors directly regulate the Parkinson's disease-linked gene alpha-synuclein. *Proc. Natl. Acad. Sci. U.S.A.* 105, 10907–10912. doi: 10.1073/pnas.0802437105

Schmitt, T. H., Frezzatti, W. A., and Schreier, S. (1993). Hemin-induced lipid membrane disorder and increased permeability: a molecular model for the mechanism of cell lysis. *Arch. Biochem. Biophys.* 307, 96–103. doi: 10.1006/abbi.1993.1566

Schoenfeld, R. A., Napoli, E., Wong, A., Zhan, S., Reutenauer, L., Morin, D., et al. (2005). Frataxin deficiency alters heme pathway transcripts and decreases mitochondrial heme metabolites in mammalian cells. *Hum. Mol. Genet.* 14, 3787–3799. doi: 10.1093/hmg/ddi393

Schulz, J. B., Dehmer, T., Schöls, L., Mende, H., Hardt, C., Vorgerd, M., et al. (2000). Oxidative stress in patients with Friedreich ataxia. *Neurology* 55, 1719–1721. doi: 10.1212/WNL.55.11.1719

Schwarz, T. L. (2013). Mitochondrial trafficking in neurons. *Cold Spring Harb. Perspect. Biol.* 5:a011304. doi: 10.1101/cshperspect.a011304

Shaibani, A., Wong, L. J., Wei Zhang, V., Lewis, R. A., and Shinawi, M. (2015). Autosomal recessive posterior column ataxia with retinitis pigmentosa caused by novel mutations in the FLVCR1 gene. *Int. J. Neurosci.* 125, 43–49. doi: 10.3109/00207454.2014.904858

Shayeghi, M., Latunde-Dada, G. O., Oakhill, J. S., Laftah, A. H., Takeuchi, K., Halliday, N., et al. (2005). Identification of an intestinal heme transporter. *Cell* 122, 789–801. doi: 10.1016/j.cell.2005.06.025

Shen, S., Callaghan, D., Juzwik, C., Xiong, H., Huang, P., and Zhang, W. (2010). ABCG2 reduces ROS-mediated toxicity and inflammation: a potential role in Alzheimer's disease. *J. Neurochem.* 114, 1590–1604. doi: 10.1111/j.1471-4159.2010.06887.x

Shi, P., Gal, J., Kwinter, D. M., Liu, X., and Zhu, H. (2010). Mitochondrial dysfunction in amyotrophic lateral sclerosis. *Biochim. Biophys. Acta* 1802, 45–51. doi: 10.1016/j.bbadis.2009.08.012

Shin, J. A., Jeong, S. I., Kim, H. W., Jang, G., Ryu, D. R., Ahn, Y. H., et al. (2018). Repression of adenosine triphosphate-binding cassette transporter ABCG2 by estrogen increases intracellular glutathione in brain endothelial cells following ischemic reperfusion injury. *Neurobiol. Aging* 66, 138–148. doi: 10.1016/j.neurobiolaging.2018.02.020

Shirendeb, U., Reddy, A. P., Manczak, M., Calkins, M. J., Mao, P., Tagle, D. A., et al. (2011). Abnormal mitochondrial dynamics, mitochondrial loss and mutant huntingtin oligomers in Huntington's disease: implications for selective neuronal damage. *Hum. Mol. Genet.* 20, 1438–1455. doi: 10.1093/hmg/ddr024

Simon, N. G., and Herkes, G. K. (2011). The neurologic manifestations of the acute porphyrias. *J. Clin. Neurosci.* 18, 1147–1153. doi: 10.1016/j.jocn.2011.01.003

Smith, A. G., Raven, E. L., and Chernova, T. (2011). The regulatory role of heme in neurons. *Metallomics* 3, 955–962. doi: 10.1039/c1mt00085c

Söderberg, C., Gillam, M. E., Ahlgren, E. C., Hunter, G. A., Gakh, O., Isaya, G., et al. (2016). The structure of the complex between yeast frataxin and ferrochelatase: characterization and pre-steady state reaction of ferrous iron delivery and heme synthesis. *J. Biol. Chem.* 291, 11887–11898. doi: 10.1074/jbc.M115.701128

Stemmler, T. L., Lesuisse, E., Pain, D., and Dancis, A. (2010). Frataxin and mitochondrial FeS cluster biogenesis. *J. Biol. Chem.* 285, 26737–26743. doi: 10.1074/jbc.R110.118679

Stockwell, B. R., Friedmann, J. P., Angeli, Bayir, H., Bush, A. I., Conrad, M., et al. (2017). Ferroptosis: a regulated cell death nexus linking metabolism, redox biology, and disease. *Cell* 171, 273–285. doi: 10.1016/j.cell.2017.09.021

Sun, J., Brand, M., Zenke, Y., Tashiro, S., Groudine, M., and Igarashi, K. (2004). Heme regulates the dynamic exchange of Bach1 and NF-E2-related factors in the Maf transcription factor network. *Proc. Natl. Acad. Sci. U.S.A.* 101, 1461–1466. doi: 10.1073/pnas.0308083100

Suzuki, H., Tashiro, S., Hira, S., Sun, J., Yamazaki, C., Zenke, Y., et al. (2004). Heme regulates gene expression by triggering Crm1-dependent nuclear export of Bach1. *EMBO J.* 23, 2544–2553. doi: 10.1038/sj.emboj.7600248

Tanaka, Y., Niwa, S., Dong, M., Farkhondeh, A., Wang, L., Zhou, R., et al. (2016). The molecular motor KIF1A transports the TrkA neurotrophin receptor and is essential for sensory neuron survival and function. *Neuron* 90, 1215–1229. doi: 10.1016/j.neuron.2016.05.002

Tang, X. D., Santarelli, L. C., Heinemann, S. H., and Hoshi, T. (2004). Metabolic regulation of potassium channels. *Annu. Rev. Physiol.* 66, 131–159. doi: 10.1146/annurev.physiol.66.041002.142720

Tang, X. D., Xu, R., Reynolds, M. F., Garcia, M. L., Heinemann, S. H., and Hoshi, T. (2003). Haem can bind to and inhibit mammalian calcium-dependent Slo1 BK channels. *Nature* 425, 531–535. doi: 10.1038/nature02003

Thomas, S., Encha-Razavi, F., Devisme, L., Etchevers, H., Bessieres-Grattagliano, B., Goudefroye, G., et al. (2010). High-throughput sequencing of a 4.1 Mb linkage interval reveals FLVCR2 deletions and mutations in lethal cerebral vasculopathy. *Hum. Mutat.* 31, 1134–1141. doi: 10.1002/humu.21329

Tiwari, A., Bahr, A., Bähr, L., Fleischhauer, J., Zinkernagel, M. S., Winkler, N., et al. (2016). Next generation sequencing based identification of disease-associated mutations in Swiss patients with retinal dystrophies. *Sci. Rep.* 6:28755. doi: 10.1038/srep28755

Tracy, J. A., and Dyck, P. J. (2014). Porphyria and its neurologic manifestations. *Handb. Clin. Neurol.* 120, 839–849. doi: 10.1016/B978-0-7020-4087-0.00056-5

Tsai, P. C., Huang, Y. H., Guo, Y. C., Wu, H. T., Lin, K. P., Tsai, Y. S., et al. (2014). A novel TFG mutation causes charcot-marie-tooth disease type 2 and impairs TFG function. *Neurology* 83, 903–912. doi: 10.1212/WNL.0000000000000758

Vallelian, F., Deuel, J. W., Opitz, L., Schaer, C. A., Puglia, M., Lönn, M., et al. (2015). Proteasome inhibition and oxidative reactions disrupt cellular homeostasis during heme stress. *Cell Death. Differ.* 22, 597–611. doi: 10.1038/cdd.2014.154

Vasconcellos, L. R., Dutra, F. F., Siqueira, M. S., Paula-Neto, H. A., Dahan, J., Kiarely, E., et al. (2016). Protein aggregation as a cellular response to oxidative stress induced by heme and iron. *Proc. Natl. Acad. Sci. U.S.A.* 113, E7474–E7482. doi: 10.1073/pnas.1608928113

Verpoorten, N., De Jonghe, P., and Timmerman, V. (2006). Disease mechanisms in hereditary sensory and autonomic neuropathies. *Neurobiol. Dis.* 21, 247–255. doi: 10.1016/j.nbd.2005.08.004

Vinchi, F., Ingoglia, G., Chiabrando, D., Mercurio, S., Turco, E., Silengo, L., et al. (2014). Heme exporter FLVCR1a regulates heme synthesis and degradation and controls activity of cytochromes P450. *Gastroenterology* 146, 1325–1338. doi: 10.1053/j.gastro.2014.01.053

Wang, J., and Doré, S. (2007). Heme oxygenase-1 exacerbates early brain injury after intracerebral haemorrhage. *Brain* 130(Pt 6), 1643–1652. doi: 10.1093/brain/awm095

Ward, R. J., Dexter, D. T., and Crichton, R. R. (2015). Neurodegenerative diseases and therapeutic strategies using iron chelators. *J. Trace Elem. Med. Biol.* 31, 267–273. doi: 10.1016/j.jtemb.2014.12.012

White, C., Yuan, X., Schmidt, P. J., Bresciani, E., Samuel, T. K., Campagna, D., et al. (2013). HRG1 is essential for heme transport from the phagolysosome of macrophages during erythrophagocytosis. *Cell Metab.* 17, 261–270. doi: 10.1016/j.cmet.2013.01.005

Williams, D., Patel, C., Fallet-Bianco, C., Kalyanasundaram, K., Yacoubi, M., Déchelotte, P., et al. (2010). Fowler syndrome-a clinical, radiological, and pathological study of 14 cases. *Am. J. Med. Genet. A* 152A, 153–160. doi: 10.1002/ajmg.a.33094

Xiang, C., Wang, Y., Zhang, H., and Han, F. (2017). The role of endoplasmic reticulum stress in neurodegenerative disease. *Apoptosis* 22, 1–26. doi: 10.1007/s10495-016-1296-4

Xiong, H., Callaghan, D., Jones, A., Bai, J., Rasquinha, I., Smith, C., et al. (2009). ABCG2 is upregulated in Alzheimer's brain with cerebral amyloid angiopathy and may act as a gatekeeper at the blood-brain barrier for Abeta(1-40) peptides. *J. Neurosci.* 29, 5463–5475. doi: 10.1523/JNEUROSCI.5103-08.2009

Yagi, T., Ito, D., and Suzuki, N. (2016). TFG-related neurologic disorders: new insights into relationships between endoplasmic reticulum and neurodegeneration. *J. Neuropathol. Exp. Neurol.* 75, 299–305. doi: 10.1093/jnen/nlw009

Yang, Y., Ouyang, Y., Yang, L., Beal, M. F., McQuibban, A., Vogel, H., et al. (2008). Pink1 regulates mitochondrial dynamics through interaction with the fission/fusion machinery. *Proc. Natl. Acad. Sci. U.S.A.* 105, 7070–7075. doi: 10.1073/pnas.0711845105

Yang, Z., Philips, J. D., Doty, R. T., Giraudi, P., Ostrow, J. D., Tiribelli, C., et al. (2010). Kinetics and specificity of feline leukemia virus subgroup C receptor (FLVCR) export function and its dependence on hemopexin. *J. Biol. Chem.* 285, 28874–28882. doi: 10.1074/jbc.M110.119131

Yoon, T., and Cowan, J. A. (2004). Frataxin-mediated iron delivery to ferrochelatase in the final step of heme biosynthesis. *J. Biol. Chem.* 279, 25943–25946. doi: 10.1074/jbc.C400107200

Yusuf, I. H., Shanks, M. E., Clouston, P., and MacLaren, R. E. (2018). A splice-site variant in FLVCR1 produces retinitis pigmentosa without posterior column ataxia. *Ophthalmic Genet.* 39, 263–267. doi: 10.1080/13816810.2017.1408848

Zeng, Y., Callaghan, D., Xiong, H., Yang, Z., Huang, P., and Zhang, W. (2012). Abcg2 deficiency augments oxidative stress and cognitive deficits in Tg-SwDI transgenic mice. *J. Neurochem.* 122, 456–469. doi: 10.1111/j.1471-4159.2012.07783.x

10

UPR Induction Prevents Iron Accumulation and Oligodendrocyte Loss in *ex vivo* Cultured Hippocampal Slices

Sinead Healy, Jill McMahon and Una FitzGerald*

Galway Neuroscience Centre, School of Natural Sciences, National University of Ireland Galway, Galway, Ireland

***Correspondence:**
Una FitzGerald
una.fitzgerald@nuigalway.ie

The accumulation of iron within the brain occurs in many chronic disorders including Alzheimer's and Parkinson's disease and multiple sclerosis. Outside the CNS, a link between levels of iron and the unfolded protein response has already been established. To determine if such a relationship operates in within the brain, we used our *ex vivo* hippocampal slice-based model of iron accumulation. Ferrocene addition caused accumulation of iron within slices and loss of oligodendrocytes, an effect that was partially inhibited when ferrocene and ER stressor tunicamycin (Tm) were added together. An upward trend (not found to be statistically significant) in the expression of UPR transcripts in response to ferrocene was demonstrated using real-time PCR, while a significant upregulation of mRNA for B cell immunoglobulin-binding protein (BiP) and C/EBP homologous binding protein (CHOP) occurred following exposure to Tm. *In silico* analysis revealed consensus DNA-binding sequences for UPR-associated transcription factors within the promoter regions of eight iron-regulatory genes. In addition, dual-staining for CHOP and oligodendrocyte transcription factor 2 (OLIG2) or Ionized calcium binding adaptor molecule 1 (Iba1) showed nuclear expression of CHOP in some oligodendrocyte-lineage cells in response to Tm or Tm+ferrocene, but CHOP was rarely found in microglia. Co-expression of UPR-associated activated transcription factor 6 (ATF6) was detected in the nuclei of some oligodendrocyte-lineage cells exposed to Tm alone, or to Tm and ferrocene, but rarely in microglia. These data highlight the therapeutic potential of targeting UPR-associated proteins when developing novel treatments for chronic brain disorders that are affected by dysregulated iron.

Keywords: iron, unfolded protein response, UPR, tunicamycin, ferrocene

INTRODUCTION

The unfolded protein response (UPR) is a 'check and balance' program activated upon disturbed homeostasis in the endoplasmic reticulum. Occasional but infrequent hints have documented an interplay between the UPR and iron metabolism (Ye and Connor, 2000; You et al., 2003; Oliveira et al., 2009; Vecchi et al., 2009). However, reports are few on the possible links between the UPR and iron within the brain (Liu and Connor, 2012; Rahman et al., 2017, 2018; Lumsden et al., 2018). A better understanding of this cross-talk might provide further clues regarding disease pathogenesis, given that aberrant iron metabolism and increased expression of markers of the UPR have been independently reported in several neurodegenerative diseases (Hetz and Mollereau, 2014), including multiple sclerosis (Stephenson et al., 2014), Alzheimer's disease and Parkinson's disease (Mercado et al., 2013; Ward et al., 2014). Researchers have exploited glial and neuronal mono- and dual-cultures *in vitro*, as well as *ex vivo* systems to investigate the regulation of iron within the brain [see (Healy et al., 2017) for comprehensive review of this topic]. As a foundation for future studies, the overall goal of this work was therefore to confirm and characterize the reciprocal relationship between UPR and iron homeostasis within our hippocampal slice-based model (Healy et al., 2016) of the accumulation of iron within the CNS.

METHODS

Ethics Statement

The research described was approved by the Animal Care Research Ethics Committee Filing ID 12/FEB/04) and was carried out in accordance with European directive 2010/63/EU.

Hippocampal Slice Culture and Reagent Exposure

Neonatal hippocampal slices were maintained as previously described (Healy et al., 2016).

Five μg/ml tunicamycin (Tm, T7765, Sigma-Aldrich, Dublin, Ireland) exposure was used to activate a UPR response, while iron loading was induced by a 12-h treatment with 1 μM ferrocene, a membrane-permeable compound that enables uptake of iron by cells (F408, Sigma-Aldrich, Dublin, Ireland). Slices were harvested immediately after iron loading.

Analysis of RNA Transcripts

RNA was isolated from control and treated slice cultures using TRIreagent (T9424, Sigma-Aldrich, Dublin, Ireland) as per the manufacturer's instructions. Following DNAse I treatment (18068-015, Thermofisher-Scientific, Dublin, Ireland) and cDNA synthesis using manufacturer protocol (1804014, Superscript II Reverse Transcriptase, Invitrogen, Dublin, Ireland), real-time PCR was accomplished using Applied Biosystems 4346906 MicroAmp®Fast Optical 96-Well Reaction Plate and Fast SYPR green master mix (applied Biosystems, 4385612) and the Step One real-time PCR System (Thermo-Fisher).

Unless otherwise indicated, oligonucleotide primer sequences (Sigma-Aldrich, Dublin, Ireland) used were designed using Primer3. Primer sequence details are summarized in the **Supplementary Table 1**. Results were quantified using the ΔΔCT method following standardization relative to β-actin as an internal control.

Tissue Viability

Tissue viability was measured as described in Healy et al. (2016), using a lactate dehydrogenase (LDH) and MTT [3-(4,5-Dimethylthiazol-2-yl)-2,5-Diphenyltetrazolium Bromide] assay.

Immunohistochemistry and Imaging

Tissue was fixed and stained as previously described (Healy et al., 2016). Briefly, slices were fixed in 4% paraformaldehyde (PFA) for 30 min followed by three washes in PBS and then blocked and permeabilised for 1 h with 10% normal goat serum and 0.4% Triton X-100 in PBS. Subsequently, the slices were incubated with primary antibody (for single and dual labeling) in 2.5% NGS (or 2.5% horse serum) and 0.1% Triton X-100 in PBS for 48 h at 4°C and then washed three times for 15 min before incubation with the appropriate secondary antibody at 4°C overnight. Source information and dilutions used for all antibodies is available in the **Supplementary Materials**. Slice cultures were mounted in Vectashield containing diamino-2-phenylindole (DAPI) (H-1200, Vector Laboratories, Peterborough, United Kingdom) to allow visualization of nuclei. Negative "no primary antibody" controls were included. Slides were stored in the dark at 4°C until imaged. All samples were imaged on a laser scanning confocal microscope (Olympus Fluoview 1000) using a 40 × oil-immersion lens (numerical aperture of 1.3).

In silico Analysis of UPR Transcription Factor Binding Sites

The ALGGEN PROMO algorithm[1] was used to determine if any UPR transcription factor consensus DNA binding sequences were present within the promoter regions of genes that encode iron homeostasis regulators. Only hits that had a dissimilarity index <15% and a random expectation <0.5 were included in this analysis.

Statistical Analysis

Data was analyzed using Prism 6 (GraphPad Software). All measurements were expressed as mean ± standard error of the mean (SEM) unless otherwise indicated. Normality was assessed using the Shapiro-Wilk test. Statistical analyses were carried out using Student's *t*-test, Mann-Whitney test or an ANOVA with Dunnet post-test, as appropriate, and as indicated in figure legends. Differences were considered statistically significant if $P<0.05$.

RESULTS

UPR Transcript Expression in Cultured Slices Exposed to Ferrocene Remains Unchanged

Real-time PCR analysis of changes in the transcripts for B-cell immunoglobulin binding protein (BiP), calreticulin (CRT), X-box binding protein 1 (XBP1), activated transcription factor

[1] http://alggen.lsi.upc.es/

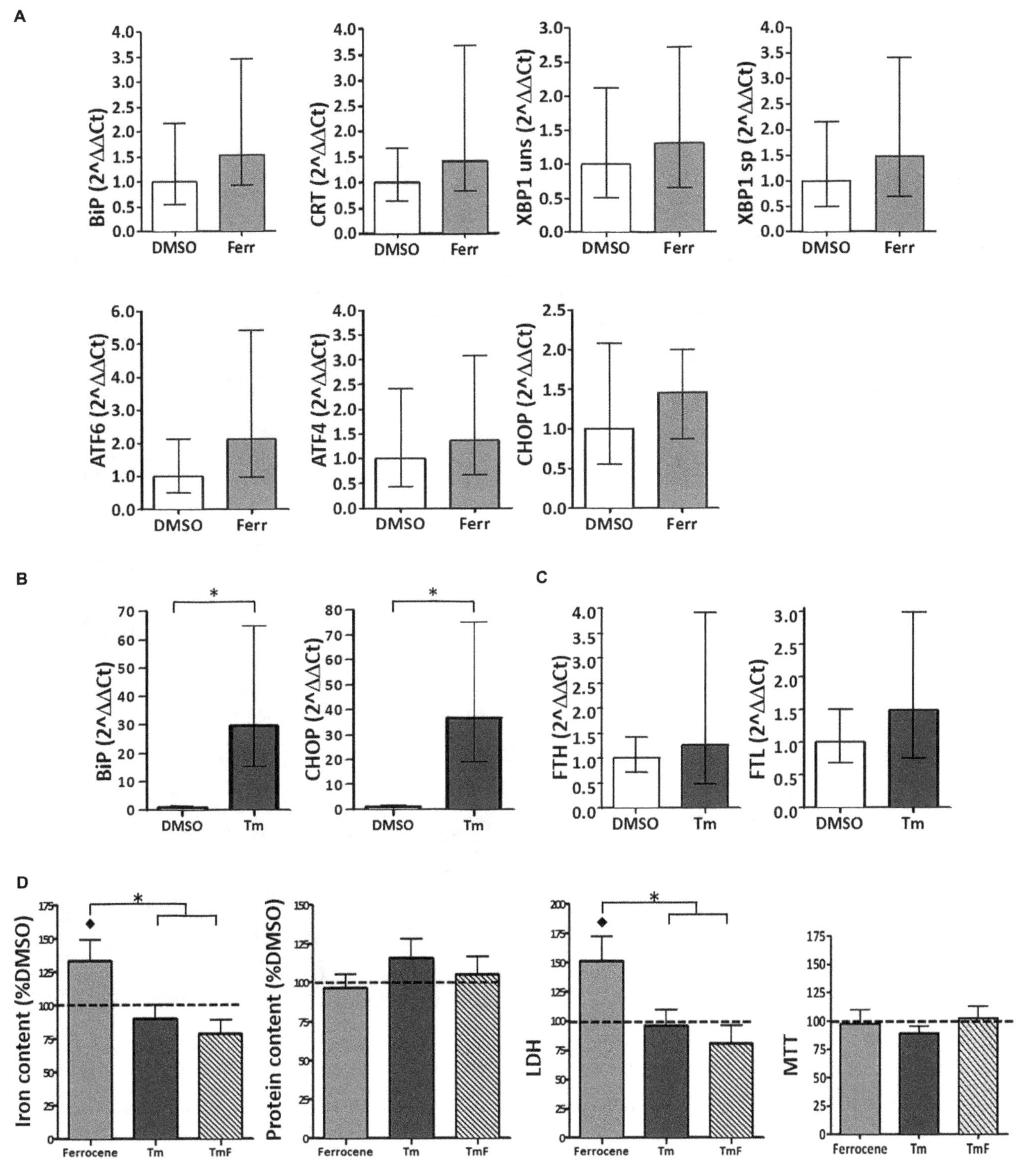

FIGURE 1 | Continued

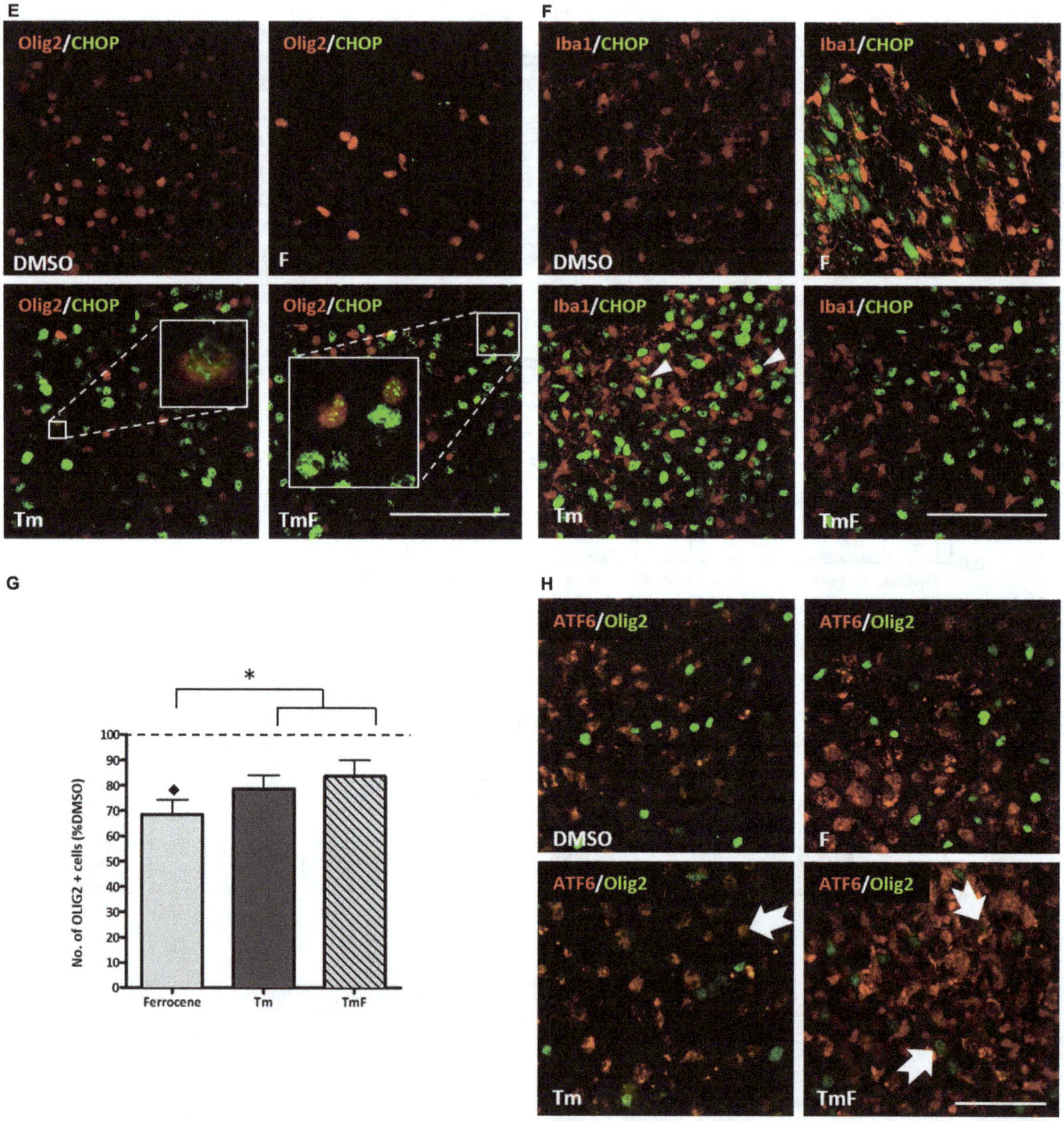

FIGURE 1 | Cross-talk between regulators of the UPR and iron homeostasis. **(A)** Real-time PCR analysis of RNA samples derived from cultured slices treated for 12 h with 1 μM ferrocene. An upward trend in the expression of BiP, CRT, XBP1, ATF6, ATF4, and CHOP was detected (*n* = 3 experimental replicates). **(B)** Increased BiP and CHOP transcripts detected following 12 h treatment with 5 μg/ml Tm (*n* = 3). Data is expressed as mean ± 95% confidence interval following completion of three experimental repeats. *denotes $p<0.05$. **(C)** Upward trend in the expression of FTL and FTH transcripts detected following 12 h Tm treatment (5 μg/ml, *n* = 2 experimental repeats). **(D)** Effect of Tm exposure (5 μg/ml, 12 h) on iron and protein content and on tissue viability (*n* = 3 experimental replicates). Cultures were loaded with 1 μM ferrocene **(F)**, 5 μg/ml Tm or both treatments concurrently (TmF). Data is expressed as percentage of DMSO control, which is indicated by the dashed line. Values are mean + SEM from three experiments. ◇ denotes a significant difference ($p<0.05$) when compared with DMSO and *denotes significant difference between F-treated slices and those treated with Tm or TMF ($p<0.05$). **(E)** CHOP expression (green) was detected within the nuclei of olig2-positive cells (red) in hippocampal slices treated with Tm or TmF (lower panels), but was not seen within the Olig2-positive population of control or F-treated slices (upper panels). Scale bar = 100 μm **(F)** When cultured slices were dual-labeled using antibodies to Iba1 (red) and CHOP (green, RH panels), CHOP was not found in DMSO-exposed slices but was seen in non-Iba1-positive slices treated with F or TmF and occasionally in Iba1-positive nuclei in slices treated with Tm alone (white arrowheads). Scale bar = 100 μm. **(G)** The significant loss of oligodendrocyte-lineage cells caused by exposure to F is partially reversed when slices are co-treated with Tm or TmF (*n* = 2 experimental replicates). ◇denotes a significant difference ($p<0.05$) when compared with DMSO; *denotes a significant difference between F-treated slices and those treated with Tm or TMF ($p<0.05$). **(H)** Cytoplasmic expression of ATF6 (red) detected in the non-olig2-expressing cells of DMSO- and F-treated hippocampal slices (top panels). Treatment with Tm or TmF led to nuclear expression of ATF6 within olig2-positive cells (green, arrows). Scale bar = 50 μm.

6 (ATF6), activated transcription factor and C/EBP homologous binding protein (CHOP) revealed an approximate 1.4–2.1-fold increase, which was not found to be statistically significant following three replicate experiments (**Figure 1A**).

UPR Induction Does Not Increase Expression of Iron Storage Protein Transcripts

The ability of cultured hippocampal slices to mount a response to ER stress was confirmed when a significant increase in BiP and CHOP transcription (approximately 30-fold for both), was detected following a 12-h treatment with 5 μg/ml tunicamycin (Tm, **Figure 1B**). Tm inhibits N-glycosylation of proteins trafficked through the ER (Foufelle and Fromenty, 2016) hence causing a build-up of mis-folded proteins and ER stress. However, Tm was not found, after two experimental repeats, to cause a significant increase in the expression of ferritin light chain (FTL) or ferritin heavy chain (FHL) transcripts (**Figure 1C**).

UPR Activation Prevents Ferrocene-Induced Iron Accumulation and Glial Perturbations

In line with our previous findings (Healy et al., 2016), 1 μM ferrocene produced a 1.3-fold increase in the levels of iron in slice cultures when compared to vehicle (**Figure 1D**). Similarly, we confirmed that ferrocene-induced a significant 1.5-fold increase in LDH release, and, once again, did not report any iron-induced loss in metabolic activity as assessed by MTT assay (**Figure 1D**). Interestingly, concurrent exposure to 5 μg/ml Tm (TmF) resulted in amelioration in iron accumulation and toxicity (**Figure 1D**). TmF treatment led to a significant reduction in iron content and a significant decrease in LDH release, when compared with ferrocene alone, but not when compared with the DMSO control. In keeping with our data relating to FTL and FTH transcriptional expression, Tm exposure alone did not lead to a significant difference in iron content. Tm treatment alone also had no effect on tissue viability when compared to DMSO control conditions. There were no significant differences in metabolic activity as measured using an MTT assay, or in protein content between groups (**Figure 1D**).

UPR Transcription Factor Expression in Glia Following Tm and Iron Exposure

Classically, CHOP is upregulated in response to phosphorylation of PERK and is frequently exploited as a marker of activation of the UPR. Immunofluorescent staining demonstrated an absence of CHOP expression in control and ferrocene-treated slice cultures, but robust upregulation of CHOP in Tm-treated tissue. Dual immunofluorescent staining confirmed CHOP expression in Olig2-positive cells within Tm-treated slices, which appeared to increase when slices were co-exposed to Tm and Ferrocene (**Figure 1E**). Less frequently, CHOP was found to be present in microglia within cultured slices exposed to Ferrocene, Tm or both (**Figure 1F**). Similar to our prior finding of significantly reduced numbers of microglial endpoints, following slice treatment with F, we also found, following two experimental repeats, fewer end-points after F treatment, which was rescued when tissue was treated with TmF (data not shown). ATF6 is the second major regulator of the UPR whose protein expression we analyzed by immunofluorescence within cultured control and treated slices. While non-nuclear ATF6 was detected in control DMSO-treated cultures, an increase in nuclear ATF6 staining was observed following treatment with Tm, F, or a combination of both reagents (not shown).

In our previous study, we reported a significant loss of oligodendrocyte-lineage cells following iron loading (Healy et al., 2016). This result was confirmed here (**Figure 1G**). Intriguingly, slice exposure to Tm or TmF reversed this loss, to the extent that Olig2-lineage cells responded by increasing their number significantly (**Figure 1G**). Dual immunofluorescence was then used to determine if the localization of ATF6 expression within Olig2-positive cells was affected by the same conditions. Our images showed that while nuclear (active) ATF6 was not detectable within DMSO-treated Olig2-lineage cells, it was present in Tm-, F- or TmF-treated cultures (**Figure 1H**).

In silico Analysis of Putative Transcription Factor Binding Sites Within Promoter Regions of Iron-Regulatory Genes

Using the ALGGEN PROMO algorithm to predict consensus transcription factor (TF) DNA binding sequences, we identified a number of putative binding sites for UPR-associated transcription within the promoter regions of iron homeostasis genes (**Table 1**). None of the TFs were found to be commonly expressed on all the promoter regions examined. Activated transcription factor 3 (ATF3) and CCAAT-enhancer-binding protein alpha (C/EBP-α) consensus-binding sequences were found on six of the eight genes (**Table 1**). Consensus sequences for XBP1, ATF and ATF2 were found within two promoter regions; the CREB consensus sequence was found on three genes and C/EBP-β was not found on any. Therefore, there was not a consistent pattern of transcription factor hits across the different genes (**Table 1**).

DISCUSSION

In an attempt to elucidate whether or not cross-talk between iron-regulatory proteins and ER stress, we exploited our rat hippocampal slice-based model of iron accumulation. Following slice exposure to Tm, F or both, real-time

PCR and fluorescent immunohistochemistry yielded the following primary findings: (1) Tm exposure does not affect the level of iron in hippocampal slices, but it triggers a UPR that appears to prevent iron overload and possibly ameliorates toxic effects of iron on oligodendrocytes and microglia; (2) iron overload causes an upward trend in the levels of transcripts encoding the major markers of the UPR, although this was not statistically significant; (3) the observation that Tm treatment led to no significant change in the expression of FTL or FTH transcripts was surprising, since the promoter regions of eight genes that encode iron-regulatory proteins, including FTL and FTH, contain putative binding sites for ER stress-associated transcription factors; (4) transcription factor ATF6 is activated following exposure of cultured hippocampal slices to Tm, F and TmF; (5) Activated ATF6 is detectable within the Tm- and TmF-treated oligodendrocycte population but rarely in similarly treated microglia.

While intriguing, it remains unclear how concurrent iron accumulation and UPR activation, demonstrated here, leads to

TABLE 1 | Putative binding sites of UPR transcription factors in the promoters of genes encoding iron homeostasis proteins.

Gene	Factor	Start	End	Dissimilarity	String	RE Equally	RE Query
Hepc	ATF3 [T01313]	23	60	6.74	tgacacaa	0.082	0.062
	ATF3 [T01313]	445	45	13.48	tgctgtca	0.164	0.132
	XBP-1 [T00902]	379	384	6.47	atgccc	0.292	0.318
	XBP-1 [T00902]	448	453	1.58	tgtcat	0.220	0.231
FTH	ATF3 [T01313]	497	504	10.12	tgacaaaa	0.222	0.225
	ATF3 [T01313]	521	528	10.12	tgacttca	0.222	0.225
	C/EBPα [T00105]	301	307	3.55	accaatc	0.137	0.225
	C/EBPα [T00105]	425	431	7.47	tgcaatg	0.273	0.290
	C/EBPα [T00105]	527	533	2.44	cattgag	0.273	0.278
	C/EBPα [T00105]	571	577	2.37	aattggg	0.273	0.279
	C/EBPα [T00105]	1063	1069	8	tccaatg	0.137	0.141
FTL	XBP-1 [T00902]	494	499	6.48	atgagg	0.401	0.434
	C/EBPα [T00105]	211	217	5.58	gtcaatt	0.401	0.283
	C/EBPα [T00105]	754	760	5.78	gccaata	0.401	0.283
TfR1	C/EBPα [T00105]	1609	1615	1.22	tattgag	0.345	0.420
	C/EBPα [T00105]	1822	1828	0	gattgag	0.345	0.334
	CREB [T00163]	2347	2355	3.08	tgacgtttg	0.086	0.091
Tf	C/EBPα [T00105]	1410	1416	4.56	gacaatc	0.280	0.270
	ATF3 [T01313]	1040	1047	8.31	gtatgtca	0.316	0.311
	ATF3 [T01313]	1397	1404	10.12	tgacctca	0.456	0.445
	ATF3 [T01313]	1887	1894	0	ttacgtca	0.035	0.033
	CREB [T00163]	1886	1894	2.66	attacgtca	0.070	0.069
	ATF-2 [T00167]	1886	1895	4.17	attacgtcaa	0.040	0.037
	ATF [T00051]	1887	1898	8.419	ttacgtcaacag	0.089	0.087
FPN	ATF3 [T01313]	2376	2383	8.31	atatgtca	0.455	0.429
	ATF3 [T01313]	2745	2752	8.31	atatgtca	0.455	0.429
	ATF3 [T01313]	3237	3244	3.37	tgacataa	0.151	0.179
	C/EBPα [T00105]	759	765	5.024	cacaatc	0.404	0.370
	C/EBPα [T00105]	777	783	3.55	gattgga	0.404	0.533
	C/EBPα [T00105]	1433	1439	4.56	gattggc	0.404	0.367
Cp	C/EBPα [T00105]	74	80	8	cattgga	0.405	0.505
	C/EBPα [T00105]	935	941	0.54	cacaatc	0.405	0.361
	C/EBPα [T00105]	1421	1427	1.22	tattgag	0.405	0.361
	C/EBPα [T00105]	1430	1436	0.54	gattggg	0.405	0.361
	ATF3 [T01313]	932	939	6.74	tgacacaa	0.456	0.519
DMT1	C/EBPα [T00105]	2	8	3.55	accaatc	0.463	0.566
	CREB [T00163]	3116	3124	2.664	tgacgtgat	0.116	0.119
	ATF3 [T01313]	2716	2723	3.372	tgacataa	0.173	0.192
	ATF-2 [T00167]	3115	3124	4.17	ttgacgtgat	0.065	0.075
	ATF [T00051]	3112	3123	5.46	gcattgacgtga	0.048	0.047

Summary of the putative binding site of the UPR-associated transcription factors in the gene sequence of an iron-homeostasis molecule with a dissimilarity index <15% and random expectation <0.5. Transcription factors tested: C/EBP-beta, C/EBP-α, CREB, XBP1, ATF, ATF3, ATF-2, and ATF1.

the ameliorated accumulation of iron. Outside the brain, the main description of the intersection between the UPR and iron metabolism is the action of CHOP on hepcidin (via modulation of C/EBPα binding and/or through CREBH) in the liver and spleen (Oliveira et al., 2009; Vecchi et al., 2009) although ER stress associated chaperones calreticulin and BiP have also been implicated in iron UPR cross-talk [reviewed in (Oliveira et al., 2011)].More recently, an increase in hepcidin expression leading to accumulated iron within the brain of rats subjected to sub-arachnoid hemorrhage, was found to be regulated by CHOP (Zhao et al., 2018).

Our observation that CHOP immunofluorescence appears to be increased in Olig-2 positive cells in slices that were co-exposed to Tm and Ferrocene compared with only Tm is consistent with these studies and it hints at the potential therapeutic benefit of UPR proteins induced by Tm to protect against iron-induced toxicity within oligodendrocyte lineage cells. However, further work is required to elucidate or reasonably speculate on such a mechanism.

AUTHOR CONTRIBUTIONS

SH carried out the PCR. SH and JM completed the tissue staining. JM and UF conceived and oversaw research described. SH, JM, and UF wrote the manuscript.

FUNDING

SH was supported by a College of Science Fellowship from The National University of Ireland, Galway. SH and JM were supported by the Foundation Office of the National University of Ireland, Galway.

REFERENCES

Foufelle, F., and Fromenty, B. (2016). Role of endoplasmic reticulum stress in drug-induced toxicity. *Pharmacol. Res. Perspect.* 4:e00211. doi: 10.1002/prp2.211

Healy, S., McMahon, J., Owens, P., and FitzGerald, U. (2016). Significant glial alterations in response to iron loading in a novel organotypic hippocampal slice culture model. *Sci. Rep.* 6:36410. doi: 10.1038/srep36410

Healy, S., McMahon, J. M., and FitzGerald, U. (2017). Modelling iron mismanagement in neurodegenerative disease in vitro: paradigms, pitfalls, possibilities & practical considerations. *Prog. Neurobiol.* 158, 1–14. doi: 10.1016/j.pneurobio.2017.08.004

Hetz, C., and Mollereau, B. (2014). Disturbance of endoplasmic reticulum proteostasis in neurodegenerative diseases. *Nat. Rev. Neurosci.* 15, 233–249. doi: 10.1038/nrn3689

Liu, Y., and Connor, J. R. (2012). Iron and ER stress in neurodegenerative disease. *Biometals* 25, 837–845. doi: 10.1007/s10534-012-9544-8

Lumsden, A. L., Rogers, J. T., Majd, S., Newman, M., Sutherland, G. T., Verdile, G., et al. (2018). Dysregulation of neuronal iron homeostasis as an alternative unifying effect of mutations causing familial Alzheimer's disease. *Front. Neurosci.* 12:533. doi: 10.3389/fnins.2018.00533

Mercado, G., Valdes, P., and Hetz, C. (2013). An ERcentric view of Parkinson's disease. *Trends Mol. Med.* 19, 165–175. doi: 10.1016/j.molmed.2012.12.005

Oliveira, S. J., de Sousa, M., and Pinto, J. P. (2011). ER stress and iron homeostasis: a new frontier for the UPR. *Biochem. Res. Int.* 2011:896474. doi: 10.1155/2011/896474

Oliveira, S. J., Pinto, J. P., Picarote, G., Costa, V. M., Carvalho, F., Rangel, M., et al. (2009). ER stress-inducible factor CHOP affects the expression of hepcidin by modulating C/EBPalpha activity. *PLoS One* 4:e6618. doi: 10.1371/journal.pone.0006618

Rahman, S., Archana, A., Jan, A. T., and Minakshi, R. (2018). Dissecting Endoplasmic Reticulum Unfolded Protein Response (UPR(ER)) in managing clandestine modus operandi of Alzheimer's disease. *Front. Aging Neurosci.* 10:30. doi: 10.3389/fnagi.2018.00030

Rahman, S., Jan, A. T., Ayyagari, A., Kim, J., Kim, J., and Minakshi, R. (2017). Entanglement of UPR(ER) in aging driven Neurodegenerative diseases. *Front. Aging Neurosci.* 9:341. doi: 10.3389/fnagi.2017.00341

Stephenson, E., Nathoo, N., Mahjoub, Y., Dunn, J. F., and Yong, V. W. (2014). Iron in multiple sclerosis: roles in neurodegeneration and repair. *Nat. Rev. Neurol.* 10, 459–468. doi: 10.1038/nrneurol.2014.118

Vecchi, C., Montosi, G., Zhang, K., Lamberti, I., Duncan, S. A., Kaufman, R. J., et al. (2009). ER stress controls iron metabolism through induction of hepcidin. *Science* 325, 877–880. doi: 10.1126/science.1176639

Ward, R. J., Zucca, F. A., Duyn, J. H., Crichton, R. R., and Zecca, L. (2014). The role of iron in brain ageing and neurodegenerative disorders. *Lancet Neurol.* 13, 1045–1060. doi: 10.1016/S1474-4422(14)701176

Ye, Z., and Connor, J. R. (2000). Identification of iron responsive genes by screening cDNA libraries from suppression subtractive hybridization with antisense probes from three iron conditions. *Nucleic Acids Res.* 28, 1802–1807. doi: 10.1093/nar/28.8.1802

You, K. R., Liu, M. J., Han, X. J., Lee, Z. W., and Kim, D. G. (2003). Transcriptional regulation of the human transferrin gene by GADD153 in hepatoma cells. *Hepatology* 38, 745–755. doi: 10.1053/jhep.2003.50367

Zhao, J., Xiang, X., Zhang, H., Jiang, D., Liang, Y., Qing, W., et al. (2018). CHOP induces apoptosis by affecting brain iron metabolism in rats with subarachnoid hemorrhage. *Exp. Neurol.* 302, 22–33. doi: 10.1016/j.expneurol.2017.12.015

11

Oxidative Stress Regulated Iron Regulatory Protein IRP2 Through FBXL5-Mediated Ubiquitination-Proteasome Way in SH-SY5Y Cells

*Qian Jiao, Xixun Du, Jie Wei, Yong Li and Hong Jiang**

Department of Physiology, Shandong Provincial Key Laboratory of Pathogenesis and Prevention of Neurological Disorders and State Key Disciplines: Physiology, School of Basic Medicine, Qingdao University, Qingdao, China

Correspondence:
Hong Jiang
hongjiang@qdu.edu.cn

Iron regulatory protein 2 (IRP2) plays a key role in the cellular iron homeostasis and could be regulated by a variety of factors, such as oxidative stress, hypoxia and iron, etc. IRP2 depletion results in neurodegenerative movement disorder with the loss of neurons and accumulations of iron. Since oxidative stress extensively exists in several neurodegenerative diseases where iron accumulation also exists, it is important to clarify the mechanisms underlying the effects of oxidative stress on IRP2 expression and its consequence. 200 and 300 μM H_2O_2 could result in the reduced cell viability in SH-SY5Y cells. The intracellular levels of reactive oxygen species (ROS) were increased by 52.2 and 87.3% with 200 and 300 μM H_2O_2 treatments, respectively. The decreased levels of mitochondrial transmembrane potential ($\Delta\Psi m$) were only observed in 300 μM H_2O_2-treated group. The protein levels of IRP2, but not for its mRNA levels, were observed decreased in both groups, which resulted in the lower TfR1 expression and decreased iron uptake in these cells. Pretreatment with MG132, the decreased IRP2 levels caused by H_2O_2 treatment could be antagonized. The protein levels of F box and leucine-rich repeat protein 5 (FBXL5), the only E3 ligase of IRP2, were observed decreased accordingly. When knockdown the intracellular FBXL5 levels by si-FBXL5, the protein levels of IRP2 were found increased with H_2O_2 treatment. Our results suggest that FBXL5 is involved in the degradation of IRP2 under oxidative stress in dopaminergic-like neuroblastoma cells, which implies that its role in the neuronal regulation of IRP2 in neurodegenerative diseases.

Keywords: oxidative stress, IRP2, FBXL5, iron metabolism, ubiquitination

INTRODUCTION

Oxidative stress occurs when the accumulated production of reactive oxygen species (ROS) and the decrease of antioxidant activity. It is thought to be one of common underlying mechanisms that lead to cellular dysfunction in neurodegenerative disease (Pong, 2003; Dias et al., 2013). As such, the substantia nigra (SN) exhibits increased levels of oxidized lipids, damaged proteins, and DNA in Parkinson's disease (PD) (Hwang, 2013). Moreover, iron levels in the SN have been reported to be elevated in patients with PD (Sofic et al., 1988; Dexter et al., 1989) and PD animal models (Wang et al., 2004; Jiang et al., 2010; You et al., 2015). Markers of oxidative stress also increase in both Alzheimer's disease (AD) patients models brain areas in which amyloid β (Aβ) is abundant (Butterfield et al., 2001). Aβ plaques can efficiently generate ROS and accelerate iron accumulation (Smith et al., 2007; van Duijn et al., 2017). Thus, the oxidative stress may play an important role in inducing iron metabolic disorder in neurodegeneration associated with several brain pathologies.

Iron homeostasis is regulated by coordination proteins that are responsible for iron uptake, storage, exports, and utilization in the cellular (Hentze et al., 2010). Iron regulatory protein(IRPs), including IRP1 and IRP2, are RNA-binding proteins that interact with RNA stem loops known as iron responsive element (IRE) to regulate the translation and stability of mRNAs that encode proteins required for iron homeostasis, including ferritin, ferroportin (Fpn), transferrin receptor (TfR) and divalent metal transporter 1 (DMT1) (Rouault, 2006; Muckenthaler et al., 2008). It has been reported that a syndrome of progressive neurodegenerative disease and anemia develops with iron deposits in white matter and a loss of Purkinje cells in $IRP2^{-/-}$ mice, whereas $IRP1^{-/-}$ mice develop polycythemia and pulmonary hypertension, indicating a prominent role of IRP2 in controlling neuronal iron metabolism (Meyron-Holtz et al., 2004; Wilkinson and Pantopoulos, 2014). But some studies considered that IRP2 deficiency without symptomatic neurodegeneration in the mouse (Galy et al., 2006). Our previous study showed that IRP2 expression is decreased in 1-Methyl-4-phenylpyridinium [MPP(+)]-induced cellular model of PD (Zhang et al., 2009), whereas IRP2 expression is increased in 6-hydroxydopamine (6- OHDA)-treated PD model (Jiang et al., 2010). In AD patients, IRP2 immunoreactivity is present in the intracellular neurofibrillary, including neurofibrillary tangles and neuropil threads, which is striking differences from the control brain (Smith et al., 1998). These suggest that IRP2 expression disruption exists in neurodegenerative diseases where oxidative stress extensively occurs. In peripheral system, such as liver and kidney, IRP2 is rapidly degraded through ubiquitin-proteasomal system in high iron and high oxygen pressure conditions (Kuhn, 2015). Additionally, hypoxia and low iron level can prevent IRP2 degradation. However, in nerve system, the underlying mechanisms of oxidative stress regulate IRP2 expression and the homeostasis of iron is not fully understood.

Iron regulatory protein 2 has unique 73-amino acid that is different from IRP1 (Iwai et al., 1995). Deletion of this sequence eliminates the rapid turnover of IRP2, and does not show a sensitivity to F box and leucine-rich repeat protein 5 (FBXL5) (Iwai et al., 1995; Salahudeen et al., 2009). FBXL5, an iron- and oxygen-regulated SCF-type ubiquitin ligase (E3), has been shown to contribute to iron-dependent degradation of IRP2 in liver or human embryonic kidney cells (Salahudeen et al., 2009; Vashisht et al., 2009; Moroishi et al., 2011). Here, we used SH-SY5Y cells, a dopaminergic-like neuroblastoma cell, to investigate the regulation mechanism of IRP2 under oxidative stress condition in nerve system. We found that oxidative stress induced by H_2O_2 reduced IRP2 protein levels through ubiquitination-proteasome way. Our results also revealed that E3 FBXL5 plays a pivotal role in the regulation of IRP2 protein levels under oxidative stress condition in nerve system.

MATERIALS AND METHODS

Cell Culture and Treatment

The SH-SY5Y cell line was purchased from the Cell Bank of the Shanghai Institute of Cell Biology and Biochemistry, Chinese Academy of Sciences (Shanghai, China). SH-SY5Y cells were cultured in DMEM/F12 (Dulbecco's modified Eagle medium and Ham's F12, 1:1, pH 7.4) with 10% fetal bovine serum (FBS), 100 U/mL of penicillin and 100 U/mL of streptomycin (all from Invitrogen, United States) at 37°C in a humidified atmosphere containing 5% CO_2. For experiments, cells were seeded in 6 well plates with 1×10^5 cells/mL and grown to 80–90% confluency before they were treated with H_2O_2 (20, 30, 50, 200, 300, 500, and 1000 μmol/L) for 24 h. After 24 h, the medium was replaced with medium containing H_2O_2, and cells were treated for another 24 h and then harvested for experiments.

Transfection of shRNA

The FBXL5 short hairpin RNA (shRNA) and the scramble shRNA control were pre-designed and purchased from Genechem (Shanghai, CN). SH-SY5Y were transfected using 1-μg plasmid and 2.5-μL Lipofectamine 2000 reagent (Invitrogen, United States) in 800-μL transfection medium per well in 12 well plate for 24 h optimal transfection and then used for the following experiments.

Cell Viability

The cell viability was detected by the conventional 3-(4,5-dimethylthiazol-2-yl) -2, 5-diphenyltetrazolium bromide (MTT) (Beyotime, CN) assay. The MTT assay is a colorimetric assay for measuring the activity of cellular enzymes that reduce the tetrazolium dye. Cells were incubated in MTT (5 mg/mL) for 3–4 h. 100 μL DMSO was added to each well after medium was removed. The formazan dye crystals were solubilized for 10 min, and absorbance was measured at 494 and 630 nm with a spectrophotometer (Molecular Device, M5, United States).

Measurement of the Mitochondrial Transmembrane Potential (ΔΨm) and the Production of Intracellular Reactive Oxygen Species (ROS)

Changes in the levels of intracellular ROS and ΔΨm with H_2O_2 (200 and 300 μmol/L) treatment of SH-SY5Y were measured using flow cytometry with Rhodamine 123 (Sigma, United States) or carboxy-H2DCFDA dye (Invitrogen, United Kingdom) as previously described (Jiang et al., 2010). After cells were washed with HEPES buffered saline (HBS, 10 mM of HEPES, 150 mM of NaCl, pH 7.4) three times, carboxy-H2DCFDA (5 μM) was added and incubated for 30 min at 37°C. Cells were washed with HBS two times, followed by centrifugation at 800 rpm for 5 min, and re-suspended in 1 mL HBS. Intracellular ROS generation was also assayed by Rhodamine 123 (5 μg/mL). Fluorescent intensity was recorded at 488 nm excitation and 525 nm emission wavelengths (Fluorescence 1, FL1). Results were demonstrated as FL1-H (Fluorescence 1-Histogram), setting the gated region M1 and M2 as a marker to observe the changing levels of fluorescence intensity using Cellquest Software.

Calcein Loading of Cells and Ferrous Iron Influx Assay

Ferrous iron influx were detected as previously described (Zhang et al., 2009; Du et al., 2016). Calcein-AM (Molecular Probes, United States) is a membrane-permeative, and forms fluorescent calcein by cytoplasmic esterases upon intracellular cleavage. This reaction is pH independent and can be quenched rapidly by divalent metals and reversed easily by chelators. The cells were planted in glass coverslips and incubated with calcein-AM (0.5 μM) in HBS at 37°C for 30 min. The excess calcein on the cell surface was washed for three times with HBS. Calcein fluorescence was recorded at an excitation wavelength of 488 nm and an emission wavelength of 525 nm and the fluorescence intensity was measured every 3 min for 30 min with continuous perfusion of 100 μM of ferrous iron (ferrous sulfate in an ascorbic acid solution, 1:44 molar ratio; prepared immediately before the experiments). Ascorbic acid maintained the reduced status of ferrous iron, in addition, ascorbate acted as a chelator to maintain the iron in solution. The mean fluorescence signal of 25–30 single cells in four separate fields was monitored at 200× magnification and processed with Fluoview 5.0 software.

Quantitative Real-Time PCR

SH-SY5Y cells were collected for the investigation of FBXL5 and IRP2 mRNA expression by quantitative real-time PCR (qRT-PCR). Total RNA was extracted by using the Trizol reagent (Invitrogen) in accordance with manufacturer's protocol and was quantified by spectrophotometry (Bio-Rad, United States). RNAs were reversely transcribed to cDNA by a reverse transcriptase kit (RevertAid First Strand Cdna Synthesis Kit, Thermo, United States). Relative abundance of each mRNA was quantified by qRT-PCR using specific primers and the SYBR Premix Ex TaqII (TaKaRa, CN). Primers for rat FBXL5 (forward 5′- TTAACTAACAAGGGCATTGGAGAAG -3′; reverse 5′- TCAGCCAAATCTTCAGCATCTAAC -3′), IRP2 (forward 5′-CGCCTTTGAGTACCTTATTGAAACA-3′; reverse 5′-CGTACAGCAGCTTCCA ACAAGA-3′) and GAPDH (forward 5′-GCACCGTCAAGGCTGAGAAC-3′; reverse 5′-TGGTGAAGACGCCAGTGGA-3′) were synthesized by TaKaRa. QRT-PCR reactions were carried out by using Real-Time PCR Detection System (Eppendorf,GER). Data were analyzed by the $2^{\Delta\Delta}$CT method, and GAPDH was taken as an internal control.

Western Blot Analysis

The SH-SY5Y cells were washed with ice-cold PBS and lysed in lysis buffer (Cwbio, CN) containing protease inhibitors cocktail (Rhoche, GER) for 30 min. The lysates were centrifuged at 12,000 × g for 10 min, and the protein concentration of the supernatants was determined with a Pierce™ BCA Protein Assay Kit (Thermo, United States). A total of 20 μg of protein was electrophoresed on 8% SDS polyacrylamide gels and transferred onto PVDF membranes (300 mA, 90 min). After blocking with 10% non-fat milk for 1 h at room temperature, the membranes were incubated overnight at 4°C with rabbit anti-FBXL5 (1:1000, Abcam, United Kingdom), rabbit anti-IRP2 (1:1000, Abcam, United Kingdom), rabbit anti-TfR1 (1:1000, Abcam, United Kingdom) and rabbit anti-β -actin monoclonal antibody (1:10000, BIOS, CN). The cross-reactivity was visualized using ECL Kit (Millopore, United States) and analyzed through scanning densitometry with a UVP image system.

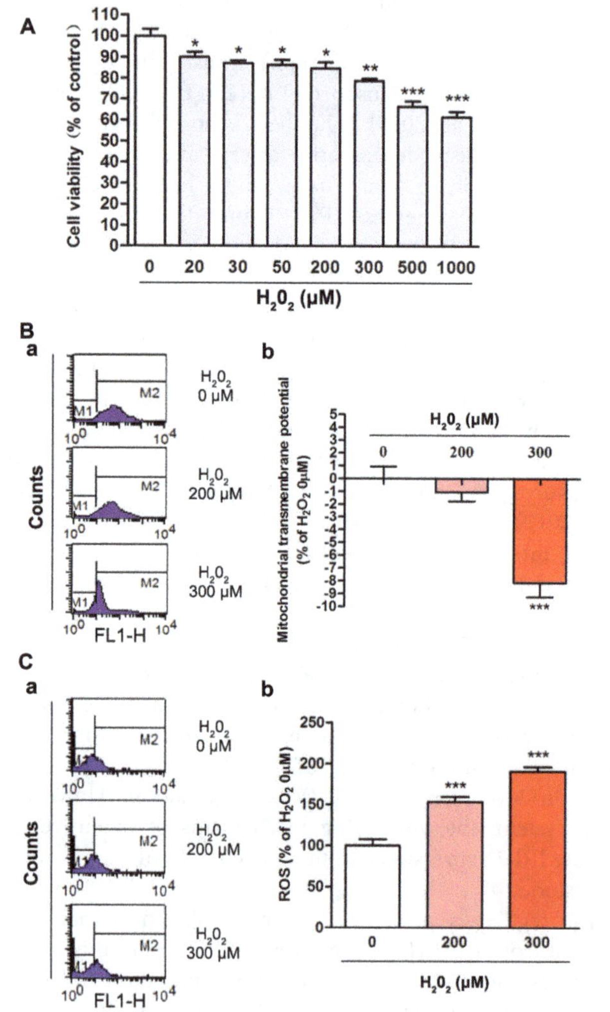

FIGURE 1 | The oxidative effects of different concentrations of H_2O_2 on SH-SY5Y cells. **(A)** Cell viability was changed with the increased concentration of H_2O_2 treatment. Cell viability of the 0 μM H_2O_2 group was set to 100%. Data were presented as mean ± SEM of 6 independent experiments. $^{*}P < 0.05$, $^{**}P < 0.01$, and $^{***}P < 0.001$ compared with 0 μM H_2O_2 group. **(B)** Fluorometric assay on $\Delta\Psi m$ in different groups **(a)** and statistical analysis **(b)**. $\Delta\Psi m$ was decreased with the increased concentration of H_2O_2. Fluorescence values of the 0 μM H_2O_2 was set to 0. Data were presented as mean ± SEM of 6 independent experiments. $^{***}P < 0.001$ compared with H_2O_2 0 μM group. **(C)** Fluorometric assay on ROS levels in different groups **(a)** and statistical analysis **(b)**. Fluorescence values of the 0 μM H_2O_2 group was set to 100%. Data were presented as mean ± SEM of 4 independent experiments. $^{***}P < 0.001$ compared with 0 μM H_2O_2 group.

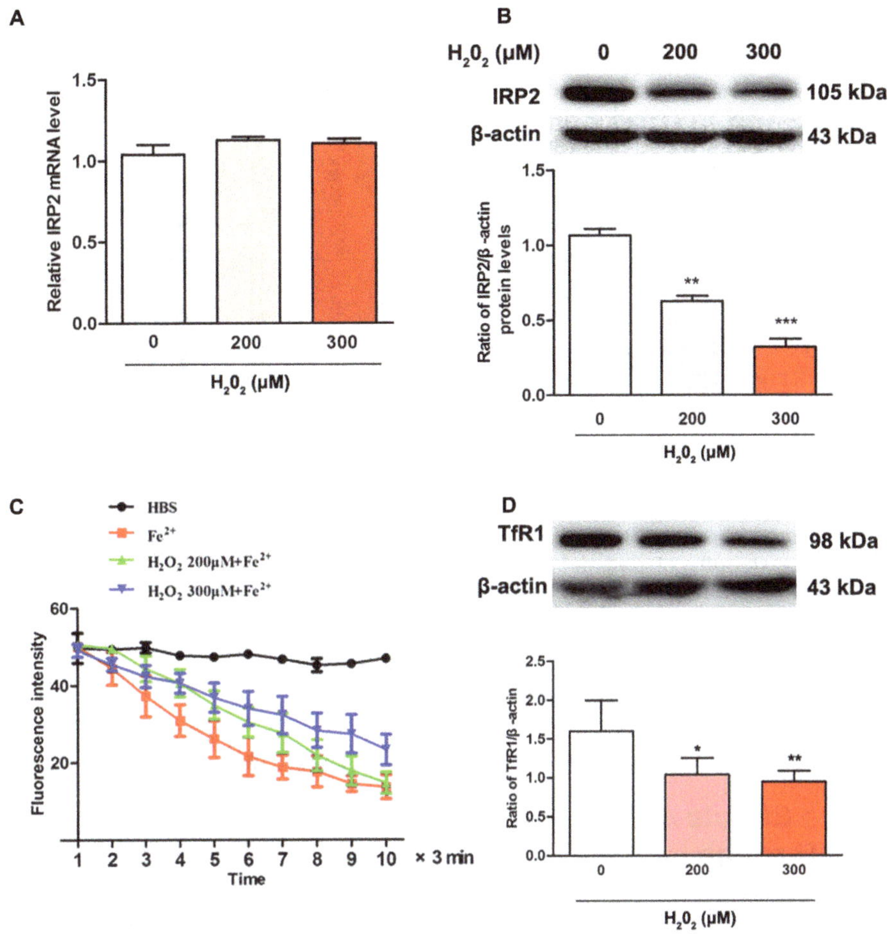

FIGURE 2 | H_2O_2 induced the changes in IRP2 levels and ferrous iron uptake in SH-SY5Y cells. **(A)** IRP2 mRNA levels were changed with H_2O_2 treatment. One-way ANOVA, data were presented as mean ± SEM of 3 independent experiments. **(B)** IRP2 protein levels were changed with H_2O_2 treatment. One-way ANOVA, data were presented as mean ± SEM of 3 independent experiments.*$P < 0.05$, **$P < 0.01$, and ***$P < 0.001$ compared with H_2O_2 0 μM group. **(C)** Calcein-indicated ferrous iron ($FeSO_4$) influx in SH-SY5Y cells. The fluorescence intensity of SH-SY5Y cells in 200 μM group and 300 μM group were significantly higher than that in 0 μM H_2O_2 group. Two-way ANOVA, *$P < 0.05$. The mean fluorescence intensity of 35 separate cells from 4 separate fields at each time point was presented as mean ± SEM of 6 independent experiments. **(D)** TfR1 protein levels were changed with H_2O_2 treatment. One-way ANOVA, data were presented as mean ± SEM of 3 independent experiments.*$P < 0.05$ and **$P < 0.01$compared with H_2O_2 0 μM group.

Statistical Analysis

Results are presented as means ± SEM. One-way analysis of variance (ANOVA) followed by the Tukey's Multiple Comparison Test was used to compare difference between means in more than two groups. The iron uptake experiment was carried out using two-way ANOVA followed by the Student-Newman-Keuls test. A probability of $P < 0.05$ was taken to indicate statistical significance.

RESULTS

The Oxidative Effects of H_2O_2 on SH-SY5Y Cells

To elucidate the oxidative effects of H_2O_2, we assessed cell viability, ΔΨm and ROS in the present study. SH-SY5Y cells were treated with different concentrations of H_2O_2 for 24 h and then MTT method was used to detect the cell viability. The results showed that the cell viability was decreased with the increased concentration of H_2O_2 (**Figure 1A**). In comparing with the 0 μM H_2O_2 group, the cell viability in 20, 30, 50, 200, 300, 500 and 1000 μM H_2O_2 group was decreased by 10.2, 12.9, 13.7, 15.3, 21.2, 33.6, and 38.6%, respectively, which displayed significant differences (**Figure 1A**, $P < 0.05$). The 200 and 300 μM effective concentration of H_2O_2 were applied for the following studies. Oxidative stress induced ΔΨm reduction and excessive generation of ROS which contribute to DNA or RNA damage. We found that the ΔΨm in cells was decreased significantly in 300 μM H_2O_2 treatment group (**Figure 1B**, $P < 0.001$). The intracellular ROS levels were increased by 52.2 and 87.3%, respectively, and the difference was statistically significant ($P < 0.001$) when compared with the 0 μM H_2O_2 group

(**Figure 1C**). Thus, these observations indicated that appropriate concentrations of H_2O_2 could induce oxidative stress in SH-SY5Y cells.

H_2O_2 Induced a Reduction in IRP2 Expression and Ferrous Iron Uptake

To test the relationship of IRP2 expression and oxidative stress induced by H_2O_2, we examined the expression of IRP2 in mRNA and protein levels. After SH-SY5Y cells were treated with 200 μM or 300 μM of H_2O_2 for 24 h, the mRNA levels of IRP2 showed that no significant difference (**Figure 2A**, $P > 0.05$), whereas the protein levels of IRP2 were decreased in comparison with the 0 μM H_2O_2 group (**Figure 2B**, $P < 0.01$). Thus, H_2O_2 regulated IRP2 expression in protein levels. The SH-SY5Y cells were incubated with 100 μM Fe^{2+} to detect the ability of cell iron uptake. Cell iron uptake ability was observed using laser confocal microscopy, and the results showed that the intracellular fluorescence intensity was increased with time, indicating a decreased Fe^{2+} uptake in both 200 μM and 300 μM H_2O_2 treatment groups (**Figure 2C**, $P < 0.05$). Moreover, the expression of TfR1in 200 and 300 μM H_2O_2 treatment groups were also decreased (**Figure 2D**, $P < 0.05$). These results suggested that H_2O_2 treatment resulted in a decrease of IRP2 protein levels rather than mRNA levels, leading to down-regulation of IRP2 targets and iron uptake ability.

The Down-Regulative Effects of H_2O_2 on IRP2 Protein Levels Through Ubiquitination Pathway

We next examined how such H_2O_2 affected IRP2 protein levels. To determine the expression of IRP2 that induced by H_2O_2 through ubiquitination pathway, we incubated SH-SY5Y cells with the ubiquitin proteasome inhibitor MG132. **Figure 3** showed that the expression levels of IRP2 levels were decreased in H_2O_2 treatment groups and were restored by MG132 treatment, the difference was statistically significant ($P < 0.05$).

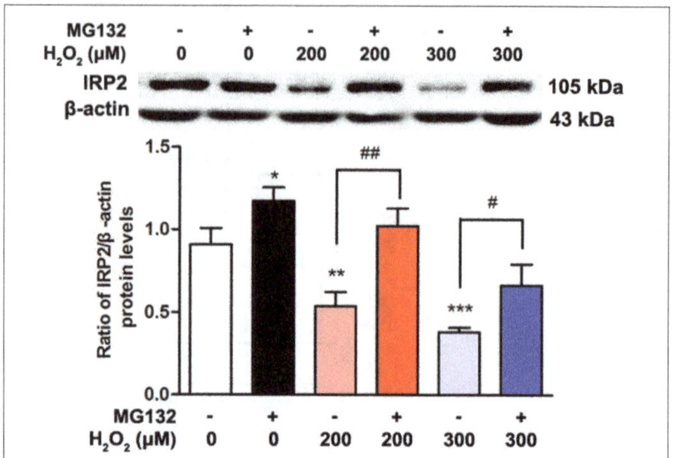

FIGURE 3 | The expression of IRP2 after treated by H_2O_2 and MG132. Data were presented as mean ± SEM of 3 independent experiments. One-way ANOVA, $^{*}P < 0.05$, $^{**}P < 0.01$, and $^{***}P < 0.001$ compared with 0 μM H_2O_2 group. *T*-test, $^{\#}P < 0.05$ and $^{\#\#}P < 0.01$.

FBXL5 Was Involved in the Degradation of IRP2 Induced by H_2O_2

F box and leucine-rich repeat protein 5, an E3 ubiquitin ligase subunit, is a key event to mediate IRP2 degradation for controlling iron homeostasis (Moroishi et al., 2011). To test our hypothesis that IRP2 reduction was raised by FBXL5 in the oxidative environment, we measured the FBXL5 expression both in mRNA and in protein levels. Results showed that the mRNA levels of FBXL5 showed no significant difference (**Figure 4A**, $P > 0.05$), whereas the protein levels of FBXL5 were increased in both H_2O_2 treatment groups (**Figure 4B**, $P < 0.05$). These data indicated that oxidative factors H_2O_2 could cause the decrease of IRP2 and the increase of FBXL5.

Sh-FBXL5 were transfected into SH-SY5Y cells, and we found that FBXL5 levels were decreased in all H_2O_2 treatment groups (**Figures 4Ca,b**, $P < 0.05$), and IRP2 levels were increased in all groups (**Figures 4Ca,c**, $P < 0.05$), the difference was statistically significant in comparing with negative control. The results suggested that H_2O_2 could down regulate IRP2 through FBXL5 mediated ubiquitination pathway.

DISCUSSION

We have shown that the oxidative stress induced by H_2O_2 in SH-SY5Y cells resulted in a down-regulation of IRP2 protein levels, which in turn leads to a decrease of iron uptake ability. The IRP2 protein stability was regulated by ubiquitination pathway. FBXL5, the E3 of IRP2, was up-regulated after treatment of H_2O_2. The knockdown of FBXL5 could attenuate the IRP2 down-regulation that induced by H_2O_2. Our findings indicate that H_2O_2 regulated IRP2 expression through FBXL5 mediated ubiquitination pathway in SH-SY5Y cells.

Molecules or molecular fragments containing one or more unpaired electrons are called free radicals. These free radicals in living systems are mostly derived from oxygen (Jomova et al., 2010). The ROS, such as (O_2^-), derived from metabolic processes, and then further interacts with other molecules via enzyme- or metal-catalyzed to generate "secondary" ROS (Jomova et al., 2010; Farina et al., 2013). Excessive exposure to ROS may induce oxidative stress particularly in mitochondria, and lead to neurodegenerative diseases. H_2O_2 generates oxygen by catalase, which lead to hyperoxia. And the free intracellular $Fe^{2+}$and H_2O_2 participate in the Fenton reaction to generate high reactive hydroxyl radical. Thus, in the present study, we used H_2O_2 mimic oxidative stress (**Figure 1**). The cell viability was reduced with the increased H_2O_2 concentrations (**Figure 1A**). The $\Delta\Psi$m reduction and excessive generation of ROS increased both in H_2O_2 (**Figures 1B,C**) treatment groups. These results indicated that cells were damaged by the artificial oxidative stress *in vitro*.

In the present study, we found that H_2O_2 reduced the expression of IRP2 just in protein levels rather than mRNA levels in the dopaminergic-like neuroblastoma cells (**Figures 2A,B**).

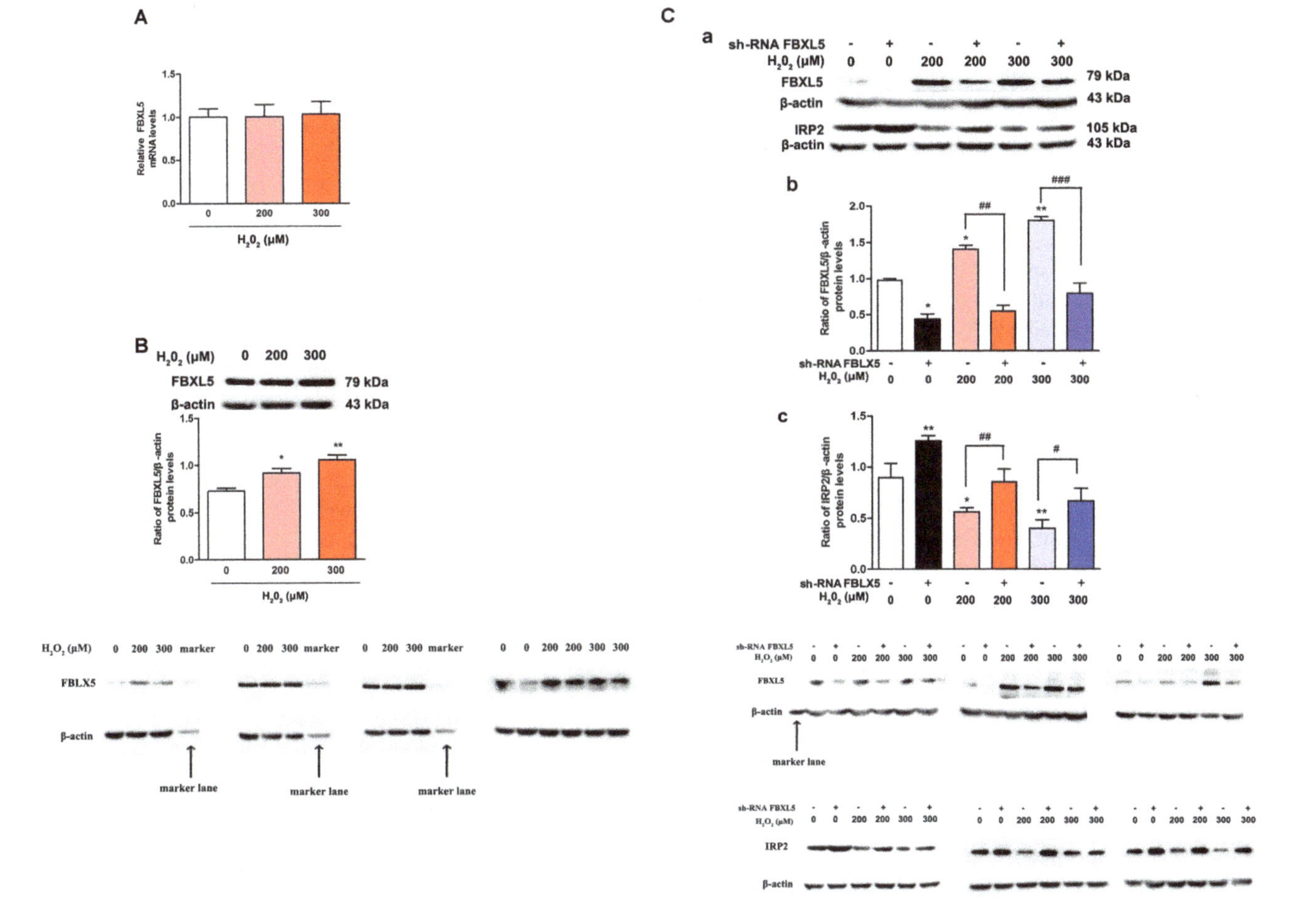

FIGURE 4 | FBXL5 was involved in the degradation of IRP2 induced by H_2O_2 treatment in SH-SY5Y cells. **(A,B)** FBXL5 mRNA **(A)** and protein **(B)** expression were observed in SH-SY5Y cells treated by H_2O_2. One-way ANOVA, data were presented as mean ± SEM of 3 independent experiments. $^{*}P < 0.05$ and $^{**}P < 0.01$ compared with 0 μM H_2O_2 group. Data were presented as mean ± SEM of 3 independent experiments. One-way ANOVA, $^{*}P < 0.05$ and $^{**}P < 0.01$ compared with 0 μM H_2O_2 group. *T*-test,$^{\#}P < 0.05$ and $^{\#\#}P < 0.01$. **(C)** Pretreatment with si-FBXL5, the expression of FBXL5 and IRP2 changed after treated by H_2O_2 and si-FBXL5. Data were presented as mean ± SEM of 3 independent experiments. One-way ANOVA, $^{*}P < 0.05$ and $^{**}P < 0.01$ compared with H_2O_2 0 μM group. *T*-test,$^{\#}P < 0.05$, $^{\#\#}P < 0.01$, and $^{\#\#\#}P < 0.001$.

Correspondingly, TfR1 expression and cell iron uptake ability were reduced. As a key regulator of brain iron metabolism, IRP2 expression is accurately modulated by the microenvironment factors, including oxygen, iron, free radicals, and cytokines. Generally, neurodegenerative diseases have high oxidative stress level (Emerit et al., 2004; Kim et al., 2015). For example, oxidative stress is especially substantiated by the complex I mitochondrial dysfunction with increased ROS production that might induced by accumulated α-synuclein and iron in the SN of PD patients (Jomova et al., 2010; Farina et al., 2013; Hwang, 2013). In our pervious study, we found that the expression of IRP2 mRNA levels was not affected by FAC at concentration of 100 μM (Zhang et al., 2009). Moreover, sodium nitroprusside, a NO donor and an oxidative generator, could inhibit the IRP2 protein expression (Wei et al., 2017). The mechanism underlying oxidative stress-mediated down-regulation of IRP2 is complex. IRP2 mRNA transcription is regulated by HIF-α of transcription factors that affected by oxygen and iron (Kaelin and Ratcliffe, 2008). In post-transcriptional regulation, IRP2 was recognized by ubiquitin ligase and then degraded by the proteasome in kidney cell line (Salahudeen et al., 2009; Takahashi-Makise et al., 2009; Vashisht et al., 2009). However, the mechanisms of oxidative stress affect IRP2 expression in neurodegenerative diseases are largely unknown. We found that MG132 treatment could prevent the reduction of IRP2 that induced by H_2O_2 (**Figure 3**), suggesting that oxidative stress regulated IRP2 expression in dopaminergic-like neuroblastoma cells might be achieved through ubiquitination pathway.

There are two E3 ubiquitin ligases for IRP2, including FBXL5 and haem-oxidized IRP2 ubiquitin ligase 1 (HOIL-1). HOIL-1 belongs to RING finger protein and recognizes IRP2 through a signal created by heme-mediated oxidative modification of the protein (Iwai et al., 2005). However, HOIL-1 is independent and is not required for iron-dependent degradation of IRP2 (Zumbrennen et al., 2008). The selective iron- and oxygen-dependent degradation of IRP2 is mediated by the Skp1/Cul1/Fbox (SCF) E3 ubiquitin ligase complex containing FBXL5 (Salahudeen et al., 2009; Vashisht et al., 2009). Disruption of the FBXL5 expression are failed to sense the increased cellular iron availability, which results in constitutional accumulation of IRP2 and the disordered expression of its target genes (Salahudeen et al., 2009; Vashisht et al., 2009). In *FBXL5* conditional deleted mice, hematopoietic stem cells are cellular iron overload and reduced in cell number (Muto et al., 2017). It is also found that $FBXL5^{-/-}$ mice die for overwhelming accumulation of oxidative stress during embryogenesis (Moroishi et al., 2011). Here, we found that FBXL5 increased and its targets IRP2 reduced when treated by H_2O_2 in SH-SY5Y cells. Thus, FBXL5 might be also referred to regulating IRP2 expression under oxidative stress condition in nerve system.

F box and leucine-rich repeat protein 5 contains a hemerythrin domain in the N-terminus that belongs to a family of iron- and oxygen-binding proteins, and contains the leucine-rich repeats in C-terminal region that binds to IRP2 (Salahudeen et al., 2009; Chollangi et al., 2012; Ruiz and Bruick, 2014). The N-terminal hemerythrin domain has iron and oxygen sensing properties for binding with Fe-O-Fe center. The Fe-O-Fe center is formed in iron replete and oxygenated cells. FBXL5 is stable when directly binds to iron in the hemerythrin domain, whereas unstable under iron-deficient conditions. With this iron-sensing ability, FBXL5 controls the abundance of IRP2 in an iron-dependent manner, and degrades IRP2 by the stabilized FBXL5 under iron-replete conditions. In addition to iron bioavailability, IRP stability and activity are regulated by oxygen. Acting as ROS sensors, the hemerythrin domain could also facilitate regulation by ROS that stabilizes FBXL5 and antagonizes the stabilization of IRP2 (Ruiz and Bruick, 2014). In our present study, oxidative stress generators H_2O_2 could up-regulate FBXL5 expression (**Figures 4A,B**) and using si-FBXL5 could alleviate the reduction of IRP2 protein levels (**Figure 4C**), suggesting that the close relationship of FBXL5 and oxidative stress in regulation nerve system cellular iron metabolism.

In conclusion, we present novel evidence that the oxidative generators H_2O_2 induced an increase of FBXL5-mediated ubiquitination degradation in dopaminergic-like neuroblastoma cells. The results of this study implicate an important role of oxidative stress in regulating iron metabolism in nerve system.

AUTHOR CONTRIBUTIONS

HJ and QJ conceived the project and designed the study. QJ, JW, and XD performed the experiments, analyzed the data, and interpreted the results. QJ wrote the manuscript. HJ and YL reviewed and edited the manuscript. All authors have read and approved the final version of the manuscript.

FUNDING

This work was supported by the NSFC (31771110, 31500837, 31471114, and 81430024), National Key Research and Development Program of China (2016YFC1306500), the Key Research and Development Program of Shandong Province (2016GSF201053), Qingdao Municipal Science and Technology Project (16-2-2-nsh) and Taishan Scholars Construction Project.

REFERENCES

Butterfield, D. A., Drake, J., Pocernich, C., and Castegna, A. (2001). Evidence of oxidative damage in Alzheimer's disease brain: central role for amyloid beta-peptide. *Trends Mol. Med.* 7, 548–554. doi: 10.1016/S1471-4914(01)02173-6

Chollangi, S., Thompson, J. W., Ruiz, J. C., Gardner, K. H., and Bruick, R. K. (2012). Hemerythrin-like domain within F-box and leucine-rich repeat protein 5 (FBXL5) communicates cellular iron and oxygen availability by distinct mechanisms. *J. Biol. Chem.* 287, 23710–23717. doi: 10.1074/jbc.M112.360404

Dexter, D. T., Wells, F. R., Lees, A. J., Agid, F., Agid, Y., Jenner, P., et al. (1989). Increased nigral iron content and alterations in other metal ions occurring in brain in Parkinson's disease. *J. Neurochem.* 52, 1830–1836. doi: 10.1111/j.1471-4159.1989.tb07264.x

Dias, V., Junn, E., and Mouradian, M. M. (2013). The role of oxidative stress in Parkinson's disease. *J. Parkinsons Dis.* 3, 461–491. doi: 10.3233/JPD-130230

Du, X., Xu, H., Shi, L., Jiang, Z., Song, N., Jiang, H., et al. (2016). Activation of ATP-sensitive potassium channels enhances DMT1-mediated iron uptake in SK-N-SH cells in vitro. *Sci. Rep.* 6:33674. doi: 10.1038/srep33674

Emerit, J., Edeas, M., and Bricaire, F. (2004). Neurodegenerative diseases and oxidative stress. *Biomed. Pharmacother.* 58, 39–46. doi: 10.1016/j.biopha.2003.11.004

Farina, M., Avila, D. S., da Rocha, J. B., and Aschner, M. (2013). Metals, oxidative stress and neurodegeneration: a focus on iron, manganese and mercury. *Neurochem. Int.* 62, 575–594. doi: 10.1016/j.neuint.2012.12.006

Galy, B., Holter, S. M., Klopstock, T., Ferring, D., Becker, L., Kaden, S., et al. (2006). Iron homeostasis in the brain: complete iron regulatory protein 2 deficiency without symptomatic neurodegeneration in the mouse. *Nat. Genet.* 38, 967–969;discussion 969–970. doi: 10.1038/ng0906-967

Hentze, M. W., Muckenthaler, M. U., Galy, B., and Camaschella, C. (2010). Two to tango: regulation of mammalian iron metabolism. *Cell* 142, 24–38. doi: 10.1016/j.cell.2010.06.028

Hwang, O. (2013). Role of oxidative stress in Parkinson's disease. *Exp. Neurobiol.* 22, 11–17. doi: 10.5607/en.2013.22.1.11

Iwai, K., Ishikawa, H., and Kirisako, T. (2005). Identification, expression, and assay of an oxidation-specific ubiquitin ligase, HOIL-1. *Methods Enzymol.* 398, 256–271. doi: 10.1016/S0076-6879(05)98021-X

Iwai, K., Klausner, R. D., and Rouault, T. A. (1995). Requirements for iron-regulated degradation of the RNA binding protein, iron regulatory protein 2. *EMBO J.* 14, 5350–5357. doi: 10.1002/j.1460-2075.1995.tb00219.x

Jiang, H., Song, N., Xu, H., Zhang, S., Wang, J., and Xie, J. (2010). Up-regulation of divalent metal transporter 1 in 6-hydroxydopamine intoxication is IRE/IRP dependent. *Cell Res.* 20, 345–356. doi: 10.1038/cr.2010.20

Jomova, K., Vondrakova, D., Lawson, M., and Valko, M. (2010). Metals, oxidative stress and neurodegenerative disorders. *Mol. Cell. Biochem.* 345, 91–104. doi: 10.1007/s11010-010-0563-x

Kaelin, W. G. Jr., and Ratcliffe, P. J. (2008). Oxygen sensing by metazoans: the central role of the HIF hydroxylase pathway. *Mol. Cell* 30, 393–402. doi: 10.1016/j.molcel.2008.04.009

Kim, G. H., Kim, J. E., Rhie, S. J., and Yoon, S. (2015). The role of oxidative stress in neurodegenerative diseases. *Exp. Neurobiol.* 24, 325–340. doi: 10.5607/en.2015.24.4.325

Kuhn, L. C. (2015). Iron regulatory proteins and their role in controlling iron metabolism. *Metallomics* 7, 232–243. doi: 10.1039/c4mt00164h

Meyron-Holtz, E. G., Ghosh, M. C., Iwai, K., LaVaute, T., Brazzolotto, X., Berger, U. V., et al. (2004). Genetic ablations of iron regulatory proteins 1 and 2 reveal why iron regulatory protein 2 dominates iron homeostasis. *EMBO J.* 23, 386–395. doi: 10.1038/sj.emboj.7600041

Moroishi, T., Nishiyama, M., Takeda, Y., Iwai, K., and Nakayama, K. I. (2011). The FBXL5-IRP2 axis is integral to control of iron metabolism in vivo. *Cell Metab.* 14, 339–351. doi: 10.1016/j.cmet.2011.07.011

Muckenthaler, M. U., Galy, B., and Hentze, M. W. (2008). Systemic iron homeostasis and the iron-responsive element/iron-regulatory protein (IRE/IRP) regulatory network. *Annu. Rev. Nutr.* 28, 197–213. doi: 10.1146/annurev.nutr.28.061807.155521

Muto, Y., Nishiyama, M., Nita, A., Moroishi, T., and Nakayama, K. I. (2017). Essential role of FBXL5-mediated cellular iron homeostasis in maintenance of hematopoietic stem cells. *Nat. Commun.* 8:16114. doi: 10.1038/ncomms16114

Pong, K. (2003). Oxidative stress in neurodegenerative diseases: therapeutic implications for superoxide dismutase mimetics. *Expert Opin. Biol. Ther.* 3, 127–139. doi: 10.1517/14712598.3.1.127

Rouault, T. A. (2006). The role of iron regulatory proteins in mammalian iron homeostasis and disease. *Nat. Chem. Biol.* 2, 406–414. doi: 10.1038/nchembio807

Ruiz, J. C., and Bruick, R. K. (2014). F-box and leucine-rich repeat protein 5 (FBXL5): sensing intracellular iron and oxygen. *J. Inorg. Biochem.* 133, 73–77. doi: 10.1016/j.jinorgbio.2014.01.015

Salahudeen, A. A., Thompson, J. W., Ruiz, J. C., Ma, H. W., Kinch, L. N., Li, Q., et al. (2009). An E3 ligase possessing an iron-responsive hemerythrin domain is a regulator of iron homeostasis. *Science* 326, 722–726. doi: 10.1126/science.1176326

Smith, D. G., Cappai, R., and Barnham, K. J. (2007). The redox chemistry of the Alzheimer's disease amyloid beta peptide. *Biochim. Biophys. Acta* 1768, 1976–1990. doi: 10.1016/j.bbamem.2007.02.002

Smith, M. A., Wehr, K., Harris, P. L., Siedlak, S. L., Connor, J. R., and Perry, G. (1998). Abnormal localization of iron regulatory protein in Alzheimer's disease. *Brain Res.* 788, 232–236. doi: 10.1016/S0006-8993(98)00002-X

Sofic, E., Riederer, P., Heinsen, H., Beckmann, H., Reynolds, G. P., Hebenstreit, G., et al. (1988). Increased iron (III) and total iron content in post mortem substantia nigra of parkinsonian brain. *J. Neural Transm.* 74, 199–205. doi: 10.1007/BF01244786

Takahashi-Makise, N., Ward, D. M., and Kaplan, J. (2009). On the mechanism of iron sensing by IRP2: new players, new paradigms. *Nat. Chem. Biol.* 5, 874–875. doi: 10.1038/nchembio.261

van Duijn, S., Bulk, M., van Duinen, S. G., Nabuurs, R. J. A., van Buchem, M. A., van der Weerd, L., et al. (2017). Cortical iron reflects severity of Alzheimer's disease. *J. Alzheimers Dis.* 60, 1533–1545. doi: 10.3233/JAD-161143

Vashisht, A. A., Zumbrennen, K. B., Huang, X., Powers, D. N., Durazo, A., Sun, D., et al. (2009). Control of iron homeostasis by an iron-regulated ubiquitin ligase. *Science* 326, 718–721. doi: 10.1126/science.1176333

Wang, J., Jiang, H., and Xie, J. X. (2004). Time dependent effects of 6-OHDA lesions on iron level and neuronal loss in rat nigrostriatal system. *Neurochem. Res.* 29, 2239–2243. doi: 10.1007/s11064-004-7031-5

Wei, J., Li, Y., Jiao, Q., Du, X. X., and Jiang, H. (2017). Influence of sodium nitroprusside on expressions of FBXL5 and IRP2 in SH-SY5Y cells. *Sheng Li Xue Bao* 69, 261–266.

Wilkinson, N., and Pantopoulos, K. (2014). The IRP/IRE system in vivo: insights from mouse models. *Front. Pharmacol.* 5:176. doi: 10.3389/fphar.2014.00176

You, L. H., Li, F., Wang, L., Zhao, S. E., Wang, S. M., Zhang, L. L., et al. (2015). Brain iron accumulation exacerbates the pathogenesis of MPTP-induced Parkinson's disease. *Neuroscience* 284, 234–246. doi: 10.1016/j.neuroscience.2014.09.071

Zhang, S., Wang, J., Song, N., Xie, J., and Jiang, H. (2009). Up-regulation of divalent metal transporter 1 is involved in 1-methyl-4-phenylpyridinium (MPP(+))-induced apoptosis in MES23.5 *cells. Neurobiol. Aging* 30, 1466–1476. doi: 10.1016/j.neurobiolaging.2007.11.025

Zumbrennen, K. B., Hanson, E. S., and Leibold, E. A. (2008). HOIL-1 is not required for iron-mediated IRP2 degradation in HEK293 cells. *Biochim. Biophys. Acta* 1783, 246–252. doi: 10.1016/j.bbamcr.2007.07.010

12

Combined Visualization of Nigrosome-1 and Neuromelanin in the Substantia Nigra Using 3T MRI for the Differential Diagnosis of Essential Tremor and *de novo* Parkinson's Disease

Lirong Jin[1†], *Jian Wang*[2,3†], *Changpeng Wang*[1†], *Danlan Lian*[4], *Ying Zhou*[5], *Yong Zhang*[6], *Minzhi Lv*[7], *Yuanfang Li*[5], *Zhen Huang*[1], *Xiaoqin Cheng*[1], *Guoqiang Fei*[1], *Kai Liu*[2,3], *Mengsu Zeng*[2,3*] and *Chunjiu Zhong*[1*]

[1] Department of Neurology, Zhongshan Hospital, Fudan University, Shanghai, China, [2] Department of Radiology, Zhongshan Hospital, Fudan University, Shanghai, China, [3] Shanghai Medical Imaging Institute, Shanghai, China, [4] Department of Radiology, Xiamen Branch, Zhongshan Hospital, Fudan University, Xiamen, China, [5] Department of Neurology, Xiamen Branch, Zhongshan Hospital, Fudan University, Xiamen, China, [6] MR Research, GE Healthcare, Shanghai, China, [7] Department of Biostatistics, Zhongshan Hospital, Fudan University, Shanghai, China

***Correspondence:**
Mengsu Zeng
zengmengsu@outlook.com
Chunjiu Zhong
zhongcj@163.com

†These authors share co-first authorship

Differentiating early-stage Parkinson's disease (PD) from essential tremor (ET) remains challenging. In the current study, we aimed to evaluate whether visual analyses of neuromelanin-sensitive magnetic resonance imaging (NM-MRI) combined with nigrosome-1 (N1) imaging using quantitative susceptibility mapping (QSM) in the substantia nigra (SN) are of diagnostic value in the differentiation of *de novo* PD from untreated ET. Sixty-eight patients with *de novo* PD, 25 patients with untreated ET, and 34 control participants underwent NM-MRI and QSM. NM and N1 signals in the SN on MR images were visually evaluated using a 3-point ordinal scale. Receiver operating characteristic (ROC) analyses were performed to determine the diagnostic values of the visual ratings of NM and N1. The diagnostic values of the predicted probabilities were calculated via logistic regression analysis using the combination of NM and N1 visual ratings, as well as their quadratic items. The proportions of invisible NM and invisible N1 were significantly higher in the PD group than those in the ET and control groups ($p < 0.001$). The sensitivity/specificity for differentiating PD from ET was 0.882/0.800 for NM and 0.794/0.920 for N1, respectively. Combining the two biomarkers, the area under the curve (AUC) of the predicted probabilities was 0.935, and the sensitivity/specificity was 0.853/0.920 when the cutoff value was set to 0.704. Our findings demonstrate that visual analyses combing NM and N1 imaging in the SN may aid in differential diagnosis of PD and ET. Furthermore, our results suggest that patients with PD exhibit larger iron deposits in the SN than those with ET.

Keywords: Parkinson's disease, essential tremor, neuromelanin, nigrosome-1, QSM, substantia nigra

INTRODUCTION

Parkinson's disease (PD) and essential tremor (ET) are common movement disorders, especially among older adults (1). PD is characterized by motor symptoms including bradykinesia, resting tremor, and rigidity, while ET often manifests as isolated tremor in the bilateral upper limbs. Although they are distinct entities, these two movement disorders may share some clinical characteristics, such as non-motor features and resting/postural tremor, as well as genetic and pathological mechanisms (2, 3). Hence, the differentiation of PD and ET remains challenging, especially early in the disease course.

Neuroimaging may aid in the differentiation of the two movement disorders. Dopamine transporter (DAT) imaging of the striatum is recommended in the differential diagnosis of PD (4). However, DAT imaging is expensive, subjects the patient to low doses of radiation, and is only available in specialized centers, limiting its clinical application. In contrast, MRI is widely available and does not subject the patient to radiation. Recent studies have provided evidence that MRI biomarkers may aid in the diagnosis of movement disorders (5, 6) and help to reveal the pathological changes correlated with motor and non-motor symptoms (7).

The pathological hallmarks of PD include progressive neurodegeneration of dopaminergic neurons and iron overload in substantia nigra (SN) (8). In contrast, whether ET is a degenerative disease is still debated, although some studies suggest that it is associated with cerebellar degeneration (9). Dopaminergic neurons in the SN contain a black pigment called neuromelanin (NM). Based on the paramagnetic properties of NM, high-resolution T1-weighted fast spin echo (FSE) imaging at high field strength (e.g., 3T) can visualize NM-generated contrast. This technique is referred to as neuromelanin-sensitive MRI (NM-MRI) (10). Previous studies have indicated that the signal intensity of NM is decreased in patients with PD (10, 11), even in the early stage of the disease (12), while it remains unchanged in patients with ET (13, 14), when compared with that in healthy controls. In addition, nigrosome-1 (N1), the largest of the five described nigrosomes, is most affected in patients with PD (~98% neuronal loss in N1) (15). N1 represents the pockets of high signal intensity in the dorsal part of the healthy SN, at intermediate and caudal levels on high resolution T2*/SWI, and can be visualized as a "swallow-tail sign" (16, 17). However, hyperintensity of N1 is absent in most patients with PD (17), possibly due to increases in iron deposition that occur in parallel to the loss of dopaminergic cells (16). Quantitative susceptibility mapping (QSM) may overcome several non-local restrictions of SWI and phase imaging, allowing for the quantification of iron content (18, 19). Indeed, this method may be more sensitive for detecting iron-related changes in patients with PD (20). To our knowledge, however, no studies have investigated N1 appearance in patients with ET.

Unlike voxel-based morphometry, diffusion tensor imaging, or blood oxygenation level-dependent imaging, which require complicated post-processing or quantitative measurements, NM on NM-MRI and N1 on QSM can be assessed visually, making these methods feasible for clinical application. To the best of our knowledge, no previous studies have investigated the combination of these two MR sequences for the differential diagnosis of PD and ET. In the current study, we aimed to evaluate whether visual analyses of NM imaging using NM-MRI combined with N1 imaging using QSM in the SN are of diagnostic value in the differentiation of *de novo* PD from untreated ET.

PARTICIPANTS AND METHODS

Participants

Sixty-eight patients with *de novo* PD, 25 patients with untreated ET, and 34 healthy controls were voluntarily recruited between September 2016 and April 2018. Patients with PD were diagnosed in accordance with MDS clinical diagnostic criteria for PD (4), while patients with ET were diagnosed in accordance with the criteria outlined in the Consensus Statement of the Movement Disorders Society on Tremor (21), by two movement specialists (J.L.R. and H.Z.). All patients were drug naïve. All control participants were recruited as volunteers from the community and had no history of neurological/psychiatric disorders. Exclusion criteria were as follows: history of other neurological/psychiatric disorders, severe infection, liver dysfunction, renal insufficiency, past/current substance abuse, tremor-related dysmetabolism including thyroid dysfunction and drug toxicity, and abnormal signals that affected further analyses on structural MRI. Unified Parkinson's Disease Rating Scale (UPDRS) motor scores were obtained for all patients with PD and ET. This study was approved by the Committee on Medical Ethics of Zhongshan Hospital, Fudan University. Written informed consent was obtained from all participants.

MRI Protocol and Imaging Analysis

Imaging Protocol

All MR images were acquired using a 3T MR unit (Discovery™ MR750, GE Healthcare, Milwaukee, WI). A T1-weighted fast spin-echo sequence was obtained for NM-MRI images, as previously described (22), and the imaging parameters were as follows: repetition time/echo time (TR/TE), 600/13 ms; echo-train length, 2; section thickness, 2.5 mm, with no intersection gap; number of slices, 16; matrix size, 512 × 320; field-of-view (FOV), 220 mm; NEX, 5. A three-dimensional multi-echo GRE sequence was used to acquire T2*-weighted images, and the scanning parameters were as follows: TR: 51.5 ms; number of echoes, 16; first TE, 2.9 ms; TE spacing, 3 ms; bandwidth, 62.50 kHz; flip angle, 12°; FOV, 22 cm; matrix, 220 × 220; slice thickness, 2 mm; acceleration factor, 2; slices, 66. Afterwards, the QSM images were reconstructed from T2*-weighted images as described in previous studies (20). In addition, conventional MRI sequences including T1-weighted images, T2-weighted fluid-attenuated inversion recovery (FLAIR) images, and diffusion-weighted images (DWI) were obtained to exclude other pathological imaging findings that may have interfered with further assessment. The axial sections were scanned parallel to the anterior commissure-posterior commissure line with whole-brain coverage for QSM and routine MRI scans, and with coverage from the posterior commissure to the pons for NM-MRI.

Visual Analysis of Imaging Data

The NM-MR images were transferred to a workstation (ADW4.6, GE Healthcare) and displayed using certain settings (window width: 400, window level: 800–900) for analysis. The method for visual analysis was based on that described in a previous study (23), with modifications. We classified NM-MR images according to an 3-point ordinal scale, as follows: 0, normal view of the SN with high signal intensity bilaterally and no volume loss, indicating a healthy SN; 1, possible abnormality with reduced signal or volume of the SN unilaterally or bilaterally, indicating possible SN pathology; 2, definite abnormality with reduced signal or volume of the SN, indicating SN pathology (**Figure 1**).

QSM data were transferred to a local computer, and images were viewed using MRIcro software (Version: 1.40 build 1). N1 was visualized as an oval-shaped area of low signal intensity surrounded by hyperintensity on QSM in the dorsal part of the healthy SN, at intermediate and caudal levels. Visual analysis of N1 was performed using a 3-point ordinal scale, as follows: 0, normal, N1 present bilaterally; 1, non-diagnostic, indecisive presence of N1 unilaterally or bilaterally; 2, pathological, N1 absent bilaterally (**Figure 1**). Two radiologists (rater 1: W.J. and rater 2: L.D.L.), who were blinded to participants information, independently performed visual analyses twice, with an interval of at least 7 days. The intra- and inter-rater agreement of visual scores was determined using weighted kappa values. For the conflicting cases between the two raters, visual analyses were conducted by a third radiologist (with 30 years of experience) to acquire a final rating for statistical analyses.

Statistical Analyses

The results were expressed as the mean ± SD. One-way analyses of variance (ANOVA), Mann-Whitney *U*-test, and chi-square test were used to compare demographic data. Logistic regression analyses were employed to estimate the combined predicted probabilities of the visual ratings for NM and N1. Diagnostic performances in visual assessments of NM and N1, separately, and in the predicted probabilities were analyzed using receiver operating characteristic (ROC) curves. The chi-square test was used to compare the area under the curve (AUC) values of the different diagnostic models. The level of significance was set to 0.05, and all tests were two-sided. Statistical analyses were performed using SPSS version 22.0 (SPSS Inc., Chicago IL) and Stata/SE version 14.0 (StataCorp LP).

RESULTS

Demographic and Clinical Data

The demographic and clinical characteristics of all participants are summarized in **Table 1**. No significant differences in gender, age, Mini Mental State Examination (MMSE) scores, or Montreal Cognitive Assessment (MoCA) scores were observed among the three groups. Disease duration was significantly longer in patients with ET than in patients with PD ($p < 0.001$), although there was no significant difference in UPDRS tremor scores between the ET and PD groups. All patients with PD had mild disease severity (Hoehn and Yahr stages 1 to 2).

Visual Analyses of the SN on NM-MRI and N1 on QSM

The proportion of conflicting cases was 22.8% (29/127) for NM-MRI analyses and 11.8% (15/127) for N1-QSM analyses for rater 1. For rater 2, the proportion of conflicting cases was 28.3% (36/127) for NM-MRI analyses and 22.0% (28/127) for N1-QSM analyses. The proportion of conflicting cases between the two observers was 25.2% (32/127) for NM-MRI analyses and 24.4% (31/127) for N1-QSM analyses. Thus, the weighted kappa coefficient was calculated to evaluate intra- and inter-rater agreement for visual analyses. For rater 1, intra-rater agreement values for NM and N1 were 0.837 and 0.903, respectively. For rater 2, intra-rater agreement values for NM and N1 were 0.828 and 0.815, respectively. Furthermore, the inter-rater agreement was 0.827 for NM and 0.777 for N1. Thus, visual analyses were highly consistent.

For NM visual analysis, scores were 0 in 8 patients with PD (11.8%), 1 in 27 patients with PD (39.7%), and 2 in 33 patients with PD (48.5%). In the ET group, NM scores were 0 in 20 patients (80.0%) and 1 in 5 patients (20.0%). In the control group, NM scores were 0 in 30 participants (88.2%) and 1 in 4 participants (11.8%) (**Figure 2A**). NM scores of 2 were not observed in the ET and control groups, and the proportion of NM ratings did not significantly differ between these two groups ($p = 0.385$). However, the proportion of NM ratings in the PD group differed significantly from that in the ET group ($p < 0.001$).

N1 scores were 0 in 3 patients with PD (4.4%), 1 in 11 patients with PD (16.2%), and 2 in 54 patients with PD (79.4%). In the ET group, N1 scores were 0 in 11 patients (44.0%), 1 in 12 patients (48.0%), and 2 in 2 patients (8.0%). In the control group, N1 scores were 0 in 10 participants (29.4%), 1 in 19 participants (55.9%), and 2 in 5 participants (14.7%) (**Figure 2B**). The proportion of N1 ratings in the ET group did not significantly differ from that in controls ($p = 0.454$). However, the proportion of patients with N1 scores of 2 was significantly lower in the ET group than in the PD group ($p < 0.001$). Representative images obtained from patients with PD and ET and controls are presented in **Figure 1**.

Diagnostic Performances of Visual Analyses of NM and N1, and of the Predicted Probabilities Combining the Two Biomarkers

Based on our findings, we then employed ROC analysis to assess the diagnostic values of several models for differentiating PD from ET. The AUC of NM-MRI (model 1) for differentiating PD from ET was 0.890 (95% CI 0.822, 0.958), and the sensitivity and specificity were 0.882 and 0.800, respectively, when the cutoff value for NM scores was set to ≥1. The AUC of N1 on QSM (model 2) for differentiating PD from ET was 0.882 (95% CI 0.802, 0.962), and the sensitivity and specificity were 0.794 and

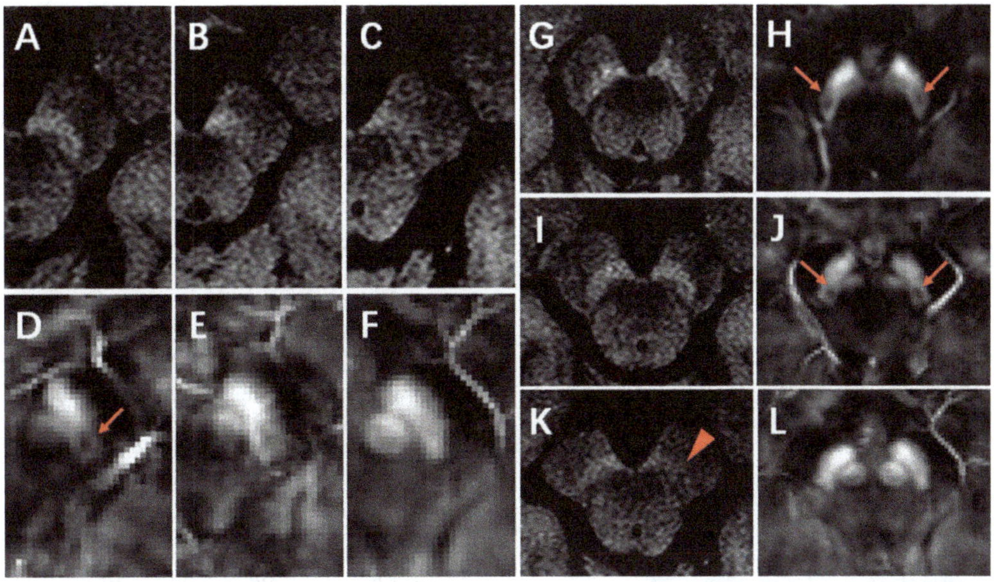

FIGURE 1 | NM-MRI and QSM images. **(A–C)** represent the normal, possibly abnormal, and definitely abnormal SN on NM-MRI, respectively. Nigrosome-1 (N1) could be visualized in the dorsal part of the healthy SN on QSM images (**D**, arrow). **(D–F)** represent that N1 was present, indecisively present and absent, respectively. **(G,H)**, a control subject, female, 65 years, neuromelanin was normal **(G)** and N1 was present (**H**, arrow) in bilateral SN. **(I,J)**, an ET patient, 59 years, female, neuromelanin was normal **(I)** and N1 was present (**J**, arrow) in bilateral SN. **(K,L)**, a *de novo* PD patient, 75 years, female, neuromelanin was definitely abnormal in unilateral SN (**K**, arrowhead) and N1 was absent in bilateral SN **(L)**.

TABLE 1 | Clinical data for patients with PD, patients with ET, and controls.

	PD group (n = 68)	ET group (n = 25)	Control group (n = 34)	p-value
Gender (M/F)	28/40	10/15	13/21	0.960
Age (years)	64.54 ± 9.67	61.12 ± 11.16	63.53 ± 7.81	0.311
MMSE score	27.75 ± 2.71	28.63 ± 1.86	28.80 ± 1.38	0.069
MoCA score	24.98 ± 3.75	25.83 ± 3.28	26.33 ± 2.28	0.165
Disease duration (years)	1.86 ± 1.68	8.60 ± 7.85		<0.001*
UPDRSIII tremor scores	2.06 ± 1.74	3.67 ± 3.27		0.063

**Significantly different; PD, Parkinson's Disease; ET, Essential Tremor; MMSE, Mini Mental State Examination; MoCA, Montreal Cognitive Assessment; UPDRS, United Parkinson's Disease Rating Scale.*

0.920, respectively, when the cutoff value for N1 scores was set to 2. No significant differences in AUC values were observed between these two models ($p > 0.05$, **Table 2**).

We calculated the predicted probabilities using logistic regression to further explore the diagnostic performance of these two biomarkers. Model 3 was established using the predicted probabilities obtained by simply combining these two biomarkers (Log $it = -2.176 + 1.923 \times \text{NM} + 1.429 \times \text{N1}$). The AUC of model 3 was 0.933 (95% CI 0.883, 0.983). The sensitivity and specificity of model 3 were 0.809 and 0.960, respectively, when the cutoff value was set to 0.848. The AUC of model 3 was significantly higher than that of model 1 ($p =$ 0.009), whereas it did not significantly differ from that of model 2 ($p =$ 0.051, **Table 2**). Furthermore, the specificity of model 3 was higher than those of model 1 and 2 while the sensitivity of model 3 was lower than that of model 1.

Model 4 was established using the predicted probabilities obtained by combining NM, N1, and N1^2 (Log $it = -1.499 + 2.014 \times \text{NM} - 1.194 \times \text{N1} + 1.267 \times \text{N1}^2$). The AUC was 0.935 (95% CI 0.884, 0.986). The sensitivity and specificity of model 4 were 0.853 and 0.920, respectively, when the cutoff value was set to 0.704. The AUC of model 4 was significantly higher than those of model 1 ($p =$ 0.041) and model 2 ($p =$ 0.014). The sensitivity and specificity of model 4 were best among the four diagnostic models (**Table 2**). We further established model 5 using the predicted probabilities obtained by combining NM, N1, NM^2, and N1^2. However, the results of model 5 were not better than those of model 4 (data not shown). The ROCs of the four diagnostic models are shown in **Figure 3**.

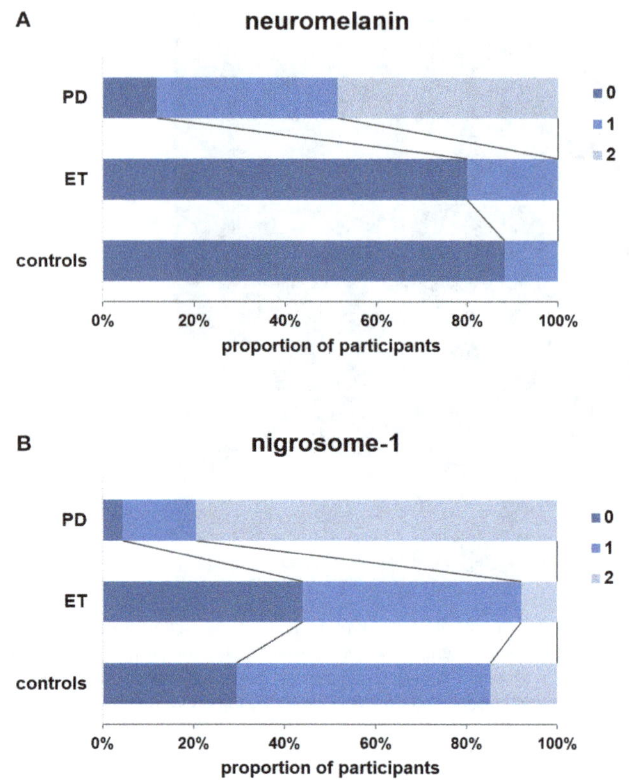

FIGURE 2 | Visual scores (3-point ordinal scale) for patients with PD, patients with ET, and controls. **(A)** Visual scores for neuromelanin. **(B)** Visual scores for nigrosome-1. Note that no definitely abnormal neuromelanin signals (score: 2) were observed in the ET and control groups, and the frequency of nigrosome-1 absence (score: 2) was significantly lower in the ET group than in the PD group ($p < 0.001$).

DISCUSSION

In the current study, we aimed to evaluate whether visual analyses of NM and N1 imaging in the SN are of diagnostic value in the differentiation of *de novo* PD from untreated ET. Patients with PD exhibited reduced signal intensity on NM imaging and an absence of N1 in the SN, relative to patients with ET and healthy controls. Moreover, when visual analyses of NM and N1 imaging were combined, the model exhibited high diagnostic accuracy for differentiating *de novo* PD from untreated ET. To date, although ET is a common neurological disease, the pathogenic mechanisms remain poorly understood (24), and there are no adequate diagnostic biomarkers. Our findings suggest that non-invasive neuroimaging studies may aid in the differential diagnosis of tremor disorders, particularly PD and ET.

NM plays an important role in the pathogenesis of PD (25). Previous MRI studies have indicated that NM signal intensity in the SN are decreased even in the early stages of PD (22, 26). NM has a high binding affinity for iron. However, Reimao et al. reported that there is no significant correlation between NM and iron content in the SN (26). A recent review demonstrated that the NM is not only directly involved in reactive oxygen species (ROS) reduction but also in Ca^{2+} homeostasis, with NM loss leading to the death of dopaminergic neurons (27). Consistent with our quantitative results, a previous analysis study (14) demonstrated that NM levels in the SN are not significantly decreased in patients with ET. Indeed, only 20% of patients with ET obtained scores of 1. All others obtained scores of 0. In contrast, 39.7 and 48.5% of patients with PD obtained scores of 1 and 2, respectively. These results may provide evidence against a possible pathogenic link between PD and ET.

Consistent with the findings of previous reports (17), our results indicated that N1 was absent on QSM images in 79.4% of patients with PD. While NM is known to participate in intracellular iron metabolism, loss of nigrosome signals may be related to iron deposition in the brain (28). At present, QSM is the optimal imaging method for quantifying iron content in the brain *in vivo* (18, 20). Thus, our findings indicated that iron overload occurs in N1 in patients with PD. Previous studies have indicated that changes in N1 can aid in the differential diagnosis of PD (29), as they can be observed in both the early and late stages of the disease (17). Our data also demonstrated the presence of N1 in most patients with ET, in contrast to our findings for patients with PD.

To date, several studies have indicated that ET is likely to be a neurodegenerative disease, especially affecting cerebellar system proven by clinical, neuroimaging, and postmortem studies (30, 31). In addition, patients with ET exhibit a 4-fold higher risk of developing PD than those without ET (32). One MRI T2*-relaxometry study revealed that ET is associated with iron deposition in the SN (33). Another functional MRI study provided further evidence of neurodegeneration in patients with ET, reporting over-activation in the parietal cortex and dorsolateral prefrontal cortex (34). Mild abnormalities in striatal DATs have also been observed in patients with ET, along with a typical PD-like pattern of uptake loss (35). However, there is no loss of DAT binding over time in patients with ET, providing evidence against the neurodegeneration hypothesis (36). To our knowledge, our study is the first to report that the rate of N1 absence is significantly lower in patients with ET than in patients with PD, suggesting that ET is associated with a lower iron deposition than PD.

By combining our NM and N1 findings for patients with PD and ET, we developed diagnostic models for the differentiation of the two disorders. Molecular imaging techniques such as DAT imaging may further improve diagnostic accuracy. Novellino et al. reported that DAT-SPECT and MIBG scintigraphy findings are abnormal in patients with probable PD, while they are normal in patients with ET (37). Another study also reported that DAT imaging can be used to differentiate early-stage PD and ET with high sensitivity (84.4%) and specificity (96.2%) (38). However, this technology is not feasible for clinical application. Several transcranial sonography (TCS) studies have also aimed to distinguish patients with PD from those with ET (38–41), achieving moderate sensitivity and high specificity. Despite these results, recording failures due to an insufficient acoustic bone window may limit the use of

TABLE 2 | Diagnostic models for differentiating PD from ET.

	AUC	Std. Err.	95% CI of AUC		Cutoff value	Sensitivity	Specificity
Model 1[a]	0.890	0.035	0.822	0.958	≥1	0.882	0.800
Model 2[b#]	0.882	0.041	0.802	0.962	=2	0.794	0.920
Model 3[c§]	0.933	0.026	0.883	0.983	0.848	0.809	0.960
Model 4[d$]	0.935	0.026	0.884	0.986	0.704	0.853	0.920

[a]Model 1: NM.
[b]Model 2: N1.
[#]No significant difference was observed between the AUCs of Model 1 and Model 2.
[c]Model 3: predicted probabilities. Log it = −2.176 + 1.923 × NM + 1.429 × N1.
[§]The AUC of model 3 was significantly higher than that of Model 1.
[d]Model 4: predicted probabilities. Log it = −1.499 + 2.014 × NM − 1.194 × N1 + 1.267 × N1^2.
[$]The AUC of model 4 was significantly higher than those of Model 1 and Model 2.
PD, Parkinson's Disease; ET, Essential Tremor; NM, Neuromelanin; N1, Nigrosome-1; AUC, Area Under the Curve.

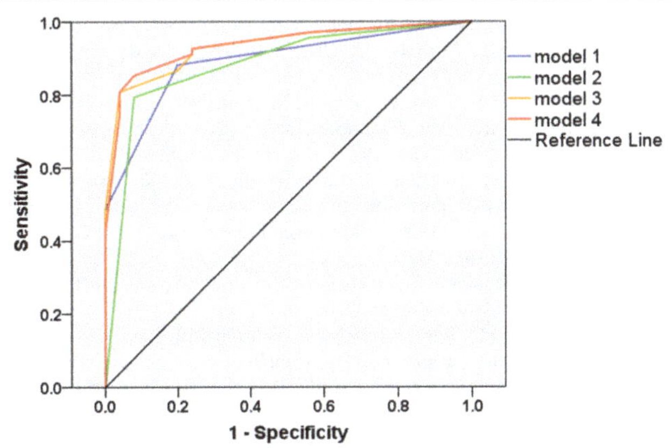

FIGURE 3 | The receiver operating characteristic (ROC) curves of the four diagnostic models.

TCS (42). A previous NM-MRI study reported sensitivity and specificity values of 67.7 and 93.3%, respectively, when high-signal areas in the SN were used to distinguish ET from PD (13). Because visual analysis is fast and more convenient for clinical applications, we performed visual analyses of NM and N1 to aid in the differential diagnosis of *de novo* PD and untreated ET. Sensitivity values were >79% for both biomarkers, while specificity values were equivalent to 80 and >90% for NM and N1, respectively. Despite the relatively good diagnostic ability of both visual assessments for NM and N1, further combining the two biomarkers may provide higher diagnostic accuracy in clinical practice for individual diagnosis. Indeed, the combination of both biomarkers achieved a sensitivity of 85.3% and specificity of 92%—values higher than those for each biomarker.

The present study possesses some limitations of note. First, the number of participants was relatively small, especially the number of patients with ET, and all participants were recruited from clinical settings. Therefore, replication in larger population-dwelling samples is warranted to confirm the effectiveness of the diagnostic models used in our study. Second, NM-MRI acquisition times were relatively long in our study, which many patients may be unable to tolerate. However, a recent study introduced a three-dimensional NM-MRI sequence that took only slightly more than 4 min, which may facilitate clinical application of this method (43). Third, the analysis in our study was qualitative, which may be more suitable for clinical application, rather than quantitative. However, QSM can be used to quantify iron content (20), while NM content can be quantified on NM-MRI based on volume/width (22, 44). Further studies should therefore focus on the quantitative differences between PD and ET. Notably, the patients recruited in this study were all drug naïve, which eliminated the undefined confounding factors associated with medication use (45).

In conclusion, our findings indicated that visual analyses combing NM and N1 may represent a diagnostic biomarker for the differentiation of tremor disorders. Furthermore, our results suggest that iron deposition is greater in patients with PD than in those with ET.

AUTHOR CONTRIBUTIONS

All authors have carefully reviewed this manuscript. In this study, each author has contributed significantly. LJ, YL, CW, YiZ, XC, ZH, ML, CZ, and GF were responsible for collecting and confirming clinical data. JW, DL, KL, MZ, and YoZ were responsible for the MRI study. CZ designed the study and wrote the manuscript.

FUNDING

This study was supported by grants from Science and Technology Commission of Shanghai Municipality (18ZR1406500), the National Key Research and Development Program Foundation of China (2016YFC1306403), and Natural Science Foundation and Major Basic Research Program of Shanghai (16JC1420502).

REFERENCES

Louis ED, Ferreira JJ. How common is the most common adult movement disorder? Update on the worldwide prevalence of essential tremor. *Mov Disord.* (2010) 25:534–41. doi: 10.1002/mds.22838

Kwon KY, Lee HM, Lee SM, Kang SH, Koh SB. Comparison of motor and non-motor features between essential tremor and tremor dominant Parkinson's disease. *J Neurol Sci.* (2016) 361:34–8. doi: 10.1016/j.jns.2015.12.016

Thenganatt MA, Jankovic J. The relationship between essential tremor and Parkinson's disease. *Parkinsonism Relat Disord.* (2016) 22(Suppl 1):S162–5. doi: 10.1016/j.parkreldis.2015.09.032

Postuma RB, Berg D, Stern M, Poewe W, Olanow CW, Oertel W, et al. MDS clinical diagnostic criteria for Parkinson's disease. *Mov Disord.* (2015) 30:1591–601. doi: 10.1002/mds.26424

Heim B, Krismer F, De Marzi R, Seppi K. Magnetic resonance imaging for the diagnosis of Parkinson's disease. *J Neural Transm.* (2017) 124:915–64. doi: 10.1007/s00702-017-1717-8

Kassubek J. MRI-based neuroimaging: atypical parkinsonisms and other movement disorders. *Curr Opin Neurol.* (2018) 31:425–30. doi: 10.1097/WCO.0000000000000578

Lehericy S, Vaillancourt DE, Seppi K, Monchi O, Rektorova I, Antonini A, et al. The role of high-field magnetic resonance imaging in parkinsonian disorders: pushing the boundaries forward. *Mov Disord.* (2017) 32:510–25. doi: 10.1002/mds.26968

Kalia LV, Lang AE. Parkinson's disease. *Lancet* (2015) 386:896–912. doi: 10.1016/S0140-6736(14)61393-3

Shill HA, Adler CH, Beach TG. Pathology in essential tremor. *Parkinsonism Relat Disord.* (2012) 18(Suppl 1):S135–7. doi: 10.1016/S1353-8020(11)70042-6

Sasaki M, Shibata E, Tohyama K, Takahashi J, Otsuka K, Tsuchiya K, et al. Neuromelanin magnetic resonance imaging of locus ceruleus and substantia nigra in Parkinson's disease. *Neuroreport* (2006) 17:1215–8. doi: 10.1097/01.wnr.0000227984.84927.a7

Matsuura K, Maeda M, Yata K, Ichiba Y, Yamaguchi T, Kanamaru K, et al. Neuromelanin magnetic resonance imaging in Parkinson's disease and multiple system atrophy. *Eur Neurol.* (2013) 70:70–7. doi: 10.1159/000350291

Reimao S, Pita Lobo P, Neutel D, Correia Guedes L, Coelho M, Rosa MM, et al. Substantia nigra neuromelanin magnetic resonance imaging in *de novo* Parkinson's disease patients. *Eur J Neurol.* (2015) 22:540–6. doi: 10.1111/ene.12613

Reimao S, Pita Lobo P, Neutel D, Guedes LC, Coelho M, Rosa MM, et al. Substantia nigra neuromelanin-MR imaging differentiates essential tremor from Parkinson's disease. *Mov Disord.* (2015) 30:953–9. doi: 10.1002/mds.26182

Wang J, Huang Z, Li Y, Ye F, Wang C, Zhang Y, et al. Neuromelanin-sensitive MRI of the substantia nigra: an imaging biomarker to differentiate essential tremor from tremor-dominant Parkinson's disease. *Parkinsonism Relat Disord.* (2018) S1353-8020(18)30309-2. doi: 10.1016/j.parkreldis.2018.07.007

Damier P, Hirsch EC, Agid Y, Graybiel AM. The substantia nigra of the human brain. II. Patterns of loss of dopamine-containing neurons in Parkinson's disease. *Brain* (1999) 122(Pt 8):1437–48.

Lehericy S, Bardinet E, Poupon C, Vidailhet M, Francois C. 7 Tesla magnetic resonance imaging: a closer look at substantia nigra anatomy in Parkinson's disease. *Mov Disord.* (2014) 29:1574–81. doi: 10.1002/mds.26043

Schwarz ST, Afzal M, Morgan PS, Bajaj N, Gowland PA, Auer DP. The 'swallow tail' appearance of the healthy nigrosome - a new accurate test of Parkinson's disease: a case-control and retrospective cross-sectional MRI study at 3T. *PLoS ONE* (2014) 9:e93814. doi: 10.1371/journal.pone.0093814

Bilgic B, Pfefferbaum A, Rohlfing T, Sullivan EV, Adalsteinsson E. MRI estimates of brain iron concentration in normal aging using quantitative susceptibility mapping. *Neuroimage* (2012) 59:2625–35. doi: 10.1016/j.neuroimage.2011.08.077

Liu T, Xu W, Spincemaille P, Avestimehr AS, Wang Y. Accuracy of the morphology enabled dipole inversion (MEDI) algorithm for quantitative susceptibility mapping in MRI. *IEEE Trans Med Imaging* (2012) 31:816–24. doi: 10.1109/TMI.2011.2182523

He N, Ling H, Ding B, Huang J, Zhang Y, Zhang Z, et al. Region-specific disturbed iron distribution in early idiopathic Parkinson's disease measured by quantitative susceptibility mapping. *Hum Brain Mapp.* (2015) 36:4407–20. doi: 10.1002/hbm.22928

Deuschl G, Bain P, Brin M. Consensus statement of the Movement Disorder Society on Tremor. *Ad hoc* scientific committee. *Mov Disord.* (1998) 13(Suppl 3):2–23.

Wang J, Li Y, Huang Z, Wan W, Zhang Y, Wang C, et al. Neuromelanin- sensitive magnetic resonance imaging features of the substantia nigra and locus coeruleus in *de novo* Parkinson's disease and its phenotypes. *Eur J Neurol.* (2018) 25:949-e973. doi: 10.1111/ene.13628

Pyatigorskaya N, Magnin B, Mongin M, Yahia-Cherif L, Valabregue R, Arnaldi D, et al. Comparative study of MRI biomarkers in the substantia nigra to discriminate idiopathic Parkinson disease. *AJNR Am J Neuroradiol.* (2018) 39:1460–7. doi: 10.3174/ajnr.A5702

Benito-Leon J, Louis ED. Clinical update: diagnosis and treatment of essential tremor. *Lancet* (2007) 369:1152–4. doi: 10.1016/S0140-6736(07)60544-3

Martin-Bastida A, Pietracupa S, Piccini P. Neuromelanin in parkinsonian disorders: an update. *Int J Neurosci.* (2017) 127:1116–23. doi: 10.1080/00207454.2017.1325883

Reimao S, Ferreira S, Nunes RG, Pita Lobo P, Neutel D, Abreu D, et al. Magnetic resonance correlation of iron content with neuromelanin in the substantia nigra of early-stage Parkinson's disease. *Eur J Neurol.* (2016) 23:368–74. doi: 10.1111/ene.12838

Knorle R. Neuromelanin in Parkinson's Disease: from Fenton Reaction to Calcium Signaling. *Neurotox Res.* (2018) 33:515–22. doi: 10.1007/s12640-017-9804-z

Massey LA, Miranda MA, Al-Helli O, Parkes HG, Thornton JS, So PW, et al. 9.4T MR microscopy of the substantia nigra with pathological validation in controls and disease. *Neuroimage Clin.* (2017) 13:154–63. doi: 10.1016/j.nicl.2016.11.015

Mahlknecht P, Krismer F, Poewe W, Seppi K. Meta-analysis of dorsolateral nigral hyperintensity on magnetic resonance imaging as a marker for Parkinson's disease. *Mov Disord.* (2017) 32:619–23. doi: 10.1002/mds.26932

Novellino F, Nicoletti G, Cherubini A, Caligiuri ME, Nistico R, Salsone M, et al. Cerebellar involvement in essential tremor with and without resting tremor: a diffusion tensor imaging study. *Parkinsonism Relat Disord.* (2016) 27:61–6. doi: 10.1016/j.parkreldis.2016.03.022

Louis ED. Essential tremor and the cerebellum. *Handb Clin Neurol.* (2018) 155:245–58. doi: 10.1016/B978-0-444-64189-2.00016-0

Benito-Leon J, Louis ED, Bermejo-Pareja F, Neurological Disorders in Central Spain Study G. Risk of incident Parkinson's disease and parkinsonism in essential tremor: a population based study. *J Neurol Neurosurg Psychiatry* (2009) 80:423–5. doi: 10.1136/jnnp.2008.147223

Novellino F, Cherubini A, Chiriaco C, Morelli M, Salsone M, Arabia G, et al. Brain iron deposition in essential tremor: a quantitative 3- Tesla magnetic resonance imaging study. *Mov Disord.* (2013) 28:196–200. doi: 10.1002/mds.25263

Cerasa A, Passamonti L, Novellino F, Salsone M, Gioia MC, Morelli M, et al. Fronto-parietal overactivation in patients with essential tremor during Stroop task. *Neuroreport* (2010) 21:148–51. doi: 10.1097/WNR.0b013e328335b42c

Isaias IU, Canesi M, Benti R, Gerundini P, Cilia R, Pezzoli G, et al. Striatal dopamine transporter abnormalities in patients with essential tremor. *Nucl Med Commun.* (2008) 29:349–53. doi: 10.1097/MNM.0b013e3282f4d307

Isaias IU, Marotta G, Hirano S, Canesi M, Benti R, Righini A, et al. Imaging essential tremor. *Mov Disord.* (2010) 25:679–86. doi: 10.1002/mds.22870

Novellino F, Arabia G, Bagnato A, Cascini GL, Salsone M, Nicoletti G, et al. Combined use of DAT-SPECT and cardiac MIBG scintigraphy in mixed tremors. *Mov Disord.* (2009) 24:2242–8. doi: 10.1002/mds.22771

Jesus-Ribeiro J, Freire A, Sargento-Freitas J, Sousa M, Silva F, Moreira F, et al. Transcranial sonography and DaTSCAN in early stage parkinson's disease and essential tremor. *Eur Neurol.* (2016) 76:252–5. doi: 10.1159/000452216

Stockner H, Sojer MKKS, Mueller J, Wenning GK, Schmidauer C, et al. Midbrain sonography in patients with essential tremor. *Mov Disord.* (2007) 22:414–7. doi: 10.1002/mds.21344

Budisic M, Trkanjec Z, Bosnjak J, Lovrencic-Huzjan A, Vukovic V, Demarin V. Distinguishing Parkinson's disease and essential tremor with transcranial sonography. *Acta Neurol Scand.* (2009) 119:17–21. doi: 10.1111/j.1600-0404.2008.01056.x

Stockner H, Wurster I. Transcranial sonography in essential tremor. *Int Rev Neurobiol.* (2010) 90:189–97. doi: 10.1016/S0074-7742(10)9 0014-7

Okawa M, Miwa H, Kajimoto Y, Hama K, Morita S, Nakanishi I, et al. Transcranial sonography of the substantia nigra in Japanese patients with Parkinson's disease or atypical parkinsonism: clinical potential and limitations. *Intern Med.* (2007) 46:1527–31. doi: 10.2169/internalmedicine.46.0271

Prasad S, Stezin A, Lenka A, George L, Saini J, Yadav R, et al. Three-dimensional neuromelanin-sensitive magnetic resonance imaging of the substantia nigra in Parkinson's disease. *Eur J Neurol.* (2018) 25:680–6. doi: 10.1111/ene. 13573

Chen X, Huddleston DE, Langley J, Ahn S, Barnum CJ, Factor SA, et al. Simultaneous imaging of locus coeruleus and substantia nigra with a quantitative neuromelanin MRI approach. *Magn Reson Imaging* (2014) 32:1301–6. doi: 10.1016/j.mri.2014. 07.003

Fahn S, Oakes D, Shoulson I, Kieburtz K, Rudolph A, Lang A, et al. Levodopa and the progression of Parkinson's disease. *N Engl J Med.* (2004) 351:2498– 508. doi: 10.1056/NEJMoa033447

13

Deciphering the Iron Side of Stroke: Neurodegeneration at the Crossroads Between Iron Dyshomeostasis, Excitotoxicity and Ferroptosis

Núria DeGregorio-Rocasolano*[1], *Octavi Martí-Sistac*[1,2]* *and Teresa Gasull*[1]

[1] Cellular and Molecular Neurobiology Research Group, Department of Neurosciences, Germans Trias i Pujol Research Institute (IGTP), Badalona, Spain, [2] Department of Cellular Biology, Physiology and Immunology, Universitat Autònoma de Barcelona, Bellaterra, Spain

***Correspondence:**
Octavi Martí-Sistac
octavi.marti@uab.cat
Teresa Gasull
tgasull@igtp.cat;
teresagasull@yahoo.com

In general, iron represents a double-edged sword in metabolism in most tissues, especially in the brain. Although the high metabolic demands of brain cells require iron as a redox-active metal for ATP-producing enzymes, the brain is highly vulnerable to the devastating consequences of excessive iron-induced oxidative stress and, as recently found, to ferroptosis as well. The blood–brain barrier (BBB) protects the brain from fluctuations in systemic iron. Under pathological conditions, especially in acute brain pathologies such as stroke, the BBB is disrupted, and iron pools from the blood gain sudden access to the brain parenchyma, which is crucial in mediating stroke-induced neurodegeneration. Each brain cell type reacts with changes in their expression of proteins involved in iron uptake, efflux, storage, and mobilization to preserve its internal iron homeostasis, with specific organelles such as mitochondria showing specialized responses. However, during ischemia, neurons are challenged with excess extracellular glutamate in the presence of high levels of extracellular iron; this causes glutamate receptor overactivation that boosts neuronal iron uptake and a subsequent overproduction of membrane peroxides. This glutamate-driven neuronal death can be attenuated by iron-chelating compounds or free radical scavenger molecules. Moreover, vascular wall rupture in hemorrhagic stroke results in the accumulation and lysis of iron-rich red blood cells at the brain parenchyma and the subsequent presence of hemoglobin and heme iron at the extracellular milieu, thereby contributing to iron-induced lipid peroxidation and cell death. This review summarizes recent progresses made in understanding the ferroptosis component underlying both ischemic and hemorrhagic stroke subtypes.

Keywords: iron, reactive oxygen species, ferroptosis, stroke, excitotoxicity, iron dyshomeostasis, neurodegeneration, transferrin saturation

---

Abbreviations: AIS, acute ischemic stroke; ALOX5: arachidonic acid lipoxygenase 5; APP, amyloid precursor protein; BBB, brain-blood barrier; CSF, cerebrospinal fluid; Dexras1, dexamethasone-induced Ras protein 1; DFO, deferoxamine; DMT1, divalent metal transporter 1; EAATs, excitatory amino acid transporters; FPN, ferroportin; FT, ferritin; FTH, ferritin heavy chain; GAPDH, glyceraldehyde-3-phosphate dehydrogenase; GPX4, glutathione peroxidase 4; GSH, glutathione; Hb, hemoglobin; HO, heme oxygenase; Hp, haptoglobin; Hpx, hemopexin; HTf, holotransferrin; ICH, intracerebral hemorrhage; I/R, ischemia/reperfusion; IREs, iron regulatory elements; IRPs, iron regulatory proteins; NAC, *N*-acetylcysteine; NMDA, *N*-methyl-D-aspartate; NTBI, non-transferrin-bound iron; OGD, oxygen and glucose deprivation; PUFA, polyunsaturated fatty acids; ROS, reactive oxygen species; TIM, T-cell immunoglobulin and mucin domain-containing receptor; Tf, transferrin; TfR1, transferrin receptor 1; TfR2, transferrin receptor 2; TSAT, saturation of transferrin with iron; UTRs, untranslated regions; X_c^-, cystine/glutamate exchanger or antiporter, i.e., SLC7A11/xCT.

IRON TRANSPORT TO THE BRAIN: THE ROLE OF THE BLOOD–BRAIN BARRIER

Iron is essential for life; numerous proteins require iron as a cofactor for their activity. Iron acts as an electron donor or acceptor, and thus is pivotal for oxygen transport (coordinated with hemoglobin), cellular respiration (as a part of heme-containing cytochromes and proteins containing Fe–S groups in the electron transport chain), and DNA synthesis (in ribonuclease reductase). Moreover, in the nervous system, iron is essential for myelinization and neurotransmitter biosynthesis.

Iron exists both as Fe^{2+} and Fe^{3+}; redox-active and cycling between these two states lead to the generation of reactive oxygen species (ROS) through the Fenton reaction. The ROS promote oxidative stress and cause extensive lipid peroxidation (Gutteridge et al., 1979). The brain is particularly vulnerable to lipid peroxidation damage because it is rich in polyunsaturated fatty acids (PUFAs) and iron, but relatively poor in antioxidant defenses (Cobley et al., 2018). The iron content remarkably differs across different brain regions: it is high in the striatum, medium in the hippocampus and cortex, and low in the pons and medulla (Ramos et al., 2014). Although it has recently attracted considerable attention, iron metabolism in the brain is yet not completely understood as that in other murine tissues (Ashraf et al., 2018). Brain imports iron from systemic circulation, and the levels of iron are determined by diet, intestinal iron absorption, release of iron initially stored in the hepatocytes, and export of iron recycled from macrophages. In addition, the levels of iron in the plasma are regulated by the hormone hepcidin through its effect on the transmembrane iron export protein ferroportin (FPN), which is mainly present at the cell membrane of macrophages, hepatocytes, and enterocytes.

In the blood and most other extracellular fluids, iron is essentially carried bound with high affinity to the iron transport protein transferrin (Tf), which shields Fe^{3+} from redox activity. In addition to Tf, iron also associates with other carrier proteins in the blood such as ferritin (FT), haptoglobin (Hp), Hpx, or albumin. Recently, half a dozen different non-proteinaceous low-molecular-weight iron species (<10 KDa) have been shown to exist in the blood (Dziuba and Lindahl, 2018); further studies are required to determine the precise identity and physiological role of these species. Once iron is bound to Tf, Fe^{3+} is rendered redox-inactive and virtually non-exchangeable or displaceable by other physiological metals or molecules. Tf–iron complexes circulate in the blood until they bind transferrin receptors (TfRs) in cellular membranes of target cells. In general, in non-iron-overload conditions, little, if any, non-transferrin-bound iron (NTBI) is found in the blood of healthy individuals (Gaasch et al., 2007). The high affinity of Tf for iron and the large amount of Tf in the blood exceed the total requirement for iron binding; in normal human blood, the saturation of transferrin with iron (TSAT) is only of around 30% (De Valk et al., 2000; Van Dijk et al., 2008). Therefore, iron transport to the brain is mainly from iron-loaded transferrin (holotransferrin, HTf) through the endothelial cells of the BBB and the epithelium of the choroid plexuses and arachnoid membrane, the blood–cerebrospinal fluid (CSF) barrier.

Although barrier cells of the brain form tight junctions laterally, epithelial cells of the choroid plexuses are fenestrated and more permeable than the endothelial cells of the BBB (Strazielle and Ghersi-Egea, 2016). The abluminal side of brain capillary endothelial cells is surrounded by pericytes and astrocytes of the neurovascular unit that provide extra structural and functional support. TfRs are abundantly expressed in the luminal side of membranes of polarized endothelial cells; once they bind Tf, the TfR–Tf complexes undergo endocytosis. The following steps are still controversial, and different pathways are thought to be involved in brain iron acquisition (Bradbury, 1997; Khan et al., 2018). Thus far, the main contribution to this process is thought to include the following pathways: (1) endocytic vesicles containing TfR–HTf traveling from the luminal membrane to fuse to the abluminal membrane and exocytose either HTf or free iron into the brain extracellular space; (2) under low pH conditions within the endosome of endothelial cells, as in most cell types, iron is extracted from Tf, converted to Fe^{2+} by endosomal ferrireductases such as the six-transmembrane epithelial antigen of prostate protein 3 (Steap3), and released to the cytosol through divalent metal transporter 1 (DMT1) or the ion channels TRPML, also known as mucolipin 1 or MCOLN1 (detailed information can be found in references Luck and Mason, 2012; Skjorringe et al., 2015). Subsequently, Fe^{2+} from the cytosol is exported through FPN present in the abluminal membrane of endothelial cells, which are in contact with astrocytes expressing ceruloplasmin, that rapidly oxidize Fe^{2+} to Fe^{3+} (this Tf/TfR endocytosis mechanism is common for endothelial and neuronal cells and is depicted in **Figures 1, 2**). A recent study performed using comprehensive mathematical models concluded that optimal iron homeostasis is dependent on the degree of saturation and the transport of HTf across the BBB from the blood (Khan et al., 2018).

In addition, in mice exposed to experimental stroke under normal iron conditions, iron deposits in the microvasculature were observed early in the border zone of the damaged areas (Desestret et al., 2009), suggesting that, when signaled, the BBB might function as an iron reservoir from which iron is released into the brain. Regarding signaling to release, in bovine retinal endothelial cells, the FPN-mediated iron export is known to be blocked by the FPN inhibitor hepcidin (Hadziahmetovic et al., 2011). In addition, new insights into the communication between systemic iron status and brain iron uptake reveal the regulation of brain iron uptake at the level of brain microvascular endothelial cells rather than the BBB acting merely as a retaining wall (Chiou et al., 2018b). In support of this regulatory hypothesis, endothelial microvascular cell distribution of TfR is altered in luminal, intracellular, and abluminal membranes depending on brain iron status (Simpson et al., 2015), and microvascular cell iron availability and efflux have been found to be tightly modulated by diffusible ceruloplasmin and hepcidin released from astrocytes surrounding the BBB (McCarthy and Kosman, 2014). Moreover, a recent study showed that inhibition of DMT1 alters the transport of iron and Tf across the endothelial cells and proposed that the levels of iron-devoid Tf (apotransferrin) and iron delivered to the brain are strongly regulated by the ratio apotransferrin:HTf as well as by

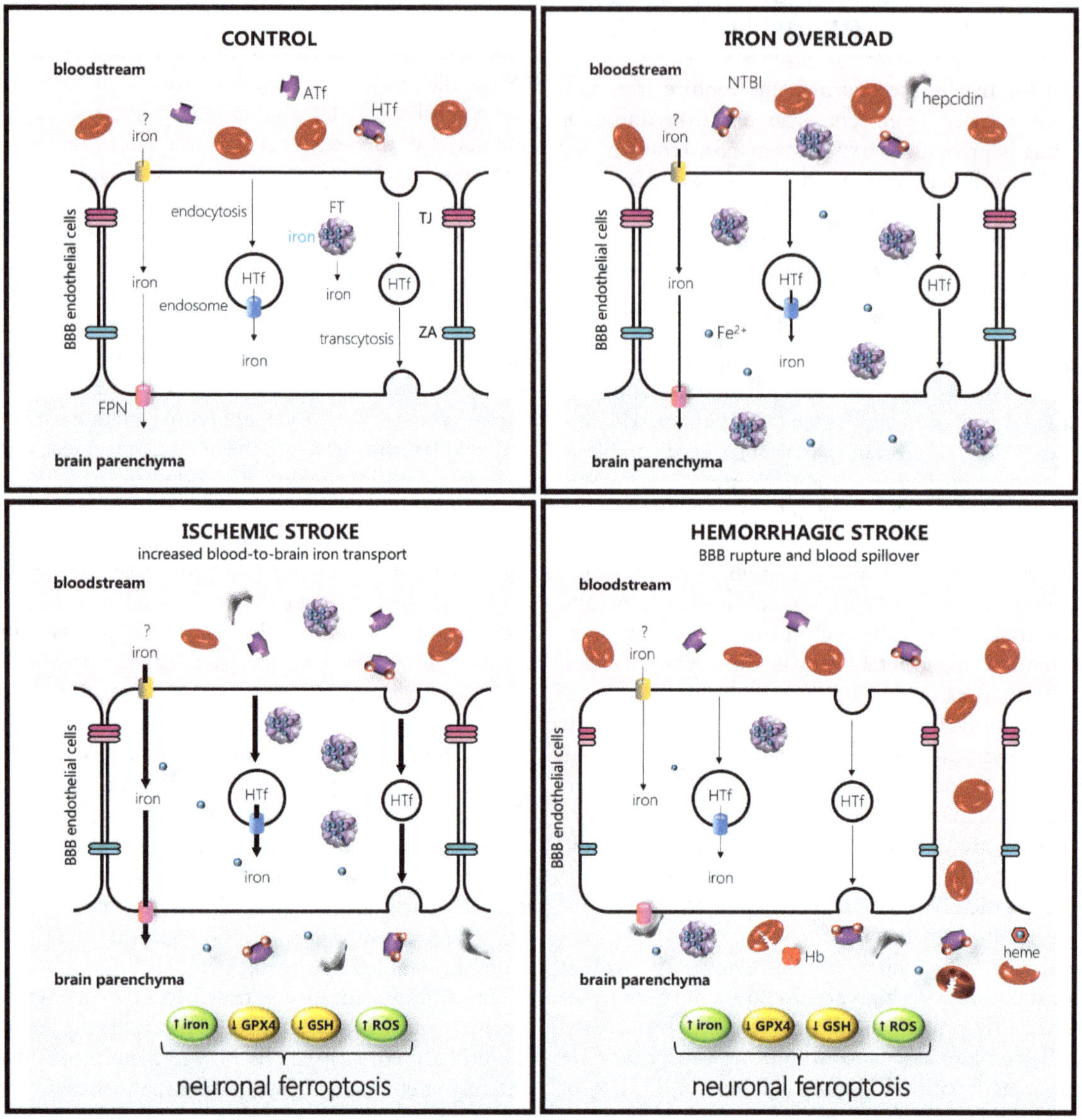

FIGURE 1 | Schematic drawing of some of the main players in iron transport to the brain in control (left hand upper side), iron overload (right-hand upper side), ischemic stroke (left-hand lower side), or intracerebral hemorrhage (right-hand lower side). The thicker the arrows the more increased the transport. Abbreviations: ATf, apotransferrin; FPN, ferroportin; HTf, holotransferrin; FT, ferritin, GPX4, glutathione peroxidase 4; GSH, glutathione; Hb, hemoglobin; NTBI, non-transferrin-bound iron; ROS, reactive oxygen species; TJ, tight junction; ZA, zonula occludens.

hepcidin levels in the extracellular fluid of each brain region (Duck et al., 2017).

Further, very recently, a new function for FT heavy chain (FTH) as a transporter of NTBI across the BBB by binding to the T-cell immunoglobulin and mucin domain-containing 1 receptor 1 (TIM-1) has been reported in human endothelial cells (Chiou et al., 2018b).

In the context of physiological iron-overload conditions found, for instance, in individuals on iron-rich diets, a significant pool of NTBI is found in the blood and might be readily absorbed by microvascular endothelial cells. This effect might be relevant considering that regional differences in the brain uptake of ^{59}Fe–NTBI versus ^{59}Fe–TfR have been reported (Deane et al., 2004), and that ^{59}Fe–NTBI seems to be transported faster than ^{59}Fe–TfR into the brain parenchyma of iron-overloaded disease-free mice. Furthermore, the iron storage protein FT has been found to be upregulated in epithelial cells of the choroid plexus and endothelial cells of the brain during systemic iron overload (Tripathi et al., 2017).

IRON UPTAKE AND HANDLING BY PARENCHYMAL BRAIN CELLS

Once in the brain interstitial fluid, both TBI and NTBI are potential iron sources for brain cells (Gaasch et al., 2007); unlike

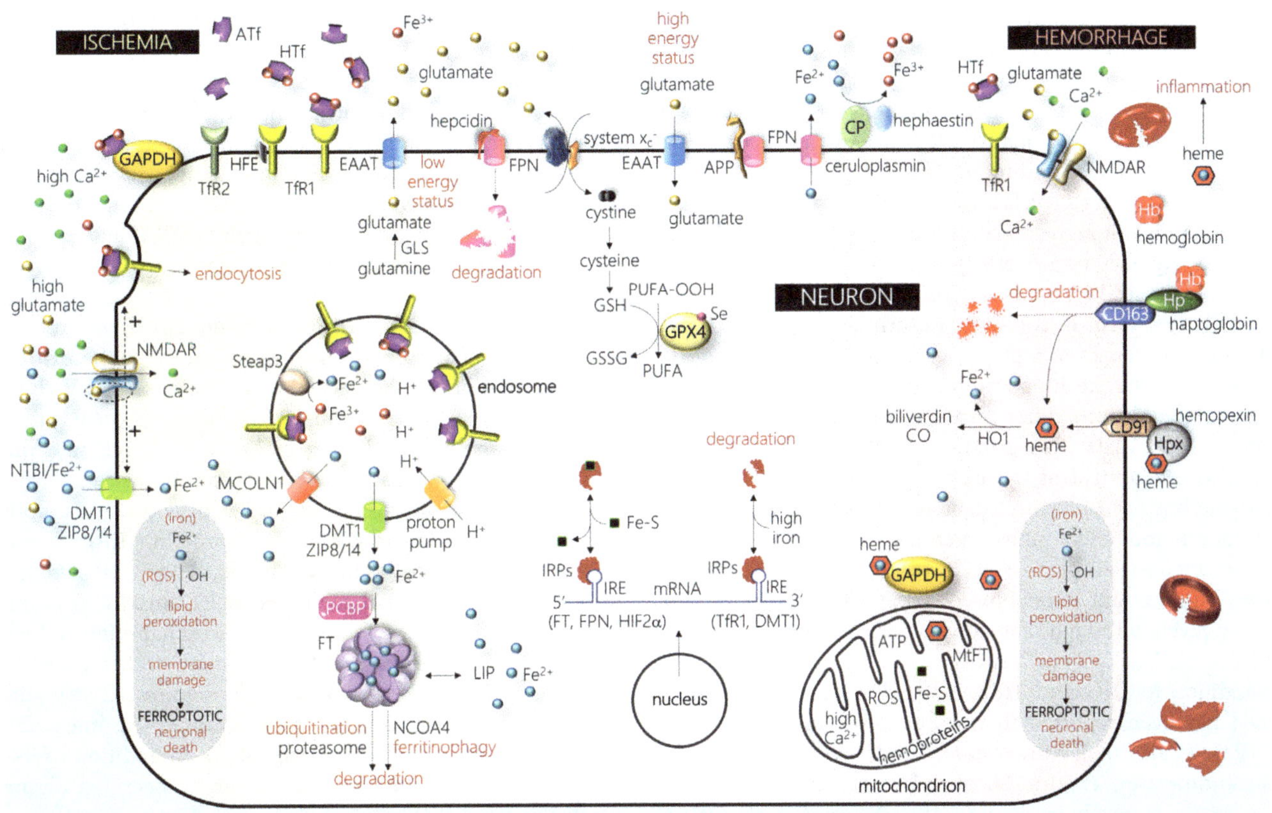

FIGURE 2 | Schematic drawing of some of the main players in a neuron under ischemic (left-hand side) and hemorrhagic (right-hand side) stress (see text for details). Abbreviations: APP, amyloid precursor protein; ATf, apotransferrin; CD163, hemoglobin/haptoglobin receptor; CD91, heme/hemopexin receptor; CO, carbon monoxide; CP, ceruloplasmin; DMT1, divalent metal transporter 1; EAAT, excitatory amino acid transporter; Fe^{2+}, ferrous iron; Fe^{3+}, ferric iron; Fe–S, iron–sulfur cluster; FPN, ferroportin; FT, ferritin; GAPDH, glyceraldehyde-3-phosphate dehydrogenase; GLS, glutaminase; GPX4, glutathione peroxidase 4; GSH, glutathione; GSSG, glutathione disulfide; Hb, hemoglobin; HFE, hereditary hemochromatosis protein; HIF, hypoxia-inducible factor; HO1, heme oxygenase 1; Hp, haptoglobin; Hpx, hemopexin; HTf, holotransferrin; IRE, iron-responsive element; IRPs, iron regulatory proteins; LIP, labile iron pool; MCOLN1, mucolipin 1; MtFT, mitochondrial ferritin; NCOA, nuclear receptor coactivator; NMDAR, NMDA receptor; NTBI, non-transferrin-bound iron; OH, hydroxyl radical; PCBP, poly(rC)-binding protein; PUFA, poly-unsaturated fatty acid; PUFA-OOH, PUFA peroxide; ROS, reactive oxygen species; Se, selenium; Steap, six-transmembrane epithelial antigen of prostate; system X_c^-, cystine–glutamate antiporter; TfR1, transferrin receptor 1; TfR2, transferrin receptor 2; ZIP8/14, zinc transporters 8/14. The picture depicts the effect of one of the major players in the pathophysiology of brain I, the disruption of glutamatergic neurotransmission homeostasis that produces elevated extracellular glutamate levels, overactivation of the NMDA subtype of glutamate receptors (NMDAR), and excitotoxic cell death. In the recent past, different authors have shown that this NMDAR overactivation boosts neuronal iron uptake and produces an iron-dependent form of neuronal death associated with massive lipid peroxidation that fits with the definition of ferroptosis. Further, in the hemorrhage type of stroke, iron derived from hemoglobin and/or heme enters neurons and produces massive lipid peroxidation. Damage by ischemic and hemorrhagic stroke is alleviated by the inhibitors of ferroptosis.

blood Tf, CSF Tf is considered to be completely saturated with iron (Bradbury, 1997). Within the extracellular milieu of the brain parenchyma, iron is carried loaded into Tf or bound to low-molecular-weight molecules such as citrate, ascorbate, or ATP. Each brain cell type uptakes extracellular TBI or NTBI depending on the iron-transport receptors and channels present in their membranes and, physiologically, safely handles iron by using the network of proteins they specifically express to import, store, traffic, and export iron. Players of cellular iron homeostasis are cell type-specific, and the list of proteins involved in iron homeostasis is still growing. As an example of iron-related new proteins, only 3 years ago, the members of the ZIP family of metal ion transporters Zip8 and Zip14, which, unlike the DMT1 transporter are only active at normal physiological pH, were reported to be expressed by hippocampal neurons, and Zip8 was found to play a major role in the accumulation of NTBI by hippocampal neurons (Ji and Kosman, 2015), whereas both Zip8 and Zip14 were considered to play a role in iron homeostasis in rat retina (Sterling et al., 2017).

Receptors Involved in Iron Uptake by Brain Cells

In addition to the well-known TfR1 as a main player of the TfR/Tf endocytic pathway in most brain cells, other proteins, e.g., transferrin receptor 2 (TfR2) (Kawabata, 2018) or glyceraldehyde-

3-phosphate dehydrogenase (GAPDH) (Raje et al., 2007), have been described as receptors for Tf and are currently being investigated. TfR1 binds HTf with a Kd of 1 nM; it is expressed in response to changes in iron levels through modulation by iron regulatory elements (IREs) present in its mRNA and binds hereditary hemochromatosis HFE protein, a molecule that competes with HTf for binding to TfR1. In contrast, TfR2 has lower affinity for HTf; its levels are not modulated by IREs (West et al., 2000) and, although still controversial, seems to bind HFE protein in a sequence non-overlapping to that of the Tf-binding site (for a review see Worthen and Enns, 2014).

The TfR2 is present in two main isoforms, TfR2α and TfR2β. The TfR2α form has been reported to be more abundant in the brain, especially in the hippocampus; brain TfR2α levels were reported to significantly differ across animals fed iron-deficient or iron-enriched diets (Pellegrino et al., 2016). A specific role for TfR2 in the control of the iron regulatory network in the brain tissue has been recently suggested, as altered brain IRPs, iron accumulation, and reactive microglia signaling were found in TfR2-KO mice (Pellegrino et al., 2016). In contrast, a previous study on TfR2 mutant mice showed changes in hepatic, but not brain iron levels, although that study reported a 30% increase in brain FT levels (Acikyol et al., 2013).

In addition to TfR1 and TfR2, the multifunctional molecule GAPDH has been reported to work as a TfR in different cell types (Raje et al., 2007; Kumar et al., 2012) with a role in iron uptake and/or iron export (Sheokand et al., 2016) and as a chaperone for intracellular heme traffic (Sweeny et al., 2018). Relevant to brain and excitotoxicity, GAPDH interacts with the α-amino-3-hydroxy-5-methyl-4-isoxazolepropionic acid subtype of glutamate receptors in the neurons without glutamate stimulation and has also been reported to be pivotal for axon development (Lee et al., 2016).

Another receptor-mediated means to import iron into brain cells, at least in oligodendrocytes, is the uptake of FTH through TIM-1/2 receptors (Todorich et al., 2008, 2011; Chiou et al., 2018a). In other non-neuronal cells, FTH internalize through TfR1 (Li et al., 2010), whereas scavenger receptor class A member 5 (SCARA5) has been found to play also a role as a receptor for FT light chain uptake (Li et al., 2009). To the best of our knowledge, the role of SCARA5 has not yet been investigated in any brain cell type.

Mechanisms and Proteins Involved in Cytosolic Iron Handling in Different Brain Cell Types

Inside the cell cytosolic and nuclear compartments, iron chaperone poly(rC)-binding proteins serve the binding and delivery of iron to iron-requiring enzymes, ubiquitous protein of iron storage FT, or the iron export membrane protein FPN (Philpott et al., 2017). In the cytosol, unused iron is stored into FT, a molecule composed of 24 subunits of a variable proportion of heavy and light chains, that shields up to 4500 iron atoms in a redox inert state. Neurons express both TfR1 and DMT1 (Pelizzoni et al., 2012; DeGregorio-Rocasolano et al., 2018); DMT1 is mainly found in the cytoplasm colocalizing with endosomes/lysosomes. Further, neurons express the iron export molecule FPN (Burdo et al., 2001; Zhou et al., 2017). Astrocytes express TfR1, DMT1, and FPN (Yang et al., 2012; Huang et al., 2014). Hence, although TfR1 is considered to be the main gate for cellular iron import, control astrocytes show low TfR1 levels, and most mature oligodendrocytes or microglial cells do not express TfR1 (Kaur and Ling, 1995; Rathnasamy et al., 2016). However, under hypoxia, both astrocytes and oligodendrocytes are found to upregulate TfR (Yang et al., 2012; Rathnasamy et al., 2016). Moreover, oligodendrocytes and cells of choroid plexuses, but not other brain cell types, express Tf under normal condition (Leitner and Connor, 2012). All the above are examples of the important heterogeneity in the expression and induction of iron homeostatic or IRPs observed in different brain cell types and situations. Most of the proteins involved in iron metabolism, including cytosolic FT levels, are mainly regulated by iron, oxidative stress, and inflammation. The iron-dependent regulation occurs mainly at the post-transcriptional level via the IREs and iron regulatory protein (IRP) machinery. When iron levels are high, iron binds to the IRP, which then loses affinity for the IRE sequence in FT mRNA, resulting in increased FT expression (the cytosolic iron handling is depicted in **Figure 2**) (Arosio et al., 2017). Several studies have shown that the mobilization of iron from FT requires FT degradation either by lysosome–autophagy or ubiquitin proteasome pathways (Asano et al., 2011; Mancias et al., 2015). In addition to its role in storing iron within the cell, FT can be secreted (Truman-Rosentsvit et al., 2018).

In addition to post-transcriptional regulation, transcriptional regulation has been reported for some of the proteins involved in iron homeostasis through the hypoxia-inducible factor family of transcription factors or the heme-dependent transcription factors (e.g., for TfR1 or FPN) (Marro et al., 2010; Man-man et al., 2017). Moreover, the master regulator of bodily iron homeostasis hepcidin is subjected to a sophisticated transcriptional regulation through the bone morphogenetic protein/SMAD pathway, interleukin 6 pathway, or erythropoietin/erythroferrone pathways when regulated according to the iron, inflammatory, or erythropoietic demands (Sangkhae and Nemeth, 2017). The regulation of cellular iron balance has been recently reviewed (Recalcati et al., 2017).

Iron also plays an important role in specific organelles; this is especially true for mitochondria. Mitochondria house the assembly of heme, the majority of the Fe–S cluster biosynthesis apparatus, and contain the respiratory complexes that need iron-containing cofactors. In addition, mitochondria are a major source of endogenous ROS. Sustained iron exposure increased mitochondrial ROS levels in dopaminergic neuroblastoma SH-SY5Y cells (Huang et al., 2017), and scavenging of mitochondrial ROS was protective against iron overload damage in hippocampal neurons, preserving mitochondrial morphological integrity and membrane potential (Pelizzoni et al., 2011). In addition, a recent study showed that sequestration of iron by mitochondrial FT was neuroprotective against oxidative stress and played an important role in preventing neuronal damage in some other conditions (You et al., 2016; Guan et al., 2017). Moreover, mitochondrial FT overexpression significantly reduced cellular labile iron pool, prevented H_2O_2-induced elevation of labile iron, and rescued cells from H_2O_2-induced damage (Gao et al., 2017).

In several cell types, although not yet studied in neurons, mitochondria–endosome interactions have been observed, suggesting a possible direct transfer of iron from endosomes to mitochondria (Das et al., 2016; Hamdi et al., 2016) through the "kiss-and-run" hypothesis.

IRON DYSHOMEOSTASIS IN THE BRAIN

Brain iron abnormalities are associated to rare, but severe, neurodegenerative conditions, and there is growing evidence that the more common systemic iron overload disorders such as hereditary hemochromatosis exert important effects on the brain iron content and pathological brain iron deposition (Nandar and Connor, 2011; Kumar et al., 2016). Moreover, the hemochromatosis H63D polymorphism of the *HFE* gene could be a disease-modifying gene in frontotemporal lobar degeneration, fostering iron deposition in the basal ganglia (Gazzina et al., 2016), or even macro- and microanatomically altering some brain structures associated with changes in Tf levels in the blood (Jahanshad et al., 2012). Recently, abnormal recycling of TfR1 due to reduced post-translational palmitoylation has been reported to be crucial to affect the iron import in the so-called neurodegeneration with brain iron accumulation disease (Drecourt et al., 2018). Further, neurodegeneration with brain iron accumulation disease-linked genes that showed altered expression in response to iron loading has been recently reported to be directly or indirectly related to myelin metabolism (Heidari et al., 2016).

A list of mild conditions, including aging (Ward et al., 2014), continuous uptake of some bioavailable iron sources (Peters et al., 2018), or obesity (Han et al., 2017), have been reported to alter brain iron content and/or distribution. In addition, a recent report showed that iron administration increases iron levels in the brains of healthy rats, which induces brain changes and triggers a hormetic response that reduces oxidative damage (Piloni et al., 2018). Moreover, other studies reveal a complex interplay between inflammation and brain iron homeostasis (Righy et al., 2018; Sankar et al., 2018), with acute inflammation increasing non-Tf iron uptake by brain microglia (McCarthy et al., 2018). This dyshomeostasis is especially important in acute pathologies such as stroke, in which the impairment of the BBB regulatory role is rapidly and massively affected following either rupture of an artery (ICH) or aberrant increase of brain microvascular endothelial permeability following ischemic stroke (AIS). Dysregulation of iron resulting in the accumulation of free iron and brain iron overload, which can increase the production of ROS, is evident in aging and stroke-related pathologies and is also a hallmark of chronic and long-term neurodegenerative pathologies. In this regard, iron overload in the brain has been reported in Huntington, Parkinson, or Alzheimer diseases [readers interested in the topic are referred to recent detailed reviews by Morris et al. (2018) and Uranga and Salvador (2018)]. Interestingly, marked age-related changes in brain iron homeostasis have also been observed in amyloid precursor protein (APP)-knockout mice (Belaidi et al., 2018).

IRON OVERLOAD WORSENS NEUROLOGICAL DAMAGE BOTH IN ISCHEMIC STROKE AND INTRACEREBRAL HEMORRHAGE

Stroke is a life-threatening disease that causes high rates of permanent disability subsequent to neuronal loss. There are two major types of strokes: ischemic stroke or AIS, which is caused by a blood clot blocking an artery and accounts for 85% of all strokes, and hemorrhagic stroke or ICH, caused by leakage or rupture of an artery and accounts for 15% of stroke cases.

Iron Overload Condition in Stroke Damage and Outcome

In ischemic stroke, neurons die because of interrelated processes that include glutamate excitotoxicity, excess of free radical production, and inflammation (Nagy and Nardai, 2017). Each of these mechanisms has already been targeted in clinical trials, although unsuccessfully (for a review see Chamorro et al., 2016). Moreover, free radical-induced oxidative stress has been for long recognized as a pathogenic factor in the ischemia/reperfusion (I/R) injury that follows reoxygenation. The hydroxyl radical, the most harmful of the free radicals, is generated through reactions catalyzed by iron (Kell, 2009; Chen H. et al., 2011). Of relevance to stroke damage and final outcome, several clinical studies indicate that a previous systemic iron overload condition, measured as high levels of serum FT at admission, is associated with increased brain damage and worse outcome induced by ischemic stroke (Davalos et al., 1994; Millan et al., 2007). A similar detrimental effect (increased ischemic damage) was observed in iron-overloaded animals exposed to experimental ischemic stroke (Castellanos et al., 2002; Gamez et al., 2003; Mehta et al., 2004; García-Yébenes et al., 2012; DeGregorio-Rocasolano et al., 2018). Iron overload is a major source of oxidative stress in ischemic brains (Carbonell and Rama, 2007). In addition, iron overload exacerbated the risk of hemorrhagic transformation in animal models of transient ischemia plus early reperfusion (García-Yébenes et al., 2012; García-Yébenes et al., 2018); therefore, in iron-overloaded animals, an initial ischemic event has higher probability to become an ICH. The contribution of iron overload to widespread the damage in the ICH is supported by the fact that systemic iron overload (estimated using high serum FT levels) was associated with higher perihematoma edema and poor outcomes in patients with ICH (Mehdiratta et al., 2008; Perez de la Ossa et al., 2010; Bakhshayesh et al., 2014; Garton et al., 2017). Further, a combination of high serum FT and low serum iron and Tf was associated with poor outcome in ICH patients (Yang et al., 2016). Therefore, systemic iron overload impacts the outcome of both ischemic and hemorrhagic stroke patients.

The brain is physiologically sheltered from fluctuations in systemic iron because of the BBB, even under experimentally induced diet iron overload conditions or intraperitoneal iron administration (Castellanos et al., 2002; Millerot et al., 2005). However, in the ischemic brain, the detrimental effect of iron overload might result from systemic iron pools reaching the brain parenchyma. Following artery occlusion, a physiological increase in transport through a still somehow intact BBB is noted, and thereafter pathological halt of the BBB function that results in leaky or broken capillaries that allow blood spill out (**Figure 1**). Some BBB impairment with aberrant exchange of brain and blood molecules occurs relatively early following ischemic stroke (within the first hours of post-symptom onset) showing a biphasic behavior in some studies (Klohs et al., 2009). Moreover, leakage through the BBB varies in different experimental stroke models (Klohs et al., 2009; Abulrob et al., 2011). Of note, post-stroke BBB leakage also varies in different areas of the brain, whereas the administration of the broadly used thrombolytic agent tissue plasminogen activator increases leakage (Jaffer et al., 2013), resulting in hemorrhagic transformation. Moreover, a recent evidence of the pivotal contribution of BBB leakage to ischemic stroke damage has been revealed by a study in which a vascular leakage blocker reduced stroke damage (Zhang et al., 2017).

Effect of Stroke on Brain Iron

Regarding iron content of the brain following ischemic stroke, an increase in total iron was observed in the ischemic areas after permanent or transient ischemic stroke (Helal, 2008; Millerot-Serrurot et al., 2008; Tuo et al., 2017). In addition, increased TfR and iron levels were observed in susceptible hippocampal areas following transient global cerebral ischemia (Park et al., 2011), or increased extravasation of iron-loaded HTf was observed following acute focal ischemic stroke (DeGregorio-Rocasolano et al., 2018). In fact, HTf from blood accumulates in the brain parenchyma of the rat ischemic brain hemisphere at 1 h after reperfusion (DeGregorio-Rocasolano et al., 2018). Subsequently, iron accumulates into the endothelial cells of brain capillaries near ischemic areas (Desestret et al., 2009), whereas increased levels of Tf were observed 24 h following a transient experimental stroke at the ischemic hemisphere (Lo et al., 2007). In fact, this Tf seems to accumulate in neurons since Tf immunoreactivity was found located at the neuronal cytoplasm 24 h after stroke onset (DeGregorio-Rocasolano et al., 2018).

In the ICH stroke type, the systemic iron pools play a direct role in brain damage since the rupture of the microvascular wall and concomitant blood release results in neurons, astrocytes, and other cells around the hemorrhagic area to become immediately exposed to blood-derived iron, either free or bound to Tf (**Figures 1, 2**). Moreover, the brain is exposed to a bulk amount of erythrocytes that undergo lysis and subsequent spill of hemoglobin (Hb). Erythrocyte lysis occurs within minutes and continues for days after the formation of brain hematoma, leading to the release of red blood cell-derived products. Cells of the brain are then sequentially exposed to aberrantly high extracellular levels of Hb, the oxidized Hb form methemoglobin, and free heme or the iron ferric heme form hemin. The main mechanisms of neurodegeneration in hemorrhagic stroke are iron- and heme-induced ROS production, amplification of an inflammatory response, direct toxic effects of iron and heme, and glutamate-induced excitotoxicity (Righy et al., 2016).

BRAIN REGULATION OF IRON METABOLISM DURING STROKE

Endogenous Mechanisms Involved in the Protection of Brain Cells From Excess Iron Following AIS

Increased brain Tf or TfR1 levels (Ding et al., 2011; DeGregorio-Rocasolano et al., 2018) were observed in lethal ischemia. Consensus exists about the protective role of increased FT expression during experimental stroke, and the same applies to hepcidin in AIS; however, the role of blunting the ischemia-induced upregulation of Tf and TfR remains controversial. Reductions of Tf and TfR were considered to be associated with neuroprotection in one specific stroke model (Lo et al., 2007). However, other neuroprotective conditions were not associated with Tf and/or TfR reductions (He et al., 2012).

Hepcidin seems to protect from neurodegeneration in AIS. It is an iron-inducible peptide hormone that is considered to be the main regulator of iron homeostasis. Hepcidin is produced as a propeptide mainly in the liver and then secreted to the blood where it interacts with the only known iron exporter FPN located at the cell membrane. Hepcidin acts as a negative regulator of cellular iron release by binding FPN and causing its internalization and degradation; this inhibits FPN-mediated iron egression from enterocytes, macrophages, hepatocytes and, as recently found, some other cell types (e.g., endothelial cells or neurons). The inhibition of iron egression, mainly from macrophages and hepatocytes, prevents the presence of NTBI in the blood as well as reduces the TSAT in the blood. In line with its main function, hepcidin deficiency leads to iron overload (Nicolas et al., 2001), and hepcidin overexpression causes severe iron deficiency (Nicolas et al., 2002a). Hepcidin has a rapid and direct impact on circulating iron pools. In fact, even a single intraperitoneal administration of hepcidin reduces the TSAT in blood to less than half the normal levels for 6–12 h (Sillerova et al., 2012). Both blood hepcidin and HTf/apotransferrin ratio might be considered as the master regulatory factors of systemic iron metabolism, since hepcidin senses iron by sensing HTf levels in the circulation and iron-FT levels inside hepatocytes. Relevant to this review on iron and stroke, hepcidin expression is also responsive to hypoxia (Nicolas et al., 2002b; Sonnweber et al., 2014) mainly by the oxygen-regulated hypoxia-inducible factor. In general, hypoxia inhibits hepcidin expression to allow the mobilization of iron to sustain erythropoietic expansion. However, a recent study showed that the exposure of mice to an hypoxic environment induces biphasic modulation of hepcidin expression with a transient increase in liver expression within the first 6 h and a reduction after 15 h of hypoxia (Ravasi et al., 2018).

Among ischemic stroke patients, who have areas of the brain exposed to oxygen and glucose deprivation (OGD), blood hepcidin levels increased within the first 6 h from symptom onset compared to those in controls; serum hepcidin levels in

ICH patients were similar to those of controls (unpublished results from our laboratory). This early increase in blood hepcidin during ischemic stroke is in agreement with the early increase reported in the hypoxic mice model (Ravasi et al., 2018) and with the two other reports on stroke patients (Petrova et al., 2015; Slomka et al., 2015) and might be a reflection of an increased expression and secretion of hepcidin from the ischemic brain cells to the extracellular medium, and a subsequent spillover out of the brain during stroke. Although hepcidin expression in the brain is thought to be low in basal conditions, hepcidin is now emerging as an important player in brain iron homeostasis (Vela, 2018). Hepcidin mRNA levels increased early in the brain in response to ischemia in a model of endothelin-induced vasoconstriction (Bickford et al., 2014), and hepcidin levels were significantly elevated in the ischemic side of the brain 24 h after occlusion in a stroke model due to middle cerebral artery occlusion; this ischemic side also showed increased TfR1 and FT levels and reduced FPN levels (Ding et al., 2011). In addition, knock-down of hepcidin slows the ischemic-mediated changes in brain FT and FPN, revealing an important contribution of this molecule to parenchyma iron regulation in cerebral ischemia. Further, normoxic iron-overloaded rats, hepcidin, either overexpressed in the brain or administrated to the brain parenchyma, reduced brain uptake of iron *in vivo* as well as reduced iron uptake in cultures of neurons or brain microvascular endothelial cells, owing to the dowregulation of iron-transport proteins (Du et al., 2015). In microglial cells, the bone morphogenetic protein antagonist noggin abrogated the OGD-induced changes in hepcidin, FPN, and FT levels, and this inhibition of bone morphogenetic protein/hepcidin axis *in vitro* shifted reactive microglia from an iron-storing to an iron-releasing phenotype after OGD plus reperfusion (Shin et al., 2018). Factors released from noggin- and OGD-exposed microglial culture medium were found to increase myelin production in oligodendrocyte cell cultures; since this effect is blunted by the iron chelator deferoxamine (DFO), iron released from the microglia is proposed to serve in the remyelination in the ischemic brain (Shin et al., 2018).

Endogenous Mechanisms Involved in the Protection of Brain Cells From Excess Iron Following ICH

Similar to that observed in AIS, subarachnoid hemorrhage has been shown to increase hepcidin expression in neurons (Zhao et al., 2018) associated with a reduction of its downstream target FPN (Tan et al., 2016). However, in this hemorrhage model, hepcidin seems to be harmful since its administration potentiated and its siRNA decreased apoptosis and early brain damage (Tan et al., 2016). In agreement with a harmful effect of hepcidin on brain hemorrhage, higher blood hepcidin levels were observed 1–7 days following ICH in patients with poorer outcomes (Xiong et al., 2015). The rationale for this harmful effect of hepcidin following ICH might be an impaired clearance of iron from brain parenchyma, since increased hepcidin expression caused by inflammation was found to inhibit intracellular iron efflux from brain microvascular endothelial cells and further draining of iron into circulation, leading to the aggravation of oxidative brain injury (Xiong et al., 2016). Conversely, addition of hepcidin or adenovirus-driven overexpression of hepcidin has been shown to protect neurons from hemin-induced injury (Zhou et al., 2017); this protection was thought to be related to the effect of hepcidin reducing hemin-induced iron uptake and reduced expression of TfR1 and DMT1.

Moreover, importantly, stroke has an inflammatory component, and some inflammatory inducers or mediators (e.g., lipopolysaccharide or interleukin 6) have been found to increase the expression of hepcidin in astrocytes, microglia, or neurons (for a recent review see Vela, 2018), although the effect on neurons is usually weaker (Ma et al., 2018).

The brain has protective mechanisms that can be activated after ICH and erythrocyte lysis, the most important one being the Hb-scavenging molecule haptoglobin (Hp) and the heme-scavenging system hemopexin (Hpx) (**Figure 2**). Hb itself is avidly bound by Hp to form a complex that prevents the release of the heme group from Hb or methemoglobin. However, Hp cannot prevent the release of the heme group from the highest oxidative Hb form ferrylHb. In the brain, Hp is almost exclusively synthesized by oligodendrocytes, and mice overexpressing Hp were more resistant, whereas Hp-knockout mice were more susceptible, to ICH injury (Zhao et al., 2011). The complex Hp:Hb binds to the Hp-specific receptor CD163 that is present in macrophages, allowing them to remove Hb from the extracellular space. In addition, CD163 is upregulated in neurons after ICH (Liu et al., 2017). The role of Hp in neuroprotection was not devoid of controversy since Hp was found to exacerbate the vulnerability of CD163-expressing neurons to Hb, an effect that was reduced by iron chelators (Chen-Roetling and Regan, 2016). However, most Hb was not bound to Hp, indicating that the CD163–Hb–Hp system is saturated, and that the primary route for Hb clearance from the CNS occurs through the BBB (Galea et al., 2012; Righy et al., 2018). A good clearance is associated with neuroprotection since lower CSF Hp levels were found in ICH patients without clinical and/or radiological evidence of delayed cerebral ischemia (Galea et al., 2012). Hb accumulated in the brain parenchyma is converted to ferrylHb, which causes the upregulation of proinflammatory adhesion molecules and increases the recruitment of inflammatory neutrophils or macrophages (Jeney et al., 2013).

Iron–hemin uptake has been reported in neurons and astrocytes and is especially high in microglial cell cultures; neurons benefit from a high export of iron following the initial iron–hemin loading, and this export was exacerbated by treatment with DFO, a compound that attenuates hemin neurotoxicity (Chen-Roetling et al., 2014). As already mentioned, the brain produces the heme scavenger protein Hpx that protects from deleterious effects of heme. In this regard, deletion/knockout of the Hpx aggravates brain injury by ICH (Chen L. et al., 2011; Ma et al., 2016) and, although endogenous levels of Hpx are insufficient to counteract the massive heme overload following ICH, increasing brain Hpx levels has been found to improve the outcome after ICH (Leclerc et al., 2018). Conversely, Hpx has recently been reported to increase the neurotoxicity of Hb in the absence of Hp (Chen-Roetling et al., 2018). Therefore, although both Hp and Hpx might provide a robust line of defense during ICH, additional knowledge on the fine tuning of this system is still required to design new possible neuroprotective treatments for ICH. The low-density lipoprotein receptor-related protein CD91 is expressed in several cell types, including macrophages and neurons, and was identified as the Hpx–heme receptor, mediating Hpx–heme uptake by endocytosis (Hvidberg et al., 2005). Once inside the cell, the heme oxygenase (HO) system is responsible for cellular heme degradation. In neurons, HO generates biliverdin, which has been reported to scavenge free radicals. Astrocytes rapidly upregulate HO1 and FT and are resistant to heme-mediated injury, and astrocyte HO1 is known to play a robust neuroprotective role after hemorrhage (Chen-Roetling et al., 2017). A recent study indicated that Hpx activates endothelial progenitor cells and reduces synaptic damage in a rodent ischemic stroke model; these effects require HO1 activity (Yang et al., 2018).

Moreover, the presence of heme groups in the extracellular milieu activates the endothelial expression of adhesion molecules and promotes the activation of neutrophil extracellular traps through a mechanism dependent on ROS generation (Chen et al., 2014). Further, inflammatory response is a well-documented mechanism of brain damage after ICH (Wang and Doré, 2007), and the mechanisms underlying heme-induced inflammation have been reviewed elsewhere (Dutra and Bozza, 2014). Iron and heme associated with pro-inflammatory mediators in the CNS following hemorrhagic stroke and inflammatory profiles are associated with poorer prognosis. Similarly, iron-induced damage following ischemic stroke in iron-overloaded animals has also been related to increased inflammatory responses associated with increased serum levels of interleukin 6 and TNF-alpha (Castellanos et al., 2002).

THE FERROPTOTIC COMPONENT OF STROKE-INDUCED NEURODEGENERATION

The Concept of Ferroptosis: Molecular Players Involved in Ferroptosis in the Neurons

The concept of ferroptosis was introduced as a form of cell death, which is morphologically, biochemically, and genetically distinct from apoptosis, necrosis, and autophagy; it is associated with excessive iron-mediated accumulation of lipid ROS in cancer cells as well as in hippocampal slice cultures exposed to glutamate excitotoxicity (Dixon et al., 2012). As excitotoxicity is the main mechanism involved in neuronal death in ischemic stroke, the involvement of ferroptosis in ischemic stroke could be suspected. In addition, the role of high systemic iron exacerbating stroke-induced damage, concomitant with increased brain iron after ischemic stroke onset (reviewed in the previous section), further suggested a possible ferroptosis component in stroke; in the recent past, mounting evidence indicated that ferroptosis plays such a pivotal role in stroke-induced neurodegeneration in both ischemic and hemorrhagic stroke subtypes. Although the concept is still evolving, ferroptosis is now considered a unique form of regulated cell death characterized by cytosolic accumulation of iron and executed by the massive peroxidation of PUFA in the plasma membrane and associated with reduced glutathione (GSH). Compounds that induce only either cytosolic or mitochondrial ROS production are not considered as ferroptosis inducers. A recent study proposed that both Fenton reactions, in which Fe^{2+} converts to Fe^{3+} producing ROS, and enzymatic lipoxygenase-mediated reactions in cellular membranes contribute to ferroptosis (Feng and Stockwell, 2018). Some authors considered that the ferroptosis concept and the previously described oxidative oxytosis concept have many common features to be regarded as independent processes (Lewerenz et al., 2018). In fact, the widely used oxidative stress stimulus *tert*-butylhydroperoxide was found to induce neuronal cell death that was blocked by ferroptosis inhibitors, thereby implying a crosstalk between the initial oxidative damage and the occurrence of ferroptosis (Wu et al., 2018). However, ferroptosis is considered a major driver of cell death in many neurodegenerative and neurological diseases (Lewerenz et al., 2018; Morris et al., 2018).

Ferroptosis can be triggered by the inhibitors of the lipid repair enzyme glutathione peroxidase 4 (GPX4), such as the RAS-selective lethal 3 compound, or depletion of the antioxidant GSH by starving the cells of GSH precursors [inhibiting the cystine/glutamate antiporter, i.e., system X_c^- (X_c^-) with erastin, sulfasalazine, sorafenib, or, alternatively, challenging the exchange capacity of X_c^- with high extracellular glutamate]. Extracellular Tf in its iron-loaded HTf form is considered as an inducer of ferroptosis as well, and inhibiting TfR expression prevents ferroptosis (Gao et al., 2015).

At present, the existence of X_c^- in neurons is still controversial, with one report showing expression lack of X_c^- in neurons (Ottestad-Hansen et al., 2018), whereas another showing neurons expressing significant X_c^- levels (Soria et al., 2016). However, neurons in culture overexpress X_c^- shortly after being exposed to OGD (Soria et al., 2014). The physiological role of X_c^- as a cystine importer is linked to its antiporter glutamate export and requires that extracellular levels of glutamate and other excitatory amino acids are maintained low by the action of excitatory amino acid transporters (EAATs). Thus, one of these glutamate transporters, the sodium-dependent EAAT3, might be selectively expressed in neurons and could also be an unidirectional cysteine import channel, with extracellular glutamate inhibiting its cysteine import capacity (Watts et al., 2014). EAAT3 might be as important as X_c^- in providing GSH precursors to neurons, considering that mice lacking EAAT3 have lower GSH levels and age prematurely (Aoyama et al., 2006). Notably, low GSH levels might also inhibit GPX4 activity since GPX4 uses GSH as a cofactor to catalyze the reduction of lipid peroxides and protect cells membranes against peroxidation (see Latunde-Dada, 2017).

Conversely, ferroptosis can be prevented by (1) iron-binding compounds such as DFO and ciclopirox; (2) small molecules, free radical scavengers, or lipophilic antioxidants such as ferrostatin-1, α-tocopherol, butylated hydroxytoluene, or liproxstatin-1; (3) treatments with molecules such as deuterated

PUFA, inhibitors of acyl-CoA synthetase long-chain family member 4, lipoxygenase inhibitors, glutaminolysis inhibitors, or cycloheximide; or (4) boosting cystine and/or cysteine import by reducing extracellular glutamate.

Glutamate is the most abundant excitatory neurotransmitters in the vertebrate nervous system, with 90% of the synaptic neurotransmission considered glutamatergic (Hofmeijer and Van Putten, 2012; Mayor and Tymianski, 2018). Under physiological conditions, extracellular glutamate levels are low, and glutamate exerts its physiological role mainly at the neuronal synapse. The ability of astrocytes near glutamatergic neurons to rapidly clear synaptic glutamate after its physiological action is critical in the functioning of synapses and neuronal circuits, and the initial increase of extracellular glutamate is inhibited mainly by glial EAAT1 and 2. Neuronal glutamate transporters, mainly EAAT3, also play a role in clearing extracellular glutamate excess. However, ischemia leads to energy failure and subsequent electrochemical gradient impairment, causing EAATs to act in a reversed manner, thereby extruding non-vesicular intracellular glutamate and resulting in large excess of extracellular glutamate and impairment of EAAT3 as a unidirectional cysteine import channel.

The impact of excess extracellular glutamate on neuronal survival is more than that on the cystine/glutamate exchanger X_c^-. In fact, most of the effect is produced by glutamate binding to specific glutamate receptors present in cell membranes of several cell types and, especially in neurons, *N*-methyl-D-aspartate (NMDA) subtype of glutamate receptors (NMDARs) (Guirao et al., 2017) that are coupled to an intracellular downstream complex of signaling effectors, which are known to initiate excitotoxic neuronal death following ischemia.

Although both glutamate and iron are essential for neuronal survival, excess glutamate can be toxic, and excess free iron through the Fenton reaction is a potentially toxic substance that can catalyze the production of extremely damaging ROS. During stroke, the impairment of BBB function allows increased access to brain of iron-carrying substances and, preceding neurodegeneration, iron accumulates in the ischemic areas (Helal, 2008); therefore, not surprisingly, iron overload conditions are associated with larger areas of brain damage in animals exposed to experimental ischemic stroke (Castellanos et al., 2002; Gamez et al., 2003; Mehta et al., 2004; García-Yébenes et al., 2012; DeGregorio-Rocasolano et al., 2018). Following experimental stroke or NMDAR overactivation, prevention of NMDA-induced neuronal iron uptake was found to be neuroprotective (DeGregorio-Rocasolano et al., 2018). Therefore, the crosstalk between neuronal homeostasis of iron and glutamatergic signaling is increasingly being supported by evidence and should not be disregarded as a therapeutic intervention target.

Glutamate-Induced Iron Uptake in Neurons and Ferroptosis

Cheah et al. (2006) from Dr. Snyder's laboratory published a study before the concept of ferroptosis was introduced and showed that the overactivation of NMDAR in neurons induces, in addition to the well-known NMDAR-mediated calcium influx, an NMDAR-mediated iron uptake. They also identified a signaling cascade whereby NMDAR regulated neuronal iron homeostasis and excitotoxicity through an NMDAR/nitric oxide/dexamethasone-induced Ras protein 1 (Dexras1) pathway that increased both non-Tf and Tf-mediated iron uptake from the extracellular medium through the neuronal plasma membrane (Cheah et al., 2006). A similar increase of iron uptake in hippocampal neurons was observed in a subsequent study in which either synaptic activity or NMDAR activity was boosted (Pelizzoni et al., 2011). Moreover, either ischemia or NMDA overactivation increased the uptake of HTf, resulting in an increase of cytosolic redox-active iron in neurons, whereas blockade of TfR1 reduced iron dyshomeostasis and NMDA-induced excitotoxicity (DeGregorio-Rocasolano et al., 2018). The original work from Snyder's laboratory hypothesized that iron in its free form gains access to the neuronal cytosol through DMT1 present in the neuronal membrane. However, this would not explain the uptake of Tf-bound iron since the DMT1 isoform endogenously overexpressed in primary cultures of hippocampal neurons exposed to NMDA is DMT1-1B/IRE(+) (Haeger et al., 2010) and is found in endosomes/lysosomes in the cytoplasm (Pelizzoni et al., 2012), thereby not supporting a direct role of DMT1 in iron entry through the neuronal membrane. Following the above rationale of crossroads between excitotoxicity and ferroptosis, several *in vitro* and *in vivo* studies showed that neurons survive otherwise lethal NMDA or glutamate concentrations when treated with iron chelators such as DFO or deferasirox (Yu et al., 2009; Tian et al., 2017; Sakamoto et al., 2018). Moreover, a study showed that the deletion of Dexras1 reduced NMDA-induced iron uptake and NMDA toxicity in cortical neurons and retinal ganglion cells (Chen et al., 2013). Moreover, Dexras1-KO mice showed increased expression of the NR2A subunit of the NMDAR (Carlson et al., 2016), a subunit that is preferentially located at synapses and related to NMDAR pro-survival signaling; this strongly suggests the existence of a functional crosstalk between the NMDA-induced iron intracellular signaling and the physiological NMDAR function. Interestingly, intracellular iron released from lysosomes has been shown to modulate NMDAR synaptic excitability via Dexras1 (White et al., 2016), and iron is needed post-synaptically to activate Ca^{2+}-dependent pathways downstream NMDAR (Muñoz et al., 2011). Further, glutamate-induced neuronal excitotoxicity was described as ferroptosis (Dixon et al., 2012).

In the widely reported scenario of elevated extracellular glutamate during ischemic stroke, NMDAR-induced iron import was upregulated in neurons associated with increased ROS production (Cheah et al., 2006), and system X_c^- and EAAT3 cystine/cysteine import are impaired by high extracellular glutamate (Conrad and Sato, 2012), thus compromising neuronal iron homeostasis and GSH-mediated free radical detoxification, eventually leading to an excess lipid oxidative stress that causes ferroptotic damage. High GSH stores are pivotal for cell survival since GSH is required for GPX4 activity and is also thought to be the only molecular species having a significant role as a cytosolic ligand for Fe^{2+} (Philpott and

Ryu, 2014). Even when ischemia is resolved in the brain owing to a successful reperfusion, other mechanisms involved in ferroptotic damage might become dangerous. In this regard, a recent study on Sertoli cells revealed that GPX4 is inactivated via GSH depletion following I/R injury (Li et al., 2018), and several studies showed that GPX4 gene inactivation causes hippocampal neurodegeneration (Seiler et al., 2008; Hambright et al., 2017) and a remarkable degeneration of motor neurons (Chen et al., 2015).

Ferroptosis in AIS and ICH Stroke Subtypes: Effect of Ferroptosis Inhibitors and Iron Chelators

In addition to a pivotal role of ferroptosis in I/R-induced damage in several peripheral organs (Friedmann Angeli et al., 2014; Linkermann et al., 2014; Gao et al., 2015), a role of ferroptosis has been specifically identified in I/R-induced brain damage in transient ischemia, as brain damage was substantially reduced by the ferroptosis inhibitor liproxstatin-1 in an AIS model (Tuo et al., 2017). These authors also showed that a reduction of tau levels, a protein that facilitates iron export by trafficking APP to membranes to stabilize FPN, was found to precede a pro-ferroptotic iron accumulation in the brain following I/R (Tuo et al., 2017). APP mRNA possesses a functional IRE with sequence homology to that of FT, and its translation is responsive to free iron levels in the cytosol (Duce et al., 2010). In addition, APP has been reported to interact with FPN to promote iron release in several brain cell types (Duce et al., 2010; McCarthy et al., 2014). APP overexpression reduces free iron content in neuroblastoma cells (Wan et al., 2012), and either preventing APP transport to the cell surface or knocking down of APP results in iron accumulation in primary cortical neurons in culture (Lei et al., 2012). The complete role of APP in ferroptosis and neurodegeneration in AIS requires additional studies. However, further evidence supporting the involvement of ferroptosis mechanisms in AIS brain damage is provided by the overexpression of lipoxygenases following brain ischemia and the protection afforded by treatment with lipoxygenase inhibitors (Cui et al., 2010; Karatas et al., 2018). Further, a recent study showed that *N*-acetylcysteine (NAC), an FDA-approved cysteine prodrug, prevents hemin-induced ferroptosis by neutralizing toxic lipids generated by arachidonate-dependent activity of 5-lipoxygenases (ALOX5) (Karuppagounder et al., 2018). They reported that ALOX5 inhibitors such as zileuton and molecules such as NAC that inhibit toxic metabolic products of ALOX5 or prevent ALOX5 recruitment to its site of action, protect against hemin or ICH-induced ferroptosis (Karuppagounder et al., 2018). Notably, NAC has been previously reported to prevent neuronal damage induced by AIS (Khan et al., 2004; Turkmen et al., 2016).

Further, the role of free iron in ferroptosis and neurodegeneration is further supported by the protective effect of treatments with exogenous iron chelators, e.g., DFO or 2,2′-dipyridyl, in animal models of stroke. After permanent ischemic stroke (Millerot-Serrurot et al., 2008), the increase in free iron, the iron form prone to induce lipid peroxidation and susceptible to be chelated, precedes the increase in total iron. In experimental models of transient ischemic stroke, DFO administered intramuscularly (Xing et al., 2009) or intranasally (Hanson et al., 2009) after the induction of ischemia significantly decreased infarct volume. Another iron chelator, the aforementioned 2,2'-dipyridyl was found to be cytoprotective after permanent arterial occlusion in rats; this was associated with reduced infarct size and preservation of GSH levels (Demougeot et al., 2004) or reduction of the apoptotic component and prevention of the enlargement of the lesion (Van Hoecke et al., 2005).

The role of iron in ICH neurodegeneration has been known for long. Recently, neuronal death following ICH was found to have features similar to those of ferroptosis, since chemical inhibitors of ferroptosis protected against Hb- and hemin-induced neurotoxicity (Zille et al., 2017). The nonheme iron present in brain parenchyma after ICH is a source of redox-active iron. The marked increase in brain nonheme iron was not cleared for weeks following the ICH event, and brain Tf, TfR, and FT levels were also increased 72 h after ICH, thereby making FT upregulation long-lasting (Wu et al., 2003). Iron chelators such as DFO reduce hemin- and iron-mediated neurotoxicity, perihematoma edema, and neuronal damage, leading to good neurologic outcomes after ICH (Nakamura et al., 2004; Hatakeyama et al., 2013). Other recent studies indicated that the specific inhibitor of ferroptosis ferrostatin-1 reduces neuron degeneration and improves neurological deficit in experimental ICH models (Li Q. et al., 2017; Zhang et al., 2018), and GPX4 levels were found to be reduced after ICH, whereas pharmacological inhibition of GPX or genetic knockdown exacerbated brain injury after ICH (Zhang et al., 2018). Moreover, inhibitors of ALOX5 or inhibition of the ALOX5 metabolic products protected against hemin- or ICH-induced ferroptosis (Karuppagounder et al., 2018).

Moreover, DFO significantly reduced hemorrhagic transformation after focal I/R (Xing et al., 2009; Li Y. et al., 2017). Some studies have shown that the effect of DFO in preventing ischemic neuronal death is related to the DFO-induced expression of hypoxia-inducible factor 1 and its downstream targets genes rather than with its iron-chelating properties or, recently, with microglial/macrophage HO1 expression in ICH (LeBlanc et al., 2016). A systematic review and meta-analysis in experimental models of ICH showed that DFO was neuroprotective, e.g., reduction of brain edema and improvement of neurobehavioral outcomes, especially when it was administered 2–4 h after ICH induction (Cui et al., 2015). In clinical studies, conclusive evidence of the benefit of DFO treatment in ICH (Zeng et al., 2018) or AIS patients is still lacking; some clinical trials of DFO in ICH and AIS are currently ongoing.

The rationale for iron chelation as a neuroprotectant relies primarily on the idea that chelation removes free iron present in the blood and enhances iron elimination in the urine. After gaining access to other body compartments, DFO could also act by chelating free extracellular and cytosolic iron, whereas its effect on blood TSAT or blood total iron levels is modest (Tauchenová et al., 2016). In fact, DFO was shown to have an extremely slow removal rate of iron from Tf (Abergel and Raymond, 2008). This, together with the fact that DFO half-life in the plasma is extremely short (20 min), poses serious doubts about the effectiveness of the treatment with intravenous DFO unless administered with continuous infusion. Recently, another iron-regulator, apotransferrin, administered after stroke AIS onset, was found to be neuroprotective because of the systemic reduction of blood TSAT and a reduction of NMDA ischemia-induced neuronal iron import (DeGregorio-Rocasolano et al., 2018).

CONCLUSION

Increasing number of studies show that ferroptosis is involved in several neurodegenerative diseases. This review summarizes the knowledge available thus far regarding the role of iron and ferroptosis in the execution of neuronal cell death during AIS and ICH. In AIS-induced cell death, the role of systemic iron, Tf, TSAT, and hepcidin on excitotoxic damage, infarct size, and neurological outcome in rodent models of stroke might have important clinical implications. Following the AIS event, high levels of extracellular glutamate and impairment of the BBB allow the NMDAR-mediated influx of iron, either bound or not to Tf, into neurons. In addition, high extracellular glutamate prevents the neuronal production of the antioxidant GSH or the function of GPX4, thereby promoting a form of cell death in which glutamate receptor overactivation boosts neuronal iron uptake, which in turn promotes an overwhelming production of membrane peroxides. The role of iron in ICH neurodegeneration has been known for long, since blood spillover results in iron-Hb and iron–heme complexes at the extracellular milieu of brain parenchymal cells, thereby contributing to iron-induced lipid peroxidation and neuronal death. The review documents the beneficial effects of iron chelators such as DFO, physiological molecules with neuroprotective potential, and specific inhibitors of ferroptosis liproxstatin-1 or ferrostatin-1 in reducing neuron degeneration and improving neurologic deficits induced by ischemic and hemorrhagic stroke subtypes.

AUTHOR CONTRIBUTIONS

The three authors have contributed in a similar way to the writing of the article.

FUNDING

This study was supported by the following grants: Instituto de Salud Carlos III (ISCIII) INVICTUS PLUS RD16/0019/0020 that was susceptible to be co-financed by FEDER funds and Agència de Gestió d'Ajuts Universitaris i de Recerca 2017 SGR 1520. We acknowledge the funding received from "la Caixa" Foundation CI15-00009 and from the European Institute of Innovation and Technology (EIT) PoC-2016-SPAIN-04. EIT receives support from the European Union's Horizon 2020 research and innovation program.

REFERENCES

Abergel, R. J., and Raymond, K. N. (2008). Terephthalamide-containing ligands: fast removal of iron from transferrin. *J. Biol. Inorg. Chem.* 13, 229–240. doi: 10.1007/s00775-007-0314-y

Abulrob, A., Brunette, E., Slinn, J., Baumann, E., and Stanimirovic, D. (2011). In vivo optical imaging of ischemic blood-brain barrier disruption. *Methods Mol. Biol.* 763, 423–429. doi: 10.1007/978-1-61779-191-8_29

Acikyol, B., Graham, R. M., Trinder, D., House, M. J., Olynyk, J. K., Scott, R. J., et al. (2013). Brain transcriptome perturbations in the transferrin receptor 2 mutant mouse support the case for brain changes in iron loading disorders, including effects relating to long-term depression and long-term potentiation. *Neuroscience* 235, 119–128. doi: 10.1016/j.neuroscience.2013.01.014

Aoyama, K., Sang, W. S., Hamby, A. M., Liu, J., Wai, Y. C., Chen, Y., et al. (2006). Neuronal glutathione deficiency and age-dependent neurodegeneration in the EAAC1 deficient mouse. *Nat. Neurosci.* 9, 119–126. doi: 10.1038/nn1609

Arosio, P., Elia, L., and Poli, M. (2017). Ferritin, cellular iron storage and regulation. *IUBMB Life* 69, 414–422. doi: 10.1002/iub.1621

Asano, T., Komatsu, M., Yamaguchi-Iwai, Y., Ishikawa, F., Mizushima, N., and Iwai, K. (2011). Distinct mechanisms of ferritin delivery to lysosomes in iron-depleted and iron-replete cells. *Mol. Cell. Biol.* 31, 2040–2052. doi: 10.1128/MCB.01437-10

Ashraf, A., Clark, M., and So, P. W. (2018). The aging of iron man. *Front. Aging Neurosci.* 10:65. doi: 10.3389/fnagi.2018.00065

Bakhshayesh, B., Hosseininezhad, M., Saadat, S., Ansar, M., Ramezani, H., and Saadat, S. (2014). Iron overload is associated with perihematoma edema growth following intracerebral hemorrhage that may contribute to in-hospital mortality and long-term functional outcome. *Curr. Neurovasc. Res.* 11, 248–253. doi: 10.2174/1567202611666140530124855

Belaidi, A. A., Gunn, A. P., Wong, B. X., Ayton, S., Appukuttan, A. T., Roberts, B. R., et al. (2018). Marked age-related changes in brain iron homeostasis in amyloid protein precursor knockout mice. *Neurotherapeutics* 15, 1055–1062. doi: 10.1007/s13311-018-0656-x

Bickford, J. S., Ali, N. F., Nick, J. A., Al-Yahia, M., Beachy, D. E., Doré, S., et al. (2014). Endothelin-1-mediated vasoconstriction alters cerebral gene expression in iron homeostasis and eicosanoid metabolism. *Brain Res.* 1588, 25–36. doi: 10.1016/j.brainres.2014.09.022

Bradbury, M. W. (1997). Transport of iron in the blood-brain-cerebrospinal fluid system. *J. Neurochem.* 69, 443–454. doi: 10.1046/j.1471-4159.1997.69020443.x

Burdo, J. R., Menzies, S. L., Simpson, I. A., Garrick, L. M., Garrick, M. D., Dolan, K. G., et al. (2001). Distribution of divalent metal transporter 1 and metal transport protein 1 in the normal and Belgrade rat. *J. Neurosci. Res.* 66, 1198–1207. doi: 10.1002/jnr.1256

Carbonell, T., and Rama, M. (2007). Iron, oxidative stress and early neurological deterioration in ischemic stroke. *Curr. Med. Chem.* 14, 857–874. doi: 10.2174/092986707780363014

Carlson, G. C., Lin, R. E., Chen, Y., Brookshire, B. R., White, R. S., Lucki, I., et al. (2016). Dexras1 a unique ras-GTPase interacts with NMDA receptor activity and provides a novel dissociation between anxiety, working memory and sensory gating. *Neuroscience* 322, 408–415. doi: 10.1016/j.neuroscience.2016.02.063

Castellanos, M., Puig, N., Carbonell, T., Castillo, J., Martinez, J. M., Rama, R., et al. (2002). Iron intake increases infarct volume after permanent middle cerebral artery occlusion in rats. *Brain Res.* 952, 1–6. doi: 10.1016/S0006-8993(02)03179-7

Chamorro, Á, Dirnagl, U., Urra, X., and Planas, A. M. (2016). Neuroprotection in acute stroke: targeting excitotoxicity, oxidative and nitrosative stress, and inflammation. *Lancet Neurol.* 15, 869–881. doi: 10.1016/S1474-4422(16)00114-9

Cheah, J. H., Kim, S. F., Hester, L. D., Clancy, K. W., Patterson, S. E., Papadopoulos, V., et al. (2006). NMDA receptor-nitric oxide transmission mediates neuronal iron homeostasis via the GTPase Dexras1. *Neuron* 51, 431–440. doi: 10.1016/j.neuron.2006.07.011

Chen, G., Zhang, D., Fuchs, T. A., Manwani, D., Wagner, D. D., and Frenette, P. S. (2014). Heme-induced neutrophil extracellular traps contribute to the pathogenesis of sickle cell disease. *Blood* 123, 3818–3827. doi: 10.1182/blood-2013-10-529982

Chen, H., Yoshioka, H., Kim, G. S., Jung, J. E., Okami, N., Sakata, H., et al. (2011). Oxidative stress in ischemic brain damage: mechanisms of cell death and potential molecular targets for neuroprotection. *Antioxid. Redox Signal.* 14, 1505–1517. doi: 10.1089/ars.2010.3576

Chen, L., Zhang, X., Chen-Roetling, J., and Regan, R. F. (2011). Increased striatal injury and behavioral deficits after intracerebral hemorrhage in hemopexin knockout mice. *J. Neurosurg.* 114, 1159–1167. doi: 10.3171/2010.10.JNS10861

Chen, L., Hambright, W. S., Na, R., and Ran, Q. (2015). Ablation of the ferroptosis inhibitor glutathione peroxidase 4 in neurons results in rapid motor neuron degeneration and paralysis. *J. Biol. Chem.* 290, 28097–28106. doi: 10.1074/jbc.M115.680090

Chen, Y., Khan, R. S., Cwanger, A., Song, Y., Steenstra, C., Bang, S., et al. (2013). Dexras1, a small GTPase, is required for glutamate-NMDA neurotoxicity. *J. Neurosci.* 33, 3582–3587. doi: 10.1523/JNEUROSCI.1497-12.2013

Chen-Roetling, J., Cai, Y., Lu, X., and Regan, R. F. (2014). Hemin uptake and release by neurons and glia. *Free Radic. Biol. Med.* 48, 200–205. doi: 10.3109/10715762.2013.859386

Chen-Roetling, J., Kamalapathy, P., Cao, Y., Song, W., Schipper, H. M., and Regan, R. F. (2017). Astrocyte heme oxygenase-1 reduces mortality and improves outcome after collagenase-induced intracerebral hemorrhage. *Neurobiol. Dis.* 102, 140–146. doi: 10.1016/j.nbd.2017.03.008

Chen-Roetling, J., Ma, S.-K., Cao, Y., Shah, A., and Regan, R. F. (2018). Hemopexin increases the neurotoxicity of hemoglobin when haptoglobin is absent. *J. Neurochem.* 145, 464–473. doi: 10.1111/jnc.14328

Chen-Roetling, J., and Regan, R. (2016). Haptoglobin increases the vulnerability of CD163-expressing neurons to hemoglobin. *J. Neurochem.* 139, 586–589. doi: 10.1111/jnc.13720

Chiou, B., Lucassen, E., Sather, M., Kallianpur, A., and Connor, J. (2018a). Semaphorin4A and H-ferritin utilize Tim-1 on human oligodendrocytes: a novel neuro-immune axis. *Glia* 66, 1317–1330. doi: 10.1002/glia.23313

Chiou, B., Neal, E. H., Bowman, A. B., Lippmann, E. S., Simpson, I. A., and Connor, J. R. (2018b). Endothelial cells are critical regulators of iron transport in a model of the human blood–brain barrier. *J. Cereb. Blood Flow Metab.* doi: 10.1177/0271678X18783372 [Epub ahead of print].

Cobley, J. N., Fiorello, M. L., and Bailey, D. M. (2018). 13 Reasons why the brain is susceptible to oxidative stress. *Redox Biol.* 15, 490–503. doi: 10.1016/j.redox.2018.01.008

Conrad, M., and Sato, H. (2012). The oxidative stress-inducible cystine/glutamate antiporter, system Xc-: cystine supplier and beyond. *Amino Acids* 42, 231–246. doi: 10.1007/s00726-011-0867-5

Cui, H. J., He, H. Y., Yang, A. L., Zhou, H. J., Wang, C., Luo, J. K., et al. (2015). Efficacy of deferoxamine in animal models of intracerebral hemorrhage: a systematic review and stratified meta-analysis. *PLoS One* 10:e0127256. doi: 10.1371/journal.pone.0127256

Cui, L., Zhang, X., Yang, R., Liu, L., Wang, L., Li, M., et al. (2010). Baicalein is neuroprotective in rat MCAO model: role of 12/15-lipoxygenase, mitogen-activated protein kinase and cytosolic phospholipase A2. *Pharmacol. Biochem. Behav.* 96, 469–475. doi: 10.1016/j.pbb.2010.07.007

Das, A., Nag, S., Mason, A. B., and Barroso, M. M. (2016). Endosome–mitochondria interactions are modulated by iron release from transferrin. *J. Cell Biol.* 214, 831–845. doi: 10.1083/jcb.201602069

Davalos, A., Fernandez-Real, J. M., Ricart, W., Soler, S., Molins, A., Planas, E., et al. (1994). Iron-related damage in acute ischemic stroke. *Stroke* 25, 1543–1546. doi: 10.1161/01.STR.25.8.1543

De Valk, B., Addicks, M. A., Gosriwatana, I., Lu, S., Hider, R. C., and Marx, J. J. M. (2000). Non-transferrin-bound iron is present in serum of hereditary haemochromatosis heterozygotes. *Eur. J. Clin. Invest.* 30, 248–251. doi: 10.1046/j.1365-2362.2000.00628.x

Deane, R., Zheng, W., and Zlokovic, B. V. (2004). Brain capillary endothelium and choroid plexus epithelium regulate transport of transferrin-bound and free iron into the rat brain. *J. Neurochem.* 88, 813–820. doi: 10.1046/j.1471-4159.2003.02221.x

DeGregorio-Rocasolano, N., Martí-Sistac, O., Ponce, J., Castelló-Ruiz, M., Millán, M., Guirao, V., et al. (2018). Iron-loaded transferrin (Tf) is detrimental whereas iron-free Tf confers protection against brain ischemia by modifying blood Tf saturation and subsequent neuronal damage. *Redox Biol.* 15, 143–158. doi: 10.1016/j.redox.2017.11.026

Demougeot, C., Van Hoecke, M., Bertrand, N., Prigent-Tessier, A., Mossiat, C., Beley, A., et al. (2004). Cytoprotective efficacy and mechanisms of the liposoluble iron chelator 2,2'-dipyridyl in the rat photothrombotic ischemic stroke model. *J. Pharmacol. Exp. Ther.* 311, 1080–1087. doi: 10.1124/jpet.104.072744

Desestret, V., Brisset, J. C., Moucharrafie, S., Devillard, E., Nataf, S., Honnorat, J., et al. (2009). Early-stage investigations of ultrasmall superparamagnetic iron oxide-induced signal change after permanent middle cerebral artery occlusion in mice. *Stroke* 40, 1834–1841. doi: 10.1161/STROKEAHA.108.531269

Ding, H., Yan, C. Z., Shi, H., Zhao, Y. S., Chang, S. Y., Yu, P., et al. (2011). Hepcidin is involved in iron regulation in the ischemic brain. *PLoS One* 6:e25324. doi: 10.1371/journal.pone.0025324

Dixon, S. J., Lemberg, K. M., Lamprecht, M. R., Skouta, R., Zaitsev, E. M., Gleason, C. E., et al. (2012). Ferroptosis: an iron-dependent form of nonapoptotic cell death. *Cell* 149, 1060–1072. doi: 10.1016/j.cell.2012.03.042

Drecourt, A., Babdor, J., Dussiot, M., Petit, F., Goudin, N., Garfa-Traoré, M., et al. (2018). Impaired transferrin receptor palmitoylation and recycling in neurodegeneration with brain iron accumulation. *Am. J. Hum. Genet.* 102, 266–277. doi: 10.1016/j.ajhg.2018.01.003

Du, F., Qian, Z. M., Luo, Q., Yung, W. H., and Ke, Y. (2015). Hepcidin suppresses brain iron accumulation by downregulating iron transport proteins in iron-overloaded rats. *Mol. Neurobiol.* 52, 101–114. doi: 10.1007/s12035-014-8847-x

Duce, J. A., Tsatsanis, A., Cater, M. A., James, S. A., Robb, E., Wikhe, K., et al. (2010). An iron-export ferroxidase activity of APP is inhibited by zinc in Alzheimer's disease. *Cell* 142, 857–867. doi: 10.1016/j.cell.2010.08.014

Duck, K. A., Simpson, I. A., and Connor, J. R. (2017). Regulatory mechanisms for iron transport across the blood-brain barrier. *Biochem. Biophys. Res. Commun.* 494, 70–75. doi: 10.1016/j.bbrc.2017.10.083

Dutra, F. F., and Bozza, M. T. (2014). Heme on innate immunity and inflammation. *Front. Pharmacol.* 5:115. doi: 10.3389/fphar.2014.00115

Dziuba, N., and Lindahl, P. A. (2018). Low-molecular-mass iron in healthy blood plasma is not predominately ferric citrate. *Metallomics* 10, 802–817. doi: 10.1039/c8mt00055g

Feng, H., and Stockwell, B. R. (2018). Unsolved mysteries: how does lipid peroxidation cause ferroptosis? *PLoS Biol.* 16:e2006203. doi: 10.1371/journal.pbio.2006203

Friedmann Angeli, J. P., Schneider, M., Proneth, B., Tyurina, Y. Y., Tyurin, V. A., Hammond, V. J., et al. (2014). Inactivation of the ferroptosis regulator Gpx4 triggers acute renal failure in mice. *Nat. Cell Biol.* 16, 1180–1191. doi: 10.1038/ncb3064

Gaasch, J. A., Lockman, P. R., Geldenhuys, W. J., Allen, D. D., and Van Der Schyf, C. J. (2007). Brain iron toxicity: differential responses of astrocytes, neurons, and endothelial cells. *Neurochem. Res.* 32, 1196–1208. doi: 10.1007/s11064-007-9290-4

Galea, J., Cruickshank, G., Teeling, J. L., Boche, D., Garland, P., Perry, V. H., et al. (2012). The intrathecal CD163-haptoglobin-hemoglobin scavenging system in subarachnoid hemorrhage. *J. Neurochem.* 121, 785–792. doi: 10.1111/j.1471-4159.2012.07716.x

Gamez, A., Carbonell, T., and Rama, R. (2003). Does nitric oxide contribute to iron-dependent brain injury after experimental cerebral ischaemia? *J. Physiol. Biochem.* 59, 249–254. doi: 10.1007/BF03179881

Gao, G., Zhang, N., Wang, Y., Wu, Q., Yu, P., Shi, Z., et al. (2017). Mitochondrial ferritin protects hydrogen peroxide-induced neuronal cell damage. *Aging Dis.* 8, 458–470. doi: 10.14336/AD.2016.1108

Gao, M., Monian, P., Quadri, N., Ramasamy, R., and Jiang, X. (2015). Glutaminolysis and transferrin regulate ferroptosis. *Mol. Cell* 59, 298–308. doi: 10.1016/j.molcel.2015.06.011

García-Yébenes, I., García-Culebras, A., Peña-Martínez, C., Fernández-López, D., Díaz-Guzmán, J., Negredo, P., et al. (2018). Iron overload exacerbates the risk of hemorrhagic transformation after tPA (tissue-type plasminogen activator) administration in thromboembolic stroke mice. *Stroke* 49, 2163–2172. doi: 10.1161/STROKEAHA.118.021540

García-Yébenes, I., Sobrado, M., Moraga, A., Zarruk, J. G., Romera, V. G., Pradillo, J. M., et al. (2012). Iron overload, measured as serum ferritin, increases brain damage induced by focal ischemia and early reperfusion. *Neurochem. Int.* 61, 1364–1369. doi: 10.1016/j.neuint.2012.09.014

Garton, A. L. A., Gupta, V. P., Christophe, B. R., and Connolly, E. S. (2017). Biomarkers of functional outcome in intracerebral hemorrhage: interplay between clinical metrics, CD163, and ferritin. *J. Stroke Cerebrovasc. Dis.* 26, 1712–1720. doi: 10.1016/j.jstrokecerebrovasdis.2017.03.035

Gazzina, S., Premi, E., Zanella, I., Biasiotto, G., Archetti, S., Cosseddu, M., et al. (2016). Iron in frontotemporal lobar degeneration: a new subcortical pathological pathway? *Neurodegener. Dis.* 16, 172–178. doi: 10.1159/000440843

Guan, H., Yang, H., Yang, M., Yanagisawa, D., Bellier, J. P., Mori, M., et al. (2017). Mitochondrial ferritin protects SH-SY5Y cells against H2O2-induced oxidative stress and modulates α-synuclein expression. *Exp. Neurol.* 291, 51–61. doi: 10.1016/j.expneurol.2017.02.001

Guirao, V., Martí-Sistac, O., DeGregorio-Rocasolano, N., Ponce, J., Dávalos, A., and Gasull, T. (2017). Specific rescue by ortho-hydroxy atorvastatin of cortical GABAergic neurons from previous oxygen/glucose deprivation: role of pCREB. *J. Neurochem.* 143, 359–374. doi: 10.1111/jnc.14210

Gutteridge, J. M., Richmond, R., and Halliwell, B. (1979). Inhibition of the iron-catalysed formation of hydroxyl radicals from superoxide and of lipid peroxidation by desferrioxamine. *Biochem. J.* 184, 469–472. doi: 10.1042/bj1840469

Hadziahmetovic, M., Song, Y., Ponnuru, P., Iacovelli, J., Hunter, A., Haddad, N., et al. (2011). Age-dependent retinal iron accumulation and degeneration in hepcidin knockout mice. *Investig. Ophthalmol. Vis. Sci.* 52, 109–118. doi: 10.1167/iovs.10-6113

Haeger, P., Alvarez, A., Leal, N., Adasme, T., Núñez, M. T., and Hidalgo, C. (2010). Increased hippocampal expression of the divalent metal transporter 1 (DMT1) mRNA variants 1B and +IRE and DMT1 protein after NMDA-receptor stimulation or spatial memory training. *Neurotox. Res.* 17, 238–247. doi: 10.1007/s12640-009-9096-z

Hambright, W. S., Fonseca, R. S., Chen, L., Na, R., and Ran, Q. (2017). Ablation of ferroptosis regulator glutathione peroxidase 4 in forebrain neurons promotes cognitive impairment and neurodegeneration. *Redox Biol.* 12, 8–17. doi: 10.1016/j.redox.2017.01.021

Hamdi, A., Roshan, T. M., Kahawita, T. M., Mason, A. B., Sheftel, A. D., and Ponka, P. (2016). Erythroid cell mitochondria receive endosomal iron by a "kiss-and-run" mechanism. *Biochim. Biophys. Acta* 1863, 2859–2867. doi: 10.1016/j.bbamcr.2016.09.008

Han, J., Plummer, J., Liu, L., Byrd, A., Aschner, M., and Erikson, K. M. (2017). The impact of obesity on brain iron levels and α-synuclein expression is regionally dependent. *Nutr. Neurosci.* doi: 10.1080/1028415X.2017.1387720 [Epub ahead of print].

Hanson, L. R., Roeytenberg, A., Martinez, P. M., Coppes, V. G., Sweet, D. C., Rao, R. J., et al. (2009). Intranasal deferoxamine provides increased brain exposure and significant protection in rat ischemic stroke. *J. Pharmacol. Exp. Ther.* 330, 679–686. doi: 10.1124/jpet.108.149807

Hatakeyama, T., Okauchi, M., Hua, Y., Keep, R. F., and Xi, G. (2013). Deferoxamine reduces neuronal death and hematoma lysis after intracerebral hemorrhage in aged rats. *Transl. Stroke Res.* 4, 546–553. doi: 10.1007/s12975-013-0270-5

He, Y., Karabiyikoglu, M., Hua, Y., Keep, R. F., and Xi, G. (2012). Ischemic preconditioning attenuates brain edema after experimental intracerebral hemorrhage. *Transl. Stroke Res.* 3, 180–187. doi: 10.1007/s12975-012-0171-z

Heidari, M., Johnstone, D. M., Bassett, B., Graham, R. M., Chua, A. C. G., House, M. J., et al. (2016). Brain iron accumulation affects myelin-related molecular systems implicated in a rare neurogenetic disease family with neuropsychiatric features. *Mol. Psychiatry* 21, 1599–1607. doi: 10.1038/mp.2015.192

Helal, G. K. (2008). Systemic administration of Zn2+during the reperfusion phase of transient cerebral ischaemia protects rat hippocampus against iron-catalysed postischaemic injury. *Clin. Exp. Pharmacol. Physiol.* 35, 775–781. doi: 10.1111/j.1440-1681.2007.04858.x

Hofmeijer, J., and Van Putten, M. J. (2012). Ischemic cerebral damage: an appraisal of synaptic failure. *Stroke* 43, 607–615. doi: 10.1161/STROKEAHA.111.632943

Huang, H., Chen, J., Lu, H., Zhou, M., Chai, Z., and Hu, Y. (2017). Iron-induced generation of mitochondrial ROS depends on AMPK activity. *BioMetals* 30, 623–628. doi: 10.1007/s10534-017-0023-0

Huang, S., Du, F., Li, L., Liu, Y., Liu, Y., Zhang, C., et al. (2014). Angiotensin II inhibits uptake of transferrin-bound iron but not non-transferrin-bound iron by cultured astrocytes. *Neuropeptides* 48, 161–166. doi: 10.1016/j.npep.2014.04.001

Hvidberg, V., Maniecki, M. B., Jacobsen, C., Højrup, P., Møller, H. J., and Moestrup, S. K. (2005). Identification of the receptor scavenging hemopexin-heme complexes. *Blood* 106, 2572–2579. doi: 10.1182/blood-2005-03-1185

Jaffer, H., Adjei, I. M., and Labhasetwar, V. (2013). Optical imaging to map blood-brain barrier leakage. *Sci. Rep.* 3:3117. doi: 10.1038/srep03117

Jahanshad, N., Kohannim, O., Hibar, D. P., Stein, J. L., McMahon, K. L., de Zubicaray, G. I., et al. (2012). Brain structure in healthy adults is related to serum transferrin and the H63D polymorphism in the HFE gene. *Proc. Natl. Acad. Sci.* 109, E851–E859. doi: 10.1073/pnas.1105543109

Jeney, V., Eaton, J. W., Balla, G., and Balla, J. (2013). Natural history of the bruise: formation, elimination, and biological effects of oxidized hemoglobin. *Oxid. Med. Cell. Longev.* 2013:703571. doi: 10.1155/2013/703571

Ji, C., and Kosman, D. J. (2015). Molecular mechanisms of non-transferrin-bound and transferring-bound iron uptake in primary hippocampal neurons. *J. Neurochem.* 133, 668–683. doi: 10.1111/jnc.13040

Karatas, H., Eun Jung, J., Lo, E. H., and van Leyen, K. (2018). Inhibiting 12/15-lipoxygenase to treat acute stroke in permanent and tPA induced thrombolysis models. *Brain Res.* 1678, 123–128. doi: 10.1016/j.brainres.2017.10.024

Karuppagounder, S. S., Alin, L., Chen, Y., Brand, D., Bourassa, M. W., Dietrich, K., et al. (2018). N-acetylcysteine targets 5 lipoxygenase-derived, toxic lipids and can synergize with PGE 2 to inhibit ferroptosis and improve outcomes following hemorrhagic stroke in mice. *Ann. Neurol.* 84, 854–872. doi: 10.1002/ana.25356

Kaur, C., and Ling, E. A. (1995). Transient expression of transferrin receptors and localisation of iron in amoeboid microglia in postnatal rats. *J. Anat.* 186, 165–173.

Kawabata, H. (2018). Transferrin and transferrin receptors update. *Free Radic. Biol. Med.* doi: 10.1016/j.freeradbiomed.2018.06.037 [Epub ahead of print].

Kell, D. B. (2009). Iron behaving badly: inappropriate iron chelation as a major contributor to the aetiology of vascular and other progressive inflammatory and degenerative diseases. *BMC Med. Genomics* 2:2. doi: 10.1186/1755-8794-2-2

Khan, A. I., Liu, J., and Dutta, P. (2018). Iron transport kinetics through blood-brain barrier endothelial cells. *Biochim. Biophys. Acta Gen. Subj.* 1862, 1168–1179. doi: 10.1016/j.bbagen.2018.02.010

Khan, M., Sekhon, B., Jatana, M., Giri, S., Gilg, A. G., Sekhon, C., et al. (2004). Administration of N-Acetylcysteine after focal cerebral ischemia protects brain and reduces inflammation in a rat model of experimental stroke. *J. Neurosci. Res.* 76, 519–527. doi: 10.1002/jnr.20087

Klohs, J., Steinbrink, J., Bourayou, R., Mueller, S., Cordell, R., Licha, K., et al. (2009). Near-infrared fluorescence imaging with fluorescently labeled albumin: a novel method for non-invasive optical imaging of blood-brain barrier impairment after focal cerebral ischemia in mice. *J. Neurosci. Methods* 180, 126–132. doi: 10.1016/j.jneumeth.2009.03.002

Kumar, N., Rizek, P., Sadikovic, B., Adams, P. C., and Jog, M. (2016). Movement disorders associated with hemochromatosis. *Can. J. Neurol. Sci.* 43, 801–808. doi: 10.1017/cjn.2016.286

Kumar, S., Sheokand, N., Mhadeshwar, M. A., Raje, C. I., and Raje, M. (2012). Characterization of glyceraldehyde-3-phosphate dehydrogenase as a novel transferrin receptor. *Int. J. Biochem. Cell Biol.* 44, 189–199. doi: 10.1016/j.biocel.2011.10.016

Latunde-Dada, G. O. (2017). Ferroptosis: role of lipid peroxidation, iron and ferritinophagy. *Biochim. Biophys. Acta Gen. Subj.* 1861, 1893–1900. doi: 10.1016/j.bbagen.2017.05.019

LeBlanc, R. H., Chen, R., Selim, M. H., and Hanafy, K. A. (2016). Heme oxygenase-1-mediated neuroprotection in subarachnoid hemorrhage via intracerebroventricular deferoxamine. *J. Neuroinflammation* 13:244. doi: 10.1186/s12974-016-0709-1

Leclerc, J. L., Santiago-Moreno, J., Dang, A., Lampert, A. S., Cruz, P. E., Rosario, A. M., et al. (2018). Increased brain hemopexin levels improve outcomes after intracerebral hemorrhage. *J. Cereb. Blood Flow Metab.* 38, 1032–1046. doi: 10.1177/0271678X16679170

Lee, F. H. F., Su, P., Xie, Y. F., Wang, K. E., Wan, Q., and Liu, F. (2016). Disrupting GluA2-GAPDH interaction affects axon and dendrite development. *Sci. Rep.* 6:30458. doi: 10.1038/srep30458

Lei, P., Ayton, S., Finkelstein, D. I., Spoerri, L., Ciccotosto, G. D., Wright, D. K., et al. (2012). Tau deficiency induces parkinsonism with dementia by impairing APP-mediated iron export. *Nat. Med.* 18, 291–295. doi: 10.1038/nm.2613

Leitner, D. F., and Connor, J. R. (2012). Functional roles of transferrin in the brain. *Biochim. Biophys. Acta Gen. Subj.* 1820, 393–402. doi: 10.1016/j.bbagen.2011.10.016

Lewerenz, J., Ates, G., Methner, A., Conrad, M., and Maher, P. (2018). Oxytosis / ferroptosis —(re-) emerging roles for oxidative cell death in diseases of the central nervous system. *Front. Neurosci.* 12:214. doi: 10.3389/fnins.2018.00214

Li, J. Y., Paragas, N., Ned, R. M., Qiu, A., Viltard, M., Leete, T., et al. (2009). Scara5 Is a ferritin receptor mediating non-transferrin iron delivery. *Dev. Cell* 16, 35–46. doi: 10.1016/j.devcel.2008.12.002

Li, L., Fang, C. J., Ryan, J. C., Niemi, E. C., Lebron, J. A., Bjorkman, P. J., et al. (2010). Binding and uptake of H-ferritin are mediated by human transferrin receptor-1. *Proc. Natl. Acad. Sci.* 107, 3505–3510. doi: 10.1073/pnas.0913192107

Li, L., Hao, Y., Zhao, Y., Wang, H., Zhao, X., Jiang, Y., et al. (2018). Ferroptosis is associated with oxygen- glucose deprivation / reoxygenation- induced Sertoli cell death. *Int. J. Mol. Med.* 41, 3051–3062. doi: 10.3892/ijmm.2018.3469

Li, Q., Han, X., Lan, X., Gao, Y., Wan, J., Durham, F., et al. (2017). Inhibition of neuronal ferroptosis protects hemorrhagic brain. *JCI Insight* 2:e90777. doi: 10.1172/jci.insight.90777

Li, Y., Yang, H., Ni, W., and Gu, Y. (2017). Effects of deferoxamine on blood-brain barrier disruption after subarachnoid hemorrhage. *PLoS One* 12:e0172784. doi: 10.1371/journal.pone.0172784

Linkermann, A., Skouta, R., Himmerkus, N., Mulay, S. R., Dewitz, C., De Zen, F., et al. (2014). Synchronized renal tubular cell death involves ferroptosis. *Proc. Natl. Acad. Sci.* 111, 16836–16841. doi: 10.1073/pnas.1415518111

Liu, R., Cao, S., Hua, Y., Keep, R. F., Huang, Y., and Xi, G. (2017). CD163 expression in neurons after experimental intracerebral hemorrhage. *Stroke* 48, 1369–1375. doi: 10.1161/STROKEAHA.117.016850

Lo, A. C. Y., Cheung, A. K. H., Hung, V. K. L., Yeung, C. M., He, Q. Y., Chiu, J. F., et al. (2007). Deletion of aldose reductase leads to protection against cerebral ischemic injury. *J. Cereb. Blood Flow Metab.* 27, 1496–1509. doi: 10.1038/sj.jcbfm.9600452

Luck, A. N., and Mason, A. B. (2012). Transferrin-mediated cellular iron delivery. *Curr. Top. Membr.* 69, 3–35. doi: 10.1016/B978-0-12-394390-3.00001-X

Ma, B., Day, J. P., Phillips, H., Slootsky, B., Tolosano, E., and Doré, S. (2016). Deletion of the hemopexin or heme oxygenase-2 gene aggravates brain injury following stroma-free hemoglobin-induced intracerebral hemorrhage. *J. Neuroinflammation* 13, 1–12. doi: 10.1186/s12974-016-0490-1

Ma, J., Li, F., Gan, Z., Yu, Z., Bao, X., Shen, Y., et al. (2018). Different characteristics of hepcidin expression in IL-6 + / + and IL- 6 - / - neurons and astrocytes treated with lipopolysaccharides. *Neurochem. Res.* 43, 1624–1630. doi: 10.1007/s11064-018-2577-9

Mancias, J. D., Vaites, L. P., Nissim, S., Biancur, D. E., Kim, A. J., Wang, X., et al. (2015). Ferritinophagy via NCOA4 is required for erythropoiesis and is regulated by iron dependent HERC2-mediated proteolysis. *eLife* 4, 1–19. doi: 10.7554/eLife.10308

Man-man, X. U., Jun, W., and Jun-xia, X. I. E. (2017). Regulation of iron metabolism by hypoxia-inducible factors. *Sheng Li Xue Bao* 69, 598–610.

Marro, S., Chiabrando, D., Messana, E., Stolte, J., Turco, E., Tolosano, E., et al. (2010). Heme controls ferroportin1 (FPN1) transcription involving Bach1, Nrf2 and a MARE/ARE sequence motif at position -7007 of the FPN1 promoter. *Haematologica* 95, 1261–1268. doi: 10.3324/haematol.2009.020123

Mayor, D., and Tymianski, M. (2018). Neurotransmitters in the mediation of cerebral ischemic injury. *Neuropharmacology* 134, 178–188. doi: 10.1016/j.neuropharm.2017.11.050

McCarthy, R. C., and Kosman, D. J. (2014). Glial cell ceruloplasmin and hepcidin differentially regulate iron efflux from brain microvascular endothelial cells. *PLoS One* 9:e89003. doi: 10.1371/journal.pone.0089003

McCarthy, R. C., Park, Y.-H., and Kosman, D. J. (2014). sAPP modulates iron efflux from brain microvascular endothelial cells by stabilizing the ferrous iron exporter ferroportin. *EMBO Rep.* 15, 809–815. doi: 10.15252/embr.201338064

McCarthy, R. C., Sosa, J. C., Gardeck, A. M., Baez, A. S., Lee, C.-H., and Wessling-Resnick, M. (2018). Inflammation-induced iron transport and metabolism by brain microglia. *J. Biol. Chem.* 293, 7853–7863. doi: 10.1074/jbc.RA118.001949

Mehdiratta, M., Kumar, S., Hackney, D., Schlaug, G., and Selim, M. (2008). Association between serum ferritin level and perihematoma edema volume in patients with spontaneous intracerebral hemorrhage. *Stroke* 39, 1165–1170. doi: 10.1161/STROKEAHA.107.501213

Mehta, S. H., Webb, R. C., Ergul, A., Tawfik, A., and Dorrance, A. M. (2004). Neuroprotection by tempol in a model of iron-induced oxidative stress in acute ischemic stroke. *Am. J. Physiol. Regul. Integr. Comp. Physiol.* 286, R283–R288. doi: 10.1152/ajpregu.00446.2002

Millan, M., Sobrino, T., Castellanos, M., Nombela, F., Arenillas, J. F., Riva, E., et al. (2007). Increased body iron stores are associated with poor outcome after thrombolytic treatment in acute stroke. *Stroke* 38, 90–95. doi: 10.1161/01.STR.0000251798.25803.e0

Millerot, E., Prigent-Tessier, A. S., Bertrand, N. M., Faure, P. J. C., Mossiat, C. M., Giroud, M. E., et al. (2005). Serum ferritin in stroke: a marker of increased body iron stores or stroke severity? *J. Cereb. Blood Flow Metab.* 25, 1386–1393. doi: 10.1038/sj.jcbfm.9600140

Millerot-Serrurot, E., Bertrand, N., Mossiat, C., Faure, P., Prigent-Tessier, A., Garnier, P., et al. (2008). Temporal changes in free iron levels after brain ischemia. Relevance to the timing of iron chelation therapy in stroke. *Neurochem. Int.* 52, 1442–1448. doi: 10.1016/j.neuint.2008.04.002

Morris, G., Berk, M., Carvalho, A. F., Maes, M., Walker, A. J., and Puri, B. K. (2018). Why should neuroscientists worry about iron? The emerging role of ferroptosis in the pathophysiology of neuroprogressive diseases. *Behav. Brain Res.* 341, 154–175. doi: 10.1016/j.bbr.2017.12.036

Muñoz, P., Humeres, A., Elgueta, C., Kirkwood, A., Hidalgo, C., and Núñez, M. T. (2011). Iron mediates N-Methyl-D-aspartate receptor-dependent stimulation of calcium-induced pathways and hippocampal synaptic plasticity. *J. Biol. Chem.* 286, 13382–13392. doi: 10.1074/jbc.M110.213785

Nagy, Z., and Nardai, S. (2017). Cerebral ischemia/repefusion injury: from bench space to bedside. *Brain Res. Bull.* 134, 30–37. doi: 10.1016/j.brainresbull.2017.06.011

Nakamura, T., Keep, R. F., Hua, Y., Schallert, T., Hoff, J. T., and Xi, G. (2004). Deferoxamine-induced attenuation of brain edema and neurological deficits in a rat model of intracerebral hemorrhage. *J. Neurosurg.* 100, 672–678. doi: 10.3171/jns.2004.100.4.0672

Nandar, W., and Connor, J. R. (2011). HFE gene variants affect iron in the brain. *J. Nutr.* 141, 729S–739S. doi: 10.3945/jn.110.130351

Nicolas, G., Bennoun, M., Devaux, I., Beaumont, C., Grandchamp, B., Kahn, A., et al. (2001). Lack of hepcidin gene expression and severe tissue iron overload in upstream stimulatory factor 2 (USF2) knockout mice. *Proc. Natl. Acad. Sci.* 98, 8780–8785. doi: 10.1073/pnas.151179498

Nicolas, G., Bennoun, M., Porteu, A., Mativet, S., Beaumont, C., Grandchamp, B., et al. (2002a). Severe iron deficiency anemia in transgenic mice expressing liver hepcidin. *Proc. Natl. Acad. Sci.* 99, 4596–4601.

Nicolas, G., Chauvet, C., Viatte, L., Danan, J. L., Bigard, X., Devaux, I., et al. (2002b). The gene encoding the iron regulatory peptide hepcidin is regulated by anemia, hypoxia, and inflammation. *J. Clin. Invest.* 110, 1037–1044.

Ottestad-Hansen, S., Hu, Q. X., Follin-Arbelet, V. V., Bentea, E., Sato, H., Massie, A., et al. (2018). The cystine-glutamate exchanger (xCT, Slc7a11) is expressed in significant concentrations in a subpopulation of astrocytes in the mouse brain. *Glia* 66, 951–970. doi: 10.1002/glia.23294

Park, U. J., Lee, Y. A., Won, S. M., Lee, J. H., Kang, S. H., Springer, J. E., et al. (2011). Blood-derived iron mediates free radical production and neuronal death in the hippocampal CA1 area following transient forebrain ischemia in rat. *Acta Neuropathol.* 121, 459–473. doi: 10.1007/s00401-010-0785-8

Pelizzoni, I., Macco, R., Morini, M. F., Zacchetti, D., Grohovaz, F., and Codazzi, F. (2011). Iron handling in hippocampal neurons: activity-dependent iron entry and mitochondria-mediated neurotoxicity. *Aging Cell* 10, 172–183. doi: 10.1111/j.1474-9726.2010.00652.x

Pelizzoni, I., Zacchetti, D., Smith, C. P., Grohovaz, F., and Codazzi, F. (2012). Expression of divalent metal transporter 1 in primary hippocampal neurons: reconsidering its role in non-transferrin-bound iron influx. *J. Neurochem.* 120, 269–278. doi: 10.1111/j.1471-4159.2011.07578.x

Pellegrino, R. M., Boda, E., Montarolo, F., Boero, M., Mezzanotte, M., Saglio, G., et al. (2016). Transferrin receptor 2 dependent alterations of brain iron metabolism affect anxiety circuits in the mouse. *Sci. Rep.* 6:30725. doi: 10.1038/srep30725

Perez de la Ossa, N., Sobrino, T., Silva, Y., Blanco, M., Millan, M., Gomis, M., et al. (2010). Iron-related brain damage in patients with intracerebral hemorrhage. *Stroke* 41, 810–813. doi: 10.1161/STROKEAHA.109.570168

Peters, D. G., Purnell, C. J., Haaf, M. P., Yang, Q. X., Connor, J. R., and Meadowcroft, M. D. (2018). Dietary lipophilic iron accelerates regional brain iron-load in C57BL6 mice. *Brain Struct. Funct.* 223, 1519–1536. doi: 10.1007/s00429-017-1565-1

Petrova, J., Manolov, V., Hadjidekova, S., Hadjiev, E., Bogov, B., Marinov, B., et al. (2015). Is there a link between changes in levels of hepcidin and stroke? *Clin. Lab.* 61, 1935–1939.

Philpott, C. C., and Ryu, M. S. (2014). Special delivery: distributing iron in the cytosol of mammalian cells. *Front. Pharmacol.* 5:173. doi: 10.3389/fphar.2014.00173

Philpott, C. C., Ryu, M. S., Frey, A., and Patel, S. (2017). Cytosolic iron chaperones: proteins delivering iron cofactors in the cytosol of mammalian cells. *J. Biol. Chem.* 292, 12764–12771. doi: 10.1074/jbc.R117.791962

Piloni, N. E., Caro, A. A., and Puntarulo, S. (2018). Iron overload prevents oxidative damage to rat brain after chlorpromazine administration. *BioMetals* doi: 10.1007/s10534-018-0104-8 [Epub ahead of print].

Raje, C. I., Kumar, S., Harle, A., Nanda, J. S., and Raje, M. (2007). The macrophage cell surface glyceraldehyde-3-phosphate dehydrogenase is a novel transferrin receptor. *J. Biol. Chem.* 282, 3252–3261. doi: 10.1074/jbc.M608328200

Ramos, P., Santos, A., Pinto, N. R., Mendes, R., Magalhães, T., and Almeida, A. (2014). Iron levels in the human brain: a post-mortem study of anatomical region differences and age-related changes. *J. Trace Elem. Med. Biol.* 28, 13–17. doi: 10.1016/j.jtemb.2013.08.001

Rathnasamy, G., Murugan, M., Ling, E. A., and Kaur, C. (2016). Hypoxia-induced iron accumulation in oligodendrocytes mediates apoptosis by eliciting endoplasmic reticulum stress. *Mol. Neurobiol.* 53, 4713–4727. doi: 10.1007/s12035-015-9389-6

Ravasi, G., Pelucchi, S., Buoli Comani, G., Greni, F., Mariani, R., Pelloni, I., et al. (2018). Hepcidin regulation in a mouse model of acute hypoxia. *Eur. J. Haematol.* 100, 636–643. doi: 10.1111/ejh.13062

Recalcati, S., Gammella, E., Buratti, P., and Cairo, G. (2017). Molecular regulation of cellular iron balance. *IUBMB Life* 69, 389–398. doi: 10.1002/iub.1628

Righy, C., Bozza, M. T., Oliveira, M. F., and Bozza, F. A. (2016). Molecular, cellular and clinical aspects of intracerebral hemorrhage: are the enemies within? *Curr. Neuropharmacol.* 14, 392–402. doi: 10.2174/1570159X14666151230110058

Righy, C., Turon, R., de Freitas, G., Japiassu, A. M., Faria Neto, H. C. C., Bozza, M., et al. (2018). Hemoglobin metabolism by-products are associated with an inflammatory response in patients with hemorrhagic stroke. *Rev. Bras. Ter. Intens.* 30, 21–27. doi: 10.5935/0103-507x.20180003

Sakamoto, K., Suzuki, T., Takahashi, K., Koguchi, T., Hirayama, T., Mori, A., et al. (2018). Iron-chelating agents attenuate NMDA-Induced neuronal injury via reduction of oxidative stress in the rat retina. *Exp. Eye Res.* 171, 30–36. doi: 10.1016/j.exer.2018.03.008

Sangkhae, V., and Nemeth, E. (2017). Regulation of the iron homeostatic hormone hepcidin. *Adv. Nutr. Int. Rev. J.* 8, 126–136. doi: 10.3945/an.116.013961

Sankar, S. B., Donegan, R. K., Shah, K. J., Reddi, A. R., and Wood, L. B. (2018). Heme and hemoglobin suppress amyloid β-mediated inflammatory activation of mouse astrocytes. *J. Biol. Chem.* 293, 11358–11373. doi: 10.1074/jbc.RA117.001050

Seiler, A., Schneider, M., Förster, H., Roth, S., Wirth, E. K., Culmsee, C., et al. (2008). Glutathione peroxidase 4 senses and translates oxidative stress into 12/15-lipoxygenase dependent- and AIF-mediated cell death. *Cell Metab.* 8, 237–248. doi: 10.1016/j.cmet.2008.07.005

Sheokand, N., Malhotra, H., Chauhan, A. S., Kumar, M., Chaudhary, S., Patidar, A., et al. (2016). Reverse overshot water-wheel retroendocytosis of apotransferrin extrudes cellular iron. *J. Cell Sci.* 129, 843–853. doi: 10.1242/jcs.180356

Shin, J. A., Kim, Y. A., Kim, H. W., Kim, H. S., Lee, K. E., Kang, J. L., et al. (2018). Iron released from reactive microglia by noggin improves myelin repair in the ischemic brain. *Neuropharmacology* 133, 202–215. doi: 10.1016/j.neuropharm.2018.01.038

Sillerova, T., Zivny, J., Vyoral, D., and Petrak, J. (2012). Nutritional hepatic iron overload is not prevented by parenteral hepcidin substitution therapy in mice. *Br. J. Nutr.* 108, 1723–1725. doi: 10.1017/S0007114512000116

Simpson, I. A., Ponnuru, P., Klinger, M. E., Myers, R. L., Devraj, K., Coe, C. L., et al. (2015). A novel model for brain iron uptake: introducing the concept of regulation. *J. Cereb. Blood Flow Metab.* 35, 48–57. doi: 10.1038/jcbfm.2014.168

Skjorringe, T., Burkhart, A., Johnsen, K. B., and Moos, T. (2015). Divalent metal transporter 1 (DMT1) in the brain: implications for a role in iron transport at the blood-brain barrier, and neuronal and glial pathology. *Front. Mol. Neurosci.* 8:19. doi: 10.3389/fnmol.2015.00019

Slomka, A., Switońska, M., and Zekanowska, E. (2015). Hepcidin levels are increased in patients with acute ischemic stroke: preliminary report. *J. Stroke Cerebrovasc. Dis.* 24, 1570–1576. doi: 10.1016/j.jstrokecerebrovasdis.2015.03.031

Sonnweber, T., Nachbaur, D., and Schroll, A. (2014). Hypoxia induced downregulation of hepcidin is mediated by platelet derived growth factor BB. *Gut* 63, 1951–1959. doi: 10.1136/gutjnl-2013-305317

Soria, F. N., Pérez-samartín, A., Martin, A., Gona, K. B., Llop, J., Szczupak, B., et al. (2014). Extrasynaptic glutamate release through cystine / glutamate antiporter contributes to ischemic damage. *J. Clin. Inverstig.* 124, 3645–3655. doi: 10.1172/JCI71886

Soria, F. N., Zabala, A., Pampliega, O., Palomino, A., Miguelez, C., Ugedo, L., et al. (2016). Cystine/glutamate antiporter blockage induces myelin degeneration. *Glia* 64, 1381–1395. doi: 10.1002/glia.23011

Sterling, J., Gutthaa, S., Song, Y., Song, D., Hadziahmetovic, M., and Dunaief, J. L. (2017). Iron importers Zip8 and Zip14 are expressed in retina and regulated by retinal iron levels JacobHHS public access. *Exp. Eye Res.* 155, 15–23. doi: 10.1016/j.exer.2016.12.008

Strazielle, N., and Ghersi-Egea, J.-F. (2016). Potential pathways for CNS drug delivery across the blood-cerebrospinal fluid barrier. *Curr. Pharm. Des.* 22, 4942–4958. doi: 10.2174/1381612822666160726112115

Sweeny, E. A., Singh, A. B., Chakravarti, R., Martinez-Guzman, O., Saini, A., Haque, M. M., et al. (2018). Glyceraldehyde 3-phosphate dehydrogenase is a chaperone that allocates labile heme in cells. *J. Biol. Chem.* 293, 14557–14568. doi: 10.1074/jbc.RA118.004169

Tan, G., Liu, L., He, Z., Sun, J., Xing, W., and Sun, X. (2016). Role of hepcidin and its downstream proteins in early brain injury after experimental subarachnoid hemorrhage in rats. *Mol. Cell. Biochem.* 418, 31–38. doi: 10.1007/s11010-016-2730-1

Tauchenová, L., Køížová, B., Kubánek, M., Fraòková, S., Melenovskı, V., Tintìra, J., et al. (2016). Successful treatment of iron-overload cardiomyopathy in hereditary hemochromatosis with deferoxamine and deferiprone. *Can. J. Cardiol.* 32, 1574.e1–1574.e3. doi: 10.1016/j.cjca.2016.07.589

Tian, Y., He, Y., Song, W., Zhang, E., and Xia, X. (2017). Neuroprotective effect of deferoxamine on N-methyl-d-aspartate-induced excitotoxicity in RGC-5 cells. *Acta Biochim. Biophys. Sin.* 49, 827–834. doi: 10.1093/abbs/gmx082

Todorich, B., Zhang, X., and Connor, J. R. (2011). H-ferritin is the major source of iron for oligodendrocytes. *Glia* 59, 927–935. doi: 10.1002/glia.21164

Todorich, B., Zhang, X., Slagle-Webb, B., Seaman, W. E., and Connor, J. R. (2008). Tim-2 is the receptor for H-ferritin on oligodendrocytes. *J. Neurochem.* 107, 1495–1505. doi: 10.1111/j.1471-4159.2008.05678.x

Tripathi, A. K., Karmakar, S., Asthana, A., Ashok, A., Desai, V., Baksi, S., et al. (2017). Transport of non-transferrin bound iron to the brain: implications for Alzheimer's disease. *J. Alzheimer's Dis.* 58, 1109–1119. doi: 10.3233/JAD-170097

Truman-Rosentsvit, M., Berenbaum, D., Spektor, L., Cohen, L. A., Belizowsky-Moshe, S., Lifshitz, L., et al. (2018). Ferritin is secreted via 2 distinct nonclassical vesicular pathways. *Blood* 131, 342–352. doi: 10.1182/blood-2017-02-768580

Tuo, Q., Lei, P., Jackman, K. A., Li, X., Xiong, H., Li, X., et al. (2017). Tau-mediated iron export prevents ferroptotic damage after ischemic stroke. *Mol. Psychiatry* 22, 1520–1530. doi: 10.1038/mp.2017.171

Turkmen, S., Gonenc, O. C., Karaca, Y., Mentese, A., Demir, S., Beyhun, E., et al. (2016). The effect of ethyl pyruvate and N -acetylcysteine on ischemia-reperfusion injury in an experimental model of ischemic stroke. *Am. J. Emerg. Med.* 34, 1804–1807. doi: 10.1016/j.ajem.2016.06.003

Uranga, R. M., and Salvador, G. A. (2018). Unraveling the burden of iron in neurodegeneration: intersections with amyloid beta peptide pathology. *Oxid. Med. Cell. Longev.* 2018:2850341. doi: 10.1155/2018/2850341

Van Dijk, B. A. C., Laarakkers, C. M. M., Klaver, S. M., Jacobs, E. M. G., Van Tits, L. J. H., Janssen, M. C. H., et al. (2008). Serum hepcidin levels are innately low in HFE-related haemochromatosis but differ between C282Y-homozygotes with elevated and normal ferritin levels. *Br. J. Haematol.* 142, 979–985. doi: 10.1111/j.1365-2141.2008.07273.x

Van Hoecke, M., Prigent-Tessier, A., Bertrand, N., Prevotat, L., Marie, C., and Beley, A. (2005). Apoptotic cell death progression after photothrombotic focal cerebral ischaemia: effects of the lipophilic iron chelator 2,2'-dipyridyl. *Eur. J. Neurosci.* 22, 1045–1056. doi: 10.1111/j.1460-9568.2005.04297.x

Vela, D. (2018). Hepcidin, an emerging and important player in brain iron homeostasis. *J. Transl. Med.* 16:25. doi: 10.1186/s12967-018-1399-5

Wan, L., Nie, G., Zhang, J., and Zhao, B. (2012). Overexpression of human wild-type amyloid-β protein precursor decreases the iron content and increases the oxidative stress of neuroblastoma SH-SY5Y cells. *J. Alzheimer's Dis.* 30, 523–530. doi: 10.3233/JAD-2012-111169

Wang, J., and Doré, S. (2007). Inflammation after intracerebral hemorrhage. *J. Cereb. Blood Flow Metab.* 27, 894–908. doi: 10.1038/sj.jcbfm.9600403

Ward, R. J., Zucca, F. A., Duyn, J. H., Crichton, R., and Zecca, L. (2014). The role of iron in brain ageing and neurodegenerative disorders. *Lancet Neurol.* 13, 1045–1060. doi: 10.1016/S1474-4422(14)70117-6

Watts, S. D., Torres-Salazar, D., Divito, C. B., and Amara, S. G. (2014). Cysteine transport through excitatory amino acid transporter 3 (EAAT3). *PLoS One* 9:e109245. doi: 10.1371/journal.pone.0109245

West, A. P., Bennett, M. J., Sellers, V. M., Andrews, N. C., Enns, C. A., and Bjorkman, P. J. (2000). Comparison of the interactions of transferrin receptor and transferrin receptor 2 with transferrin and the hereditary hemochromatosis protein HFE. *J. Biol. Chem.* 275, 38135–38138. doi: 10.1074/jbc.C000664200

White, R. S., Bhattacharya, A. K., Chen, Y., Byrd, M., McMullen, M. F., Siegel, S. J., et al. (2016). Lysosomal iron modulates NMDA receptor-mediated excitation via small GTPase, Dexras1. *Mol. Brain* 9:38. doi: 10.1186/s13041-016-0220-8

Worthen, C. A., and Enns, C. A. (2014). The role of hepatic transferrin receptor 2 in the regulation of iron homeostasis in the body. *Front. Pharmacol.* 5:34. doi: 10.3389/fphar.2014.00034

Wu, C., Zhao, W., Yu, J., Li, S., Lin, L., and Chen, X. (2018). Induction of ferroptosis and mitochondrial dysfunction by oxidative stress in PC12 cells. *Sci. Rep.* 8:574. doi: 10.1038/s41598-017-18935-1

Wu, J., Hua, Y., Keep, R. F., Nakamura, T., Hoff, J. T., and Xi, G. (2003). Iron and iron-handling proteins in the brain after intracerebral hemorrhage. *Stroke* 34, 2964–2969. doi: 10.1161/01.STR.0000103140.52838.45

Xing, Y., Hua, Y., Keep, R. F., and Xi, G. (2009). Effects of deferoxamine on brain injury after transient focal cerebral ischemia in rats with hyperglycemia. *Brain Res.* 1291, 113–121. doi: 10.1016/j.brainres.2009.07.032

Xiong, X. Y., Chen, J., Zhu, W. Y., Zhao, T., Zhong, Q., Zhou, K., et al. (2015). Serum hepcidin concentrations correlate with serum iron level and outcome in patients with intracerebral hemorrhage. *Neurol. Sci.* 36, 1843–1849. doi: 10.1007/s10072-015-2266-2

Xiong, X. Y., Liu, L., Wang, F. X., Yang, Y. R., Hao, J. W., Wang, P. F., et al. (2016). Toll-like receptor 4/MyD88-mediated signaling of hepcidin expression causing brain iron accumulation, oxidative injury, and cognitive impairment after intracerebral hemorrhage. *Circulation* 134, 1025–1038. doi: 10.1161/CIRCULATIONAHA.116.021881

Yang, G., Hu, R., Zhang, C., Qian, C., and Luo, Q. (2016). A combination of serum iron, ferritin and transferrin predicts outcome in patients with intracerebral hemorrhage. *Sci. Rep.* 6:21970. doi: 10.1038/srep21970

Yang, L., Fan, M., Du, F., Gong, Q., Bi, Z. G., Zhu, Z. J., et al. (2012). Hypoxic preconditioning increases iron transport rate in astrocytes. *Biochim. Biophys. Acta Mol. Basis Dis.* 1822, 500–508. doi: 10.1016/j.bbadis.2011.12.004

Yang, Y., Dong, B., Lu, J., Wang, G., and Yu, Y. (2018). Hemopexin reduces blood-brain barrier injury and protects synaptic plasticity in cerebral ischemic rats by promoting EPCs through the HO-1 pathway. *Brain Res.* 1699, 177–185. doi: 10.1016/j.brainres.2018.08.008

You, L. H., Li, Z., Duan, X. L., Zhao, B. L., Chang, Y. Z., and Shi, Z. H. (2016). Mitochondrial ferritin suppresses MPTP-induced cell damage by regulating iron metabolism and attenuating oxidative stress. *Brain Res.* 1642, 33–42. doi: 10.1016/j.brainres.2016.03.023

Yu, J., Guo, Y., Sun, M., Li, B., Zhang, Y., and Li, C. (2009). Iron is a potential key mediator of glutamate excitotoxicity in spinal cord motor neurons. *Brain Res.* 1257, 102–107. doi: 10.1016/j.brainres.2008.12.030

Zeng, L., Tan, L., Li, H., Zhang, Q., Li, Y., and Guo, J. (2018). Deferoxamine therapy for intracerebral hemorrhage: a systematic review. *PLoS One* 13:e0193615. doi: 10.1371/journal.pone.0193615

Zhang, H., Park, J. H., Maharjan, S., Park, J. A., Choi, K. S., Park, H., et al. (2017). Sac-1004, a vascular leakage blocker, reduces cerebral ischemia-reperfusion injury by suppressing blood-brain barrier disruption and inflammation. *J. Neuroinflammation* 14:122. doi: 10.1186/s12974-017-0897-3

Zhang, Z., Wu, Y., Yuan, S., Zhang, P., Zhang, J., Li, H., et al. (2018). Glutathione peroxidase 4 participates in secondary brain injury through mediating ferroptosis in a rat model of intracerebral hemorrhage. *Brain Res.* 1701, 112–125. doi: 10.1016/j.brainres.2018.09.012

Zhao, J., Xiang, X., Zhang, H., Jiang, D., Liang, Y., Qing, W., et al. (2018). CHOP induces apoptosis by affecting brain iron metabolism in rats with subarachnoid hemorrhage. *Exp. Neurol.* 302, 22–33. doi: 10.1016/j.expneurol.2017.12.015

Zhao, X., Song, S., Sun, G., Zhang, J., Strong, R., Zhang, L., et al. (2011). Cytoprotective role of haptoglobin in brain after experimental intracerebral hemorrhage. *Acta Neurochir. Suppl.* 111, 107–112. doi: 10.1007/978-3-7091-0693-8_17

Zhou, Y. F., Zhang, C., Yang, G., Qian, Z. M., Zhang, M. W., Ma, J., et al. (2017). Hepcidin protects neuron from hemin-mediated injury by reducing iron. *Front. Physiol.* 8:332. doi: 10.3389/fphys.2017.00332

Zille, M., Karuppagounder, S. S., Chen, Y., Gough, P. J., Bertin, J., Finger, J., et al. (2017). Neuronal death after hemorrhagic stroke in vitro and in vivo shares features of ferroptosis and necroptosis. *Stroke* 48, 1033–1043. doi: 10.1161/STROKEAHA.116.015609

14

Ceruloplasmin Plays a Neuroprotective Role in Cerebral Ischemia

*Fari Ryan, Juan G. Zarruk, Lena Lößlein and Samuel David**

Centre for Research in Neuroscience, The Research Institute of the McGill University Health Centre, Montreal, QC, Canada

***Correspondence:**
Samuel David
sam.david@mcgill.ca

Ceruloplasmin (Cp) is a ferroxidase that also plays a role in iron efflux from cells. It can thus help to regulate cellular iron homeostasis. In the CNS, Cp is expressed as a membrane-anchored form by astrocytes. Here, we assessed the role of Cp in permanent middle cerebral artery occlusion (pMCAO) comparing wildtype and Cp null mice. Our studies show that the lesion size is larger and functional recovery impaired in Cp null mice compared to wildtype mice. Expression of Cp increased ninefold at 72 h after pMCAO and remained elevated about twofold at day 14. We also assessed changes in mRNA and protein expression of molecules involved in iron homeostasis. As expected there was a reduction in ferroportin in Cp null mice at 72 h. There was also a remarkable increase in DMT1 protein in both genotypes at 72 h, being much higher in wildtype mice (19.5-fold), that then remained elevated about twofold at 14 days. No difference was seen in transferrin receptor 1 (TfR1) expression, except a small reduction in wildtype mice at 72 h, suggesting that the increase in DMT1 may underlie iron uptake independent of TfR1-endosomal uptake. There was also an increase of ferritin light chain in both genotypes. Iron histochemistry showed increased iron accumulation after pMCAO, initially along the lesion border and later throughout the lesion. Immunofluorescence labeling for ferritin (a surrogate marker for iron) and GFAP or CD11b showed increased ferritin in GFAP+ astrocytes along the lesion border in Cp null mice, while CD11b+ macrophages expressed ferritin equally in both genotypes. Increased lipid peroxidation assessed by 4HNE staining was increased threefold in Cp null mice at 72 h after pMCAO; and 3-nitrotyrosine labeling showed a similar trend. Three key pro-inflammatory cytokines (IL-1β, TNFα, and IL-6) were markedly increased at 24 h after pMCAO equally in both genotypes, and remained elevated at lower levels later, indicating that the lack of Cp does not alter key inflammatory cytokine expression after pMCAO. These data indicate that Cp expression is rapidly upregulated after pMCAO, and loss of Cp results in dysregulation of iron homeostasis, increased oxidative damage, greater lesion size and impaired recovery of function.

Keywords: stroke, ferroxidase, iron, oxidative damage, ferritin

INTRODUCTION

Dysregulation of cellular iron homeostasis is considered to contribute to neural damage after ischemic stroke (Millerot-Serrurot et al., 2008; Texel et al., 2011; Garcia-Yebenes et al., 2012). Iron plays an important role in many physiological processes by catalyzing a variety of enzymatic reactions (Rouault and Tong, 2005). The reason for these various functions is the redox active nature of iron, which can transition between the ferrous (Fe2+) and ferric (Fe3+) states. Divalent ferrous iron (Fe2+) can react with hydrogen peroxide in the Fenton reaction to catalyze the formation of free radicals, which cause oxidative damage (Crielaard et al., 2017). Therefore, the levels of cellular iron needs to be tightly regulated via a complex system of interactions involving several cell surface and intracellular proteins (Hentze et al., 2004; Crielaard et al., 2017).

Ceruloplasmin (Cp) is a ferroxidase that safely converts ferrous (Fe2+) iron to its ferric (Fe3+) form (Williams et al., 1974; Calabrese et al., 1989). The soluble form of Cp is expressed by the liver and found in serum (Gitlin, 1988). We identified a glycosylphosphatidylinositol-anchored form of Cp (GPI-Cp) in the central nervous system (CNS) that is expressed by astrocytes (Patel and David, 1997; Patel et al., 2000; Jeong and David, 2003). We have also reported that GPI-Cp is expressed abundantly by meningeal cells that surround the brain and spinal cord (Mittal et al., 2003). The choroid plexus located in the ventricular spaces in the CNS, and which produces cerebrospinal fluid, expresses the soluble form of Cp (Patel and David, 1997). We provided early evidence that GPI-Cp partners with the iron efflux transporter ferroportin to regulate iron efflux from astrocytes (Jeong and David, 2003). We and others have reported that Cp gene knockout mice show disruption of iron homeostasis in the CNS and other tissues such as the liver (Harris et al., 1999; Patel et al., 2002) and lead to iron accumulation in the CNS with age (> 18 months of age), resulting in free-radical mediated neuronal loss (Patel et al., 2002; Jeong and David, 2006). Other work also indicates that the absence of GPI-Cp results in the internalization and degradation of the iron exporter, ferroportin (Fpn), from the cell surface, which results in iron accumulation (De Domenico et al., 2007). Iron accumulation in the CNS and other organs, which increases with age is a characteristic feature of humans with aceruloplasminemia, which results from mutations in the Cp gene (Harris et al., 1995; Morita et al., 1995; Yoshida et al., 1995; Xu et al., 2004). We have also reported a slow accumulation of iron in the brain in Cp null mice with age (> 18 months of age) (Patel et al., 2002; Jeong and David, 2006).

Mechanisms that lead to iron accumulation in cells in the CNS in different neurological conditions are not fully understood but can give rise to oxidative damage and neurodegeneration. In CNS injury and disease, increased iron loading of cells occurs either when dying cells release their intracellular iron content into the extracellular space (as in cell necrosis or physical damage) and/or are taken up by microglia and macrophages (phagocytosis) as occurs in ischemic stroke. Increased iron load in the CNS also occurs acutely after hemorrhage and uptake of red blood cells by phagocytes, as occurs in hemorrhagic stroke. In addition, dysregulation of molecules involved in maintaining cellular iron homeostasis can also result in iron accumulation, i.e., increased iron uptake or reduce iron efflux. The extent of iron-mediated free-radical damage will depend on how well excess iron is taken up and safely sequestered in ferritin or exported/effluxed out of the cells (Finazzi and Arosio, 2014). Moreover, in CNS disorders such as multiple sclerosis (MS), iron accumulation is seen in microglia that eventually appear to become dystrophic and undergo cell death (Hametner et al., 2013), which could lead to further cycles of iron uptake and cell death. We have reported recently, that iron accumulation in macrophages in a mouse model of MS [experimental autoimmune encephalomyelitis (EAE)] may be due to hepcidin-mediated internalization of Fpn (Zarruk et al., 2015).

In the present study, we examined the role of Cp in ischemic stroke using wildtype and Cp null mice. We examined the role of Cp on lesion size and functional recovery, as well as changes in the expression of various molecules involved in iron homeostasis in the ischemic brain. We also studied the extent of iron deposition, free radical damage and changes in the expression of inflammatory cytokines. This work suggests that Cp plays a significant role in functional recovery and tissue neuroprotection after permanent cerebral ischemia.

MATERIALS AND METHODS

Induction of Permanent Middle Cerebral Artery Occlusion (pMCAO)

Male Cp−/− and Cp+/+ mice on a C57BL/6 background, 8–12 weeks of age, were used. Ceruloplasmin knockout mice were generated in our lab several years ago as previously described (Patel et al., 2002). All surgical procedures were approved by the Animal Care Committee of the Research Institute of the McGill University Health Centre and followed the guidelines of the Canadian Council on Animal Care, and the ARRIVE guidelines for reporting animal research (Kilkenny et al., 2010). The pMCAO surgery was done as described previously (Zarruk et al., 2012) and is a variant of an earlier model (Chen et al., 1986). Briefly, animals were deeply anesthetized with isoflurane in O_2 (0.5–1 L/min; inhalation) during the entire procedure. During surgery, body temperature was maintained at $37.0 \pm 0.5°C$ using a homeothermic system with a rectal probe (Harvard apparatus). A small craniotomy was made over the region of the trunk of the left middle cerebral artery (MCA) above the rhinal fissure. The pMCAO was done by ligating the trunk of the MCA just before its bifurcation between the frontal and parietal branches using a 9-0 suture. Complete interruption of blood flow was confirmed under visual inspection under the operating microscope. In addition, the left common carotid artery was then occluded. After surgery, animals were returned to their cages with free access to water and food. Spontaneous mortality was not observed after the surgical procedure.

Infarct Volume

Nissl stained tissue sections (30 μm) spanning the entire lesion were assessed to estimate the infarct volume using the ImageJ software. To calculate the infarct volume, two measurements

TABLE 1 | Primer sequences used for qPCR.

Gene	Forward sequence	Reverse sequence
Ceruloplasmin	ACATTGCTGCTGAGG AGGTCATCT	TGTTCCTCATCAGGG CCTCTTTGT
Ferroportin	AACCAGAGTCACTG TCATCAGCCA	TCGGCCCAAGTCA GTGAAGGTAAA
DMT1	TGAATCGGGCGAA TAAGCAGGA	TCAGCAAAGACGGC AACGACAA
Ferritin HC	TAAAGAACTGGGTGA CCACGTGAC	AAGTCAGCTTAGC TCTCATCACCG
Ferritin LC	GGCTTTCCAGGAAG TCACAGAGAT	TGGCCATGGAG AAGAACCTGAATC
TfR1	AAACTGGCTGAAACG GAGGAGACA	GCTGCTTGATGGTG TCAGCAAACT
TNF-α	TTGCTCTGTGAAGGG AATGG	GGCTCTGAGGAGT AGACAATAAAG
IL-1β	ATGGGCAACCACTTA CCTATTT	GTTCTAGAGAGT GCTGCCTAATG
IL-6	CTTCCATC CAGTTGCCTTCT	CTCCGACTTGTGAAG TGGTATAG
IL-10	ACAGCCGGGAAGACA ATAAC	CAGCTGGTCCTTTGT TTGAAAG
GAPDH	GGAGAAACCTGCCAA GTATGA	TCCTCAGTGTAGCCC AAGA

were taken: the whole ipsilateral hemisphere and the ipsilateral hemisphere excluding the lesion. The 2 values were used to calculate the % of infarcted hemisphere. This is done to accurately estimate the lesion in each animal and to exclude any variations in brain size or distortions due to histological preparation. These values were used for statistical analysis.

Functional Assay

The "adhesive-tape removal" assay was used to assess functional recovery. This test assesses the integrity of motor and sensory function. It was originally described for rats and then adapted to mice (Bouet et al., 2009; Zarruk et al., 2011). In brief, a small piece of adhesive tape is placed over the hairless parts of the forepaw (pads, thenar, and hypothenar). This is repeated on both sides. Habituation and training was done for 5 days before surgery, each time alternating the order in which the tape was placed (left or right paw). The test was done on 1, 2, 7, and 14-days post-surgery (n = 13–15 mice per group). Three trials were done per day per mouse and the mean of each day was calculated. On the evaluation day, after the adhesive tape was placed, the mice were placed back into the evaluation box/cage, and the time taken to remove the tape is measured. Sham surgery animals were used as controls. The asymmetry between the right and left sides was calculated by dividing the time taken to remove the tape on the affected side (right) versus the non-affected side (left). The higher the number meant greater disability which is explained because ischemic lesions will affect the sensorimotor abilities of the mice on the contralateral side, impairing their ability to feel and/or remove the tape.

Collection of Tissue for mRNA and Western Blotting

Under deep anesthesia the mice were perfused via the heart with phosphate buffered saline and the brain rapidly exposed and removed; and the cortex dissected out and rapidly frozen in liquid nitrogen. The most rostral and caudal parts of the brain (1-mm thick) were excluded to avoid regions that lack the infarct. The ipsi and contralateral sides of the cerebral hemisphere were taken for analysis. Samples were taken for mRNA and protein at different time intervals as indicated in the results section.

Quantitative Real Time Polymerase Chain Reaction (qPCR)

Total RNA was extracted using RNeasy Mini Kit (Qiagen, Mississauga, ON, Canada) following manufacturer's instructions. cDNA was reverse transcribed with the Qiagen Quantinova Kit (Cat. No. 205411) and amplified using an ABI OneStep cycler (Applied Biosystems) using specific primer pairs as indicated in **Table 1**. GAPDH was used as an internal control gene. The results were quantified using the $\Delta\Delta$CT method following standardization relative to GAPDH (Livak and Schmittgen, 2001).

Western Blotting

Brain tissue was obtained after intracardiac perfusion with PBS as described above. Total protein was extracted with 1% Nonidet P-40 (Sigma), 1% sodium deoxycholate (BDH Chemicals), 2% SDS, 0.15 M sodium phosphate (pH 7.2), and 2 mM EDTA, containing a mixture of protease inhibitors (Roche Diagnostics) as described previously (Jeong and David, 2003). Protein concentrations were estimated using the Bio-Rad DC protein assay following manufacturer's instructions (Cat. No 500-0121). Then 25 μg of proteins per sample were separated by sodium dodecyl sulfate polyacrylamide electrophoresis (SDS–PAGE) gels 4–12% (Novex, life Technologies), transferred to polyvinylidene fluoride membrane (PVDF) (Millipore, Billerica, MA). Membranes were blocked in 5% milk in 0.05% PBS Tween-20 and incubated overnight at 4°C with the following primary antibodies: rabbit anti-ferritin (1:500; Sigma-Aldrich Inc.; F5012), rabbit anti-DMT1 (1:1000; Alpha Diagnostics), mouse anti-TfR1 (1:1000; Invitrogen; 13–6800), rabbit anti-Cp (1:1000 DakoCytomation; Q 0121), or rabbit anti-Fpn (1:300 Alpha Diagnostic; MTP11-A). Blots were washed and incubated with horseradish peroxidase-conjugated IgG (1:10,000 –100,000; Jackson ImmunoResearch, West Grove, PA, United States) and visualized with enhanced chemiluminescence (PerkinElmer). Equal loading of proteins was estimated by re-probing the membranes with rabbit anti-β-actin antibodies (1:1000; Sigma-Aldrich). The blots were quantified using ImageJ software (version 1.48r NIH-USA).

Immunofluorescence and Confocal Microscopy

Mice were perfused with phosphate buffer saline followed by 4% paraformaldehyde in 0.1 M phosphate buffer. After post-fixation in the same fixative for 24 h, the tissue was cryoprotected in

30% sucrose and 14 μm thick coronal sections of the brain cut with a cryostat and used for the immunofluorescence labeling. Tissue sections were incubated with 0.3% Triton X-100 (Sigma-Aldrich), 5% normal goat serum (Jackson ImmunoResearch Inc.), 2% ovalbumin (Sigma-Aldrich) in phosphate buffer for 3 h room temperature (RT) to block non-specific binding of antibodies. Sections were then incubated overnight at 4°C with primary antibodies against ferritin (1:200). These primary antibodies were combined with the following cell type specific antibodies: rat anti CD11b (for macrophages/microglia; 1:200; Serotec; MCA711), guinea pig anti-glial acidic protein (GFAP) (for astrocytes; 1:500; Synaptic Systems cat No. 173004). Sections were washed in 0.05% PBS-Tween-20 and incubated with appropriate fluorescent-conjugated secondary antibodies, anti-rabbit Alexa Fluor 488, anti-rat Alexa Fluor 568 or anti-guinea pig Alexa Fluor 568 (all 1:500, Invitrogen). Tissue sections were viewed with a confocal laser scanning microscope (FluoView FV1000, Olympus) and micrographs taken with the FV10-ASW 3.0 software (Olympus). For comparing between groups, the same setting was applied in all images of each immunostaining. The quantification of the double labeling of GFAP and ferritin at 72 h after pMCAO was assessed using the Image J software to estimate Pearson's correlation coefficient as described previously (Dunn et al., 2011).

Diaminobenzidine-Enhanced Turnbull's Blue Staining for Iron

Turnbull's blue iron histochemistry was done to detect ferric and ferrous iron as previously described (Meguro et al., 2007). Briefly, at different times after pMCAO mice were perfused with 0.1 M phosphate buffer followed by 4% paraformaldehyde. The brains were dissected out, and cryoprotected in 30% sucrose and 14 μm sections cut with a cryostat (Leica CM 3050 S). Sections were incubated in 10% ammonium sulfide for 90 min at RT, washed with distilled water (dH_2O) and incubated for 30 min in a solution of 20% potassium ferricyanide (Sigma-Aldrich) and 1% hydrochloric acid. Sections were then washed in double distilled water and endogenous peroxidase blocked for 60 min at room temperature in 99 ml PBS + 0.01 M NaN3 (65 mg) + 1 ml 30% H_2O_2. After washes in 0.1 M phosphate buffer, iron staining in the tissue sections was visualized by incubation with 0.025% 3,3′ diaminobenzidine with 0.005% H_2O_2 in 0.1 M phosphate buffer (20 min at RT). The reaction was stopped with tap water and sections were counterstained with Mayer's hemalum solution (EMD Millipore, 1.09249.1000) and mounted with Entellan (Electron Microscopy Sciences). For quantification of iron labeled cell at 72 h post-pMCAO, the number of labeled cells were counted and estimated per μm^2. Direct cell counts of iron labeled cells could not be done at 14 days because the cells were densely packed in the lesion. Therefore, for quantification of iron staining at 14 days, we used densitometry to estimate the integrated density as follows: microscope images were prepared and analyzed with Image J (version 1.48r NIH-USA). The background was first subtracted with a rolling ball of 200 pixels. Staining intensity was then quantified using the densitometry 1 channel plug-in with a tolerance of 100 and the mean of integrated density was calculated for each animal and each group and plotted on the *y*-axis.

Immunohistochemistry for 4HNE and 3-NT

Brain cryostat sections (14 μm thick) from 4% paraformaldehyde perfused-fixed mice, 72 h post-pMCAO were used for DAB immunohistochemistry for 4HNE (4-Hydroxynonenal) and 3-NT (3-Nitrotyrosine) as described previously (Zarruk et al., 2015). In brief, endogenous peroxidase was blocked with 0.2% H_2O_2 in PBS for 30 min at RT. Then non-specific binding was blocked for 3 h at RT in blocking solution (3% Triton, 5% normal goat serum, in PBS) with avidin D solution (Vector laboratories; SP2001) followed by overnight incubation with primary rabbit anti-4HNE antibody (1:300; Abcam; AB46545) or rabbit anti-3NT antibody (1:500; Invitrogen; A21285), with the biotin solution (Vector laboratories; SP2001). The Avidin/Biotin blocking kit (Vector) was used as an extra step to block non-specific avidin/biotin binding. Sections were washed in 0.05% PBS-Tween and incubated for 1 h at RT with secondary goat anti-rabbit biotinylated (1:1000; Jackson ImmunoResearch), washed and incubated with avidin peroxidase 1 h (RT) (1:100; Sigma #A-2693151). Labeling was visualized with 3,3′ diaminobenzidine-tetrahydro chloride using the ImmPACT DAB peroxidase substrate kit according to manufacturer instructions (Vector; SK-4105) and counterstained with Mayer's hemalum. The number of cells per μm^2 was quantify in each group from 10x images taken with a Zeiss Axioskop II light microscope using Image J (version 1.48r NIH-USA).

Statistical Analyses

All types of analyses were carried out blind, so the evaluator was not aware of the groups. Data are shown as mean ± Standard Error of the Mean (SEM). Two-way ANOVA followed by Bonferroni's *post hoc* test was used to analyze the results from "adhesive tape removal" test at different time points. The colocalization of GFAP and ferritin was quantified using Pearson's colocalization coefficient (Dunn et al., 2011) with the ImageJ colocalization Threshold plug-in. A zero value is given for the pixels below the thresholds. That means that all the pixels which have intensities above the two thresholds have greater than zero correlation, and the pixels below the thresholds have none or negative correlated intensities. Therefore, the closest the value is to 1 the better the colocalization (1 = full colocalization, 0 = no colocalization). Mann–Whitney non-parametric test was used to compare two groups. A value of $p \leq 0.05$ was considered significant.

RESULTS

Decreased Functional Recovery in Cp Null Mice After pMCAO

We first assessed functional recovery after pMCAO using the "adhesive-tape removal" test. In this test, a small piece of adhesive tape is stuck on the paw of each forelimb, and the time taken

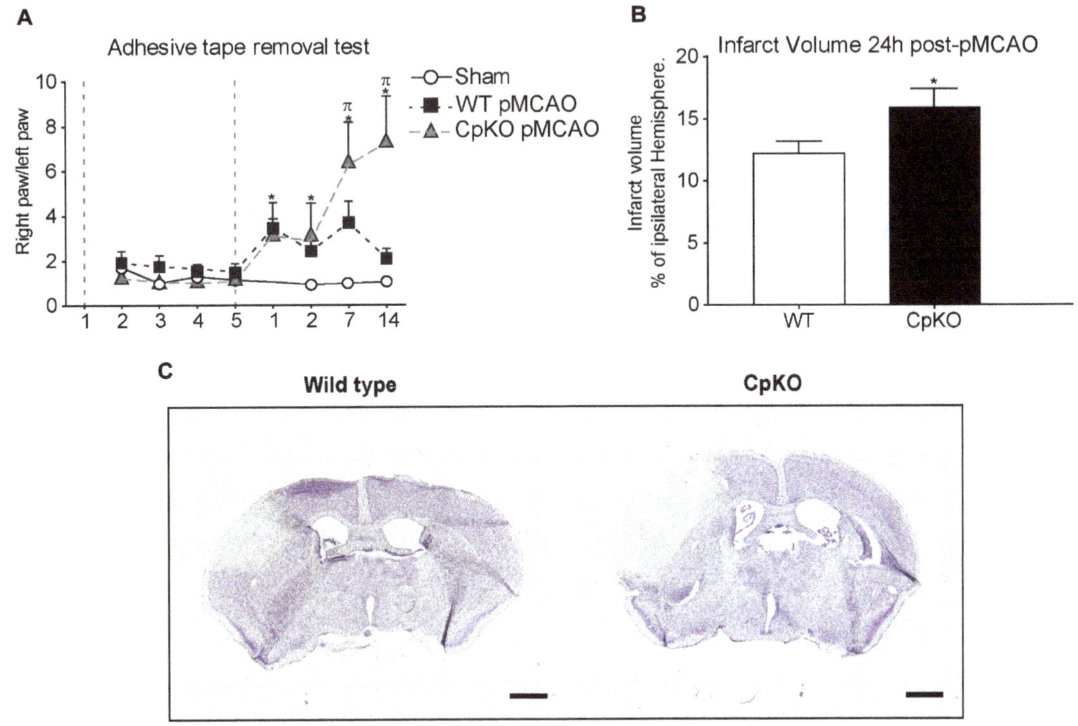

FIGURE 1 | (A) Graph showing functional recovery assessed with the "adhesive-tape removal" test. Mice were trained for 5 days prior to the surgery for pMCAO (period indicated between the two vertical dashed lines). At days 1 and 2 after pMCAO wildtype and Cp KO mice both show similar deficits. Wildtype mice recover to normal values by day 14, while CpKO mice show increasing functional deficits at 7 and 14 days. The sham animals show no deficits. **(B)** Cp null mice show significantly larger lesion size as compared to wildtype mice at 24 h after pMCAO. **(C)** Nissl stained sections showing the ischemic lesion in wildtype and Cp KO mice 24 h after pMCAO. $n = 13–15$ per group in **A**; and 9 per group in **B**. Two-way ANOVA was used to analyze results in A, followed by Bonferroni's *post hoc* test. *p-value ≤ 0.05 compared to sham-control group; πp-value ≤ 0.05 compared to wild-type group. Mann–Whitney test was used to compare WT vs. CpKO in B. *p-value ≤ 0.05; scale bar = 100 μm.

by the mouse to remove the tape is estimated. This test showed that Cp KO mice took a longer time to remove the tape as compared to wildtype mice (**Figure 1A**). Interestingly, the Cp KO and wildtype mice showed similar levels of deficit at 1 and 2 days after pMCAO. However, at 7 and 14 days, the two groups diverged with the Cp null mice showing increasingly worse deficits, while the wildtype mice showed recovery to normal values at 14 days. The latter may be due to neural plasticity in wildtype mice, which appears to be impaired in Cp null mice, possibly due to free radical mediated secondary damage to neurons (e.g., dendritic spine formation) and glia (microglia and astrocytes). For example, pruning of synaptic arbors by microglia is required for establishment of proper function (Stephan et al., 2012). Astrocytes are also required for recycling of neurotransmitters and the proper functioning of synapses (Allen, 2014). We have reported previously that Cp null mice show changes in CNS glia with reduction of astrocytes with age (Jeong and David, 2006). Sham controls did not show any deficits.

Infarct Size Is Larger in Cp Null Mice

We next determined the infarct size using Nissl stained tissue sections obtained from mice 24 h and 14 days after pMCAO. The ImageJ software was used to measure the total infarct volume and presented as a percentage of the ipsilateral hemisphere (**Figure 1B**). This analysis showed a significant increase in the size of the lesion in Cp null mice 24 h after pMCAO (17.5 mm^3) as compared to wildtype mice (15.8 mm^3) (**Figures 1B,C**). At 14 days post-pMCAO there was a trend to an increase in the Cp null mice, but these differences were not statistically significant (data not shown). This may be because by 14 days there is marked shrinkage of the lesion leading eventually to a scar, making the differences less prominent.

Changes in the Expression of Iron Homeostasis Proteins at the mRNA and Protein Levels

Ceruloplasmin

In wildtype mice, there is a modest but significant increase in Cp mRNA expression in the ipsilateral ischemic hemisphere as compared to the uninjured contralateral hemisphere at both 72 h and 14 days after pMCAO (**Figure 2A**). Interestingly, Western blot analysis showed an 8.8-fold increase in Cp expression at 72 h after pMCAO and remained significantly elevated at about twofold at day 14 (**Figures 2B,C**). These findings suggest up-regulation of Cp expression at the protein level in ischemic stroke. This increase in Cp expression is in keeping with its protective

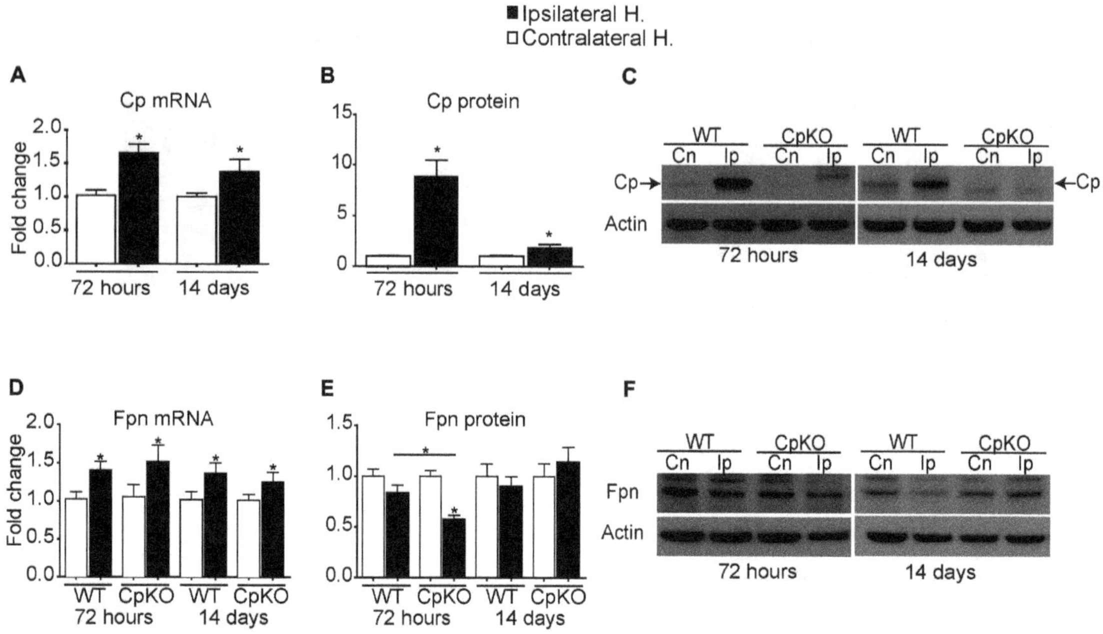

FIGURE 2 | Changes in mRNA detected by q-PCR and protein expression detected by Western blot analysis of Cp **(A–C)** and Fpn **(D–F)** in the ipsilateral ischemic side as compared to the contralateral uninjured side at 72 h and 14 days after pMCAO. Changes in the ipsilateral ischemic side are represented as fold-change as compared to contralateral uninjured side. Changes in expression of Cp mRNA **(A)**, and protein **(B)** quantified from Western blots; a representative example of the Western blot for Cp is shown **(C)**. Note the marked increase in Cp protein at 72 h (8.8-fold) and which remains significantly elevated (twofold) at 14 days. **(C)** The weak bands seen on the ipsilateral side in the Cp null mice are non-specific bands that are not at the expected 135 kDa GPI-Cp band (arrows). Changes in Fpn mRNA **(D)** and protein **(E)** and representative Western blots **(F)**. Fpn is significantly reduced on the ipsilateral side in Cp null mice at 72 h. β actin was used as a loading control. *n* = 6 per group; **p*-value ≤ 0.05.

role as a ferroxidase to reduce the toxic effects of ferrous iron and to export iron out of cells, particularly astrocytes in the CNS, and thus prevent intracellular iron accumulation.

Ferroportin

Cp partners with ferroportin (Fpn), the ubiquitously expressed iron efflux transporter, to export iron out of cells. We therefore assessed the expression of Fpn at the mRNA and protein levels. At the mRNA level there was a modest increase in Fpn expression on the ipsilateral ischemic cortex in both genotypes at 72 h and 14 days (**Figure 2D**). However, at the protein level there was about a 50% reduction in Fpn expression at 72 h in the ipsilateral side in Cp null mice versus the contralateral uninjured cortex (**Figures 2E,F**), as well as a significant reduction in the ipsilateral side in Cp null mice compared to wildtype mice at 72 h (**Figures 2E,F**). Our previous studies have shown that GPI-Cp is required for the stability of Fpn on the cell surface (De Domenico et al., 2007). In the absence of GPI-Cp, Fpn gets internalized and eventually degraded. This may account for the reduction of Fpn protein acutely in Cp null mice at 72 h. In addition, the partial reduction in Fpn protein may be because Cp is only expressed by astrocytes but no other cell types in the CNS (Patel and David, 1997). No differences in Fpn protein were seen in wildtype mice at 72 h and between any of the groups at 14 days post-pMCAO despite increases in Fpn mRNA on the ipsilateral side. Why the increase in mRNA levels on the ipsilateral side are not reflected in increase in protein levels in the Western blots is not known at present but may involve regulated internalization and degradation of the protein.

Transferrin Receptor 1 (TfR1) and Divalent Metal Ion Transporter 1 (DMT1)

There was a small but significant reduction in TfR1 mRNA and protein in the ipsilateral cortex in wildtype mice at 14 days post-ischemia. No other differences were seen (**Figures 3A–C**).

No differences were observed in the mRNA level of DMT1 after pMCAO in either genotype (**Figure 3D**). In contrast, Western blot analysis of tissue taken at 72 h post-pMCAO showed a large almost 19.5-fold increase in DMT1 protein in the ipsilateral ischemic cortex in wildtype mice and a smaller (sixfold) increase in the ipsilateral cortex in Cp null mice (**Figures 3E,F**). A smaller (twofold) significant increase in DMT1 protein continued to be detected in the ipsilateral cortex of both genotypes at 14 days (**Figures 3E,F**). DMT1 is known to be involved in release of endosomal iron taken up via the Tf-TfR1 complex. DMTI is also expressed on the surface of astrocytes (Jeong and David, 2003) and so may be involved in transferrin-independent iron uptake into cells. Our data showing no increases in TfR1 expression would suggest that the increase in DMT1 might contribute to direct uptake of iron into astrocytes after cerebral ischemia. It is also important to note that DMT1 protein expression was 3 times

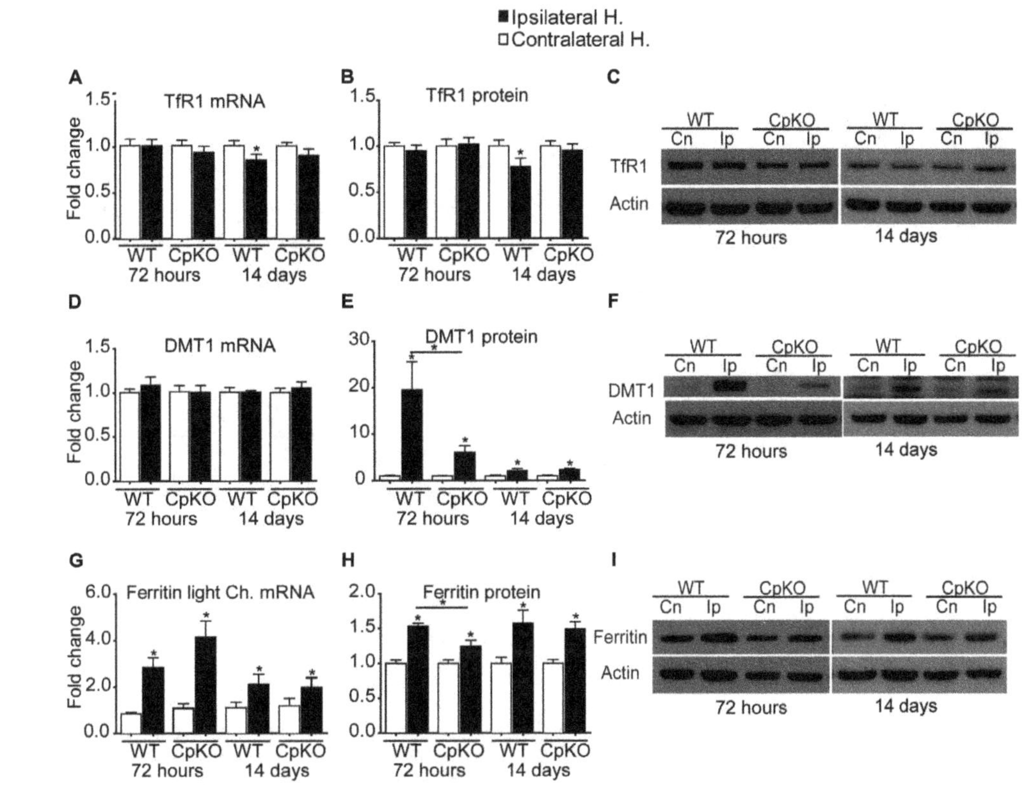

FIGURE 3 | Changes in mRNA and protein expression of TfR1 **(A–C)**, DMT1 **(D–F)**, and ferritin **(G–I)** shown as fold-change in the ipsilateral ischemic side as compared to the contralateral uninjured side at 72 h and 14 days after pMCAO. No changes are seen in TfR1 mRNA **(A)** or protein **(B)** except for a small but significant reduction in the ipsilateral side in wildtype mice at 14 days. Representative Western blot shown in **C**. Changes in expression of DMT1 mRNA **(D)**, and protein **(E)** quantified from Western blots; representative Western blot shown in **F**. Note the marked increase in DMT1 protein on the ipsilateral side in wildtype (19.5-fold) and Cp null (sixfold) mice at 72 h, which remain elevated at twofold at 14 days in both genotypes. Changes in mRNA expression of ferritin light chain **(G)** and ferritin protein **(H)** and a representative Western blot **(I)**. Note the increase in mRNA and protein levels in the ipsilateral side in all groups. β actin was used as a loading control; note that the same blot was used to probe DMT1 **(F)** and Cp (**Figure 2C**) hence the actin blots for these are the same. $n = 6$ per group; *p-value ≤ 0.05.

lower in Cp null mice compared to wildtype mice at 72 h (**Figure 3E**).

Ferritin

Ferritin is the iron storage protein in cells. Each molecule of ferritin consists of 24 heavy and light chain subunits that form a sphere in which iron is stored. Each molecule of ferritin can store up to 4,500 atoms of iron and so is a very efficient iron storage protein (Arosio and Levi, 2002, 2010). Excess iron is stored in ferritin. There is a significant increase at the mRNA level of ferritin light chain (the major iron storage form) in the ipsilateral hemispheres in both genotypes compared to the contralateral hemispheres. The mRNA increase at 72 h in wildtype mice is about threefold and in Cp null mice about fourfold (**Figure 3G**). In contrast, mRNA expression of ferritin heavy chain, which has ferroxidase activity, showed no difference after ischemia in either genotype, except for a small but significant increase in the ipsilateral side in Cp null mice at 72 h (data not shown). At the protein level in Western blots, the antibody does not distinguish between heavy and light chains, so the results are a summation of the levels of both chains. In the ipsilateral ischemic cortex there is a significant increase in ferritin protein at 72 h and 14 days in both genotypes (**Figures 3H,I**).

Iron Histochemistry and Ferritin Immunofluorescence Labeling

To investigate further the changes in iron accumulation in ischemic stroke, we performed diaminobenzidine (DAB)-enhanced Turnbull's blue iron histochemistry. These studies showed that iron labeled cells are seen in the lesion along the lesion border at 72 h after pMCAO in both wildtype and Cp knockout mice (**Figures 4A,B**). The cell counts of labeled cells did not differ between the two genotypes at 72 h (**Figure 4C**). However, at 14 days after pMCAO, there was a marked increase in iron staining throughout the lesion in both genotypes (**Figures 4D,E**). The labeled cells were densely packed in the lesion making it difficult to obtain cell counts. Densitometry analysis, however, showed a significant increase in Cp null mice compared to wildtype mice (**Figure 4F**).

Iron histochemistry is not compatible with immunostaining, therefore, to assess which cell types accumulate iron in the ischemic brain, we carried out double immunofluorescence

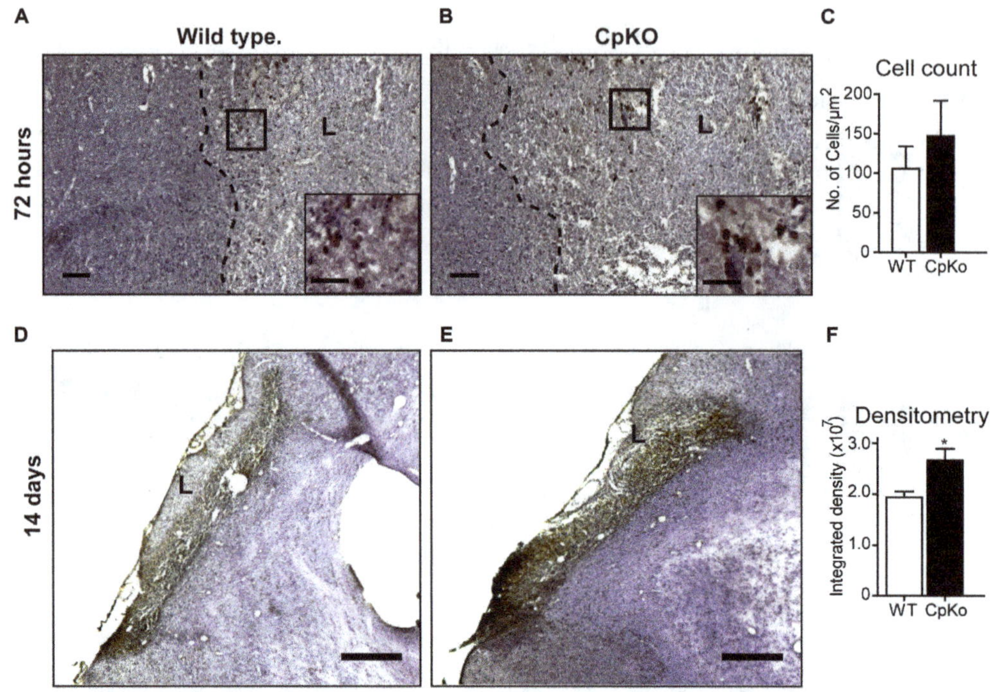

FIGURE 4 | Iron histochemistry. Detected by the enhanced Turnbull's staining of tissue sections taken 72 h **(A–C)** and 14 days **(D–F)** after pMCAO. At 72 h the cells labeled for iron (stained dark brown; see insets in **A** and **B**) are located in the lesion and distributed along the lesion border in both wildtype **(A)** and CpKO **(B)** mice; L = lesion; areas in the black squares in **A,B** are shown at higher magnification in the insets. **(C)** Graph shows that the number of iron+ cells is not significantly different in the two genotypes. At 14 days **(D,E)** the iron labeled cells are densely packed in the lesion (L) making it difficult to do cell counts. Densitometric analysis **(F)** showed higher levels of iron deposition in CpKO mice compared to wildtype mice at 14 days. All sections counterstained with Mayer's hemalum stain. Scale bars in **A–E** = 100 μm, inset = 50 μm; $n = 6$ per group; *p-value ≤ 0.05.

labeling for ferritin, a good surrogate marker for iron, and co-labeled the sections with antibodies to GFAP (astrocytes) (**Figure 5**) and CD11b (macrophages/microglia) (**Figure 6**) at 72 h after pMCAO. The double labeling showed that in the ipsilateral ischemic cortex of Cp null mice, ferritin expression is more intense (**Figures 5E,K**) and co-localizes to significantly more GFAP-positive astrocytes as compared to wildtype mice (**Figures 5F,L,M**). Colocalization of ferritin and GFAP was quantified using Pearson's correlation coefficient, as the two labels are in the cytoplasmic compartment (**Figure 5M**). These ferritin+ astrocytes are located in the intact CNS tissue along the border region of the infarct. Co-localization of ferritin in CD11b+ macrophages/microglia is seen in the ischemic lesioned tissue along the border region of the infarct (**Figures 6A–F**). The number of ferritin+/CD11b+ macrophages/microglia at 72 h post-pMCAO was similar in Cp null and wildtype mice (**Figure 6G**).

These results suggest that at 72 h post-pMCAO, the iron labeled cells seen by the Turnbull's stain along the lesion border are likely to include both astrocytes and macrophage/microglia.

Changes in Markers of Oxidative Stress

Two indicators of lipid and protein oxidative damage were assessed. Lipid peroxidation in tissue sections was evaluated by immunohistochemical detection of changes in 4-hydroxynonenal (4HNE). Protein oxidation was assessed by immunohistochemical labeling for 3-nitrotyrosine (3-NT) a product of tyrosine nitration that is mediated by peroxynitrite. Immunohistochemical staining for 4HNE and 3-NT was done on tissue sections of the brain taken at 72 h after pMCAO. The expression of 4HNE was visualized with the DAB technique and appeared as dark brown staining of cells along the border of the infarct region (**Figures 7A–D**). Adjacent intact regions of the cortex did not show such labeling. The number of 4HNE+ cells in the ipsilateral cortex was significantly higher in Cp null mice as compared to wildtype mice (**Figure 7E**).

Immunohistochemistry for 3-nitrotyrosine occurred in the infarct area and there appeared to be a trend to an increase in CpKO mice compared to wildtype mice but this did not reach statistical significance (**Figure 8**).

Expression of Inflammatory Cytokines

It is known that the iron status of cells can affect their inflammatory profile (Kroner et al., 2014; Rathore et al., 2012). We therefore assessed whether changes in iron homeostasis after cerebral ischemia also influenced the inflammatory response in Cp null mice. We assessed the expression of four key cytokines that include IL-1β, TNFα, IL-6, and IL-10. Changes in these cytokines was assessed at 24, 72 h, and 14 days after pMCAO. There were marked increases in the mRNA expression of the three proinflammatory cytokines (IL-1β, TNFα, and IL-6) at 24 h, which remained elevated at lower levels at 72 h after pMCAO

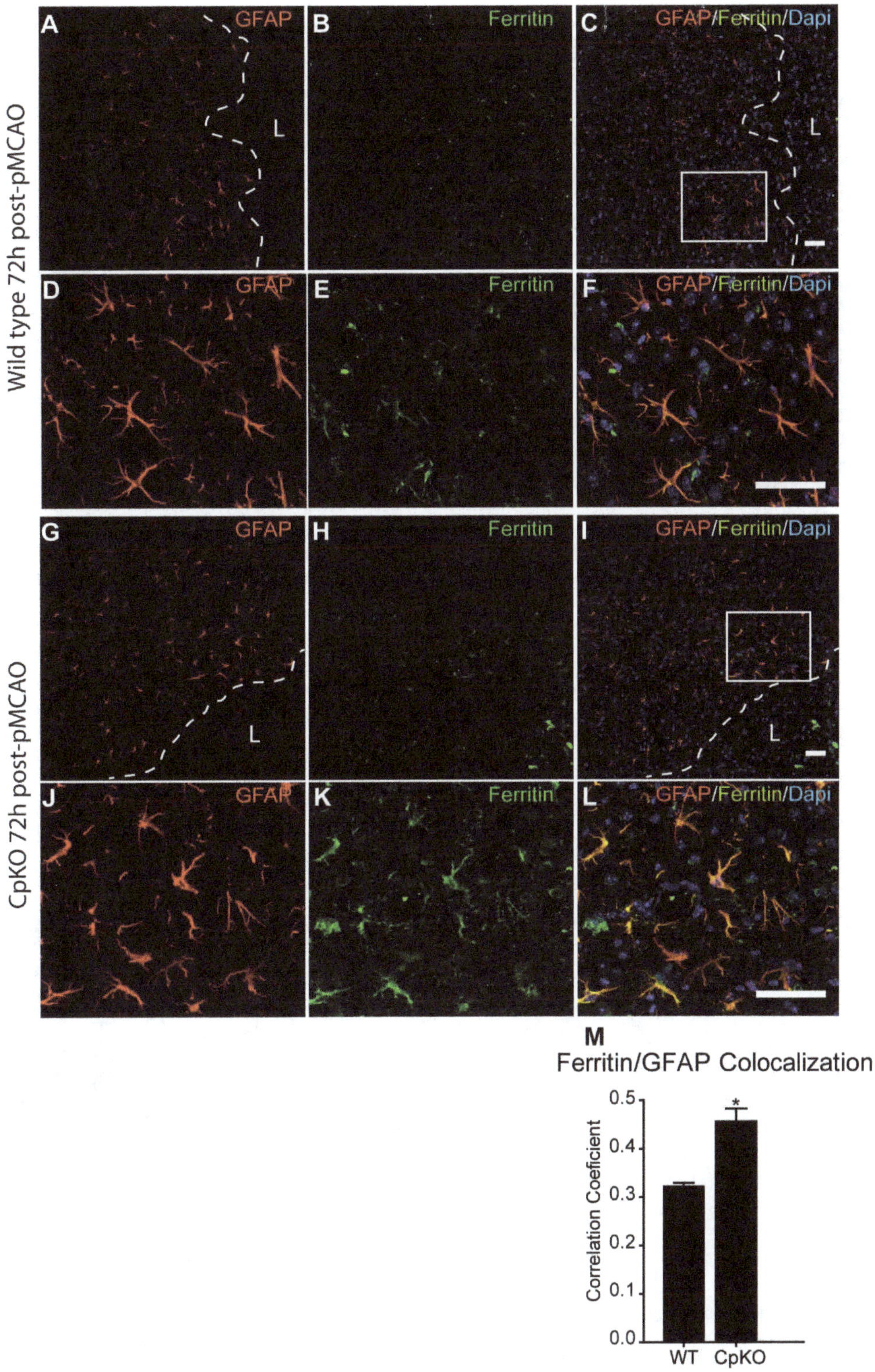

FIGURE 5 | Immunofluorescence labeling for ferritin in astrocytes. Low magnification images of the border region of the infarct and the peri-infarct region in wildtype **(A–C)** and Cp KO **(G–I)** mice 72 h after pMCAO. Dotted line demarcates the lesion boundary and L marks the lesion site. The area in the white square in panels **C,I** are shown at higher magnification in panels **D–F** and **J–L**. Note increase in the number and intensity of the ferritin labeling in CpKO mice **(K)** as compared to the wildtype mice **(E)**. The number of astrocytes that are double labeled for ferritin is higher in the Cp KO **(K)** than in wildtype mice **(E)**. The merged images **(C,F,I,L)** show GFAP, ferritin and DAPI nuclear staining. **(M)** Graph showing the extent of double labeling of GFAP and ferritin estimated using Pearson's correlation coefficient ($n = 4$). Scale bar = 50 μm, *p-value ≤ 0.05.

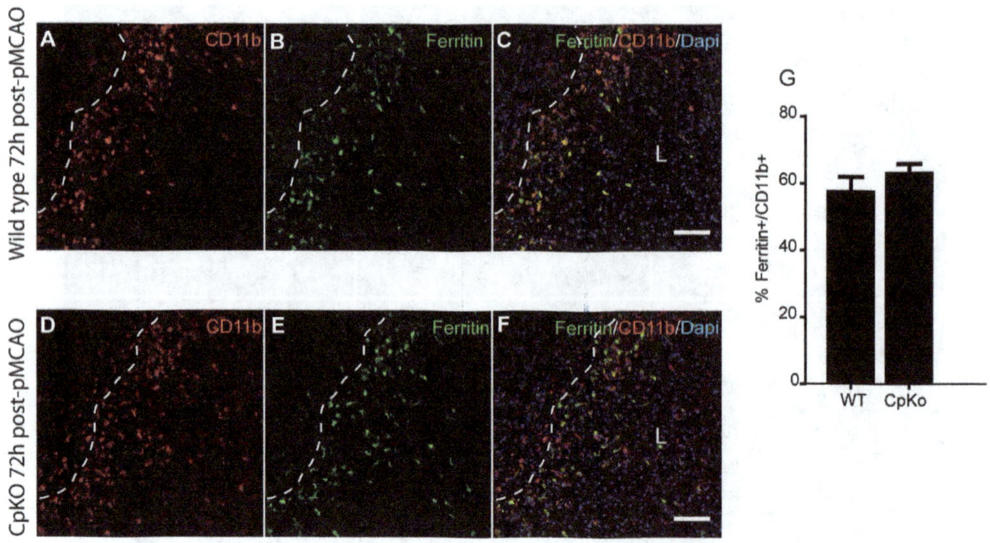

FIGURE 6 | Immunofluorescence labeling for ferritin in macrophage/microglia. Double immunofluorescence labeling show that ferritin+/CD11b+ macrophage/microglia are located mainly in the lesion (L) along the lesion border in both wildtype **(A–C)** and CpKO **(D–F)** mice 72 h after pMCAO. Dotted line demarcates the lesion boundary. The merged images **(C,F)** show CD11b, ferritin and DAPI nuclear staining. Note that the number of CD11b+/ferritin+ doubled labeled cells are not significantly different in the two genotypes **(G)**. Scale bar = 100 μm.

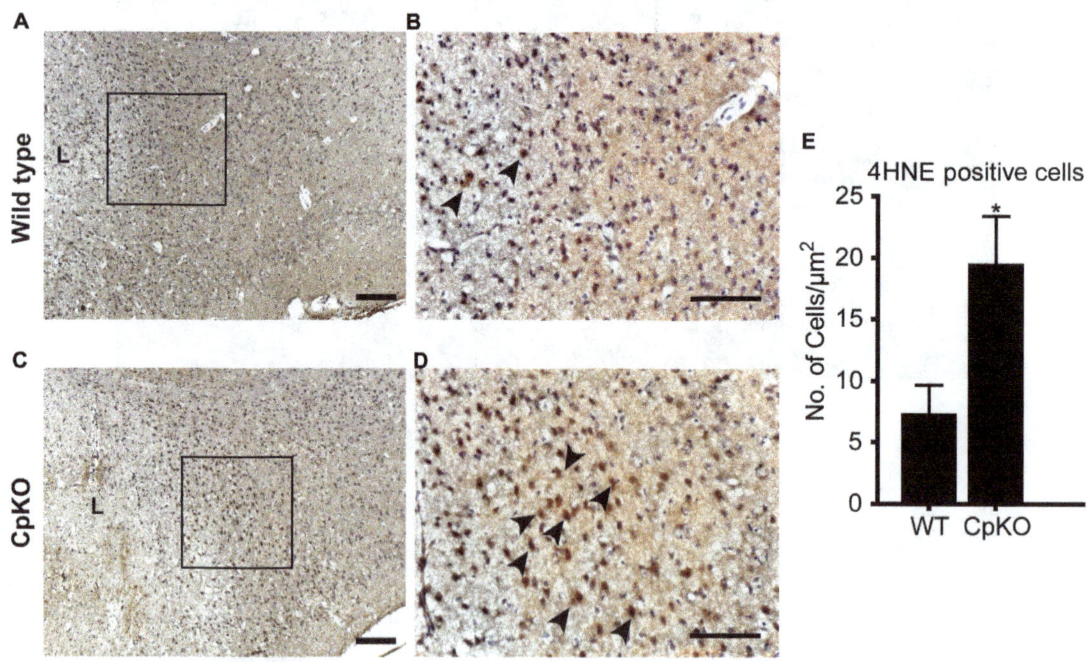

FIGURE 7 | Changes in lipid peroxidation detected by 4-HNE labeling. Tissue sections of wildtype **(A,B)** and CpKO **(C,D)** mice showing immunohistochemical staining for 4HNE. The area demarcated by the black squares in **A** and **C** are shown at higher magnification in panels **B,D**. The lesion area in **A,C** are indicated by "L." The 4HNE staining is seen as a brown reaction product (arrowheads); the tissue sections were counterstained with Mayer's hemalaum which labels the cell nuclei blue. **(E)** Graph shows that the number of 4HNE+ cells is significantly higher in CpKO as compared to wildtype mice. Scale bar = 100 μm, *p-value ≤ 0.05.

(**Figure 9**). No differences were noted between genotypes. The highest increases were detected at 24 h when IL-1β increased by 15-fold, TNFα by 10-fold and IL-6 by about 55-fold. These values dropped markedly by 72 h but were still significantly higher in the lesioned side versus the unlesioned side. By 14 days the values had almost returned to unlesioned control levels (**Figure 9**). IL-10 levels were not significantly changed but there appeared to be a trend to an increase at 72 h and 14 days. The important point to

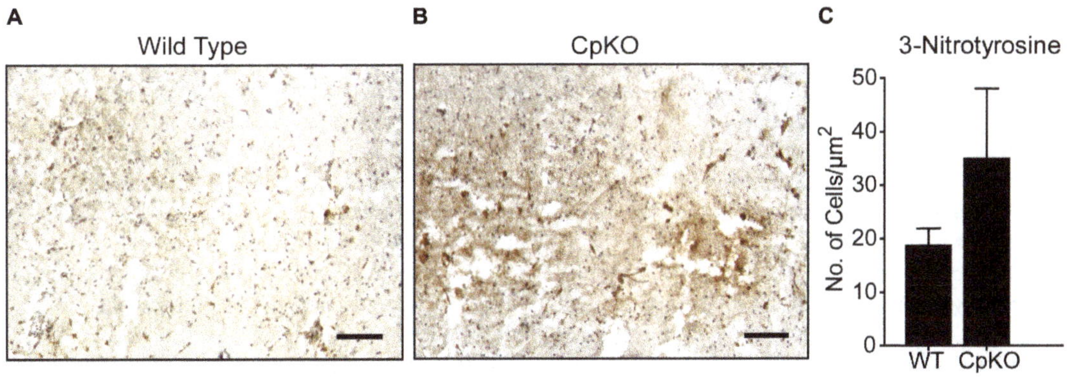

FIGURE 8 | Changes in protein oxidation detected by 3-nitrotyrosine labeling. Tissue sections of wildtype **(A)** and CpKO **(B)** mice showing immunohistochemical staining for 3-NT. The 3-NT staining is seen as a brown reaction product. **(C)** Graph shows that the number of 3-NT+ cells shows a trend to be higher in CpKO compared to wildtype mice but does not reach statistical significance. The tissue sections were counterstained with Mayer's hemalum which labels the cell nuclei blue. $n = 4$; scale bar = 100 μm.

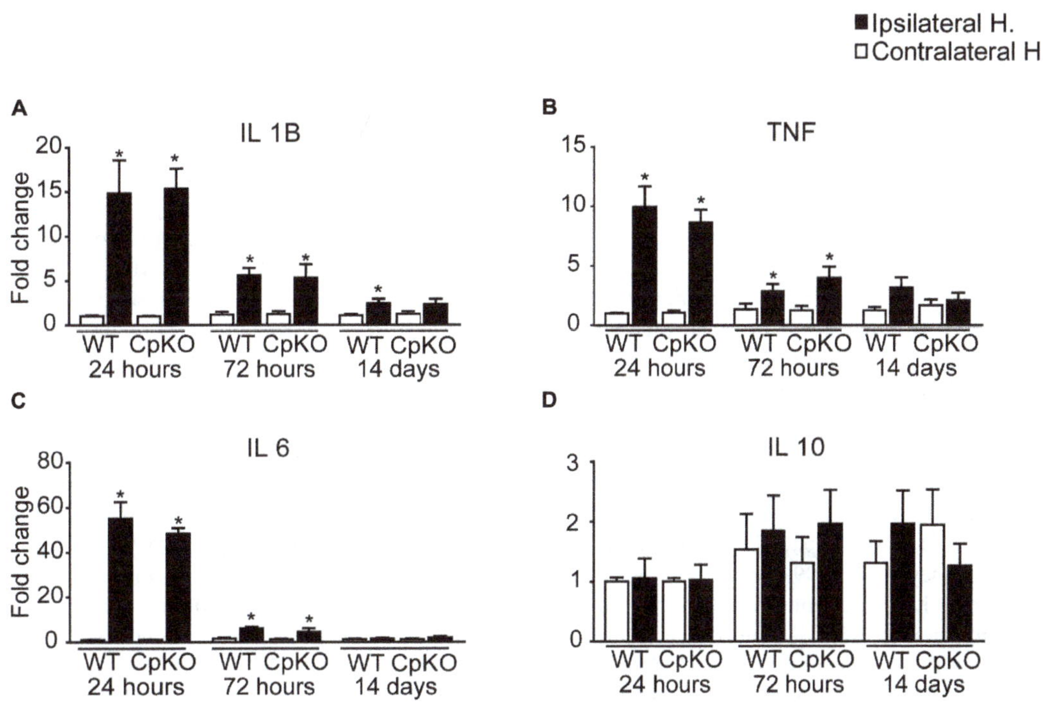

FIGURE 9 | Changes in expression of inflammatory cytokines after pMCAO. The change in the mRNA expression of four key inflammatory cytokines in the brain were assessed by qPCR at 24, 72 h and 14 days after pMCAO in wildtype and CpKO mice. Data are plotted as fold-change on the ipsilateral ischemic side as compared to the uninjured contralateral side. Note the marked increases in IL-1β **(A)**, TNF **(B)** and IL-6 **(C)** at 24 h in both genotypes. They remained elevated at lower levels at 72 h. There were no significant changes in expression of IL-10 **(D)**. $*p$-value ≤ 0.05.

note here is that the absence of Cp does not alter the expression of key inflammatory cytokines after pMCAO as compared to wildtype mice.

DISCUSSION

We provide evidence that the lack of Cp leads to loss of functional recovery and greater lesion size after pMCAO in mice. This was accompanied by alterations in expression of molecules involved in regulating iron homeostasis in the CNS, including reduction in expression of iron efflux transporter (ferroportin), increase in iron uptake transporter (DMT1) and increased iron accumulation (ferritin). Iron histochemistry showed deposition of iron in cells along the border of the lesion at early timepoints after pMCAO and throughout the infarct area by 14 days. Double immunofluorescence labeling for ferritin (a surrogate marker for iron) and cell type specific markers revealed that macrophage/microglia and astrocytes along the lesion border accumulate iron. The labeling in astrocytes being greater in Cp null mice. These changes were also accompanied by increased lipid peroxidation (4HNE staining) and greater nitration of tyrosine residues in proteins as evidenced by increased 3-nitrotyrosine labeling. Increases in key inflammatory cytokines in both genotypes early after pMCAO indicate that inflammation contributes to the evolving pathology but is not influenced by the lack of Cp.

This study provides clear evidence that lack of Cp results in larger lesions and worsening of functional recovery as determined by the "sticky-tape" removal test. Wildtype mice take longer time to remove the adhesive tape between 1 and 7 days after pMCAO as compared to sham-control mice, and subsequently return to almost normal values at day 14. This may be due to neural plasticity-mediated reorganization of neural circuits that lead to recovery of function (Carmichael et al., 2001; Arvidsson et al., 2002; Winship and Murphy, 2009). Of interest to note is that function worsens in Cp null mice as compared to wildtype mice at 7 and 14 days, suggesting that the lack of Cp may induce neurogenerative processes during the second week after pMCAO in Cp null mice. This may be related to free radical mediated damage triggered by the absence of the two major functions of Cp, namely (i) its ability as a ferroxidase to safely convert ferrous iron ($Fe2+$) to its ferric ($Fe3+$) form; (ii) its ability to partner with Fpn to export iron out of cells (Calabrese et al., 1989; Patel et al., 2002).

Ferrous iron can react with hydrogen peroxide, which is produced in mitochondria through normal cellular metabolism and via the Fenton reaction produce highly toxic hydroxyl radicals that can damage lipids, proteins and DNA (Hentze et al., 2004; Rouault and Tong, 2005). Ceruloplasmin has six domains with three mononuclear type 1 coppers in domains 2, 4 and 6, as well as a trinuclear copper center that lies between domains 1 and 6 (Calabrese et al., 1989; Zaitsev et al., 1999). The mononuclear coppers in domains 4 and 6 participate in the oxidation of ferrous to ferric iron (Zaitsev et al., 1999; Quintanar et al., 2004, 2007). This ferroxidase activity is coupled via electron transfer to the reduction of dioxygen to $2H_2O$ at the trinuclear copper center (Calabrese et al., 1989; Zaitsev et al., 1999; Quintanar et al., 2004; Bento et al., 2007). Ceruloplasmin, therefore, safely oxidizes ferrous iron without the generation of free radicals as would happen with the Fenton reaction. Mutations in the trinuclear copper center lead to loss of ferroxidase activity and the degradation of Cp as seen in patients with aceruloplasminemia (Kono, 2013). These patients show iron accumulation in the CNS which increases with age. We have seen increased oxidative stress and iron deposition in the CNS in the Cp null mice with age (Patel et al., 2002; Jeong and David, 2006). On the other hand, iron accumulation occurs because Cp partners with Fpn, the iron efflux transporter, to oxidize ferrous iron that is exported via Fpn (Jeong and David, 2003). In the absence of Cp, Fpn is internalized and degraded (De Domenico et al., 2007), leading to lack of iron efflux and thus iron accumulation. It therefore makes sense that we see significant reduction in the expression of Fpn in the ischemic brain of mice that lack Cp, as well as see increased oxidative damage (4HNE and 3NT) in these mice.

Using ferritin immunofluorescence labeling as a surrogate marker for iron we previously reported that iron accumulation in normally aging Cp null mice occurs in astrocytes, and that the neuronal loss seen may be due to the inability of astrocytes to deliver iron to neurons (Jeong and David, 2006). This may be because unlike neurons which do not directly contact CNS blood vessels, astrocytes are intimately associated with blood vessels via their astrocytic end-feet (Jeong and David, 2006; McCarthy and Kosman, 2015). In other words, astrocytes are equipped to acquire iron from blood vessels in the CNS and deliver it to neurons (McCarthy and Kosman, 2015). After CNS injury, such as spinal cord injury, Cp null mice show greater iron accumulation that is localized to macrophages/microglia at the site of injury (Rathore et al., 2008). These are mainly macrophages that have phagocytosed red blood cells (Rathore et al., 2008). However, in CNS lesions in which hemorrhage does not occur, as in multiple sclerosis or its animal model (EAE), macrophages and microglia accumulate iron likely from phagocytosis of dead and dying cells (Hametner et al., 2013; Zarruk et al., 2015). In the present study, we also see iron accumulation in CD11b+ macrophages/microglia initially around the border of the lesion and later throughout the infarcted area, suggesting that these iron laden cells may be infiltrating macrophages and resident microglia that have phagocytosed dying cells. Interestingly, in Cp null mice, increased ferritin staining was seen in GFAP+ astrocytes lining the lesion border as GPI-Cp is normally expressed selectively by astrocytes in the CNS (Patel and David, 1997). This may add to the iron burden in Cp null mice compared to wildtype mice with pMCAO.

It is not clear at present what might underlie the dysregulated massive 19.5-fold increase in DMT1 protein expression in wildtype mice 72 h after pMCAO. Interestingly, the increase in DMT1 at this time point in Cp null mice was 3 times less (sixfold). The latter might be a way to counteract reduced iron efflux and resultant increase in iron accumulation in Cp null mice due to the reduction in Fpn (50%). The retention of Fpn on the cell surface requires the presence of GPI-Cp (De Domenico et al., 2007). Given that Cp is expressed only in astrocytes in the CNS, the 50% reduction in Fpn seen by Western blot is likely to largely affect astrocytes. In fact, the immunofluorescence labeling experiments showed that there is increased ferritin expression in GFAP+ astrocytes in Cp null mice compared to wildtype mice. So, the lower level of increase in DMT1 in Cp null mice could be a compensatory mechanism that prevents even greater increases in intracellular iron in astrocytes. As mentioned earlier, since the increase in DMT1 in both genotypes is not accompanied by increases in TfR1 expression, it is unlikely that the increased DMT1 is involved in the release of endosomal iron from Tf-TfR1-dependent iron uptake but instead is likely to be involved in Tf-independent cellular iron uptake. We have previously reported that astrocytes express DMT1 on their cell surface but not TfR1, and so can take up iron independent of TfR1 (Jeong and David, 2003) as seen in other non-neural cell types (Wessling-Resnick, 2000).

Inflammation is a well-recognize feature of ischemic stroke (Offner et al., 2006; Wang et al., 2007; Denes et al., 2010; Zarruk et al., 2012; Amantea et al., 2015) in which there is rapid upregulation of pro-inflammatory cytokines. It is important to note that we see a rapid increase in expression in pro-inflammatory cytokines IL-1β, TNFα and IL-6 in both genotypes with no differences between them over the first 14 days after pMCAO. This suggests that the lack of Cp has no influence on the expression of these key inflammatory mediators after ischemic stroke. Recent studies have reported that parenteral treatment with soluble Cp improved lesion size and functional outcome after transient ischemic stroke in mice and rats (Tuo et al., 2017). What we show here is that in addition, the normal levels of Cp present in wildtype mice already has a significant beneficial effect, since lack of this Cp leads to worsening of functional recovery and to larger lesion size.

CONCLUDING REMARKS

This study further elucidates the role of Cp in ischemic stroke. Ceruloplasmin has two fundamental roles (i) in oxidizing ferrous iron and (ii) in the egress of ferrous iron out of cells via Fpn. Lack of Cp, therefore, leads to excess iron buildup in cells. Using wildtype and Cp null mice, we provide clear evidence that Cp has tissue protective effects in the acute phase (24 h) as the ischemic lesion size is larger in Cp null mice. Further evidence of the importance of this antioxidant in the acute phase after pMCAO is suggested by the ninefold increase in its expression at 72 h. In addition, our functional analysis revealed that the absence of Cp leads to worsening of functional recovery at 7 and 14 days after onset of ischemia. This suggests a late effect which could be due to detrimental effects on synaptic reorganization and circuitry via free-radical mediated effects on neurons, astrocytes and microglia. Future work will need to address if Cp influences microglial and astrocyte responses after ischemic stroke that can impact on functional recovery. Analysis of dendritic arborizations and dendritic spines in the penumbral regions of the cortex in wildtype and Cp null mice will also be worth assessing. Evidence of increased iron in the ischemic tissue was detected by iron histochemistry. Furthermore, immunofluorescence staining for ferritin (a surrogate marker for iron) showed increased ferritin in both astrocytes and macrophages/microglia after pMCAO in wildtype mice but this is significantly higher in astrocytes in Cp null mice. These perturbations in iron levels in the tissue was accompanied by increased oxidative damage to lipids and proteins. There is evidence that systemic treatment with Cp improves outcome after ischemic stroke in rodents. Our current study shows that the increased expression of Cp in the ischemic cortex of wildtype mice has important neuroprotective effects after cerebral ischemia.

AUTHOR CONTRIBUTIONS

JZ, FR, and SD planned the study and interpreted the results. JZ, FR, and LL carried out the experiments. JZ and FR analyzed the data and edited the manuscript. SD wrote the manuscript.

FUNDING

This work was supported by a grant from the Canadian Institutes of Health Research (CIHR) (MOP-142231) to SD. JZ was supported by Postdoctoral Fellowships (PDF) from the Heart and Stroke Foundation of Canada, and the Fonds de Recherche du Québec - Santé.

ACKNOWLEDGMENTS

We thank Ourania Tsatas and Laura Curran for technical assistance.

REFERENCES

Allen, N. J. (2014). Astrocyte regulation of synaptic behavior. *Annu. Rev. Cell Dev. Biol.* 30, 439–463. doi: 10.1146/annurev-cellbio-100913-013053

Amantea, D., Micieli, G., Tassorelli, C., Cuartero, M. I., Ballesteros, I., Certo, M., et al. (2015). Rational modulation of the innate immune system for neuroprotection in ischemic stroke. *Front. Neurosci.* 9:147. doi: 10.3389/fnins.2015.00147

Arosio, P., and Levi, S. (2002). Ferritin, iron homeostasis, and oxidative damage. *Free Radic. Biol. Med.* 33, 457–463. doi: 10.1016/S0891-5849(02)00842-0

Arosio, P., and Levi, S. (2010). Cytosolic and mitochondrial ferritins in the regulation of cellular iron homeostasis and oxidative damage. *Biochim. Biophys. Acta* 1800, 783–792. doi: 10.1016/j.bbagen.2010.02.005

Arvidsson, A., Collin, T., Kirik, D., Kokaia, Z., and Lindvall, O. (2002). Neuronal replacement from endogenous precursors in the adult brain after stroke. *Nat. Med.* 8, 963–970. doi: 10.1038/nm747

Bento, I., Peixoto, C., Zaitsev, V. N., and Lindley, P. F. (2007). Ceruloplasmin revisited: structural and functional roles of various metal cation-binding sites. *Acta Crystallogr. D. Biol. Crystallogr.* 63, 240–248. doi: 10.1107/S090744490604947X

Bouet, V., Boulouard, M., Toutain, J., Divoux, D., Bernaudin, M., Schumann-Bard, P., et al. (2009). The adhesive removal test: a sensitive method to assess sensorimotor deficits in mice. *Nat. Protoc.* 4, 1560–1564. doi: 10.1038/nprot.2009.125

Calabrese, L., Carbonaro, M., and Musci, G. (1989). Presence of coupled trinuclear copper cluster in mammalian ceruloplasmin is essential for efficient electron transfer to oxygen. *J. Biol. Chem.* 264, 6183–6187.

Carmichael, S. T., Wei, L., Rovainen, C. M., and Woolsey, T. A. (2001). New patterns of intracortical projections after focal cortical stroke. *Neurobiol. Dis.* 8, 910–922. doi: 10.1006/nbdi.2001.0425

Chen, S. T., Hsu, C. Y., Hogan, E. L., Maricq, H., and Balentine, J. D. (1986). A model of focal ischemic stroke in the rat: reproducible extensive cortical infarction. *Stroke* 17, 738–743. doi: 10.1161/01.STR.17.4.738

Crielaard, B. J., Lammers, T., and Rivella, S. (2017). Targeting iron metabolism in drug discovery and delivery. *Nat. Rev. Drug Discov.* 16, 400–423. doi: 10.1038/nrd.2016.248

De Domenico, I., Ward, D. M., di Patti, M. C., Jeong, S. Y., David, S., Musci, G., et al. (2007). Ferroxidase activity is required for the stability of cell surface ferroportin in cells expressing GPI-ceruloplasmin. *EMBO J.* 26, 2823–2831. doi: 10.1038/sj.emboj.7601735

Denes, A., Thornton, P., Rothwell, N. J., and Allan, S. M. (2010). Inflammation and brain injury: acute cerebral ischaemia, peripheral and central inflammation. *Brain Behav. Immun.* 24, 708–723. doi: 10.1016/j.bbi.2009.09.010

Dunn, K. W., Kamocka, M. M., and McDonald, J. H. (2011). A practical guide to evaluating colocalization in biological microscopy. *Am. J. Physiol. Cell Physiol.* 300, C723–C742. doi: 10.1152/ajpcell.00462.2010

Finazzi, D., and Arosio, P. (2014). Biology of ferritin in mammals: an update on iron storage, oxidative damage and neurodegeneration. *Arch. Toxicol.* 88, 1787–1802. doi: 10.1007/s00204-014-1329-0

Garcia-Yebenes, I., Sobrado, M., Moraga, A., Zarruk, J. G., Romera, V. G., Pradillo, J. M., et al. (2012). Iron overload, measured as serum ferritin, increases brain damage induced by focal ischemia and early reperfusion. *Neurochem. Int.* 61, 1364–1369. doi: 10.1016/j.neuint.2012.09.014

Gitlin, J. D. (1988). Transcriptional regulation of ceruloplasmin gene expression during inflammation. *J. Biol. Chem.* 263, 6281–6287.

Hametner, S., Wimmer, I., Haider, L., Pfeifenbring, S., Bruck, W., and Lassmann, H. (2013). Iron and neurodegeneration in the multiple sclerosis brain. *Ann. Neurol.* 74, 848–861. doi: 10.1002/ana.23974

Harris, Z. L., Durley, A. P., Man, T. K., and Gitlin, J. D. (1999). Targeted gene disruption reveals an essential role for ceruloplasmin in cellular iron efflux. *Proc. Natl. Acad. Sci. U.S.A.* 96, 10812–10817. doi: 10.1073/pnas.96.19.10812

Harris, Z. L., Takahashi, Y., Miyajima, H., Serizawa, M., MacGillivray, R. T., and Gitlin, J. D. (1995). Aceruloplasminemia: molecular characterization of this disorder of iron metabolism. *Proc. Natl. Acad. Sci. U.S.A.* 92, 2539–2543. doi: 10.1073/pnas.92.7.2539

Hentze, M. W., Muckenthaler, M. U., and Andrews, N. C. (2004). Balancing acts: molecular control of mammalian iron metabolism. *Cell* 117, 285–297. doi: 10.1016/S0092-8674(04)00343-5

Jeong, S. Y., and David, S. (2003). Glycosylphosphatidylinositol-anchored ceruloplasmin is required for iron efflux from cells in the central nervous system. *J. Biol. Chem.* 278, 27144–27148. doi: 10.1074/jbc.M301988200

Jeong, S. Y., and David, S. (2006). Age-related changes in iron homeostasis and cell death in the cerebellum of ceruloplasmin-deficient mice. *J. Neurosci.* 26, 9810–9819. doi: 10.1523/JNEUROSCI.2922-06.2006

Kilkenny, C., Browne, W. J., Cuthill, I. C., Emerson, M., and Altman, D. G. (2010). Improving bioscience research reporting: the ARRIVE guidelines for reporting animal research. *PLoS Biol.* 8:e1000412. doi: 10.1371/journal.pbio.1000412

Kono, S. (2013). Aceruloplasminemia: an update. *Int. Rev. Neurobiol.* 110, 125–151. doi: 10.1016/B978-0-12-410502-7.00007-7

Kroner, A., Greenhalgh, A. D., Zarruk, J. G., Passos Dos Santos, R., Gaestel, M., David, S., et al. (2014). TNF and increased intracellular iron alter macrophage polarization to a detrimental M1 phenotype in the injured spinal cord. *Neuron* 83, 1098–1116. doi: 10.1016/j.neuron.2014.07.027

Livak, K. J., and Schmittgen, T. D. (2001). Analysis of relative gene expression data using real-time quantitative PCR and the 2(-Delta Delta C(T)) Method. *Methods* 25, 402–408. doi: 10.1006/meth.2001.1262

McCarthy, R. C., and Kosman, D. J. (2015). Mechanisms and regulation of iron trafficking across the capillary endothelial cells of the blood-brain barrier. *Front. Mol. Neurosci.* 8:31. doi: 10.3389/fnmol.2015.00031

Meguro, R., Asano, Y., Odagiri, S., Li, C., Iwatsuki, H., and Shoumura, K. (2007). Nonheme-iron histochemistry for light and electron microscopy: a historical, theoretical and technical review. *Arch. Histol. Cytol.* 70, 1–19. doi: 10.1679/aohc.70.1

Millerot-Serrurot, E., Bertrand, N., Mossiat, C., Faure, P., Prigent-Tessier, A., Garnier, P., et al. (2008). Temporal changes in free iron levels after brain ischemia Relevance to the timing of iron chelation therapy in stroke. *Neurochem. Int.* 52, 1442–1448. doi: 10.1016/j.neuint.2008.04.002

Mittal, B., Doroudchi, M. M., Jeong, S. Y., Patel, B. N., and David, S. (2003). Expression of a membrane-bound form of the ferroxidase ceruloplasmin by leptomeningeal cells. *Glia* 41, 337–346. doi: 10.1002/glia.10158

Morita, H., Ikeda, S., Yamamoto, K., Morita, S., Yoshida, K., Nomoto, S., et al. (1995). Hereditary ceruloplasmin deficiency with hemosiderosis: a clinicopathological study of a Japanese family. *Ann. Neurol.* 37, 646–656. doi: 10.1002/ana.410370515

Offner, H., Subramanian, S., Parker, S. M., Afentoulis, M. E., Vandenbark, A. A., and Hurn, P. D. (2006). Experimental stroke induces massive, rapid activation of the peripheral immune system. *J. Cereb. Blood Flow Metab.* 26, 654–665. doi: 10.1038/sj.jcbfm.9600217

Patel, B. N., and David, S. (1997). A novel glycosylphosphatidylinositol-anchored form of ceruloplasmin is expressed by mammalian astrocytes. *J. Biol. Chem.* 272, 20185–20190. doi: 10.1074/jbc.272.32.20185

Patel, B. N., Dunn, R. J., and David, S. (2000). Alternative RNA splicing generates a glycosylphosphatidylinositol-anchored form of ceruloplasmin in mammalian brain. *J. Biol. Chem.* 275, 4305–4310. doi: 10.1074/jbc.275.6.4305

Patel, B. N., Dunn, R. J., Jeong, S. Y., Zhu, Q., Julien, J. P., and David, S. (2002). Ceruloplasmin regulates iron levels in the CNS and prevents free radical injury. *J. Neurosci.* 22, 6578–6586. doi: 10.1523/JNEUROSCI.22-15-06578.2002

Quintanar, L., Gebhard, M., Wang, T. P., Kosman, D. J., and Solomon, E. I. (2004). Ferrous binding to the multicopper oxidases *Saccharomyces cerevisiae* Fet3p and human ceruloplasmin: contributions to ferroxidase activity. *J. Am. Chem. Soc.* 126, 6579–6589. doi: 10.1021/ja049220t

Quintanar, L., Stoj, C., Taylor, A. B., Hart, P. J., Kosman, D. J., and Solomon, E. I. (2007). Shall we dance? How a multicopper oxidase chooses its electron transfer partner. *Acc. Chem. Res.* 40, 445–452. doi: 10.1021/ar600051a

Rathore, K. I., Kerr, B. J., Redensek, A., Lopez-Vales, R., Jeong, S. Y., Ponka, P., et al. (2008). Ceruloplasmin protects injured spinal cord from iron-mediated oxidative damage. *J. Neurosci.* 28, 12736–12747. doi: 10.1523/JNEUROSCI.3649-08.2008

Rathore, K. I., Redensek, A., and David, S. (2012). Iron homeostasis in astrocytes and microglia is differentially regulated by TNF-alpha and TGF-beta1. *Glia* 60, 738–750. doi: 10.1002/glia.22303

Rouault, T. A., and Tong, W. H. (2005). Iron-sulphur cluster biogenesis and mitochondrial iron homeostasis. *Nat. Rev. Mol. Cell Biol.* 6, 345–351. doi: 10.1038/nrm1620

Stephan, A. H., Barres, B. A., and Stevens, B. (2012). The complement system: an unexpected role in synaptic pruning during development and disease. *Annu. Rev. Neurosci.* 35, 369–389. doi: 10.1146/annurev-neuro-061010-113810

Texel, S. J., Zhang, J., Camandola, S., Unger, E. L., Taub, D. D., Koehler, R. C., et al. (2011). Ceruloplasmin deficiency reduces levels of iron and BDNF in the cortex and striatum of young mice and increases their vulnerability to stroke. *PLoS One* 6:e25077. doi: 10.1371/journal.pone.0025077

Tuo, Q. Z., Lei, P., Jackman, K. A., Li, X. L., Xiong, H., Li, X. L., et al. (2017). Tau-mediated iron export prevents ferroptotic damage after ischemic stroke. *Mol. Psychiatry* 22, 1520–1530. doi: 10.1038/mp.2017.171

Wang, Q., Tang, X. N., and Yenari, M. A. (2007). The inflammatory response in stroke. *J. Neuroimmunol.* 184, 53–68. doi: 10.1016/j.jneuroim.2006.11.014

Wessling-Resnick, M. (2000). Iron transport. *Annu. Rev. Nutr.* 20, 129–151. doi: 10.1146/annurev.nutr.20.1.129

Williams, D. M., Lee, G. R., and Cartwright, G. E. (1974). Ferroxidase activity of rat ceruloplasmin. *Am. J. Physiol.* 227, 1094–1097. doi: 10.1152/ajplegacy.1974.227.5.1094

Winship, I. R., and Murphy, T. H. (2009). Remapping the somatosensory cortex after stroke: insight from imaging the synapse to network. *Neuroscientist* 15, 507–524. doi: 10.1177/1073858409333076

Xu, X., Pin, S., Gathinji, M., Fuchs, R., and Harris, Z. L. (2004). Aceruloplasminemia: an inherited neurodegenerative disease with impairment of iron homeostasis. *Ann. N. Y. Acad. Sci.* 1012, 299–305. doi: 10.1196/annals.1306.024

Yoshida, K., Furihata, K., Takeda, S., Nakamura, A., Yamamoto, K., Morita, H., et al. (1995). A mutation in the ceruloplasmin gene is associated with systemic hemosiderosis in humans. *Nat. Genet.* 9, 267–272. doi: 10.1038/ng0395-267

Zaitsev, V. N., Zaitseva, I., Papiz, M., and Lindley, P. F. (1999). An X-ray crystallographic study of the binding sites of the azide inhibitor and organic substrates to ceruloplasmin, a multi-copper oxidase in the plasma. *J. Biol. Inorg. Chem.* 4, 579–587. doi: 10.1007/s007750050380

Zarruk, J. G., Berard, J. L., Passos dos Santos, R., Kroner, A., Arosio, P., Lee, J., et al. (2015). Expression of iron homeostasis proteins in the spinal cord in experimental autoimmune encephalomyelitis and their implications for iron accumulation. *Neurobiol. Dis.* 81, 93–107. doi: 10.1016/j.nbd.2015.02.001

Zarruk, J. G., Fernandez-Lopez, D., Garcia-Yebenes, I., Garcia-Gutierrez, M. S., Vivancos, J., Nombela, F., et al. (2012). Cannabinoid type 2 receptor activation downregulates stroke-induced classic and alternative brain macrophage/microglial activation concomitant to neuroprotection. *Stroke* 43, 211–219. doi: 10.1161/STROKEAHA.111.631044

Zarruk, J. G., Garcia-Yebenes, I., Romera, V. G., Ballesteros, I., Moraga, A., Cuartero, M. I., et al. (2011). Neurological tests for functional outcome assessment in rodent models of ischaemic stroke. *Rev. Neurol.* 53, 607–618.

15

Brain Iron Accumulation in Atypical Parkinsonian Syndromes: *In vivo* MRI Evidences for Distinctive Patterns

Jae-Hyeok Lee [1] and Myung-Sik Lee [2]**

[1] Department of Neurology, Research Institute for Convergence of Biomedical Science and Technology, Pusan National University Yangsan Hospital, Pusan National University School of Medicine, Yangsan, South Korea, [2] Department of Neurology, Gangnam Severance Hospital, Yonsei University College of Medicine, Seoul, South Korea

***Correspondence:**
Jae-Hyeok Lee
jhlee.neuro@pusan.ac.kr
Myung-Sik Lee
mslee@yuhs.ac

Recent data suggest mechanistic links among perturbed iron homeostasis, oxidative stress, and misfolded protein aggregation in neurodegenerative diseases. Iron overload and toxicity toward dopaminergic neurons have been established as playing a role in the pathogenesis of Parkinson's disease (PD). Brain iron accumulation has also been documented in atypical parkinsonian syndromes (APS), mainly comprising multiple system atrophy (MSA), and progressive supranuclear palsy (PSP). Iron-sensitive magnetic resonance imaging (MRI) has been applied to identify iron-related signal changes for the diagnosis and differentiation of these disorders. Topographic patterns of widespread iron deposition in deep brain nuclei have been described as differing between patients with MSA and PSP and those with PD. A disease-specific increase of iron occurs in the brain regions mainly affected by underlying disease pathologies. However, whether iron changes are a primary pathogenic factor or an epiphenomenon of neuronal degeneration has not been fully elucidated. Moreover, the clinical implications of iron-related pathology in APS remain unclear. In this review study, we collected data from qualitative and quantitative MRI studies on brain iron accumulation in APS to identify disease-related patterns and the potential role of iron-sensitive MRI.

Keywords: iron, neurodegeneration, magnetic resonance imaging, atypical parkinsonian syndromes, multiple system atrophy, progressive supranuclear palsy

INTRODUCTION

Iron overload in the substantia nigra and its toxicity toward dopaminergic neurons has been suggested to play a key role in the pathogenesis of Parkinson's disease (PD) (1). Brain iron accumulation has also been repeatedly documented in atypical parkinsonian syndromes (APS), mainly comprising multiple system atrophy (MSA), and progressive supranuclear palsy (PSP). Pathological studies have shown that iron levels in the putamen, globus pallidus, and substantia nigra are higher in MSA patients than in PD and control patients, and resembles the levels found in PSP patients (2–4).

Iron-sensitive magnetic resonance imaging (MRI) has been applied to identify iron-related signal changes for the diagnosis and differentiation of these disorders. However, the clinical and pathogenic implications of iron-related pathology detected by MRI in APS remain unclear. In this review study, we collected data from qualitative and quantitative MRI studies on brain iron accumulation in APS to identify disease-related patterns and the potential role of iron-sensitive MRI.

Potential Pathogenic Mechanisms of Iron Accumulation in APS

Brain iron accumulation can be caused by several factors, such as impaired iron homoeostasis, neuroinflammation, and increased blood–brain barrier permeability (1). The key proteins associated with degenerative parkinsonism, α-synuclein and tau, are believed to play roles in iron homeostasis (5). α-synuclein is a cellular ferrireductase responsible for reducing ferric iron (Fe^{3+}) to ferrous iron (Fe^{2+}) (6). In the presence of functional tau, the export of ferrous iron in neurons is controlled by the binding of the amyloid precursor protein (APP) to tau, which results in the trafficking of the protein complex to the neuronal surface, where APP interacts with ferroportin (7). Changes in these proteins might result in altered cellular iron homeostasis (5).

Dysregulation of the proteins involved in iron homeostasis has been reported in APS patients. In PSP patients, the amount of ferritin, an iron-storing protein, has been reported to be considerably lower than that in control patients, which is the opposite trend of increasing iron burden (8). High levels of iron might exceed the iron-buffering capacity of complexes, such as neuromelanin and ferritin in the substantia nigra (1, 9). In MSA, an increase in ferritin iron coupled with a reduction in ferroportin expression has been detected in the pons and putamen (10). These findings suggest a potential deficit in bioavailable iron despite an excess of tissue iron.

Impaired iron homeostasis can induce toxic protein oligomers and abnormal intracellular aggregates under pathological conditions. The aggregation of α-synuclein and tau has been shown to be triggered by iron *in vitro* (1). Iron promotes α-synuclein aggregation by inducing β-sheet conformational changes and increasing oxidative stress and microglial activation (4, 11). Abundant evidence has demonstrated the role of iron in tau hyperphosphorylation and aggregation into fibrils (12, 13).

In postmortem brain tissues, high concentrations of iron have been colocalized with α-synuclein and hyperphosphorylated tau aggregates. Notably, the highest iron content in the putamen, as assessed by histochemistry, is correlated with the highest density of glial cytoplasmic inclusions and α-synuclein aggregation in MSA brains (14). Hyperphosphorylated tau aggregates from the brains of PSP patients have been shown to colocalize with ferritin (15).

Iron overload in brain regions that undergo protein misfolding and aggregation can promote oxidative stress and neuroinflammation (4). In turn, iron-induced oxidative stress leads to apoptosis and ferroptosis, a novel mode of regulated cell death dependent on iron and lipid peroxidation (1, 16). Scavenging of accumulated labile iron by chelation can protect against iron-mediated neuronal damage (17).

CURRENT MRI METHODS FOR DETECTION AND QUANTIFICATION OF BRAIN IRON

Iron-Sensitive MRI Techniques

Iron-sensitive MRI techniques have been used to differentiate parkinsonian disorders and monitor disease progression (18–20). Various methods have been used to study iron content, including R2 ($1/T_2$), R_2^* ($1/T_2^*$), R′2 ($1/T'_2$), susceptibility weighted imaging (SWI), and quantitative susceptibility mapping (QSM) (20, 21). SWI enhances image contrast by using the susceptibility differences between tissues; images are obtained by combining T2*-weighted magnitude images with filtered phase images in the gradient echo data. SWI further enhances the contrast between tissues of different susceptibilities (22). Because of its high degree of sensitivity in detecting and visualizing iron deposition, SWI has been applied in the diagnosis and differentiation of parkinsonian disorders (23). However, SWI does not provide quantitative measurement of magnetic susceptibility, which is a limitation that has been addressed by the recent development of QSM (22, 23). Both QSM and the transverse relaxation rate (R2*) are highly sensitive and represent the most accurate measurement of iron content in the brain (20); results have been shown to correlate closely with iron concentrations measured in postmortem brain tissues (24, 25). QSM can also overcome the confounding effect of increased water content influencing relaxation values, thus counteracting the effect of increased iron levels (20). Recent studies have shown that QSM achieves stronger diagnostic performance than R2* for detecting iron deposition in the subcortical gray matter (26, 27). However, the opposite effect of myelin on QSM may impede its positive correlation with iron. A histological validation study found lower correlation coefficients for QSM and iron in white matter and cortical gray matter regions than in the basal ganglia when correlating R2* and iron (28).

Quantitative MRI Measurements of Brain Iron

The region-of-interest (ROI) method is commonly used to calculate regional iron content. The method is based on the manual or automated segmentation of target structures (29). Automated ROI analysis eliminates bias in the process of selecting images and drawing ROIs (30). Computer-based MRI analyses using machine learning techniques and support vector machine (SVM) classification have proven potential in the discrimination of parkinsonian syndromes and the tracking of disease progression (31, 32). SVM pattern recognition of SWI data can accurately discriminate PD from APS (32).

Focal or unevenly increased iron deposition should be considered in determining the iron concentration within a structure (23, 33). Single or two consecutive ROIs in two-dimensional images without delineation of the exact boundaries of a structure may not sufficiently reflect unevenly or focally increased iron content of the whole three-dimensional structure. Voxel-based analysis can provide additional information about the topographic distribution of sub-regional iron deposition (34).

The multimodal MRI approach combines MRI techniques for imaging iron and other MRI sequences that are sensitive to complementary tissue characteristics, including volume atrophy and microstructural damage (35). This approach may aid early diagnosis, monitoring of disease progression, and highlighting of pathogenic mechanisms (36, 37).

IRON-DEPOSITION PATTERNS IN APS: THE DETERMINANTS OF REGION SPECIFICITY

Age-Related and Structure-Specific Patterns

The regional distribution of iron is heterogeneous in normal adult brains. The basal ganglia have the highest iron concentrations, whereas low concentrations are detected in the cortical gray matter, white matter, brainstem, and cerebellum (1). Typically, total iron concentrations increase with age in the substantia nigra, putamen, globus pallidus, caudate nucleus, and cortices. However, the rate of iron accumulation varies among strictures throughout the adult life span (38, 39). For example, a previous study found high iron concentration in the globus pallidus regardless of age, but a significantly greater presence of iron in the putamen with advancing age (38). Regional heterogeneity of brain iron and its changes with age have been confirmed *in vivo* by MRI (1).

The region- or structure-specific pattern of iron deposition in normal aging can be enhanced in pathologic conditions. In the parkinsonian variant of MSA (MSA-P), iron deposition predominantly in the posterolateral part of the putamen is in line with the aging pattern (40, 41). The motor-related subcortical structures may present with different patterns in both volume and iron level. In previous MRI studies, the putamen demonstrated a decrease in volume and an increase in iron level, whereas the thalamus did not show iron deposition despite volume shrinkage (42, 43).

Pathoanatomy-Related Distribution

Total iron levels have been found to be elevated in most areas of the basal ganglia in the postmortem brain tissue of patients with APS (2). However, *in vivo* iron-sensitive MRI has shown topographical differences in excessive iron accumulation among the distinct subtypes of parkinsonism (23, 33, 34, 43–46). Significant increases in iron-related signals (SWI phase and QSM susceptibility) have been found in the midbrain and globus pallidus of patients with PSP, and in the putamen of patients with MSA (**Figure 1**) (34, 46).

Regions of higher iron content are correlated with the main sites of underlying pathology. Increased iron in the putamen is the most consistent finding in MSA (23, 33, 34, 43–47), and specifically in MSA-P (48, 49), as well as being correlated with hypometabolism on ^{18}F-flurodeoxyglucose positron-emission tomography (PET) (50). In a previous study, *in vivo* ^{18}F-flortaucipir tau PET revealed that PSP patients had the highest overall uptake in the globus pallidus with the greatest discriminant power (51).

The multimodal MRI approach combining volumetry and iron estimation has shown that excessive iron accumulation is associated with advanced atrophy in a region-specific manner (4, 43, 49). R2* values are negatively correlated with volumes in the putamen and globus pallidus (43). In a longitudinal study, iron accumulation in the putamen increased in parallel with the extent of atrophy (49).

Uneven or Sub-structural Distribution

Iron distribution can be uneven across the entire structure of the brain. Iron concentrations in MSA-P are highest in the posterolateral subregion of the putamen (33, 41, 44, 48). Sub-structural differences have also been demonstrated by voxel-based analysis (34, 43). A previous study reported significant increases in SWI hypointensity in the posterolateral putamen and adjacent lateral aspect of the globus pallidus in patients with MSA-P, and in the anterior and medial aspects of the globus pallidus in patients with PSP (34). Similarly, higher R2* values have been reported in more atrophic sub-regions (43). In MSA-P, increases in R2* values in the putamen and globus pallidus have been noted more posteriorly and dorsally than those in PSP.

Conventional MRI techniques are insufficient to delineate the inner structure of the substantia nigra and measure the loss of melanized dopaminergic neurons and the increase of iron deposition (52). Recently, iron-sensitive MRI sequences at high field strengths have been reported to consistently display a hyperintense ovoid area within the dorsolateral border of the otherwise hypointense substantia nigra pars compacta, which is referred to as dorsolateral nigral hyperintensity (53–55). A postmortem 9.4 T MRI study with histopathological correlation indicated that this MRI feature corresponds to nigrosome-1 (56). Loss of dorsolateral nigral hyperintensity, a typical finding for patients with PD, is also observed in the majority of patients with MSA or PSP (53–55).

CLINICAL IMPLICATIONS OF BRAIN IRON DEPOSITION IN APS

Discriminant Markers

Distinctive patterns of iron deposition detected on iron-sensitive MRI can be used in clinical practice to differentiate PD, MSA, and PSP (see **Table 1**). Patients with PSP have more widespread iron deposition in the motor-related subcortical nuclei than patients with other parkinsonian disorders (**Figure 1**) (34, 61). In receiver operating characteristic (ROC) analyses, the putamen has been consistently demonstrated to have the highest area under the curve (AUC) values (~0.8–0.9) in differentiating MSA-p from PSP and PD (34, 45, 46, 58, 59, 63). Furthermore, the red nucleus and globus pallidus are the two most valuable nuclei in the diagnosis of PSP (34, 46). However, direct comparisons among studies are difficult because of differences in patient characteristics (e.g., clinical severity and clinical subtypes) and methodology (e.g., MRI parameters, selected brain structures, and analysis methods) (31). The role of iron-sensitive MRI in other APS, such as diffuse Lewy body disease and corticobasal degeneration, has not yet been determined.

SWI can provide improved diagnostic accuracy through assessment of the degree and distribution of hypointensity in the putamen using a visual rating scale (**Supplementary Figure 1**) (41). A pattern of posterolateral putaminal hypointensity with a striking lateral-to-medial gradient on SWI is a highly specific sign of MSA-P (**Supplementary Figures 1D–F**). However, grading of putaminal hypointensity focused only on the signal intensity without consideration of the distributional

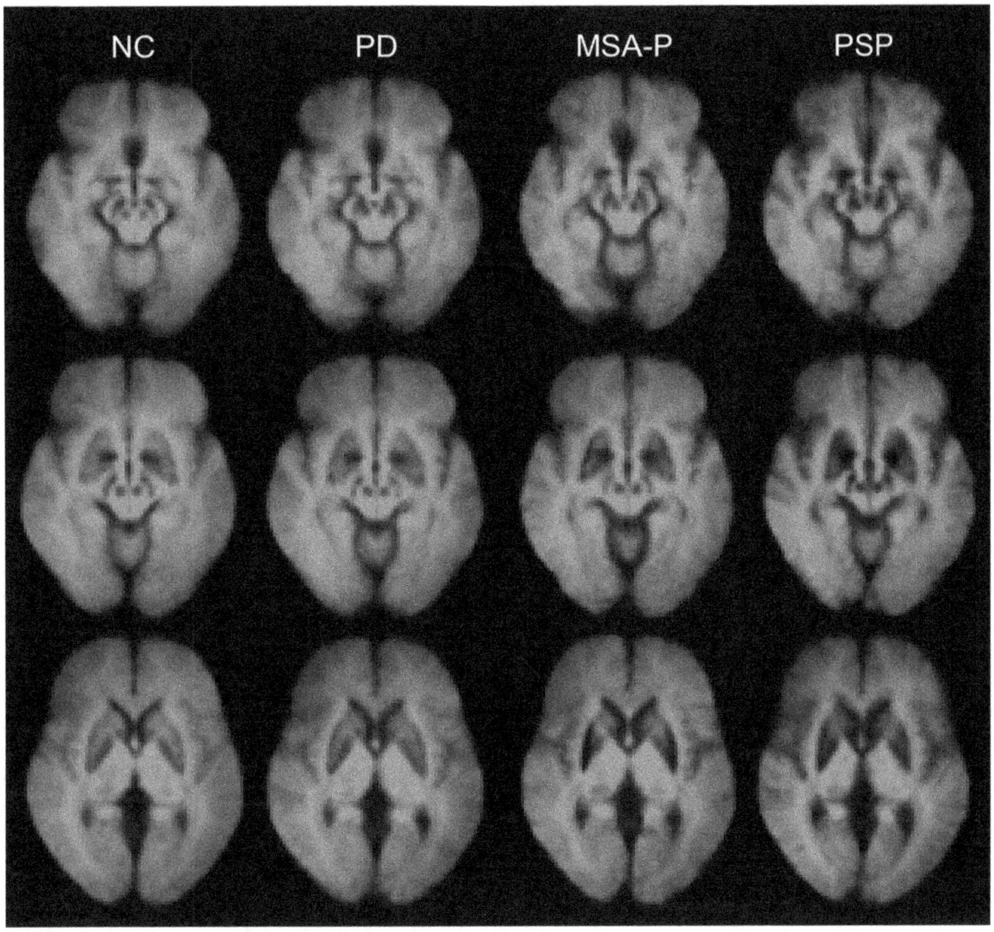

FIGURE 1 | Disease-specific susceptibility weighted imaging maps generated using the mean images of normal control (NC), patients with Parkinson's disease (PD), the parkinsonian variant of multiple system atrophy (MSA-P), and progressive supranuclear palsy (PSP). The images were obtained from the Pusan National University Yangsan Hospital using protocols approved by the institutional review board. Written informed consent was obtained from all participants.

pattern fails to differentiate MSA-P from PD (57). Slit-like hypointensity along the lateral margin of the putamen or evenly distributed hypointensity throughout the putamen can be a nonspecific and age-related sign of physiological mineralization (**Supplementary Figures 1A–C**) (40, 41). Compared with SWI, T2- or T2*-weighted images have limited diagnostic value with lower sensitivity (66, 67).

Because of uneven and focal accumulation of iron within the structure of the brain, subregional analyses could have higher diagnostic value than total average iron calculations (33). The posterior and inner subregion of the putamen is the most valuable among four subregional ROIs in differentiating MSA-P from PD. Moreover, high iron deposition percentages can be used to detect smaller increases in iron with higher sensitivity than average SWI phase shifts.

Multimodal MRI can identify specific markers to discriminate patients with PD from patients with MSA with high accuracy (37). The combination of T2* relaxation rates and mean diffusivity (MD) in the putamen achieves discrimination of >95% between patients with MSA-P and PD (65).

Clinical Correlates

Increased iron content in motor-related subcortical nuclei may be associated with the severity of parkinsonian motor deficits. Nigral iron accumulation in PD correlated with symptoms linked to dopaminergic neurodegeneration (68). A recent study identified a significant correlation between Unified MSA Rating Scale II scores and putaminal R2* values in patients with MSA (65). The phase-shift value of the posterior aspect of the putamen has demonstrated significantly higher asymmetry in MSA-P patients than in PD patients (60). These findings are frequently detected in the contralateral symptomatic side of patients.

In a recent study of correlations between R2* values and the degree of Unified Parkinson's Disease Rating Scale scores in PSP, the burden of iron-related PSP pathologies in the lenticular nucleus was associated with the severity of rigidity, and nigro-striato-pallidal and dentate iron content were associated with the severity of tremors (62). Other studies have failed to show a correlation of iron-sensitive MRI markers with clinical severity scale scores in MSA and PSP (34, 43, 49, 64), but have instead reported that diffusion tensor metrics, such as MD values, are

TABLE 1 | Summary of studies using iron-sensitive MRI in atypical parkinsonian syndromes.

Study	References	Number of subjects	MRI methods	Selected structures	Analysis methods	Main findings
Signal intensity grading	Gupta et al. (57)	12 MSA-P, 12 PSP, 11 PD, 11 NC	SWI, 1.5T	RN, SN, DN, PUT	Grade 0–3 on the basis of the mean SI values	1. Hypointensity score of SN and RN: higher in PSP than that of MSA-P and PD. 2. Hypointensity score of PUT: higher in PSP than that of PD.
	Sakurai et al. (44)	10 MSA-P, 10 PD, 10 NC	PRESTO, T2*WI, 3T	PUT	PUT SI scored in comparison with that of the GP	1. PUT signal changes: the posterolateral part with a striking lateral to medial gradient. 2. PRESTO: lower intensity and better than T2*WI.
	Lee and Baik (41)	11 MSA-P, 30 PD, 30 NC	SWI, 3T	PUT	Grade 0-3 on the basis of the pattern of hypointensity	The pattern of posterolateral PUT: a striking lateral to medial gradient (a grade of ≥2) differentiated MSA-P from PD and NC.
	Sugiyama et al. (58)	15 MSA, 9 PSP, 16 PD, 10 NC	T2WI, T2*WI, 1.5T	PUT	PUT abnormality scores on visual analog scale	1. PUT hypointensity on T2*WI: the highest diagnostic accuracy. 2. AUCs of 0.797 (vs. PSP), 0.867 (vs. PD), and 0.896 (vs. NC) for differentiating MSA from PSP, PD and NC.
	Wang et al. (59)	18 MSA-P, 21 MSA-C, 18 PD, 31 NC	SWI, 3T	PUT, SN	Grade 0-3 on the basis of the mean SI values of PUT; "Swallow-tail" sign (nigrosome 1) of SN	AUC of combined signs: increased from 0.85 (swallow tail) or 0.68 (PUT hypointensity) to 0.93.
ROI-based quantification of iron	Wang et al. (33)	8 MSA-P, 16 PD, 44 NC	SWI, 1.5T	SN, RN, CN, PUT, GP, TH (PT)	Manually-drawn ROI (2D); Average-total-iron-deposition values (phase shift) and high-iron-content area percentages; 4 subregions of the PUT	1. The high-iron-deposition-percentage area: superior to the average phase shift in differentiating MSA-P from PD (PUT: AUC = 0.88 vs. 0.78; PT: AUC = 0.79 vs. 0.62). 2. Lower inner region of the putamen: the most valuable subregion.
	Han et al. (34)	12 MSA-P, 11 PSP, 15 PD, 20 NC	SWI, 3T	RN, SN, CN, GP, PUT, TH	Group comparisons of mean phase shift values in the manually-drawn ROI (2D); Voxel-based analysis of the processed SWI	1. PUT (AUC = 0.836): the most valuable nucleus in differentiating MSA-P from PSP and PD. 2. GP (AUC = 0.869) and TH (AUC = 0.884): the two most valuable nuclei in differentiating PSP from MSA-P and PD. 3. Sub-regional differences in SWI hypointensity in the PUT, GP, and TH between MSA-P and PSP.
	Sakurai et al. (45)	13 MSA-P, 12 PSP, 12 PD, 13 NC	PRESTO, 1.5T	RN, SN, DN, STN, PUT	Volume of interest (VOI) analysis of normalized images; Comparison of SI ratio in target VOIs	1, PUT: the highest AUCs of 0.83 (vs. PSP) and 0.91 (vs. NC) in the diagnosis of MSA-P. 2. RN: the highest AUCs of 0.87 (vs. MSA-P), 0.90 (vs. PD), and 0.89 (vs. NC) in the diagnosis of PSP.
	Sjöström et al. (46)	11 MSA, 15 PSP, 62 PD, 14 NC	QSM, 1.5/3T	SN, RN, PUT, GP	Group comparisons of susceptibility in the manually-drawn ROI (2D)	1. RN: the most promising biomarker for separating groups, especially for PSP (AUC of 0.97 for PSP vs. PD, 0.86 for MSA vs. PD and 0.75 for PSP vs. MSA). 2. GP: a similar accuracy in separating PSP from MSA of 0.73.
	Yoon et al. (50)	17 MSA-P, 30 PD	SWI, 3T	PUT	Group comparisons of mean SI values of the anterior and posterior halves of the PUT in the manually-drawn ROI; Correlation of the ROI SI values of SWI and SUVR on 18F-FDG PET	1. The values of dominant-side of the posterior half of the PUT: high AUC values (AUC of 18F-FDG PET = 1; AUC of SWI = 0.947) to differentiate MSA-P and PD. 2. The low SI in the putamen on SWI correlated with hypometabolism on 18F-FDG PET in MSA-P.

(Continued)

TABLE 1 | Continued

Study	References	Number of subjects	MRI methods	Selected structures	Analysis methods	Main findings
	Hwang et al. (60)	27 MSA-P, 50 PD, 27 NC	SWI, 3T	PUT	Quantitatively measured PUT width and phase-shift values	1. Significantly higher asymmetric phase-shift value of the posterior PUT in MSA-P. 2. A contralateral correlation between the symptomatic side and the marked hypointense signal side.
	Boelmans et al. (61)	12 PSP, 30 PD, 24 NC	T2, T2*, T2′, 1.5T	CN, PUT, GP, TH, WM	Group comparisons of mean T2′ values in the manually-drawn ROI; A stepwise linear discriminant analysis to predict the clinical diagnosis	1. Shortened T2′ values in the CN, PUT, and GP in PSP compared to PD and NC. 2.T2′ mean values: excellent discrimination between PSP and PD patients.
	Lee et al. (62)	24 PSP, 20 NC	R2*, 3T	SN, STN, DN, PUT, GP	Correlations between R2* values and UPDRS	1. Significantly higher R2* values in all of the five brain regions in PSP patients. 2. UPDRS subscores correlated with R2* values.
Multimodal MRI analysis	Focke et al. (63)	10 MSA-P, 9 PSP, 12 PD, 13 NC	R2*, R2, R1, DTI, MT, 3T	SN, CN, PUT, GP	Group comparisons of quantitative MRI data in the manually-drawn ROI (3D)	R2* mapping in the PUT: the best separation of MSA from PD patients and controls with a good predictive power (AUC of ≤0.96).
	Lee et al. (43)	15 MSA-P, 13 PSP, 29 PD, 22 NC	R2*, T1-Vol., 3T	CN, PUT, GP, TH	Automated ROI (3D) analysis for R2* and volume calculation; Voxel-based analysis to visualize a topographical correlation of R2* and volume	1. Negative correlation between R2* values and volumes in the PUT ($r = -0.777$, $p < 0.001$) and GP ($r = -0.409$, $p = 0.025$) of MSA-P, and GP ($r = -0.4$, $p = 0.043$) of PSP. 2. Higher R2* values in more severely atrophic sub-regions.
	Lee et al. (49)	8 MSA-P, 9 MSA-C, 15 PD	R2*, T1-Vol., 3T	CN, PUT, GP, TH	Automated ROI (3D) analysis; Longitudinal, two serial MRIs	1. Greater annual rates of progression of R2* and volume in the PUT of MSA-P than MSA-C and PD patients. 2. Significant correlation between the R2* and volume changes.
	Lee et al. (64)	21 MSA-P, 18 MSA-C, 22 NC	R2*,T1-Vol., DTI, 3T	CN, PUT, GP, TH, Brainstem, cerebellum	Automated ROI (3D) analysis; Principal component analysis and structural equation modeling to show a model consisting of multiple inter-dependencies	1. No significant correlation between alterations in the R2* of the basal ganglia region and the MRI variables associated with brainstem–cerebellar degeneration. 2. Significant correlation between the PUT MD values and the UPDRS and UMSARS scores.
	Barbagallo et al. (65)	16, MSA-P, 13 MSA-C, 26 PD	R2*,T1-Vol., DTI, 3T	SN, CN, PUT	Automated ROI (3D) analysis; Correlation analyses between MRI findings and clinical variables	1. The combination of PUT R2* and MD: >95% discrimination between patients with MSA-P and PD (AUC = 96). 2. The UMSARS-II scores correlated with PUT R2* values of the MSA (total) patients, with the PUT MD values of the MSA-P patients, and with the PUT volumes of the MSA-C patients.
	Péran et al. (37)	16 MSA-P, 13 MSA-C, 26 PD, 26 NC	R2*, T1, DTI, 3T	Whole brain	Voxel-based analysis of the gray density, MD, fractional anisotropy, and R2* maps; Unsupervised machine-learning method to classify patients.	1. Several combinations of 2 different markers: >95% discrimination between MSA and PD patients. 2. Specific single marker allowed for 95% of discriminant power. 3. The unsupervised analysis could regroup individuals according to their clinical diagnosis.

AUC, area under the curve; CN, caudate nucleus; D, dimensional; DN, dentate nucleus; DTI, diffusion tensor imaging; FDG, Fluorodeoxyglucose; GP, globus pallidus; MD, mean diffusivity; MSA, multiple system atrophy; MSA-P, parkinsonian variant of MSA; MSA-C. cerebellar variant of MSA; MT, magnetization transfer; NC, normal control; PD, Parkinson's disease; PRESTO, principles of echo shifting using a train of observations; PSP, progressive supranuclear palsy; PT, pulvinar thalamus; PUT, putamen; QSM, quantitative susceptibility mapping; RN, red nucleus; ROI, region-of-interest; SI, signal intensity; SN, substantia nigra; SUVR, standardized uptake value; SWI, susceptibility-weighted imaging; T, tesla; TH, thalamus; T1-Vol., T1 volumetry; UMSARS, unified multiple system atrophy rating scale; UPDRS, unified Parkinson's disease rating scale; WM, white matter.

closely correlated with clinical severity (63, 64). Iron-sensitive MRI markers may have less sensitivity to reflect clinical status than diffusion tensor metrics.

Structural MRI abnormalities in MSA are segregated into basal ganglia and brainstem-cerebellar factors (64). Alterations in the R2* of the basal ganglia region are not significantly correlated with the MRI variables associated with brainstem-cerebellar degeneration. In a longitudinal study, a higher rate of iron accumulation was observed in the putamen of MSA-P patients compared to patients with the cerebellar variant of MSA and PD (49). These findings may underlie the stratification of the motor subtype of MSA. Thus, far, no attempt has been made to correlate regional iron deposition with the severity of motor deficits according to the subtypes of PSP.

A recent *post-hoc* analysis demonstrated that MSA-specific MRI abnormalities are associated with more rapid progression and worse overall prognosis (69). In a longitudinal study, greater baseline iron content in the putamen was correlated with smaller volumes at follow-up in MSA patients (49). Similarly, accumulation of iron in the putamen predicts volume loss in healthy older adults (70). Excessive iron accumulation in the putamen may serve as a marker for impending progression of neurodegeneration in MSA.

Current Limitations and Future Directions

Although recent data suggest a mechanistic link between perturbed iron homeostasis, oxidative stress, and misfolded protein aggregation, whether iron accumulation is a primary pathogenic factor or an epiphenomenon of neuronal degeneration remains to be elucidated. In a single case report, putaminal iron deposition preceded the occurrence of the initial symptoms of MSA-P (71). However, when iron deposition appears during the course of disease is unknown. A longitudinal study on the relationship between multimodal MRI abnormalities at earlier stages of the disease is necessary to identify the spatiotemporal patterns of iron-related neurodegeneration.

High-field MRI developments have advanced the ability to map the distribution of iron *in vivo* (1). However, studies that have investigated the pathological correlates of iron-sensitive MRI measurements are rare. Signal hypointensities observed using T2 or T2* methods are correlated with iron deposits (Fe^{3+}) and ferritin in histologic analysis (8, 48, 72). A recent study showed that R2* is significantly associated with nigral α-synuclein. Iron-sensitive MRI may capture the pathological aspects of disorders other than iron (73). Further research is needed to verify the exact underlying pathology of MRI signal alterations.

CONCLUSION

A distinctive pattern of iron deposition in MSA and PSP has been described. We highlighted the main factors that can determine region specificity. Disease-specific increases of iron occur in the brain regions mainly affected by underlying disease pathologies. Therefore, *in vivo* MRI mapping of brain iron deposition may serve as an indirect marker of neurodegenerative changes in pathoanatomically relevant sites. Age-related, structure-specific, and sub-structural patterns of iron accumulation should be considered when investigating iron-related neurodegeneration using MRI.

AUTHOR CONTRIBUTIONS

All authors listed have made a substantial, direct and intellectual contribution to the work, and approved it for publication.

FUNDING

This research was supported by a grant of the Korea Health Technology R&D Project through the Korea Health Industry Development Institute (KHIDI), funded by the Ministry of Health & Welfare, Republic of Korea (grant number: HI18C0713).

REFERENCES

Ward RJ, Zucca FA, Duyn JH, Crichton RR, Zecca L. The role of iron in brain ageing and neurodegenerative disorders. *Lancet Neurol.* (2014) 13:1045–60. doi: 10.1016/S1474-4422(14)70117-6

Dexter DT, Carayon A, Javoy-Agid F, Agid Y, Wells FR, Daniel SE, et al. Alterations in the levels of iron, ferritin and other trace metals in Parkinson's disease and other neurodegenerative diseases affecting the basal ganglia. *Brain* (1991) 114:1953–75.

Jellinger KA. Neuropathological spectrum of synucleinopathies. *Mov Disord.* (2003) 18:2–12. doi: 10.1002/mds.10557

Kaindlstorfer C, Jellinger KA, Eschlböck S, Stefanova N, Weiss G, Wenning GK. The relevance of iron in the pathogenesis of multiple system atrophy: a viewpoint. *J Alzheimers Dis.* (2018) 61:1253–73. doi: 10.3233/JAD-170601

Angelova DM, Brown DR. Iron, aging, and neurodegeneration. *Metals* (2015) 5:2070–92. doi: 10.3390/met5042070

Davies P, Moualla D, Brown DR. Alpha-synuclein is a cellular ferrireductase. *PLoS ONE* (2011) 6:e15814. doi: 10.1371/journal.pone.0015814

Stankowski JN, Dawson VL, Dawson TM. Ironing out tau's role in *parkinsonism*. *Nat Med.* (2012) 18:197–8. doi: 10.1038/nm.2668

Foroutan P, Murray ME, Fujioka S, Schweitzer KJ, Dickson DW, Wszolek ZK et al. Progressive supranuclear palsy: high-field-strength MR microscopy in the human substantia nigra and globus pallidus. *Radiology* (2013) 266:280–8. doi: 10.1148/radiol.12102273

Zucca FA, Segura-Aguilar J, Ferrari E, Muñoz P, Paris I, Sulzer D, et al. Interactions of iron, dopamine and neuromelanin pathways in brain aging and Parkinson's disease. *Prog Neurobiol.* (2017) 155:96–119. doi: 10.1016/j.pneurobio.2015.09.012.

Visanji NP, Collingwood JF, Finnegan ME, Tandon A, House E, Hazrati LN. Iron deficiency in *parkinsonism*: region-specific iron dysregulation in Parkinson's disease and multiple system atrophy. *J Parkinsons Dis.* (2013) 3:523–37. doi: 10.3233/JPD-130197

Ostrerova-Golts N, Petrucelli L, Hardy J, Lee JM, Farer M, Wolozin B. The A53T alpha-synuclein mutation increases iron- dependent aggregation and toxicity. *J Neurosci.* (2000) 20:6048–54. doi: 10.1523/JNEUROSCI.20-16-06048.2000

Kim AC, Lim S, Kim YK. Metal ion effects on Aβ and tau aggregation. *Int J Mol Sci.* (2018) 19:128. doi: 10.3390/ijms19010128

Yamamoto A, Shin RW, Hasegawa K, Naiki H, Sato H, Yoshimasu F, et al. Iron (III) induces aggregation of hyperphosphorylated tau and its reduction to iron (II) reverses the aggregation: implications in the formation of neurofibrillary tangles of Alzheimer's disease. *J Neurochem.* (2002) 82:1137– 47. doi: 10.1046/j.1471-4159.2002.t01-1-01061.x

Jellinger KA. Neuropathology of multiple system atrophy: new thoughts about pathogenesis. *Mov Disord.* (2014) 29:1720–41. doi: 10.1002/mds.26052

Pérez M, Valpuesta JM, de Garcini EM, Quintana C, Arrasate M, López Carrascosa JL, et al. Ferritin is associated with the aberrant tau filaments present in progressive supranuclear palsy. *Am J Pathol.* (1998) 152:1531–9.

Masaldan S, Bush AI, Devos D, Rolland AS, Moreau C. Striking while the iron is hot: Iron metabolism and ferroptosis in neurodegeneration. *Free Radic Biol Med.* (2018). doi: 10.1016/j.freeradbiomed.2018.09.033. [Epub ahead of print].

Devos D, Moreau C, Devedjian JC, Kluza J, Petrault M, Laloux C, et al. Targeting chelatable iron as a therapeutic modality in Parkinson's disease. *Antioxid Redox Signal* (2014) 21:195–210. doi: 10.1089/ars.2013.5593.

Pietracupa S, Martin-Bastida A, Piccini P. Iron metabolism and its detection through MRI in *parkinsonian* disorders: a systematic review. *Neurol Sci.* (2017) 38:2095–101. doi: 10.1007/s10072-017-3099-y

Lehericy S, Vaillancourt DE, Seppi K, Monchi O, Rektorova I, Antonini A, et al. The role of high-field magnetic resonance imaging in parkinsonian disorders: Pushing the boundaries forward. *Mov Disord.* (2017) 32:510–25. doi: 10.1002/mds.26968

Yan F, He N, Lin H, Li R. Iron deposition quantification: Applications in the brain and liver. *J Magn Reson Imag.* (2018) 48:301–17. doi: 10.1002/jmri.26161

Ghassaban K, Liu S, Jiang C, Haacke EM. Quantifying iron content in magnetic resonance imaging. *Neuroimage* (2018). doi: 10.1016/j.neuroimage.2018.04.047. [Epub ahead of print].

Liu C, Li W, Tong KA, Yeom KW, Kuzminski S. Susceptibility-weighted imaging and quantitative susceptibility mapping in the brain. *J Magn Reson Imag.* (2015) 42:23–41. doi: 10.1002/jmri.24768

Wang Z, Luo XG, Gao C. Utility of susceptibility-weighted imagingin Parkinson's disease and atypical Parkinsonian disorders. *Transl Neurodegener* (2016) 5:17. doi: 10.1186/s40035-016-0064-2

Langkammer C, Krebs N, Goessler W, Scheurer E, Ebner F, Yen K, et al. Quantitative MR imaging of brain iron: a postmortem validation study. *Radiology* (2010) 257:455–62. doi: 10.1148/radiol.10100495

Sun H, Walsh AJ, Lebel RM, Blevins G, Catz I, Lu JQ, et al. Validation of quantitative susceptibility mapping with Perls' iron staining for subcortical gray matter. *Neuroimage* (2015) 105:486–92. doi: 10.1016/j.neuroimage.2014.11.010

Barbosa JH, Santos AC, Tumas V, Liu M, Zheng W, Haacke EM, et al.. Quantifying brain iron deposition in patients with Parkinson's disease using quantitative susceptibility mapping, R2 and R2⊠. *Magn Reson Imag.* (2015) 33:559–65. doi: 10.1016/j.mri.2015.02.021

Murakami Y, Kakeda S, Watanabe K, Ueda I, Ogasawara A, Moriya J, et al. Usefulness of quantitative susceptibility mapping for the diagnosis of Parkinson disease. *Am J Neuroradiol.* (2015) 36:1102–8. doi: 10.3174/ajnr.A4260

Hametner S, Endmayr V, Deistung A, Palmrich P, Prihoda M, Haimburger E et al.. The influence of brain iron and myelin on magnetic susceptibility and effective transverse relaxation - A biochemical and histological validation study. *Neuroimage* (2018) 179:117–33. doi: 10.1016/j.neuroimage.2018. 06.007

Despotović I, Goossens B, Philips W. MRI segmentation of the human brain: challenges, methods, and applications. *Comput Math Methods Med.* (2015) 2015:450341. doi: 10.1155/2015/450341

Smith SM1, Jenkinson M, Woolrich MW, Beckmann CF, Behrens TE, Johansen-Berg H, et al. Advances in functional and structural MR image analysis and implementation as FSL. *Neuroimage* (2004) 23:S208–19. doi: 10.1016/j.neuroimage.2004.07.051

Kassubek J. MRI-based neuroimaging: atypical parkinsonisms and other movement disorders. *Curr Opin Neurol.* (2018) 31:425–30. doi: 10.1097/WCO.0000000000000578

Haller S, Badoud S, Nguyen D, Barnaure I, Montandon ML, Lovblad KO, et al. Differentiation between Parkinson disease and other forms of Parkinsonism using support vector machine analysis of susceptibility- weighted imaging (SWI): initial results. *Eur Radiol.* (2013) 23:12–9. doi: 10.1007/s00330-012-2579-y

Wang Y, Butros SR, Shuai X, Dai Y, Chen C, Liu M, et al.. Different iron-deposition patterns of multiple system atrophy with predominant parkinsonism and idiopathetic Parkinson diseases demonstrated by phase- corrected susceptibility-weighted imaging. *Am J Neuroradiol.* (2012) 33:266–73. doi: 10.3174/ajnr.A2765

Han YH, Lee JH, Kang BM, Mun CW, Baik SK, Shin YI, et al. Topographical differences of brain iron deposition between progressive supranuclear palsy and parkinsonian variant multiple system atrophy. *J Neurol Sci.* (2013) 325:29–35. doi: 10.1016/j.jns.2012.11.009

Cerasa A, Cherubini A, Peran P. Multimodal MRI in neurodegenerative disorders. *Neurol Res Int.* (2012) 2012:287891. doi: 10.1155/2012/287891

Péran P, Cherubini A, Assogna F, Piras F, Quattrocchi C, Peppe A, et al. Magnetic resonance imaging markers of Parkinson's disease nigrostriatal signature. *Brain* (2010) 133:3423–33. doi: 10.1093/brain/awq212

Péran P, Barbagallo G, Nemmi F, Sierra M, Galitzky M, Traon AP, et al. MRI supervised and unsupervised classification of Parkinson's disease and multiple system atrophy. *Mov Disord.* (2018) 33:600–8. doi: 10.1002/mds.27307

Pfefferbaum A, Adalsteinsson E, Rohlfing T, Sullivan EV. MRI estimates of brain iron concentration in normal aging: comparison of field- dependent (FDRI) and phase (SWI) methods. *Neuroimage* (2009) 47:493–500. doi: 10.1016/j.neuroimage.2009.05.006

Bilgic B, Pfefferbaum A, Rohlfing T, Sullivan EV, Adalsteinsson E. MRI estimates of brain iron concentration in normal aging using quantitative susceptibility mapping. *Neuroimage* (2012) 59:2625–35. doi: 10.1016/j.neuroimage.2011.08.077

Harder SL, Hopp KM, Ward H, Neglio H, Gitlin J, Kido D. Mineralization of the deep gray matter with age: a retrospective review with susceptibility-weighted MR imaging. *Am J Neuroradiol.* (2008) 29:176–83. doi: 10.3174/ajnr.A0770

Lee JH, Baik SK. Putaminal hypointensity in the parkinsonian variant of multiple system atrophy: simple visual assessment using susceptibility-weighted imaging. *J Mov Disord.* (2011) 4:60–3. doi: 10.14802/jmd. 11012

Péran P, Cherubini A, Luccichenti G, Hagberg G, Démonet JF, Rascol O, et al. Volume and iron content in basal ganglia and thalamus. *Hum Brain Mapp.* (2009) 30:2667–75. doi: 10.1002/hbm.20698

Lee JH, Han YH, Kang BM, Mun CW, Lee SJ, Baik SK. Quantitative assessment of subcortical atrophy and iron content in progressive supranuclear palsy and parkinsonian variant of multiple system atrophy. *J Neurol.* (2013) 260:2094–101. doi: 10.1007/s00415-013-6951-x

Sakurai K, Kawaguchi T, Kawai T, Ogino H, Hara M, Okita K, et al. Usefulness of 3D-PRESTO imaging in evaluating putaminal abnormality in parkinsonian variant of multiple system atrophy. *Neuroradiology* (2010) 52:809–14. doi: 10.1007/s00234-009-0621-9

Sakurai K, Imabayashi E, Tokumaru AM, Ito K, Shimoji K, Nakagawa M, et al. Volume of interest analysis of spatially normalized PRESTO imaging to differentiate between parkinson disease and atypical parkinsonian syndrome. *Magn Reson Med Sci.* (2017) 16:16–22. doi: 10.2463/mrms.mp.2015-0132

Sjöström H, Granberg T, Westman E, Svenningsson P. Quantitative susceptibility mapping differentiates between parkinsonian disorders. *Parkinsonism Relat Disord.* (2017) 44:51–57. doi: 10.1016/j.parkreldis.2017.08.029

Ozawa T, Paviour D, Quinn NP, Josephs KA, Sangha H, Kilford L, et al. The spectrum of pathological involvement of the striatonigral and olivopontocerebellar systems in multiple system atrophy: clinicopathological correlations. *Brain* (2004) 127:2657–71. doi: 10.1093/brain/awh303

Matsusue E, Fujii S, Kanasaki Y, Sugihara S, Miyata H, Ohama E, et al. Putaminal lesion in multiple system atrophy: postmortem MR-pathological correlations. *Neuroradiology* (2008) 50:559–67. doi: 10.1007/s00234-008-0381-y

6. Lee JH, Kim TH, Mun CW, Kim TH, Han YH. Progression of subcortical atrophy and iron deposition in multiple system atrophy: a comparison between clinical subtypes. *J Neurol.* (2015) 262:1876–82. doi: 10.1007/s00415-015-7785-5

Yoon RG, Kim SJ, Kim HS, Choi CG, Kim JS, Oh J, et al. The utility of susceptibility-weighted imaging for differentiating Parkinsonism- predominant multiple system atrophy from Parkinson's disease: correlation with 18F-flurodeoxyglucose positron-emission tomography. *Neurosci Lett.* (2015) 584:296–301. doi: 10.1016/j.neulet.2014. 10.046

Schonhaut DR, McMillan CT, Spina S, Dickerson BC, Siderowf A, Devous MD Sr, et al. 18 F-flortaucipir tau positron emission tomography distinguishes established progressive supranuclear palsy from controls and Parkinson disease: a multicenter study. *Ann Neurol.* (2017) 82:622–34. doi: 10.1002/ana.25060

Cosottini M, Frosini D, Pesaresi I, Costagli M, Biagi L, Ceravolo R, et al. MR imaging of the substantia nigra at 7 T enables diagnosis of Parkinson disease. *Radiology* (2014) 271:831–8. doi: 10.1148/radiol.14131448

Reiter E, Mueller C, Pinter B, Krismer F, Scherfler C, Esterhammer R, et al. Dorsolateral nigral hyperintensity on 3.0T susceptibility-weighted imaging in neurodegenerative Parkinsonism. *Mov Disord.* (2015) 30:1068–76. doi: 10.1002/mds.26171

Bae YJ, Kim JM, Kim E, Lee KM, Kang SY, Park HS, et al. Loss of Nigral Hyperintensity on 3 Tesla MRI of Parkinsonism: comparison with (123) I-FP-CIT SPECT. *Mov Disord.* (2016) 31:684–92. doi: 10.1002/mds.26584

Mahlknecht P, Krismer F, Poewe W, Seppi K. Meta-analysis of dorsolateral nigral hyperintensity on magnetic resonance imaging as a marker for Parkinson's disease. *Mov Disord.* (2017) 32:619–23. doi: 10.1002/mds. 26932

Massey LA, Miranda MA, Al-Helli O, Parkes HG, Thornton JS, So PW, et al. 9.4 T MR microscopy of the substantia nigra with pathological validation in controls and disease. *Neuroimage Clin.* (2016) 13:154–63. doi: 10.1016/j.nicl.2016.11.015

Gupta D, Saini J, Kesavadas C, Sarma PS, Kishore A. Utility of susceptibility-weighted MRI in differentiating Parkinson's disease and atypical parkinsonism. *Neuroradiology* (2010) 52:1087–94. doi: 10.1007/s00234-010-0677-6

Sugiyama A, Ito S, Suichi T, Sakurai T, Mukai H, Yokota H, et al. Putaminal hypointensity on T2⊠-weighted MR imaging is the most practically useful sign in diagnosing multiple system atrophy: a preliminary study. *J Neurol Sci.* (2015) 349:174–8. doi: 10.1016/j.jns.2015.01.013

Wang N, Yang H, Li C, Fan G, Luo X. Using 'swallow-tail' sign and putaminal hypointensity as biomarkers to distinguish multiple system atrophy from idiopathic Parkinson's disease: a susceptibility-weighted imaging study. *Eur Radiol.* (2017) 27:3174–80. doi: 10.1007/s00330-017-4743-x

Hwang I, Sohn CH, Kang KM, Jeon BS, Kim HJ, Choi SH, et al. Differentiation of parkinsonism-predominant multiple system atrophy from idiopathic parkinson disease using 3T susceptibility-weighted MR imaging, focusing on putaminal change and lesion asymmetry. *Am J Neuroradiol.* (2015) 36:2227–34. doi: 10.3174/ajnr.A4442

Boelmans K, Holst B, Hackius M, Finsterbusch J, Gerloff C, Fiehler J, et al. Brain iron deposition fingerprints in Parkinson's disease and progressive supranuclear palsy. *Mov Disord.* (2012) 27:421–7. doi: 10.1002/mds. 24926

Lee SH, Lyoo CH, Ahn SJ, Rinne JO, Lee MS. Brain regional iron contents in progressive supranuclear palsy. *Parkinsonism Relat Disord.* (2017) 45:28–32. doi: 10.1016/j.parkreldis.2017.09.020

Focke NK, Helms G, Pantel PM, Scheewe S, Knauth M, Bachmann CG, et al. Differentiation of typical and atypical Parkinson syndromes by quantitative MR imaging. *Am J Neuroradiol.* (2011) 32:2087–92. doi: 10.3174/ajnr.A2865

Lee MJ, Kim TH, Mun CW, Shin HK, Son J, Lee JH. Spatial correlation and segregation of multimodal MRI abnormalities in multiple system atrophy. *J Neurol.* (2018) 265:1540–7. doi: 10.1007/s00415-018-8874-z

Barbagallo G, Sierra-Peña M, Nemmi F, Traon AP, Meissner WG, Rascol O, et al. Multimodal MRI assessment of nigro-striatal pathway in multiple system atrophy and Parkinson disease. *Mov Disord.* (2016) 31:325–34. doi: 10.1002/mds.26471

Feng JY, Huang B, Yang WQ, Zhang YH, Wang LM, Wang LJ, et al. The putaminal abnormalities on 3.0T magnetic resonance imaging: can they separate parkinsonism-predominant multiple system atrophy from Parkinson's disease? *Acta Radiol.* (2015) 56:322–8. doi: 10.1177/0284185114524090

Arabia G, Morelli M, Paglionico S, Novellino F, Salsone M, Giofrè L, et al. An magnetic resonance imaging T2⊠-weighted sequence at short echo time to detect putaminal hypointensity in Parkinsonisms. *Mov Disord.* (2010) 25:2728–34. doi: 10.1002/mds.23173

Martin-Bastida A, Lao-Kaim NP, Loane C, Politis M, Roussakis AA, Valle- Guzman N, et al. Motor associations of iron accumulation in deep grey matter nuclei in Parkinson's disease: a cross-sectional study of iron-related magnetic resonance imaging susceptibility. *Eur J Neurol.* (2017) 24:357–365. doi: 10.1111/ene.13208

Krismer F, Seppi K, Wenning GK, Papapetropoulos S, Abler V, Goebel G, et al. Abnormalities on structural MRI associate with faster disease progression in multiple system atrophy. *Parkinsonism Relat Disord.* (2018). doi: 10.1016/j.parkreldis.2018.08.004. [Epub ahead of print].

Daugherty AM, Raz N. Accumulation of iron in the putamen predicts its shrinkage in healthy older adults: a multi-occasion longitudinal study. *Neuroimage* (2016) 128:11–20. doi: 10.1016/j.neuroimage.2015.12.045

Kikuchi Y, Shibata M, Hirayanagi K, Nagashima K, Mihara B, Ikeda Y. Putaminal iron deposition precedes MSA-P onset by 2 years. *Neurology* (2018) 90:1071–72. doi: 10.1212/WNL.0000000000005637

Matsusue E, Fujii S, Kanasaki Y, Kaminou T, Ohama E, Ogawa T. Cerebellar lesions in multiple system atrophy: Postmortem MR imaging-pathologic correlations. *Am J Neuroradiol.* (2009) 30:1725–30. doi: 10.3174/ajnr.A1662

Lewis MM, Du G, Baccon J, Snyder AM, Murie B, Cooper F, et al. Susceptibility MRI captures nigral pathology in patients with parkinsonian syndromes. *Mov Disord.* (2018) 33:1432–9. doi: 10.1002/mds.27381

16

Iron and Alzheimer's Disease: From Pathogenesis to Therapeutic Implications

Jun-Lin Liu[1†], Yong-Gang Fan[1†], Zheng-Sheng Yang[2], Zhan-You Wang[1,3] and Chuang Guo[1*]*

[1] College of Life and Health Sciences, Northeastern University, Shenyang, China, [2] Department of Dermatology, First Hospital of Qinhuangdao, Qinhuangdao, China, [3] Key Laboratory of Medical Cell Biology of Ministry of Education, Institute of Health Sciences, China Medical University, Shenyang, China

***Correspondence:**
Zhan-You Wang
wangzy@mail.neu.edu.cn
Chuang Guo
guoc@mail.neu.edu.cn

† These authors have contributed equally to this work

As people age, iron deposits in different areas of the brain may impair normal cognitive function and behavior. Abnormal iron metabolism generates hydroxyl radicals through the Fenton reaction, triggers oxidative stress reactions, damages cell lipids, protein and DNA structure and function, and ultimately leads to cell death. There is an imbalance in iron homeostasis in Alzheimer's disease (AD). Excessive iron contributes to the deposition of β-amyloid and the formation of neurofibrillary tangles, which in turn, promotes the development of AD. Therefore, iron-targeted therapeutic strategies have become a new direction. Iron chelators, such as desferoxamine, deferiprone, deferasirox, and clioquinol, have received a great deal of attention and have obtained good results in scientific experiments and some clinical trials. Given the limitations and side effects of the long-term application of traditional iron chelators, alpha-lipoic acid and lactoferrin, as self-synthesized naturally small molecules, have shown very intriguing biological activities in blocking Aβ-aggregation, tauopathy and neuronal damage. Despite a lack of evidence for any clinical benefits, the conjecture that therapeutic chelation, with a special focus on iron ions, is a valuable approach for treating AD remains widespread.

Keywords: Alzheimer's disease, iron, chelation, alpha-lipoic acid, lactoferrin

INTRODUCTION

Alzheimer's disease (AD) is a neurodegenerative disease that occurs in the elderly population. Most patients show early loss of memory, and as the condition worsens, language disorders, loss of directionality, and anxiety behaviors will also be present (Cheng et al., 2013). Regarding late-stage patients, their mental activities, such as cognition, emotion and behavior, are abnormal, and their bodily functions are gradually lost (Ikonomovic et al., 2011). With the development of society and changes in the human environment, the incidence of AD has increased year by year. In the epidemiological survey performed by the Alzheimer's Association in the United States in 2017, the number of AD patients in the United States exceeded 5.5 million, and people over the age of 65 were found to be twice as likely to suffer from AD. However, the pathogenesis of AD remains unclear, and drugs that can completely cure AD or relieve symptoms have not yet been developed (Blennow et al., 2006; Huang and Mucke, 2012; Mullard, 2012; Reese et al., 2012; Selkoe, 2012).

THE PATHOGENIC HYPOTHESIS OF ALZHEIMER'S DISEASE

The two major histopathological features of AD in the brain are senile plaques (SPs), formed by the deposition of extracellular β-amyloid protein (Aβ), and neurofibrillary tangles (NFTs), formed by hyperphosphorylation of tau proteins associated with microtubules in neurons (Colvez et al., 2002). Based on these obvious pathological features, scholars have proposed two hypotheses about the developmental mechanism of AD: the amyloid cascade hypothesis and the NFTs hypothesis. With the deepening of research, more recent scholars also proposed the hypothesis of inflammation and the metal ion hypothesis and continuously enriched the developmental mechanism of AD.

The amyloid cascade hypothesis stems from the amyloid degradation pathway of β-amyloid precursor protein (APP). This hypothesis states that Aβ1-42, produced by the amyloid degradation pathway of APP, has significant neurotoxicity, can induce aggregation and hyperphosphorylation of tau protein, form NFTs, cause neuronal damage, and eventually lead to dementia (Klein et al., 2001). The NFTs hypothesis originates from the presence of a large number of fiber tangles formed by the aggregation of hyperphosphorylated tau proteins in the neurons of AD patients. This hypothesis suggests that hyperphosphorylated tau protein competes with normal tau protein for binding to tubulin, disrupting the dynamic balance of microtubule assembly and disaggregation (Cardenas-Aguayo Mdel et al., 2014) and resulting in impaired axonal transport and accumulation of intracellular waste. Neurons gradually degenerate and cause dementia. In addition to amyloid plaques and NFTs, the researchers found a large amount of activated astrocytes and microglia in the brains of AD patients, accompanied by increased expression levels of TNF-α, IL-1β, IL-6 and other inflammatory factors (Cunningham et al., 2005). Therefore, the neuroinflammation hypothesis was proposed. This hypothesis suggests that neuroinflammation is not a passive system in AD that is activated by SPs and NFTs, but, like plaques and tangles, plays an important role in the development of diseases (Zhang et al., 2013).

Interestingly, substantial evidence has indicated that the steady-state dysregulation of metal ion metabolism *in vivo* can be involved in the pathology of AD (Kim et al., 2018). An imbalance in the metal levels in the brains of AD patients has been identified and is accompanied by metal-catalyzed oxidative damage (Nunomura et al., 2001; Perry et al., 2003). A large number of studies have shown that metal ions, such as copper, iron, zinc, magnesium and aluminum, are involved in the occurrence and development of AD (Wang and Wang, 2017). Clinical studies have also shown elevated levels of copper, iron and zinc in the brains of AD patients (Bush, 2013). Metal ions can affect neuronal metabolism, cause oxidative stress, and promote the deposition of Aβ and the formation of SPs (Lovell et al., 1998). At the same time, studies have also shown that the deposition of Aβ in the brain and its toxicity are directly related to metabolic disorders of zinc, copper, iron, and other metal ions in the cortex and the hippocampus (Liu et al., 2006). Studies have also shown that an imbalance of metal homeostasis can directly cause neuronal dysfunction (Myhre et al., 2013) and lead to neuronal cell death (Wright and Baccarelli, 2007). Moreover, the successful application of metal (zinc, copper, iron) chelators in several animal models of AD and patients with early AD provided strong evidence that AD is a transition metal-overloading disease (Guo et al., 2013b, 2015, 2017; Dusek et al., 2016; Giampietro et al., 2018; Kawahara et al., 2018; Zhang et al., 2018). Based on the research described above, the metal ion hypothesis was proposed to emphasize the role of metal ions in the pathogenesis of AD, which further complemented the pathogenesis of AD.

BRAIN IRON DYSHOMEOSTASIS AND THE PATHOPHYSIOLOGY OF ALZHEIMER'S DISEASE

Iron is the second most abundant metal on earth, second only to aluminum, and it is also an essential element for the survival of all living things on earth (Crielaard et al., 2017). The biological activity of iron depends, to a large extent, on its effective electron transfer properties, allowing it to accept or provide electrons during the transition between divalent, ferric and tetravalent iron states of ferrous iron, thus serving as a catalytic cofactor in a variety of biochemical reactions (Hohenberger et al., 2012). Iron also promotes the activity of various biological enzymes in the process of DNA replication and repair in the form of iron–sulfur clusters (Fe-S). Simultaneously, iron is also a component of hemoglobin and myoglobin, which is involved in the transport of oxygen and carbon dioxide in organisms (Takeda, 2004).

Many important physiological activities in the brain involve iron. If iron is absent during the development of the brain, it will cause irreversible developmental delays; however, if the iron overload in the brain also has a neurotoxic effect, this will damage the normal physiological activities of the brain. The iron content in the brain gradually increases with age. Interestingly, using magnetic resonance imaging (MRI), it was found that the iron content in the brains of AD patients was significantly increased (Du et al., 2018). This finding was also confirmed in a comparative study of APP/PS1E9 double transgenic AD mice and wild-type mice of the same age (Dwyer et al., 2009). Besides, some scholars believe that an iron metabolism disorder is an important cause of late-onset AD formation (Corder et al., 1995). Based on the various discoveries related to iron, researchers realized that iron plays an extremely important role in the occurrence of AD. Therefore, research on iron as a target has gradually become a new direction for scientists to explore the pathogenesis of AD.

Iron Absorption and Transport Into the Brain

Iron mainly exists in non-heme iron and heme iron in foods, and non-heme iron accounts for 90% of them. Non-heme iron is reduced to Fe^{2+} in the upper part of the small intestine and enters mucosal epithelial cells via a divalent metal ion transporter (DMT1) on the membrane of the small intestine epithelium.

The remaining 10% of heme iron reacts with heme oxygenase (HO) in the proximal part of the small intestine, releasing Fe^{2+} and is directly taken up by small intestinal mucosa epithelial cells via DMT1 (Krishnamurthy et al., 2007; Horl, 2008). Fe^{2+} uptake by epithelial cells can be used directly by cells, while unutilized Fe^{2+} is oxidized by ferrous oxidase (hephaestin) or ceruloplasmin to Fe^{3+}. The resulting Fe^{3+} is transported out of the cell via the ferroportin 1 (FPN1) of the basolateral membrane of the intestinal mucosal epithelium. The transferred out Fe^{3+} is mainly combined with the transferrin (Tf) in the blood to form the iron-transferrin complex and can also be combined with lactoferrin to form a non-transferrin-bound iron into the peripheral blood circulation (Frazer and Anderson, 2005; Garrick and Garrick, 2009).

The iron-transferrin complex circulating in the peripheral blood to the brain enters the cells through endocytosis of brain capillary endothelial cells. This endocytosis is mediated mainly by transferrin receptor (TfR) on the surface of endothelial cells. Non-transferrin-bound iron in peripheral blood can enter the brain through the lactoferrin/lactoferrin receptor pathway (Ke and Qian, 2007). Iron-transferrin complexes form endosomes into cells via endocytosis. Due to the action of the proton pump on the endosome membrane, the PH in the endosome is reduced, which leads to the dissociation of iron and Tf/TfR complexes, at the same time Fe^{3+} is reduced to Fe^{2+}. Fe^{2+} enters the endothelial cytoplasm through DMT1 on the endosome membrane (**Figure 1**). The detached iron Tf/TfR complex exudes from the vesicle to the lateral lumen of the endothelial cells. In the pH 7.4 environment, Tf dissociates from TfR and re-enters the blood (Dringen et al., 2007).

Iron Regulation in the Brain

According to autopsy reports, total iron deposition in the human brain is positively related to age and contains high concentrations of iron in the basal ganglia of the putamen, globus pallidus, and substantia nigra (Connor et al., 1995), whereas the cerebral cortex, the brainstem and cerebellum contain low concentrations of iron (Zecca et al., 2004; Ramos et al., 2014). Iron homeostasis in nerve cells is mainly regulated by the transcriptional levels of mRNAs involved in iron metabolism. The proteins involved in brain iron metabolism mainly include iron regulatory proteins (IRPs), Tf, TfR1, ferritin, FPN1, DMT1,

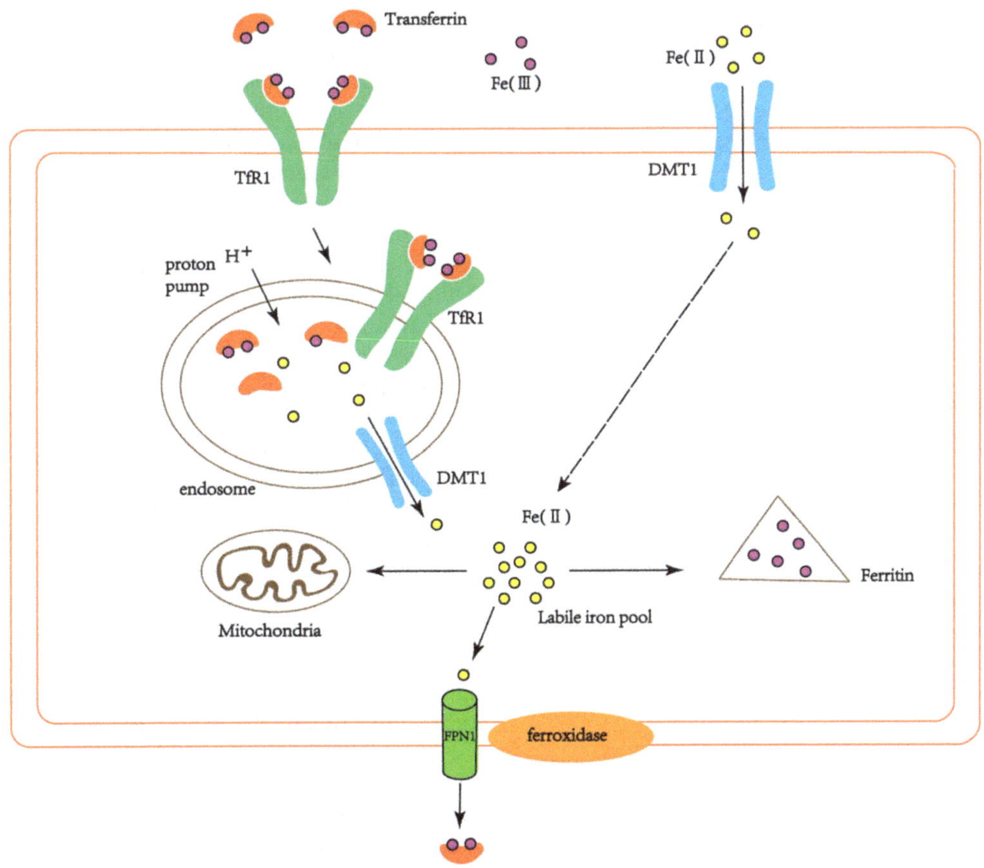

FIGURE 1 | The schematic diagram of iron transport into cells. Part of the extracellular bivalent iron can be directly transferred into cells through DMT1. Transferrin-bound iron binds TfR1 through endocytosis to form endosomes in the cells. Due to the action of the proton pump on the endosome, trivalent iron dissociates from the Tf/TfR1 complex and is reduced to divalent iron, which enters the cytoplasm via DMT1. Part of the ferrous iron that enters the cytoplasm is used by the cell itself (such as mitochondria), and part of it is oxidized to ferrous iron by ferritin and stored. Another part is oxidized to ferric iron by the ferroxidase on the cell membrane, and the cells are exported by FPN1 and recombined with extracellular Tf.

and so on (Crielaard et al., 2017) The mRNAs encoding TfR1, ferritin, FPN1 and DMT1 all contain a special amino acid sequence called the iron regulatory element (IRE). Iron regulates the transcription of iron-related proteins by controlling the binding of IRPs to IRE, thereby maintaining intracellular iron homeostasis (Zhou and Tan, 2017). After continuous in-depth research, people further realized that hepcidin, an antibacterial peptide, is an important factor in iron homeostasis, particularly brain iron homeostasis (Vela, 2018). FPN1 is the major receptor for hepcidin *in vivo*. A series of studies demonstrated that hepcidin regulates iron homeostasis via direct interaction between hepcidin and FPN1, inducing the internalization and degradation of FPN1 reducing the ability of cells to export iron (De Domenico et al., 2008), and thereby increasing the possibility of intracellular iron overload (Daher et al., 2017). Later, cell experiments showed that hepcidin not only downregulated the expression of FPN1 in astrocytes and neurons but also downregulated the expression of TfR and DMT1 (Du et al., 2011, 2015). The above results suggested that hepcidin regulates iron homeostasis not only by controlling the iron output of cells but also by regulating the iron input of cells.

In addition to iron-related proteins that regulate iron, APP and tau also act to regulate iron. Studies have shown that APP is a certain regulator for iron homeostasis, which can interact with FPN1 to regulate the efflux of ferrous ions (Kawahara et al., 2017). Indeed, APP knockout or haplo-insufficiency preferentially mediates brain iron accumulation in mice (Duce et al., 2010). Tau acts as an intracellular microtubule-associated protein, which can transport the produced APP to the cell surface to promote iron output (Li et al., 2015). Interestingly, tau knockout mice develop age-dependent iron accumulation and brain atrophy, and iron retention in the primary cultured neurons is caused by decreasing surface trafficking of APP, indicating that tau-mediated iron homeostasis might be APP-dependent(Lei et al., 2012; Tuo et al., 2017).

Iron Participates in the Occurrence of Alzheimer's Disease

In the brain, iron is not only involved in the synthesis of myelin and neurotransmitter synthesis and metabolism but also plays an important role in maintaining the high metabolic capacity of neurons (Gerlach et al., 1994). Under normal physiological conditions, iron metabolism maintains homeostasis in the brain. Once iron metabolism is out of balance, it will have different effects on brain function. As early as Goodman (1953) found that iron was increased in the SPs in the brains of AD patients. Later, the use of quantitative susceptibility map (QSM) once again confirmed the co-localization of brain iron and Aβ plaques, and showed that the co-localization of brain iron deposition and Aβ plaques promoted the development of the disease (van Bergen et al., 2016). In fact, there are also progressive iron deposits that occur in the normal aging process of the brain, particularly in the substantia nigra, globus pallidus, caudate nucleus, and cortex, and these brain regions are closely related to neurodegenerative diseases (Rodrigue et al., 2011; Callaghan et al., 2014; Collingwood and Davidson, 2014; Ward et al., 2014). Compared with healthy people of the same age, the iron deposition in patients with AD is more serious in these areas. Further, the APP mRNA of peripheral blood mononuclear cells of AD patients was significantly lower than that of the control group by fluorescence quantitative PCR, which indirectly indicated the iron dyshomeostasis in AD (Guerreiro et al., 2015).

Iron Participates in the Deposition of Aβ Plaques and Tau Tangles

Studies have demonstrated that iron metabolic disorders can induce the production and accumulation of Aβ because iron can act on the IRE site of APP mRNA, thereby enhancing the translation and expression of endogenous APP (Cahill et al., 2009). It has also been found that long-term administration of high concentrations of iron in APP/PS1E9 double transgenic mice results in an increase in the number of SPs in the brain (Smith et al., 1997). When extended iron exposure to 12 months, the increased brain iron with 3,5,5-trimethylhexanoyl ferrocene diet accelerated the formation of SPs and microglial iron inclusions in APP mice (Peters et al., 2018).

Although there is a lot of evidence that iron and Aβ plaques co-localize, it is not known what form iron is present in plaques. Recently, Plascencia-Villa et al. (2016) used transmission electron microscopy (TEM) to confirm that iron is present in the core of SPs in the form of iron oxide (Fe_3O_4) magnetite nanoparticles. This provides evidence of metal biology associated with iron accumulation and Aβ aggregation. Later, using *in situ* X-ray magnetic circular dichroism again revealed the existence of magnetite in human SPs (Everett et al., 2018). Magnetite, as a polycrystalline iron oxide, is not a normal feature in the human brain, and its elevated content indicates that the anomalous iron redox chemistry affects AD (Ayton et al., 2017b). Furthermore, Telling et al. (2017) used advanced sub-microscopic resolution of X-ray microscopy to find evidence of the direct correlation between the morphology of SPs and iron and the formation of iron-amyloid complexes. Importantly, Aβ binds to iron through three histidine residues and one tyrosine residue in the hydrophilic N-terminal region of the peptide, which helps to stabilize these iron ions (Lane et al., 2018). In turn, studies also found that the binding of ferrous ions to Aβ reduced the peptide helix structure and increased the β-sheet content of the peptide, indicating that ferrous ions promote amyloid monomers to form oligomers and fibrils by enhancing the interaction between peptide-peptides (Boopathi and Kolandaivel, 2016; Tahirbegi et al., 2016). Except promoting Aβ aggregation, high iron levels can impact amyloidogenic processing of APP. Early studies found that iron had a modulatory effect on the α-secretase cleavage activity of APP (Bodovitz et al., 1995). Later, studies found that the process of converting α-secretase and β-secretase from the inactive state to the active state was regulated by furin, and iron could regulate the expression of furin at the transcriptional level (Silvestri and Camaschella, 2008). Excessive iron inhibits the expression of furin, which favors the activation of β-secretase, thereby promoting the production of Aβ from the amyloid pathway (Ward et al., 2014). Another study found that presenilin enhancer 2 (PEN-2), a γ-secretase components, could bind to iron through the ferritin light chain, enhancing

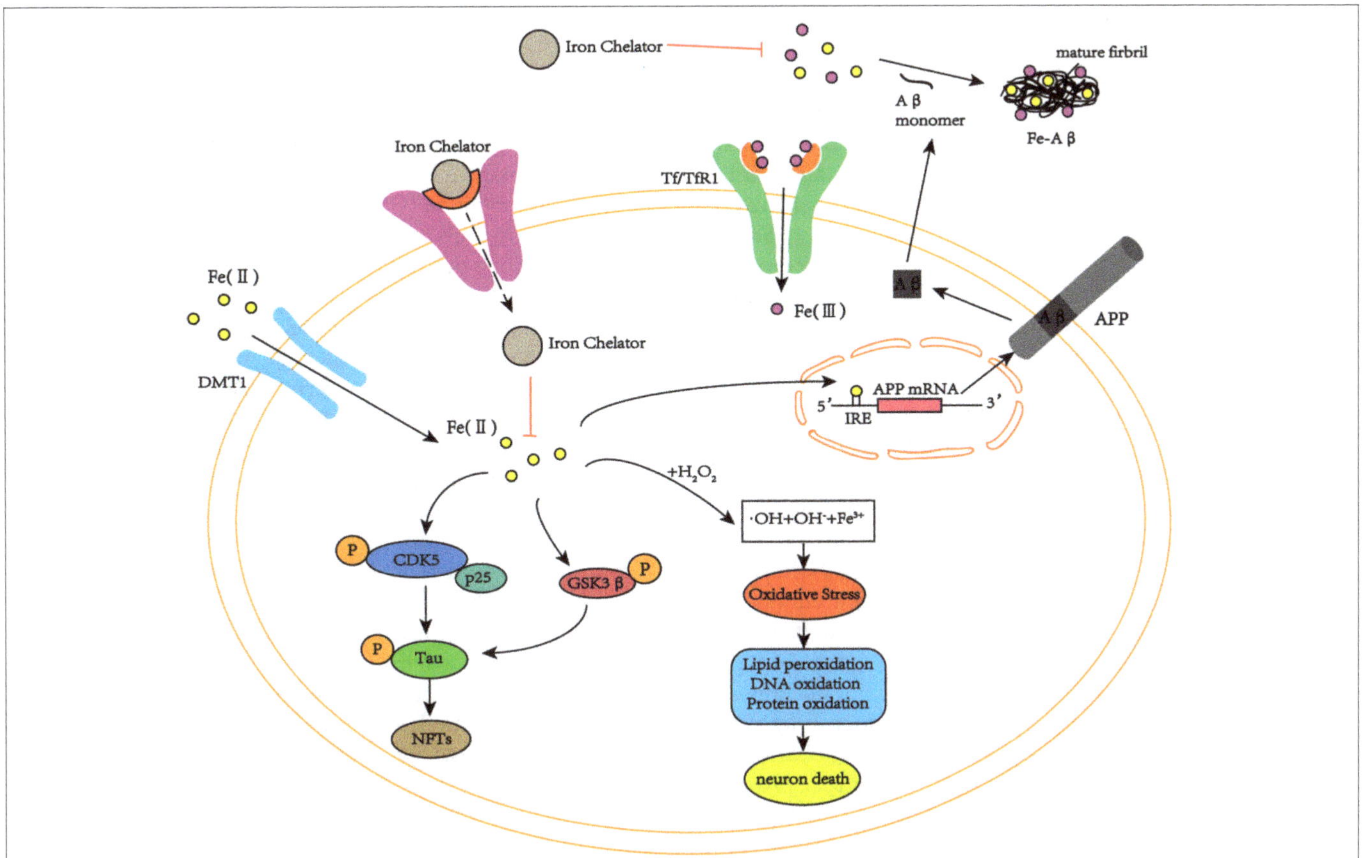

FIGURE 2 | The schematic diagram of iron participation in the deposition of Aβ plaques and tau tangles. In neurons, iron interacts with Aβ and promotes Aβ aggregation into fibrous forms. Iron can also act on the IRE site of APP mRNA, increasing the expression of endogenous APP. In addition to the interaction with Aβ, iron can also promote the phosphorylation of tau by activating the CDK5/p25 complex and GSK3β to form NFTs. At the same time, iron can also cause oxidative stress through the Fenton reaction, damaging DNA, lipids and proteins and eventually leading to cell death. The iron chelators reduce the phosphorylation of tau and inhibit the production of NFTs by inhibiting the activation of the CDK5/p25 complex and GSK3β by iron. Simultaneously, iron chelators inhibit the aggregation of Aβ monomers into toxic fibrous forms by chelating iron, delaying cell death.

γ-secretase activity, thereby increasing Aβ formation (Li et al., 2013).

In vitro studies have also found that iron can promote aggregation of Aβ peptides and increase their cytotoxicity (Tahmasebinia and Emadi, 2017; Galante et al., 2018). However, there are different opinions on the role of iron and Aβ. Earlier studies have found that Fe^{2+} and Fe^{3+} interacted with APP and Aβ to promote aggregation of Aβ into fibrous forms (Ha et al., 2007). Fe^{2+} can also interact with the amino acids of the Aβ protein, which may impart changes in the form of amyloid in a different manner than copper and zinc (Dahms et al., 2012). Fe^{3+} bound to Aβ is easily reduced to Fe^{2+} and increases reactive oxygen species (ROS) production, which causes β-secretase to cleave monomer Aβ42 into more toxic Aβ oligomers, accelerating neuronal death (Cohen et al., 2013; Balejcikova et al., 2018). Importantly, Aβ can damage mitochondrial function, convert Fe^{3+} into Fe^{2+} with redox activity, and induce oxidative stress, thereby aggravating iron overload and aggravating the AD condition (Everett et al., 2014; Mena et al., 2015). Further, it has been shown that iron exposure promotes the accumulation of APP in cultured SHSY5Y cells, along with the increase of β-secretase activity and Aβ42 in the medium (Banerjee et al., 2014). Inconsistently, a recent study showed that iron treatment of neurons promoted the APP non-amyloid pathway, altered the distribution of sAPPα and retained it in cell lysates rather than secreted outside the cell, while iron did not change β-secretion enzyme expression, but significantly inhibits its activity (Chen et al., 2018). Another study also found that Aβ can significantly reduce the redox ability of iron, which may indicate neuroprotection and metal chelation of Aβ during the pathogenesis of AD, but becomes toxic under certain conditions (Lane et al., 2018).

Neurofibrillary tangles are another major pathological feature of AD, and phosphorylated tau protein is the main component of NFTs. Studies have found iron deposition in neurons with NFTs (Smith et al., 1997). In addition to Aβ peptides, iron can bind to tau protein, induce tau protein phosphorylation, and aggregate phosphorylated tau protein, whereas this phenomenon can be reversed by iron chelators (Amit et al., 2008). Fe^{3+} induces the aggregation of hyperphosphorylated tau protein, and when Fe^{3+} is reduced to Fe^{2+}, its induced aggregation can be reversed (Yamamoto et al., 2002). These results reveal that iron may play an important role in the accumulation of hyperphosphorylated tau protein to form NFTs. Recent studies have shown that tau protein indirectly participates in the transmission of iron ions in brain neurons during the pathogenesis of AD (Lei et al., 2012). Moreover, *in vitro* and *in vivo* experiments have shown that iron is involved in the hyperphosphorylation of tau protein through the activation of the cyclin-dependent kinase (CDK5)/P25 complex and glycogen synthase kinase-3β (GSK-3β) (Xie et al., 2012; Guo et al., 2013a), but no relevant experiments have reported whether iron is also related to the inactivation of the protein phosphatase PP2A (**Figure 2**). Additionally, Fe^{3+} can promote the reduction of superoxide radicals released by mitochondria (Kudin et al., 2004; Aliaga et al., 2011). The reduction of Fe^{3+} can lead to the production of superoxide, and the reaction of superoxide with nitric oxide (NO) to produce per-nitrate can damage tyrosine residues that function normally (Nakamura and Lipton, 2011). In AD, nitration of tau prevents its stabilization of the microtubule lattice, and nitrating tau protein has been observed in tau entanglement and SPs (Reynolds et al., 2006; Kummer et al., 2011). Interestingly, the accumulation of tau in NFTs is also associated with increased induction of HO1 (Wang et al., 2015). HO1 is a potent antioxidant that can metabolize heme released from damaged mitochondria, and it also promotes the release of Fe^{2+}, which may cause free radicals to initiate additional oxidative stress (Ward et al., 2014). Thus, iron-induced oxidative stress may also promote hyperphosphorylation and aggregation of tau (Lane et al., 2018).

To date, although the specific mechanism of iron involvement in the aggregation of Aβ plaques and hyperphosphorylated tau protein is not yet clear, it has been shown that iron can accelerate this process by affecting related signaling pathways and the three-dimensional conformation of proteins. Nevertheless, the changes in iron levels in AD need to be emphasized, and homeostatic imbalance may have dual effects through iron induction. On the one hand, iron overload areas in the brain contribute to oxidative stress and cell death around SPs and NFTs; on the other hand, other areas of the brain may suffer from impaired neuronal function due to iron deficiency (Belaidi and Bush, 2016).

Ferroptosis and AD

Cell death plays an important role in the growth and development of organism and tissue homeostasis. Studies have found that cell death is dysregulated in AD (Yang and Stockwell, 2016). Based on the unique pathological state caused by iron overload, scholars have also proposed a fourth cell death mode that differs from apoptosis, necrosis, and autophagy, namely, ferroptosis (Dixon et al., 2012).

Ferroptosis refers to iron-dependent lipid peroxidation-induced cell death that depends on ROS production and iron availability, with severe lipid peroxidation (Dixon, 2017). One of the hallmarks of ferroptosis is the iron-dependent accumulation of lipid ROS, a form of death that is dependent on intracellular iron rather than other metals (Abdalkader et al., 2018). The morphological features of ferroptosis are mainly reflected in intracellular mitochondria. Compared to the mitochondria of normal cells, the mitochondrial volume of ferroptosis cells is smaller, the density of mitochondrial membranes is reduced, mitochondrial hemorrhoids are reduced or have disappeared, and the mitochondrial outer membrane ruptures (Xie et al., 2016). Moreover, studies have found that the occurrence of ferroptosis consists of the accumulation of lipid ROS triggered by the inactivation of the intracellular antioxidant glutathione (GSH). Therefore, ferroptosis is caused by the imbalance in cellular redox homeostasis (Gao et al., 2016). Glutathione peroxidase 4 (GPx4), an antioxidant defense enzyme that repairs oxidative damage to lipids, is a central endogenous suppressor of ferroptosis (Chen et al., 2015). Studies have found that the GPx4 gene knockout mice involve in both three pronounced hallmarks of ferroptosis (iron dysregulation, lipid peroxidation, inflammation) and prodromal indices of AD (behavior dysfunction, hippocampal neurodegeneration), and these pathological changes can be ameliorated or prevented by a ferroptosis inhibitor (Seiler et al., 2008; Hambright et al., 2017). Intriguingly, erastin, a ferroptosis attractant, can induce neuronal death accompanied by ferroptosis (Hirata et al., 2018). Conversely, iron chelators and antioxidants specifically involved in protecting cells against ferroptosis (Hambright et al., 2017). Taken together, although the physiological function of ferroptosis is still unclear, its role in age-related neurodegenerative diseases (including AD) has been established. This suggests that considering ferroptosis the center, the development of ferroptosis inhibitors may be a new direction to alleviate the symptoms of AD.

BIOMARKERS FOR CLINICAL DIAGNOSIS OF AD PROGRESSION

The pathogenesis of AD has not yet been fully explained. If special methods can be used to detect AD in the early stage, it is very important to increase our understanding of the disease and active prevention of the disease. Currently, the clinical diagnosis of AD is based primarily on family history and certain cognitive dysfunctions (Alzheimer's, 2016). Other methods mainly detect the levels of Aβ1-42 and phosphorylated tau and total tau in cerebrospinal fluid to predict the development and severity of AD (Bulk et al., 2018). A common method for detecting Aβ plaques is positron emission tomography (PET). With the deepening of research, more and more new technologies are used to identify changes in the Alzheimer brain, and gradient echo multiple contrast imaging (GEPCI) technology is one of them. The study confirmed a strong correlation between the GEPCI brain tissue index and the Aβ load defined by PET, providing a new method for assessing AD-related histopathology in the preclinical and early symptom stages of AD (Zhao et al., 2017).

Although Aβ and tau degeneration are considered to be key factors in AD, iron dyshomeostasis is increasingly reported as a potential cause of AD pathophysiology. Can iron be used as a biomarker for the progression of AD to detect the occurrence of AD and reflect the severity of AD? For this reason, iron as a biomarker of AD has become a research hotspot for scientists. The current effective method for detecting brain iron levels is QSM. QSM has better specificity and can be used to non-invasively assess tissue magnetic susceptibility, which has been confirmed to have a good correlation with brain iron levels (Du et al., 2018). Through QSM, Du et al. (2018)found that the magnetic susceptibility values of the caudate nucleus on the left side of the brain may be used as biomarkers for the severity of mild and moderate AD disease. As early as Moon et al. (2016) have found that the magnetic susceptibility values of the core and caudate nucleus of AD patients are significantly different from those of the control group. Later, van Bergen et al. (2018) jointly used QSM and PET to show that the local correlation of Aβ plaque load and iron deposition can provide relevant information about the cognitive performance of healthy elderly people. Studies have shown that AD patients have higher iron accumulation in the frontal cortex, and the degree is related to the number of Aβ plaques and NFT, and there is a different iron distribution, and these changes appear to occur after the development of AD pathology markers (van Duijn et al., 2017). These findings suggest that changes in iron-based magnetic resonance (MRI) contrast can be used to indirectly determine the extent of AD pathology. Although iron concentration was identified as the main source of comparison in QSM in the brain, O'Callaghan et al. (2017) found a correlation between QSM and tau concentration, suggesting that QSM may be a useful biomarker for early detection of tau pathology in AD.

As a major iron storage protein in the body, ferritin is closely related to AD. Elevated ferritin in CSF has been shown to be associated with poor cognitive function and increases the risk of mild cognitive impairment to AD (Ayton et al., 2015). Moreover, research has shown ferritin's potential to contribute to a blood biomarker panel for preclinical AD (Goozee et al., 2017). CSF ferritin levels were negatively correlated with cognitive performance and strongly correlated with apolipoprotein E (ApoE) in CSF, suggesting that CSF ferritin as an indicator of brain iron load may be a biomarker of AD cognitive function (Ayton et al., 2015). However, another study combining QSM and PET to predict the value of longitudinal cognitive deterioration found that iron can worsen cognitive function in the presence of Aβ pathology. There is no Aβ pathology, and iron has no correlation with cognitive function (Ayton et al., 2017a). More advanced, Ayton et al. (2018) further found that high concentrations of CSF ferritin can accelerate the decrease of Aβ in CSF of 296 participants, which supports the possibility that iron may promote Aβ deposition and accelerate disease progression. This is the first clinical evidence that iron is associated with amyloid plaque formation.

Due to the invasiveness of lumbar puncture, the use of this CSF biomarker limits the widespread clinical application, while serum or plasma biomarkers are relatively simple to acquire and less invasive, and thus have great potential for application in AD. Studies have shown that serum and iron-related protein levels in AD patients are significantly elevated (Sternberg et al., 2017). Unlike Aβ peptides, iron and iron-related proteins are significantly associated with cognitive assessment tests, neuroimaging and clinical data (Sternberg et al., 2017). This at least partly indicates that iron can act as a biomarker for AD.

IRON-TARGETING TREATMENT STRATEGIES

Metal-chelating agents can bind metal ions to the inside of a chelating agent through the strong binding action of a chelating agent molecule with a metal ion to become a stable compound with a larger molecular weight, thereby preventing metal ions from acting. Since iron overload plays an important role in the occurrence and development of AD, the use of metal chelators to reduce excessive iron in certain areas of the brain of AD patients, to achieve the strategy of relieving or even treating AD, has received an increased amount of attention. For a metal chelator to effectively exert chelation, it must have the following characteristics: (1) easy to penetrate the cell membrane and blood-brain barrier (BBB); (2) target iron-enriched areas without depleting transferrin-bound iron from plasma; (3) remove chelated iron from iron accumulation sites or transfer it to other biological proteins, such as circulating transferrin; and (4) no side effects or minor side effects on the body (Boddaert et al., 2007).

Clioquinol

Clioquinol (CQ) has the chemical name 5-chloro-7-iodo-8-hydroxyquinoline and is an effective metal (iron, copper, and zinc) chelating agent. Studies have found that treatment of animal models of AD with CQ can reduce the deposition of amyloid in the brain and improve memory impairment (Cherny et al., 2001; Grossi et al., 2009). The probable cause of this phenomenon is that the high binding affinity of CQ to iron, zinc and copper ions allows it to competitively seize these metals from Aβ and prevent aggregation of Aβ (Opazo et al., 2006). Another study showed that 15-month-old APP Tg2576AD mice treated with CQ demonstrated a significantly reduced number and sizes of SPs in the brain compared with those of the sham-treated littermates (Cherny et al., 2001). Simultaneously, an *in vivo* experiment also found that, compared with the control group, CQ reduced the expression of APP by inhibiting the expression of β-secretase (BACE1) and γ-secretase (PS1) in the brains of APP/PS1 double transgenic mice (Wang et al., 2012). In coincidence with the results in animal models of AD, a small phase 2 clinical trial, it was also found that, compared with the control group, patients with moderately severe AD after oral CQ demonstrated slower decline in cognitive function and decreased Aβ42 levels in cerebrospinal fluid (Ritchie et al., 2003). However, it still lacks of the direct evidences supporting that CQ rescues the AD-like phenotypes via targeting iron *in vivo*. As is well known that tau deficiency induced age-dependent iron accumulation can be prevented by oral treatment with CQ (Lei et al., 2012, 2015). Moreover, CQ treatment can effectively prevent an iron-synuclein interaction in hA53T transgenic mice (Billings et al., 2016), as well as reverse the Fe^{3+}-induced fibrin formation *in vitro* (Pretorius et al., 2013). Importantly, the formation of Aβ40 and Aβ42 aggregates in the presence of Fe^{3+} and Cu^{2+} were investigated, the study demonstrated that Fe^{3+}, but not Cu^{2+}, promotes the aggregation of Aβ40 and Aβ42, and CQ significantly reduces the Fe^{3+}-induced Aβ42 aggregation (Tahmasebinia and Emadi, 2017). These researches provide the evidence that the anti-AD ability of CQ may, at least in part, via targeting iron and, surely, the underlying mechanism need to be further elucidated, Although it is now thought that CQ is toxic to the body, it at least opens up a promising direction for us.

Desferoxamine, Deferasirox and Deferiprone

Desferoxamine (DFO) is a well-proven iron chelator that inhibits the toxicity of iron or aluminum and the ROS that it induces on the body. It was first thought that DFO was a chelating agent for aluminum ions, and aluminum was thought to be an independent factor that increased the risk of AD (Campbell and Bondy, 2000). The results of Crapper McLachlan et al. (1991) showed that the degree of decline in the daily living abilities of AD patients given intramuscular injections of DFO was alleviated compared with AD patients given a placebo. *In vitro* experiments showed that DFO can inhibit the formation of β-sheets of Aβ1-42 and dissolve preformed plaque-like amyloid plaques (House et al., 2004). There are also studies that have shown that DFO can inhibit the translation of APP mRNA and the expression of APP whole protein and reduce the secretion of Aβ peptides (Rogers et al., 2002; Morse et al., 2004). Our research revealed that nasal feeding of DFO can reverse iron-induced memory deficits in AD mice and inhibit the formation of APP (Guo et al., 2013b). In addition to its effect on APP, DFO also influences the phosphorylation of tau protein. Fine et al. (2012) have found that DFO has the ability to phosphorylate GSK-3β, which in turn reduces the level of phosphorylated tau, but the mechanism of its inhibition of tau protein phosphorylation is not yet clear. Although DFO can inhibit the phosphorylation of tau protein in the brain of AD model mice, the effect of DFO on the phosphorylation of tau protein has not been determined in the presence of iron. Our previous experiments, which involved feeding APP/PS1 transgenic mice high concentrations of iron and then nasally administered DFO to the mice, showed that intranasal DFO treatment inhibited iron-induced tau phosphorylation through the CDK5 and GSK-3β pathways (Guo et al., 2013a). We also found that DFO can also attenuate synaptic loss in the brain of APP/PS1 transgenic mice through the P38/HIF-1α pathway (Guo et al., 2015).

Although DFO has achieved certain results in a variety of experimental mouse models and has been approved by the Federal Drug Administration (FDA) for the treatment of iron overload disease, there are still many problems in the clinical application of DFO. First, the bioavailability of DFO is poor, and the molecular size and hydrophilicity of DFO prevent it from freely crossing the BBB, reducing its availability in the central nervous system; Second, DFO cannot be taken orally and must be given by injection. The time of a single injection is long (up to 10 h) and the frequency of injections is high (5–7 times per week), resulting in low patient compliance (Crielaard et al., 2017); Again, there are many side effects, including neurotoxicity after long-term treatment and systemic metal ion depletion accompanied by anemia (Cuajungco et al., 2000), gastrointestinal malabsorption and rapid degradation (May and Bulman, 1983).

Deferasirox is the first FDA-approved oral iron repellent that can be routinely used. Its chemical name is 4-[3,5-bis(2-hydroxyphenyl)-1,2,4-tris Oxazol-1-yl]benzoic acid, and it is commonly used as a treatment for patients with thalassemia iron overload. Deferasirox's ability to bind iron is limited. This drug can only bind part of the iron and supply it to the extracellular and intracellular iron receptors. It is not easy to induce iron deficiency, but the efficacy of reducing iron accumulation is also relatively low. At present, studies have found that deferasirox plays a role in reducing brain iron accumulation. However, some studies have shown that deferasirox does not reduce brain iron accumulation or reduce iron toxicity in the brain (Sripetchwandee et al., 2016). This may be because deferasirox does not easily pass through the BBB, and its ability to bind iron is also weak. Three molecules of deferasirox are required for each binding molecule of iron, and thus higher doses are required.

The chemical name of deferiprone is 3-hydroxy-l,2-dimethyl-4-(lH)-pyridone. Like deferasirox, deferiprone is also approved for the treatment of patients with thalassemia iron overload. Deferiprone can bind almost all of the iron in the body to make it unable to further induce the production of ROS, and can also supply the bound iron to the iron receptors inside and outside the cell. Since deferiprone has a high iron-binding capacity, two molecules of deferiprone are required for each binding of one molecule of iron, and thus iron aggregation can be effectively reduced. Studies have found that deferiprone and DFO exert protective effects by reducing the rate of BBB disintegration, reducing brain iron accumulation and brain mitochondrial dysfunction in the presence of iron overload (Sripetchwandee et al., 2016). Although both deferiprone and DFO exert a protective effect, deferiprone can achieve greater advantages by oral administration.

Currently, DFO, deferasirox and deferiprone are recommended as iron overloaded first-line iron chelators, but they all have certain side effects, including allergic reactions, liver and renal dysfunction, and neuronal hearing loss (Borgna-Pignatti and Marsella, 2015). This requires further development of iron chelation therapy.

α-lipoic Acid

α-lipoic acid (LA) is a small molecule compound that can be naturally synthesized in mammals. It is a coenzyme that exists in mitochondria. Its structure contains hydroxyl and disulfide bonds, so it has both fat-soluble and water-soluble properties, and it easily crosses the BBB. The study found that, after 60 min of intravenous injection of LA in mice, the traces of LA were observed in the mouse cerebral cortex (Panigrahi et al., 1996). After a continuous injection over 7–14 days, the presence of LA was detected in multiple parts of the mouse brain (Arivazhagan et al., 2002). Surprisingly, however, when a certain amount of LA was administered to mice daily by gavage, LA accumulation was not detected in the mouse brain after a period of time (Chng et al., 2009). The most likely reason for this is that LA is quickly reduced to dihydro-lipoic acid (DHLA) in the stomach and is transported through the blood circulation to tissues throughout the body to participate in metabolism and is eventually excreted in urine.

In Europe, LA has been used as a therapeutic drug for more than 50 years, and it is mainly used for the treatment of diabetic polyneuropathy. Later, in a clinical study, it was found that the decline in cognitive abilities of 129 patients who may have been suffering from AD was effectively alleviated after LA treatment for some time (Fava et al., 2013). However, the sample size of this study was relatively small, and there was no randomized sample. The study subjects were likely AD patients and were not confirmed by neuropathology. Therefore, the results were not very convincing. Several studies have shown that supplementation with LA can increase the activity of acetylcholine transferase (ChAT) in the brains of rodents and relieve their cognitive impairment (de Freitas, 2010; Dwivedi et al., 2014). The activation of ChAT positively regulates the content of acetylcholine in the brain, and the decreased expression of acetylcholine is closely related to the impairment of cognitive function in AD. Therefore, LA may increase the expression of acetylcholine by activating ChAT and improve the cognitive function of AD patients. At the same time, studies have shown that the activation of ChAT is also beneficial to the neurogenesis of cholinergic neurons (Park et al., 2013), which further demonstrates that LA may improve the severity of central nervous system diseases. A large number of studies have shown that LA can reduce the release of IL-1β, IL-6, and TNFα by inhibiting the activity of the NF-κB and MAPK signaling pathways (Bierhaus et al., 1997; Wong et al., 2001; Zhang and Frei, 2001). Simultaneously, LA also inhibits the infiltration of inflammatory cells into the central nervous system and downregulates the expression of vascular cell adhesion molecule-1 (Kunt et al., 1999; Guo et al., 2016). In addition to its ability to chelate metal ions, LA can also play a role in anti-inflammation, antioxidant and activated glucose uptake and utilization. So far, no serious side effects of LA treatment have been observed, which also indicates that LA may become a trend for clinical drug development for AD treatment.

In vitro studies have shown that LA can bind with metal ions, such as Cu^{2+}, Zn^{2+}, and DHLA, and can form complexes with Cu^{2+}, Zn^{2+}, Pb^{2+}, Hg^{2+}, and Fe^{3+}, thereby exerting metal chelation (Ou et al., 1995). Treatment of lens epithelial cells with LA causes a significant decrease in iron uptake rates and dynamic iron pools within the cells (Goralska et al., 2003). These results suggested that LA not only reduces the level of iron that enters the cell but also reduces the dynamic iron pool within the cell by increasing iron stores. *In vivo* studies have shown that feeding of LA for 2 weeks in aged rats can reduce iron accumulation in the age-related cortical regions (Suh et al., 2005). The results of Fonte et al. (2001) showed that LA enhances the solubility of Aβ in the frontal cortex of APP-overexpressing transgenic mice, confirming that LA, like other metal ion chelators, can successfully resolubilize Aβ and reduce amyloid deposition in the brains of AD patients. However, in another study, learning and memory retention of LA-treated AD mice was significantly improved, but there was no significant changes in soluble or insoluble Aβ levels in the brain (Quinn et al., 2007). Although the metal chelation of LA has been proven by many experimental results, there is controversy as to whether it can inhibit the deposition of Aβ and increase the solubility of Aβ by chelating iron. Most recently, our group also found that chronic treatment with LA effectively inhibited tau hyperphosphorylation and alleviated neuronal degeneration and abnormal behavior in P301S tau transgenic mice; the improvement is accompanied by alleviation of oxidative stress, inflammation and ferroptosis in the brains of transgenic mice (Zhang et al., 2018).

Lactoferrin

Lactoferrin (LF) is a non-heme iron-binding glycoprotein with a molecular weight of 80 kDa that is widely present in various secretions, such as milk, saliva, and urine. Because its amino acid sequence is 60% identical to that of transferrin, it is classified as a transferrin family member (Metz-Boutigue et al., 1984). LF is composed of two spherical leaves folded from a polypeptide chain of 703 amino acids. Each molecule can bind reversibly with two iron, zinc, copper or other metal ions. The binding site is located on the two globular domains of the protein. The affinity of LF for iron is 300 times that of transferrin, and the affinity is further enhanced in weakly acidic environments, which may be related to the transfer of iron from transferrin to LF when inflammation occurs (Dhennin-Duthille et al., 2000). It has also been found that, in the central nervous system, activated microglia can also generate and release LF (Xu et al., 2017). The results of immunohistochemistry studies showed that LF accumulated in the brain tissue of patients with neurodegenerative diseases. Further studies have found abnormal LF content and distribution in the brains of AD patients (Brown et al., 1985), with a large amount of LF deposition in the SP- and NFT-enriched areas (Valverde et al., 1990). Wang et al. (2010) detected LF deposition in the brains of AD model mice, but no LF deposition was found in wild mice, and the formation of SPs preceded LF. Further studies showed that LF deposition was localized in SPs and amyloid lesions. LF deposition increased with the age of transgenic mice, but after 18 months of age, most SPs showed a decrease in LF positives (Wang et al., 2010). Using laser confocal technology in AD transgenic mice to colocalize LF and Aβ in the brain, it was found that LF is expressed on Aβ, Aβ formation precedes deposition of LF, and Aβ plaques develop as the age of the rat increases and as both the size and number of LF accumulations increase, indicating that there is a close relationship between LF and AD (van de Looij et al., 2014). In combination with other biological functions of LF, such as its participation in metal ion metabolism and the regulation of cell proliferation and apoptosis, we hypothesize that LF may delay the occurrence of active AD.

With the presence of LF receptors (LFR) on the blood membrane of BBB vascular endothelial cells, exogenous LF can easily cross the BBB; thus, in recent years, LF has been widely used as a carrier for drug targeting of the brain. Interestingly, Kamalinia et al. (2013) used the PC12 cell line to demonstrate that lactoferrin-DFO conjugates are able to interfere with apoptosis. The expression levels of autophagy markers, including Atg7, Atg12-Atg5 and LC3-II/LC3-I, increased, and the LF-conjugated peritoneal cavity mainly affected the expression levels of Capsase-3, PARP, Bax and bcl-2. Furthermore, intraperitoneal injection of LF conjugates can significantly improve the learning abilities of AD rats and reduce Aβ (Kamalinia et al., 2013), which provides a theoretical basis for the use of LF in the treatment of neurodegenerative diseases.

Therefore, the use of exogenous LF as a therapeutic agent has been investigated to identify its roles in AD. Our group was the first to investigate whether exogenous LF administration could stimulate the non-amyloidogenic processing of APP and α-secretase catalytic activity and expression, which consequently reduce Aβ deposition and ameliorate cognitive decline in AD model mice (Guo et al., 2017). We also addressed the molecular mechanisms by which LF modulates APP processing. In fact, it has been reported in the literature that the function of human LF is similar to that of the iron chelator DFO, and it can also induce the neuroprotective effect of hypoxia-inducible factor (HIF-1α) expression under hypoxic conditions (Kawamata et al., 1993). Specifically, our results suggested that LF can enhance the α-secretase-dependent APP process through the ERK1/2-CREB and HIF-1α pathways *in vitro* and *in vivo* (Guo et al., 2017), once again proving that LF plays an active role in the treatment of AD. Consistent with previous observations, Aizawa et al. (2017) recently reported that the binding of LF to low-density lipoprotein receptor-associated protein-1 (LRP1) leads to the activation of the AMP-activated protein kinase signaling pathway, which in turn, promotes cell autophagy. This shows that LF may regulate the production of Aβ and NFTs through anti-inflammation, regulation of immunity, chelation of metal ions, regulation of cell autophagy, and may ultimately affect the occurrence and development of AD.

CONCLUSION

The pathogenesis of AD has been studied for decades, and although it is clear that SPs formed by Aβ deposition and NFTs formed by hyperphosphorylation of tau protein are two major pathological features of AD pathogenesis, there are many opinions about the inducing factors of SPs and NFTs that have not been clearly clarified yet. In light of the complex causes of AD, the study of its pathogenesis from multiple perspectives has been accepted by the public and has achieved good results. The study of the pathogenesis of AD using iron as a target has become a research hotspot in recent years. The use of iron chelators to chelate excess iron in the brains of AD patients has also become a new strategy for the treatment of AD. However, unlike other tissues and organs, there is a BBB in the brain that has strict specificity for the entry of drugs. Therefore, finding an iron chelator that easily crosses the BBB and that can function effectively must be sought from the body's self-synthesizing substances. There are many proteins or molecules that bind to iron in the body, and LA and LF are among these candidate drugs. *In vitro* and *in vivo* experiments have confirmed that direct administration of LA and LF can alleviate the symptoms of AD (Guo et al., 2017; Zhang et al., 2018), but the relevant mechanism of action on them has not been clarified, and further studies are needed. At the same time, LF-based nano-drug molecules are also under study. This drug molecule attaches to the LF molecule and can easily cross the BBB, thereby exerting a therapeutic effect on lesions and achieving better therapeutic effect. Future research will also use iron as an opportunity to study the mechanism of the occurrence and development of AD from the iron steady state to more fully explain the causes of AD.

AUTHOR CONTRIBUTIONS

J-LL and Y-GF wrote the manuscript. Z-SY, Z-YW, and CG approved and revised the final manuscript. All the authors have read and approved the final manuscript.

FUNDING

This work was supported by the Natural Science Foundation of China (U1608282).

REFERENCES

Abdalkader, M., Lampinen, R., Kanninen, K. M., Malm, T. M., and Liddell, J. R. (2018). Targeting Nrf2 to suppress ferroptosis and mitochondrial dysfunction in neurodegeneration. *Front. Neurosci.* 12:466. doi: 10.3389/fnins.2018.00466

Aizawa, S., Hoki, M., and Yamamuro, Y. (2017). Lactoferrin promotes autophagy via AMP-activated protein kinase activation through low-density lipoprotein receptor-related protein 1. *Biochem. Biophys. Res. Commun.* 493, 509–513. doi: 10.1016/j.bbrc.2017.08.160

Aliaga, M. E., Carrasco-Pozo, C., Lopez-Alarcon, C., Olea-Azar, C., and Speisky, H. (2011). Superoxide-dependent reduction of free Fe(3+) and release of Fe(2+) from ferritin by the physiologically-occurring Cu(I)-glutathione complex. *Bioorg. Med. Chem.* 19, 534–541. doi: 10.1016/j.bmc.2010.10.064

Alzheimer's Association (2016). 2016 Alzheimer's disease facts and figures. *Alzheimers Dement.* 12, 459–509.

Amit, T., Avramovich-Tirosh, Y., Youdim, M. B., and Mandel, S. (2008). Targeting multiple Alzheimer's disease etiologies with multimodal neuroprotective and neurorestorative iron chelators. *FASEB J.* 22, 1296–1305. doi: 10.1096/fj.07-8627rev

Arivazhagan, P., Shila, S., Kumaran, S., and Panneerselvam, C. (2002). Effect of DL-alpha-lipoic acid on the status of lipid peroxidation and antioxidant enzymes in various brain regions of aged rats. *Exp. Gerontol.* 37, 803–811. doi: 10.1016/S0531-5565(02)00015-3

Ayton, S., Diouf, I., Bush, A. I., and Alzheimer's disease Neuroimaging Initiative (2018). Evidence that iron accelerates Alzheimer's pathology: a CSF biomarker study. *J. Neurol. Neurosurg. Psychiatry* 89, 456–460. doi: 10.1136/jnnp-2017-316551

Ayton, S., Faux, N. G., Bush, A. I., and Alzheimer's Disease Neuroimaging Initiative (2015). Ferritin levels in the cerebrospinal fluid predict Alzheimer's disease outcomes and are regulated by APOE. *Nat. Commun.* 6:6760. doi: 10.1038/ncomms7760

Ayton, S., Fazlollahi, A., Bourgeat, P., Raniga, P., Ng, A., Lim, Y. Y., et al. (2017a). Cerebral quantitative susceptibility mapping predicts amyloid-beta-related cognitive decline. *Brain* 140, 2112–2119. doi: 10.1093/brain/awx137

Ayton, S., James, S. A., and Bush, A. I. (2017b). Nanoscale imaging reveals big role for iron in Alzheimer's disease. *Cell Chem. Biol.* 24, 1192–1194. doi: 10.1016/j.chembiol.2017.10.002

Balejcikova, L., Siposova, K., Kopcansky, P., and Safarik, I. (2018). Fe(II) formation after interaction of the amyloid beta-peptide with iron-storage protein ferritin. *J. Biol. Phys.* doi: 10.1007/s10867-018-9498-3 [Epub ahead of print].

Banerjee, P., Sahoo, A., Anand, S., Ganguly, A., Righi, G., Bovicelli, P., et al. (2014). Multiple mechanisms of iron-induced amyloid beta-peptide accumulation in

SHSY5Y cells: protective action of negletein. *Neuromolecular Med.* 16, 787–798. doi: 10.1007/s12017-014-8328-4

Belaidi, A. A., and Bush, A. I. (2016). Iron neurochemistry in Alzheimer's disease and Parkinson's disease: targets for therapeutics. *J. Neurochem.* 139(Suppl. 1), 179–197. doi: 10.1111/jnc.13425

Bierhaus, A., Chevion, S., Chevion, M., Hofmann, M., Quehenberger, P., Illmer, T., et al. (1997). Advanced glycation end product-induced activation of NF-kappaB is suppressed by alpha-lipoic acid in cultured endothelial cells. *Diabetes Metab. Res. Rev.* 46, 1481–1490. doi: 10.2337/diabetes.46.9.1481

Billings, J. L., Hare, D. J., Nurjono, M., Volitakis, I., Cherny, R. A., Bush, A. I., et al. (2016). Effects of neonatal iron feeding and chronic clioquinol administration on the parkinsonian human A53T transgenic mouse. *ACS Chem. Neurosci.* 7, 360–366. doi: 10.1021/acschemneuro.5b00305

Blennow, K., De Leon, M. J., and Zetterberg, H. (2006). Alzheimer's disease. *Lancet* 368, 387–403. doi: 10.1016/S0140-6736(06)69113-7

Boddaert, N., Le Quan Sang, K. H., Rotig, A., Leroy-Willig, A., Gallet, S., Brunelle, F., et al. (2007). Selective iron chelation in Friedreich ataxia: biologic and clinical implications. *Blood* 110, 401–408. doi: 10.1182/blood-2006-12-065433

Bodovitz, S., Falduto, M. T., Frail, D. E., and Klein, W. L. (1995). Iron levels modulate alpha-secretase cleavage of amyloid precursor protein. *J. Neurochem.* 64, 307–315. doi: 10.1046/j.1471-4159.1995.64010307.x

Boopathi, S., and Kolandaivel, P. (2016). Fe(2+) binding on amyloid beta-peptide promotes aggregation. *Proteins* 84, 1257–1274. doi: 10.1002/prot.25075

Borgna-Pignatti, C., and Marsella, M. (2015). Iron chelation in thalassemia major. *Clin. Ther.* 37, 2866–2877. doi: 10.1016/j.clinthera.2015.10.001

Brown, R. D., Rickard, K. A., and Kronenberg, H. (1985). Lactoferrin in the myeloproliferative disorders: a search for granulopoietic regulator defects. *Br. J. Haematol.* 59, 617–626. doi: 10.1111/j.1365-2141.1985.tb07356.x

Bulk, M., Abdelmoula, W. M., Nabuurs, R. J. A., Van Der Graaf, L. M., Mulders, C. W. H., Mulder, A. A., et al. (2018). Postmortem MRI and histology demonstrate differential iron accumulation and cortical myelin organization in early- and late-onset Alzheimer's disease. *Neurobiol. Aging* 62, 231–242. doi: 10.1016/j.neurobiolaging.2017.10.017

Bush, A. I. (2013). The metal theory of Alzheimer's disease. *J. Alzheimers Dis.* 33(Suppl. 1), S277–S281. doi: 10.3233/JAD-2012-129011

Cahill, C. M., Lahiri, D. K., Huang, X., and Rogers, J. T. (2009). Amyloid precursor protein and alpha synuclein translation, implications for iron and inflammation in neurodegenerative diseases. *Biochim. Biophys. Acta* 1790, 615–628. doi: 10.1016/j.bbagen.2008.12.001

Callaghan, M. F., Freund, P., Draganski, B., Anderson, E., Cappelletti, M., Chowdhury, R., et al. (2014). Widespread age-related differences in the human brain microstructure revealed by quantitative magnetic resonance imaging. *Neurobiol. Aging* 35, 1862–1872. doi: 10.1016/j.neurobiolaging.2014.02.008

Campbell, A., and Bondy, S. C. (2000). Aluminum induced oxidative events and its relation to inflammation: a role for the metal in Alzheimer's disease. *Cell. Mol. Biol.* 46, 721–730.

Cardenas-Aguayo Mdel, C., Gomez-Virgilio, L., Derosa, S., and Meraz-Rios, M. A. (2014). The role of tau oligomers in the onset of Alzheimer's disease neuropathology. *ACS Chem. Neurosci.* 5, 1178–1191. doi: 10.1021/cn500148z

Chen, L., Hambright, W. S., Na, R., and Ran, Q. (2015). Ablation of the ferroptosis inhibitor glutathione peroxidase 4 in neurons results in rapid motor neuron degeneration and paralysis. *J. Biol. Chem.* 290, 28097–28106. doi: 10.1074/jbc.M115.680090

Chen, Y. T., Chen, W. Y., Huang, X. T., Xu, Y. C., and Zhang, H. Y. (2018). Iron dysregulates APP processing accompanying with sAPPalpha cellular retention and beta-secretase inhibition in rat cortical neurons. *Acta Pharmacol. Sin.* 39, 177–183. doi: 10.1038/aps.2017.113

Cheng, X. S., Zhao, K. P., Jiang, X., Du, L. L., Li, X. H., Ma, Z. W., et al. (2013). Nmnat2 attenuates Tau phosphorylation through activation of PP2A. *J. Alzheimers Dis.* 36, 185–195. doi: 10.3233/JAD-122173

Cherny, R. A., Atwood, C. S., Xilinas, M. E., Gray, D. N., Jones, W. D., Mclean, C. A., et al. (2001). Treatment with a copper-zinc chelator markedly and rapidly inhibits beta-amyloid accumulation in Alzheimer's disease transgenic mice. *Neuron* 30, 665–676. doi: 10.1016/S0896-6273(01)00317-8

Chng, H. T., New, L. S., Neo, A. H., Goh, C. W., Browne, E. R., and Chan, E. C. (2009). Distribution study of orally administered lipoic acid in rat brain tissues. *Brain Res.* 1251, 80–86. doi: 10.1016/j.brainres.2008.11.025

Cohen, S. I., Linse, S., Luheshi, L. M., Hellstrand, E., White, D. A., Rajah, L., et al. (2013). Proliferation of amyloid-beta42 aggregates occurs through a secondary nucleation mechanism. *Proc. Natl. Acad. Sci. U.S.A.* 110, 9758–9763. doi: 10.1073/pnas.1218402110

Collingwood, J. F., and Davidson, M. R. (2014). The role of iron in neurodegenerative disorders: insights and opportunities with synchrotron light. *Front. Pharmacol.* 5:191. doi: 10.3389/fphar.2014.00191

Colvez, A., Joel, M. E., Ponton-Sanchez, A., and Royer, A. C. (2002). Health status and work burden of Alzheimer patients' informal caregivers: comparisons of five different care programs in the European Union. *Health Policy* 60, 219–233. doi: 10.1016/S0168-8510(01)00215-9

Connor, J. R., Snyder, B. S., Arosio, P., Loeffler, D. A., and Lewitt, P. (1995). A quantitative analysis of isoferritins in select regions of aged, parkinsonian, and Alzheimer's diseased brains. *J. Neurochem.* 65, 717–724. doi: 10.1046/j.1471-4159.1995.65020717.x

Corder, E. H., Saunders, A. M., Strittmatter, W. J., Schmechel, D. E., Gaskell, P. C. Jr., Rimmler, J. B., et al. (1995). Apolipoprotein E, survival in Alzheimer's disease patients, and the competing risks of death and Alzheimer's disease. *Neurology* 45, 1323–1328. doi: 10.1212/WNL.45.7.1323

Crapper McLachlan, D. R., Dalton, A. J., Kruck, T. P., Bell, M. Y., Smith, W. L., Kalow, W., et al. (1991). Intramuscular desferrioxamine in patients with Alzheimer's disease. *Lancet* 337, 1304–1308. doi: 10.1016/0140-6736(91)92978-B

Crielaard, B. J., Lammers, T., and Rivella, S. (2017). Targeting iron metabolism in drug discovery and delivery. *Nat. Rev. Drug Discov.* 16, 400–423. doi: 10.1038/nrd.2016.248

Cuajungco, M. P., Faget, K. Y., Huang, X., Tanzi, R. E., and Bush, A. I. (2000). Metal chelation as a potential therapy for Alzheimer's disease. *Ann. N. Y. Acad. Sci.* 920, 292–304. doi: 10.1111/j.1749-6632.2000.tb06938.x

Cunningham, C., Wilcockson, D. C., Campion, S., Lunnon, K., and Perry, V. H. (2005). Central and systemic endotoxin challenges exacerbate the local inflammatory response and increase neuronal death during chronic neurodegeneration. *J. Neurosci.* 25, 9275–9284. doi: 10.1523/JNEUROSCI.2614-05.2005

Daher, R., Manceau, H., and Karim, Z. (2017). Iron metabolism and the role of the iron-regulating hormone hepcidin in health and disease. *Presse Med.* 46(12 Pt 2), e272–e278. doi: 10.1016/j.lpm.2017.10.006

Dahms, S. O., Konnig, I., Roeser, D., Guhrs, K. H., Mayer, M. C., Kaden, D., et al. (2012). Metal binding dictates conformation and function of the amyloid precursor protein (APP) E2 domain. *J. Mol. Biol.* 416, 438–452. doi: 10.1016/j.jmb.2011.12.057

De Domenico, I., Nemeth, E., Nelson, J. M., Phillips, J. D., Ajioka, R. S., Kay, M. S., et al. (2008). The hepcidin-binding site on ferroportin is evolutionarily conserved. *Cell Metab.* 8, 146–156. doi: 10.1016/j.cmet.2008.07.002

de Freitas, R. M. (2010). Lipoic acid increases hippocampal choline acetyltransferase and acetylcholinesterase activities and improvement memory in epileptic rats. *Neurochem. Res.* 35, 162–170. doi: 10.1007/s11064-009-0041-6

Dhennin-Duthille, I., Masson, M., Damiens, E., Fillebeen, C., Spik, G., and Mazurier, J. (2000). Lactoferrin upregulates the expression of CD4 antigen through the stimulation of the mitogen-activated protein kinase in the human lymphoblastic T Jurkat cell line. *J. Cell. Biochem.* 79, 583–593. doi: 10.1002/1097-4644(20001215)79:4<583::AID-JCB70>3.0.CO;2-9

Dixon, S. J. (2017). Ferroptosis: bug or feature? *Immunol. Rev.* 277, 150–157. doi: 10.1111/imr.12533

Dixon, S. J., Lemberg, K. M., Lamprecht, M. R., Skouta, R., Zaitsev, E. M., Gleason, C. E., et al. (2012). Ferroptosis: an iron-dependent form of nonapoptotic cell death. *Cell* 149, 1060–1072. doi: 10.1016/j.cell.2012.03.042

Dringen, R., Bishop, G. M., Koeppe, M., Dang, T. N., and Robinson, S. R. (2007). The pivotal role of astrocytes in the metabolism of iron in the brain. *Neurochem. Res.* 32, 1884–1890. doi: 10.1007/s11064-007-9375-0

Du, F., Qian, C., Qian, Z. M., Wu, X. M., Xie, H., Yung, W. H., et al. (2011). Hepcidin directly inhibits transferrin receptor 1 expression in astrocytes via a cyclic AMP-protein kinase A pathway. *Glia* 59, 936–945. doi: 10.1002/glia.21166

Du, F., Qian, Z. M., Luo, Q., Yung, W. H., and Ke, Y. (2015). Hepcidin suppresses brain iron accumulation by downregulating iron transport proteins in iron-overloaded rats. *Mol. Neurobiol.* 52, 101–114. doi: 10.1007/s12035-014-8847-x

Du, L., Zhao, Z., Cui, A., Zhu, Y., Zhang, L., Liu, J., et al. (2018). increased iron deposition on brain quantitative susceptibility mapping correlates with decreased cognitive function in Alzheimer's disease. *ACS Chem. Neurosci.* 9, 1849–1857. doi: 10.1021/acschemneuro.8b00194

Duce, J. A., Tsatsanis, A., Cater, M. A., James, S. A., Robb, E., Wikhe, K., et al. (2010). Iron-export ferroxidase activity of beta-amyloid precursor protein is inhibited by zinc in Alzheimer's disease. *Cell* 142, 857–867. doi: 10.1016/j.cell.2010.08.014

Dusek, P., Schneider, S. A., and Aaseth, J. (2016). Iron chelation in the treatment of neurodegenerative diseases. *J. Trace Elem. Med. Biol.* 38, 81–92. doi: 10.1016/j.jtemb.2016.03.010

Dwivedi, N., Flora, G., Kushwaha, P., and Flora, S. J. (2014). Alpha-lipoic acid protects oxidative stress, changes in cholinergic system and tissue histopathology during co-exposure to arsenic-dichlorvos in rats. *Environ. Toxicol. Pharmacol.* 37, 7–23. doi: 10.1016/j.etap.2013.10.010

Dwyer, B. E., Zacharski, L. R., Balestra, D. J., Lerner, A. J., Perry, G., Zhu, X., et al. (2009). Getting the iron out: phlebotomy for Alzheimer's disease? *Med. Hypotheses* 72, 504–509. doi: 10.1016/j.mehy.2008.12.029

Everett, J., Cespedes, E., Shelford, L. R., Exley, C., Collingwood, J. F., Dobson, J., et al. (2014). Ferrous iron formation following the co-aggregation of ferric iron and the Alzheimer's disease peptide beta-amyloid (1-42). *J. R. Soc. Interface* 11:20140165. doi: 10.1098/rsif.2014.0165

Everett, J., Collingwood, J. F., Tjendana-Tjhin, V., Brooks, J., Lermyte, F., Plascencia-Villa, G., et al. (2018). Nanoscale synchrotron X-ray speciation of iron and calcium compounds in amyloid plaque cores from Alzheimer's disease subjects. *Nanoscale* 10, 11782–11796. doi: 10.1039/c7nr06794a

Fava, A., Pirritano, D., Plastino, M., Cristiano, D., Puccio, G., Colica, C., et al. (2013). The effect of lipoic acid therapy on cognitive functioning in patients with Alzheimer's disease. *J. Neurodegener. Dis.* 2013, 454253. doi: 10.1155/2013/454253

Fine, J. M., Baillargeon, A. M., Renner, D. B., Hoerster, N. S., Tokarev, J., Colton, S., et al. (2012). Intranasal deferoxamine improves performance in radial arm water maze, stabilizes HIF-1alpha, and phosphorylates GSK3beta in P301L tau transgenic mice. *Exp. Brain Res.* 219, 381–390. doi: 10.1007/s00221-012-3101-0

Fonte, J., Miklossy, J., Atwood, C., and Martins, R. (2001). The severity of cortical Alzheimer's type changes is positively correlated with increased amyloid-β Levels: Resolubilization of amyloid-β with transition metal ion chelators. *J. Alzheimers Dis.* 3, 209–219. doi: 10.3233/JAD-2001-3206

Frazer, D. M., and Anderson, G. J. (2005). Iron imports. I. Intestinal iron absorption and its regulation. *Am. J. Physiol. Gastrointest. Liver Physiol.* 289, G631–G635. doi: 10.1152/ajpgi.00220.2005

Galante, D., Cavallo, E., Perico, A., and D'arrigo, C. (2018). Effect of ferric citrate on amyloid-beta peptides behavior. *Biopolymers* 109:e23224. doi: 10.1002/bip.23224

Gao, M., Monian, P., Pan, Q., Zhang, W., Xiang, J., and Jiang, X. (2016). Ferroptosis is an autophagic cell death process. *Cell Res.* 26, 1021–1032. doi: 10.1038/cr.2016.95

Garrick, M. D., and Garrick, L. M. (2009). Cellular iron transport. *Biochim. Biophys. Acta* 1790, 309–325. doi: 10.1016/j.bbagen.2009.03.018

Gerlach, M., Ben-Shachar, D., Riederer, P., and Youdim, M. B. (1994). Altered brain metabolism of iron as a cause of neurodegenerative diseases? *J. Neurochem.* 63, 793–807. doi: 10.1046/j.1471-4159.1994.63030793.x

Giampietro, R., Spinelli, F., Contino, M., and Colabufo, N. A. (2018). The pivotal role of copper in neurodegeneration: a new strategy for the therapy of neurodegenerative disorders. *Mol. Pharm.* 15, 808–820. doi: 10.1021/acs.molpharmaceut.7b00841

Goodman, L. (1953). Alzheimer's disease; a clinico-pathologic analysis of twenty-three cases with a theory on pathogenesis. *J. Nerv. Ment. Dis.* 118, 97–130. doi: 10.1097/00005053-195308000-00001

Goozee, K., Chatterjee, P., James, I., Shen, K., Sohrabi, H. R., Asih, P. R., et al. (2017). Elevated plasma ferritin in elderly individuals with high neocortical amyloid-beta load. *Mol. Psychiatry* doi: 10.1038/mp.2017.146 [Epub ahead of print].

Goralska, M., Dackor, R., Holley, B., and Mcgahan, M. C. (2003). Alpha lipoic acid changes iron uptake and storage in lens epithelial cells. *Exp. Eye Res.* 76, 241–248. doi: 10.1016/S0014-4835(02)00307-X

Grossi, C., Francese, S., Casini, A., Rosi, M. C., Luccarini, I., Fiorentini, A., et al. (2009). Clioquinol decreases amyloid-beta burden and reduces working memory impairment in a transgenic mouse model of Alzheimer's disease. *J. Alzheimers Dis.* 17, 423–440. doi: 10.3233/JAD-2009-1063

Guerreiro, C., Silva, B., Crespo, A. C., Marques, L., Costa, S., Timoteo, A., et al. (2015). Decrease in APP and CP mRNA expression supports impairment of iron export in Alzheimer's disease patients. *Biochim. Biophys. Acta* 1852, 2116–2122. doi: 10.1016/j.bbadis.2015.07.017

Guo, C., Wang, P., Zhong, M. L., Wang, T., Huang, X. S., Li, J. Y., et al. (2013a). Deferoxamine inhibits iron induced hippocampal tau phosphorylation in the Alzheimer transgenic mouse brain. *Neurochem. Int.* 62, 165–172. doi: 10.1016/j.neuint.2012.12.005

Guo, C., Wang, T., Zheng, W., Shan, Z. Y., Teng, W. P., and Wang, Z. Y. (2013b). Intranasal deferoxamine reverses iron-induced memory deficits and inhibits amyloidogenic APP processing in a transgenic mouse model of Alzheimer's disease. *Neurobiol. Aging* 34, 562–575. doi: 10.1016/j.neurobiolaging.2012.05.009

Guo, C., Yang, Z. H., Zhang, S., Chai, R., Xue, H., Zhang, Y. H., et al. (2017). Intranasal lactoferrin enhances alpha-secretase-dependent amyloid precursor protein processing via the ERK1/2-CREB and HIF-1alpha pathways in an Alzheimer's disease mouse model. *Neuropsychopharmacology* 42, 2504–2515. doi: 10.1038/npp.2017.8

Guo, C., Zhang, Y. X., Wang, T., Zhong, M. L., Yang, Z. H., Hao, L. J., et al. (2015). Intranasal deferoxamine attenuates synapse loss via up-regulating the P38/HIF-1alpha pathway on the brain of APP/PS1 transgenic mice. *Front. Aging Neurosci.* 7:104. doi: 10.3389/fnagi.2015.00104

Guo, J., Gao, S., Liu, Z., Zhao, R., and Yang, X. (2016). Alpha-lipoic acid alleviates acute inflammation and promotes lipid mobilization during the inflammatory response in white adipose tissue of mice. *Lipids* 51, 1145–1152. doi: 10.1007/s11745-016-4185-2

Ha, C., Ryu, J., and Park, C. B. (2007). Metal ions differentially influence the aggregation and deposition of Alzheimer's beta-amyloid on a solid template. *Biochemistry* 46, 6118–6125. doi: 10.1021/bi7000032

Hambright, W. S., Fonseca, R. S., Chen, L., Na, R., and Ran, Q. (2017). Ablation of ferroptosis regulator glutathione peroxidase 4 in forebrain neurons promotes cognitive impairment and neurodegeneration. *Redox Biol.* 12, 8–17. doi: 10.1016/j.redox.2017.01.021

Hirata, Y., Yamada, C., Ito, Y., Yamamoto, S., Nagase, H., Oh-Hashi, K., et al. (2018). Novel oxindole derivatives prevent oxidative stress-induced cell death in mouse hippocampal HT22cells. *Neuropharmacology* 135, 242–252. doi: 10.1016/j.neuropharm.2018.03.015

Hohenberger, J., Ray, K., and Meyer, K. (2012). The biology and chemistry of high-valent iron-oxo and iron-nitrido complexes. *Nat. Commun.* 3:720. doi: 10.1038/ncomms1718

Horl, W. H. (2008). New insights into intestinal iron absorption. *Nephrol. Dial. Transplant.* 23, 3063–3064. doi: 10.1093/ndt/gfn458

House, E., Collingwood, J., Khan, A., Korchazkina, O., Berthon, G., and Exley, C. (2004). Aluminium, iron, zinc and copper influence the in vitro formation of amyloid fibrils of Abeta42 in a manner which may have consequences for metal chelation therapy in Alzheimer's disease. *J. Alzheimers Dis.* 6, 291–301. doi: 10.3233/JAD-2004-6310

Huang, Y., and Mucke, L. (2012). Alzheimer mechanisms and therapeutic strategies. *Cell* 148, 1204–1222. doi: 10.1016/j.cell.2012.02.040

Ikonomovic, M. D., Klunk, W. E., Abrahamson, E. E., Wuu, J., Mathis, C. A., Scheff, S. W., et al. (2011). Precuneus amyloid burden is associated with reduced cholinergic activity in Alzheimer disease. *Neurology* 77, 39–47. doi: 10.1212/WNL.0b013e3182231419

Kamalinia, G., Khodagholi, F., Atyabi, F., Amini, M., Shaerzadeh, F., Sharifzadeh, M., et al. (2013). Enhanced brain delivery of deferasirox-lactoferrin conjugates for iron chelation therapy in neurodegenerative disorders: in vitro and in vivo studies. *Mol. Pharm.* 10, 4418–4431. doi: 10.1021/mp4002014

Kawahara, M., Kato-Negishi, M., and Tanaka, K. (2017). Cross talk between neurometals and amyloidogenic proteins at the synapse and the pathogenesis of neurodegenerative diseases. *Metallomics* 9, 619–633. doi: 10.1039/c7mt00046d

Kawahara, M., Tanaka, K. I., and Kato-Negishi, M. (2018). Zinc, carnosine, and neurodegenerative diseases. *Nutrients* 10:E147. doi: 10.3390/nu10020147

Kawamata, T., Tooyama, I., Yamada, T., Walker, D. G., and Mcgeer, P. L. (1993). Lactotransferrin immunocytochemistry in Alzheimer and normal human brain. *Am. J. Pathol.* 142, 1574–1585.

Ke, Y., and Qian, Z. M. (2007). Brain iron metabolism: neurobiology and neurochemistry. *Prog. Neurobiol.* 83, 149–173. doi: 10.1016/j.pneurobio.2007.07.009

Kim, A. C., Lim, S., and Kim, Y. K. (2018). Metal ion effects on abeta and tau aggregation. *Int. J. Mol. Sci.* 19:128. doi: 10.3390/ijms19010128

Klein, W. L., Krafft, G. A., and Finch, C. E. (2001). Targeting small Abeta oligomers: the solution to an Alzheimer's disease conundrum? *Trends Neurosci.* 24, 219–224.

Krishnamurthy, P., Xie, T., and Schuetz, J. D. (2007). The role of transporters in cellular heme and porphyrin homeostasis. *Pharmacol. Ther.* 114, 345–358. doi: 10.1016/j.pharmthera.2007.02.001

Kudin, A. P., Bimpong-Buta, N. Y., Vielhaber, S., Elger, C. E., and Kunz, W. S. (2004). Characterization of superoxide-producing sites in isolated brain mitochondria. *J. Biol. Chem.* 279, 4127–4135. doi: 10.1074/jbc.M310341200

Kummer, M. P., Hermes, M., Delekarte, A., Hammerschmidt, T., Kumar, S., Terwel, D., et al. (2011). Nitration of tyrosine 10 critically enhances amyloid beta aggregation and plaque formation. *Neuron* 71, 833–844. doi: 10.1016/j.neuron.2011.07.001

Kunt, T., Forst, T., Wilhelm, A., Tritschler, H., Pfuetzner, A., Harzer, O., et al. (1999). Alpha-lipoic acid reduces expression of vascular cell adhesion molecule-1 and endothelial adhesion of human monocytes after stimulation with advanced glycation end products. *Clin. Sci.* 96, 75–82. doi: 10.1042/cs0960075

Lane, D. J. R., Ayton, S., and Bush, A. I. (2018). Iron and Alzheimer's disease: an update on emerging mechanisms. *J. Alzheimers Dis.* 64, S379–S395. doi: 10.3233/JAD-179944

Lei, P., Ayton, S., Appukuttan, A. T., Volitakis, I., Adlard, P. A., Finkelstein, D. I., et al. (2015). Clioquinol rescues Parkinsonism and dementia phenotypes of the tau knockout mouse. *Neurobiol. Dis.* 81, 168–175. doi: 10.1016/j.nbd.2015.03.015

Lei, P., Ayton, S., Finkelstein, D. I., Spoerri, L., Ciccotosto, G. D., Wright, D. K., et al. (2012). Tau deficiency induces parkinsonism with dementia by impairing APP-mediated iron export. *Nat. Med.* 18, 291–295. doi: 10.1038/nm.2613

Li, X., Lei, P., Tuo, Q., Ayton, S., Li, Q. X., Moon, S., et al. (2015). Enduring elevations of hippocampal amyloid precursor protein and iron are features of beta-amyloid toxicity and are mediated by Tau. *Neurotherapeutics* 12, 862–873. doi: 10.1007/s13311-015-0378-2

Li, X., Liu, Y., Zheng, Q., Yao, G., Cheng, P., Bu, G., et al. (2013). Ferritin light chain interacts with PEN-2 and affects gamma-secretase activity. *Neurosci. Lett.* 548, 90–94. doi: 10.1016/j.neulet.2013.05.018

Liu, G., Huang, W., Moir, R. D., Vanderburg, C. R., Lai, B., Peng, Z., et al. (2006). Metal exposure and Alzheimer's pathogenesis. *J. Struct. Biol.* 155, 45–51. doi: 10.1016/j.jsb.2005.12.011

Lovell, M. A., Robertson, J. D., Teesdale, W. J., Campbell, J. L., and Markesbery, W. R. (1998). Copper, iron and zinc in Alzheimer's disease senile plaques. *J. Neurol. Sci.* 158, 47–52. doi: 10.1016/S0022-510X(98)00092-6

May, P. M., and Bulman, R. A. (1983). The present status of chelating agents in medicine. *Prog. Med. Chem.* 20, 225–336. doi: 10.1016/S0079-6468(08)70220-0

Mena, N. P., Urrutia, P. J., Lourido, F., Carrasco, C. M., and Nunez, M. T. (2015). Mitochondrial iron homeostasis and its dysfunctions in neurodegenerative disorders. *Mitochondrion* 21, 92–105. doi: 10.1016/j.mito.2015.02.001

Metz-Boutigue, M. H., Jolles, J., Mazurier, J., Schoentgen, F., Legrand, D., Spik, G., et al. (1984). Human lactotransferrin: amino acid sequence and structural comparisons with other transferrins. *Eur. J. Biochem.* 145, 659–676. doi: 10.1111/j.1432-1033.1984.tb08607.x

Moon, Y., Han, S. H., and Moon, W. J. (2016). Patterns of brain iron accumulation in vascular dementia and Alzheimer's dementia using quantitative susceptibility mapping imaging. *J. Alzheimers Dis.* 51, 737–745. doi: 10.3233/JAD-151037

Morse, L. J., Payton, S. M., Cuny, G. D., and Rogers, J. T. (2004). FDA-preapproved drugs targeted to the translational regulation and processing of the amyloid precursor protein. *J. Mol. Neurosci.* 24, 129–136. doi: 10.1385/JMN:24:1:129

Mullard, A. (2012). Sting of Alzheimer's failures offset by upcoming prevention trials. *Nat. Rev. Drug Discov.* 11, 657–660. doi: 10.1038/nrd3842

Myhre, O., Utkilen, H., Duale, N., Brunborg, G., and Hofer, T. (2013). Metal dyshomeostasis and inflammation in Alzheimer's and Parkinson's diseases: possible impact of environmental exposures. *Oxid. Med. Cell. Longev.* 2013:726954. doi: 10.1155/2013/726954

Nakamura, T., and Lipton, S. A. (2011). S-nitrosylation of critical protein thiols mediates protein misfolding and mitochondrial dysfunction in neurodegenerative diseases. *Antioxid. Redox. Signal.* 14, 1479–1492. doi: 10.1089/ars.2010.3570

Nunomura, A., Perry, G., Aliev, G., Hirai, K., Takeda, A., Balraj, E. K., et al. (2001). Oxidative damage is the earliest event in Alzheimer disease. *J. Neuropathol. Exp. Neurol.* 60, 759–767. doi: 10.1093/jnen/60.8.759

O'Callaghan, J., Holmes, H., Powell, N., Wells, J. A., Ismail, O., Harrison, I. F., et al. (2017). Tissue magnetic susceptibility mapping as a marker of tau pathology in Alzheimer's disease. *Neuroimage* 159, 334–345. doi: 10.1016/j.neuroimage.2017.08.003

Opazo, C., Luza, S., Villemagne, V. L., Volitakis, I., Rowe, C., Barnham, K. J., et al. (2006). Radioiodinated clioquinol as a biomarker for beta-amyloid: Zn complexes in Alzheimer's disease. *Aging Cell* 5, 69–79. doi: 10.1111/j.1474-9726.2006.00196.x

Ou, P., Tritschler, H. J., and Wolff, S. P. (1995). Thioctic (lipoic) acid: a therapeutic metal-chelating antioxidant? *Biochem. Pharmacol.* 50, 123–126. doi: 10.1016/0006-2952(95)00116-H

Panigrahi, M., Sadguna, Y., Shivakumar, B. R., Kolluri, S. V., Roy, S., Packer, L., et al. (1996). Alpha-Lipoic acid protects against reperfusion injury following cerebral ischemia in rats. *Brain Res.* 717, 184–188. doi: 10.1016/0006-8993(96)00009-1

Park, D., Yang, Y. H., Bae, D. K., Lee, S. H., Yang, G., Kyung, J., et al. (2013). Improvement of cognitive function and physical activity of aging mice by human neural stem cells over-expressing choline acetyltransferase. *Neurobiol. Aging* 34, 2639–2646. doi: 10.1016/j.neurobiolaging.2013.04.026

Perry, G., Taddeo, M. A., Petersen, R. B., Castellani, R. J., Harris, P. L., Siedlak, S. L., et al. (2003). Adventiously-bound redox active iron and copper are at the center of oxidative damage in Alzheimer disease. *Biometals* 16, 77–81. doi: 10.1023/A:1020731021276

Peters, D. G., Pollack, A. N., Cheng, K. C., Sun, D., Saido, T., Haaf, M. P., et al. (2018). Dietary lipophilic iron alters amyloidogenesis and microglial morphology in Alzheimer's disease knock-in APP mice. *Metallomics* 10, 426–443. doi: 10.1039/c8mt00004b

Plascencia-Villa, G., Ponce, A., Collingwood, J. F., Arellano-Jimenez, M. J., Zhu, X., Rogers, J. T., et al. (2016). High-resolution analytical imaging and electron holography of magnetite particles in amyloid cores of Alzheimer's disease. *Sci. Rep.* 6:24873. doi: 10.1038/srep24873

Pretorius, E., Vermeulen, N., Bester, J., Lipinski, B., and Kell, D. B. (2013). A novel method for assessing the role of iron and its functional chelation in fibrin fibril formation: the use of scanning electron microscopy. *Toxicol. Mech. Methods* 23, 352–359. doi: 10.3109/15376516.2012.762082

Quinn, J. F., Bussiere, J. R., Hammond, R. S., Montine, T. J., Henson, E., Jones, R. E., et al. (2007). Chronic dietary alpha-lipoic acid reduces deficits in hippocampal memory of aged Tg2576 mice. *Neurobiol. Aging* 28, 213–225. doi: 10.1016/j.neurobiolaging.2005.12.014

Ramos, P., Santos, A., Pinto, N. R., Mendes, R., Magalhaes, T., and Almeida, A. (2014). Iron levels in the human brain: a post-mortem study of anatomical region differences and age-related changes. *J. Trace Elem. Med. Biol.* 28, 13–17. doi: 10.1016/j.jtemb.2013.08.001

Reese, J. P., Dams, J., Winter, Y., Balzer-Geldsetzer, M., Oertel, W. H., and Dodel, R. (2012). Pharmacoeconomic considerations of treating patients with advanced Parkinson's disease. *Expert Opin. Pharmacother.* 13, 939–958. doi: 10.1517/14656566.2012.677435

Reynolds, M. R., Reyes, J. F., Fu, Y., Bigio, E. H., Guillozet-Bongaarts, A. L., Berry, R. W., et al. (2006). Tau nitration occurs at tyrosine 29 in the fibrillar lesions of Alzheimer's disease and other tauopathies. *J. Neurosci.* 26, 10636–10645. doi: 10.1523/JNEUROSCI.2143-06.2006

Ritchie, C. W., Bush, A. I., Mackinnon, A., Macfarlane, S., Mastwyk, M., Macgregor, L., et al. (2003). Metal-protein attenuation with iodochlorhydroxyquin (clioquinol) targeting Abeta amyloid deposition and toxicity in Alzheimer disease: a pilot phase 2 clinical trial. *Arch. Neurol.* 60, 1685–1691. doi: 10.1001/archneur.60.12.1685

Rodrigue, K. M., Haacke, E. M., and Raz, N. (2011). Differential effects of age and history of hypertension on regional brain volumes and iron. *Neuroimage* 54, 750–759. doi: 10.1016/j.neuroimage.2010.09.068

Rogers, J. T., Randall, J. D., Cahill, C. M., Eder, P. S., Huang, X., Gunshin, H., et al. (2002). An iron-responsive element type II in the 5′-untranslated region of the Alzheimer's amyloid precursor protein transcript. *J. Biol. Chem.* 277, 45518–45528. doi: 10.1074/jbc.M207435200

Seiler, A., Schneider, M., Forster, H., Roth, S., Wirth, E. K., Culmsee, C., et al. (2008). Glutathione peroxidase 4 senses and translates oxidative stress into 12/15-lipoxygenase dependent- and AIF-mediated cell death. *Cell Metab.* 8, 237–248. doi: 10.1016/j.cmet.2008.07.005

Selkoe, D. J. (2012). Preventing Alzheimer's disease. *Science* 337, 1488–1492. doi: 10.1126/science.1228541

Silvestri, L., and Camaschella, C. (2008). A potential pathogenetic role of iron in Alzheimer's disease. *J. Cell. Mol. Med.* 12, 1548–1550. doi: 10.1111/j.1582-4934.2008.00356.x

Smith, M. A., Harris, P. L., Sayre, L. M., and Perry, G. (1997). Iron accumulation in Alzheimer disease is a source of redox-generated free radicals. *Proc. Natl. Acad. Sci. U.S.A.* 94, 9866–9868. doi: 10.1073/pnas.94.18.9866

Sripetchwandee, J., Wongjaikam, S., Krintratun, W., Chattipakorn, N., and Chattipakorn, S. C. (2016). A combination of an iron chelator with an antioxidant effectively diminishes the dendritic loss, tau-hyperphosphorylation, amyloids-beta accumulation and brain mitochondrial dynamic disruption in rats with chronic iron-overload. *Neuroscience* 332, 191–202. doi: 10.1016/j.neuroscience.2016.07.003

Sternberg, Z., Hu, Z., Sternberg, D., Waseh, S., Quinn, J. F., Wild, K., et al. (2017). Serum hepcidin levels, iron dyshomeostasis and cognitive loss in Alzheimer's disease. *Aging Dis.* 8, 215–227. doi: 10.14336/AD.2016.0811

Suh, J. H., Moreau, R., Heath, S. H., and Hagen, T. M. (2005). Dietary supplementation with (R)-alpha-lipoic acid reverses the age-related accumulation of iron and depletion of antioxidants in the rat cerebral cortex. *Redox Rep.* 10, 52–60. doi: 10.1179/135100005X21624

Tahirbegi, I. B., Pardo, W. A., Alvira, M., Mir, M., and Samitier, J. (2016). Amyloid Abeta 42, a promoter of magnetite nanoparticle formation in Alzheimer's disease. *Nanotechnology* 27:465102. doi: 10.1088/0957-4484/27/46/465102

Tahmasebinia, F., and Emadi, S. (2017). Effect of metal chelators on the aggregation of beta-amyloid peptides in the presence of copper and iron. *Biometals* 30, 285–293. doi: 10.1007/s10534-017-0005-2

Takeda, A. (2004). Essential trace metals and brain function. *Yakugaku Zasshi* 124, 577–585. doi: 10.1248/yakushi.124.577

Telling, N. D., Everett, J., Collingwood, J. F., Dobson, J., Van Der Laan, G., Gallagher, J. J., et al. (2017). Iron biochemistry is correlated with amyloid plaque morphology in an established mouse model of Alzheimer's disease. *Cell Chem. Biol.* 24, e1203. doi: 10.1016/j.chembiol.2017.07.014

Tuo, Q. Z., Lei, P., Jackman, K. A., Li, X. L., Xiong, H., Li, X. L., et al. (2017). Tau-mediated iron export prevents ferroptotic damage after ischemic stroke. *Mol. Psychiatry* 22, 1520–1530. doi: 10.1038/mp.2017.171

Valverde, F., Lopez-Mascaraque, L., and De Carlos, J. A. (1990). Distribution and morphology of Alz-50-immunoreactive cells in the developing visual cortex of kittens. *J. Neurocytol.* 19, 662–671. doi: 10.1007/BF01188035

van Bergen, J. M., Li, X., Hua, J., Schreiner, S. J., Steininger, S. C., Quevenco, F. C., et al. (2016). Colocalization of cerebral iron with amyloid beta in mild cognitive impairment. *Sci. Rep.* 6:35514. doi: 10.1038/srep35514

van Bergen, J. M. G., Li, X., Quevenco, F. C., Gietl, A. F., Treyer, V., Meyer, R., et al. (2018). Simultaneous quantitative susceptibility mapping and Flutemetamol-PET suggests local correlation of iron and beta-amyloid as an indicator of cognitive performance at high age. *Neuroimage* 174, 308–316. doi: 10.1016/j.neuroimage.2018.03.021

van de Looij, Y., Ginet, V., Chatagner, A., Toulotte, A., Somm, E., Huppi, P. S., et al. (2014). Lactoferrin during lactation protects the immature hypoxic-ischemic rat brain. *Ann. Clin. Transl. Neurol.* 1, 955–967. doi: 10.1002/acn3.138

van Duijn, S., Bulk, M., Van Duinen, S. G., Nabuurs, R. J. A., Van Buchem, M. A., Van Der Weerd, L., et al. (2017). Cortical iron reflects severity of Alzheimer's disease. *J. Alzheimers Dis.* 60, 1533–1545. doi: 10.3233/JAD-161143

Vela, D. (2018). Hepcidin, an emerging and important player in brain iron homeostasis. *J. Transl. Med.* 16:25. doi: 10.1186/s12967-018-1399-5

Wang, D., Hui, Y., Peng, Y., Tang, L., Jin, J., He, R., et al. (2015). Overexpression of heme oxygenase 1 causes cognitive decline and affects pathways for tauopathy in mice. *J. Alzheimers Dis.* 43, 519–534. doi: 10.3233/JAD-140567

Wang, L., Sato, H., Zhao, S., and Tooyama, I. (2010). Deposition of lactoferrin in fibrillar-type senile plaques in the brains of transgenic mouse models of Alzheimer's disease. *Neurosci. Lett.* 481, 164–167. doi: 10.1016/j.neulet.2010.06.079

Wang, P., and Wang, Z. Y. (2017). Metal ions influx is a double edged sword for the pathogenesis of Alzheimer's disease. *Ageing Res. Rev.* 35, 265–290. doi: 10.1016/j.arr.2016.10.003

Wang, T., Wang, C. Y., Shan, Z. Y., Teng, W. P., and Wang, Z. Y. (2012). Clioquinol reduces zinc accumulation in neuritic plaques and inhibits the amyloidogenic pathway in AbetaPP/PS1 transgenic mouse brain. *J. Alzheimers Dis.* 29, 549–559. doi: 10.3233/JAD-2011-111874

Ward, R. J., Zucca, F. A., Duyn, J. H., Crichton, R. R., and Zecca, L. (2014). The role of iron in brain ageing and neurodegenerative disorders. *Lancet Neurol.* 13, 1045–1060. doi: 10.1016/S1474-4422(14)70117-6

Wong, A., Dukic-Stefanovic, S., Gasic-Milenkovic, J., Schinzel, R., Wiesinger, H., Riederer, P., et al. (2001). Anti-inflammatory antioxidants attenuate the expression of inducible nitric oxide synthase mediated by advanced glycation end products in murine microglia. *Eur. J. Neurosci.* 14, 1961–1967. doi: 10.1046/j.0953-816x.2001.01820.x

Wright, R. O., and Baccarelli, A. (2007). Metals and neurotoxicology. *J. Nutr.* 137, 2809–2813. doi: 10.1093/jn/137.12.2809

Xie, L., Zheng, W., Xin, N., Xie, J. W., Wang, T., and Wang, Z. Y. (2012). Ebselen inhibits iron-induced tau phosphorylation by attenuating DMT1 up-regulation and cellular iron uptake. *Neurochem. Int.* 61, 334–340. doi: 10.1016/j.neuint.2012.05.016

Xie, Y., Hou, W., Song, X., Yu, Y., Huang, J., Sun, X., et al. (2016). Ferroptosis: process and function. *Cell Death Differ.* 23, 369–379. doi: 10.1038/cdd.2015.158

Xu, H., Wang, Y., Song, N., Wang, J., Jiang, H., and Xie, J. (2017). New progress on the role of glia in iron metabolism and iron-induced degeneration of dopamine neurons in Parkinson's disease. *Front. Mol. Neurosci.* 10:455. doi: 10.3389/fnmol.2017.00455

Yamamoto, A., Shin, R. W., Hasegawa, K., Naiki, H., Sato, H., Yoshimasu, F., et al. (2002). Iron (III) induces aggregation of hyperphosphorylated tau and its reduction to iron (II) reverses the aggregation: implications in the formation of neurofibrillary tangles of Alzheimer's disease. *J. Neurochem.* 82, 1137–1147. doi: 10.1046/j.1471-4159.2002.t01-1-01061.x

Yang, W. S., and Stockwell, B. R. (2016). Ferroptosis: death by lipid peroxidation. *Trends Cell Biol.* 26, 165–176. doi: 10.1016/j.tcb.2015.10.014

Zecca, L., Stroppolo, A., Gatti, A., Tampellini, D., Toscani, M., Gallorini, M., et al. (2004). The role of iron and copper molecules in the neuronal vulnerability of locus coeruleus and substantia nigra during aging. *Proc. Natl. Acad. Sci. U.S.A.* 101, 9843–9848. doi: 10.1073/pnas.0403495101

Zhang, B., Gaiteri, C., Bodea, L. G., Wang, Z., Mcelwee, J., Podtelezhnikov, A. A., et al. (2013). Integrated systems approach identifies genetic nodes and networks in late-onset Alzheimer's disease. *Cell* 153, 707–720. doi: 10.1016/j.cell.2013.03.030

Zhang, W. J., and Frei, B. (2001). Alpha-lipoic acid inhibits TNF-alpha-induced NF-kappaB activation and adhesion molecule expression in human aortic endothelial cells. *FASEB J.* 15, 2423–2432. doi: 10.1096/fj.01-0260com

Zhang, Y. H., Wang, D. W., Xu, S. F., Zhang, S., Fan, Y. G., Yang, Y. Y., et al. (2018). alpha-Lipoic acid improves abnormal behavior by mitigation of oxidative stress, inflammation, ferroptosis, and tauopathy in P301S Tau transgenic mice. *Redox Biol.* 14, 535–548. doi: 10.1016/j.redox.2017.11.001

Zhao, Y., Raichle, M. E., Wen, J., Benzinger, T. L., Fagan, A. M., Hassenstab, J., et al. (2017). In vivo detection of microstructural correlates of brain pathology in preclinical and early Alzheimer Disease with magnetic resonance imaging. *Neuroimage* 148, 296–304. doi: 10.1016/j.neuroimage.2016.12.026

Zhou, Z. D., and Tan, E. K. (2017). Iron regulatory protein (IRP)-iron responsive element (IRE) signaling pathway in human neurodegenerative diseases. *Mol. Neurodegener.* 12:75. doi: 10.1186/s13024-017-0218-4

17

Iron Dysregulation and Dormant Microbes as Causative Agents for Impaired Blood Rheology and Pathological Clotting in Alzheimer's Type Dementia

Lesha Pretorius[1], Douglas B. Kell[2,3†] and Etheresia Pretorius[1*]*

[1] Department of Physiological Sciences, Stellenbosch University, Stellenbosch, South Africa, [2] School of Chemistry, The University of Manchester, Manchester, United Kingdom, [3] The Manchester Institute of Biotechnology, The University of Manchester, Manchester, United Kingdom

***Correspondence:**
Douglas B. Kell
dbk@manchester.ac.uk
orcid.org/0000-0001-5838-7963
Etheresia Pretorius
resiap@sun.ac.za
orcid.org/0000-0002-9108-2384

†Present address:
Douglas B. Kell,
Dept of Biochemistry, Institute of Integrative Biology, University of Liverpool, Liverpool, United Kingdom

Alzheimer's disease and other similar dementias are debilitating neurodegenerative disorders whose etiology and pathogenesis remain largely unknown, even after decades of research. With the anticipated increase in prevalence of Alzheimer's type dementias among the more susceptible aging population, the need for disease-modifying treatments is urgent. While various hypotheses have been put forward over the last few decades, we suggest that Alzheimer's type dementias are triggered by external environmental factors, co-expressing in individuals with specific genetic susceptibilities. These external stressors are defined in the Iron Dysregulation and Dormant Microbes (IDDM) hypothesis, previously put forward. This hypothesis is consistent with current literature in which serum ferritin levels of individuals diagnosed with Alzheimer's disease are significantly higher compared those of age- and gender-matched controls. While iron dysregulation contributes to oxidative stress, it also causes microbial reactivation and virulence of the so-called dormant blood (and tissue) microbiome. Dysbiosis (changes in the microbiome) or previous infections can contribute to the dormant blood microbiome (atopobiosis[1]), and also directly promotes systemic inflammation via the amyloidogenic formation and shedding of potent inflammagens such as lipopolysaccharides. The simultaneous iron dysregulation and microbial aberrations affect the hematological system, promoting fibrin amylodiogenesis, and pathological clotting. Systemic inflammation and oxidative stress can contribute to blood brain barrier permeability and the ensuing neuro-inflammation, characteristic of Alzheimer's type dementias. While large inter-individual variability exists, especially concerning disease pathogenesis, the IDDM hypothesis acknowledges primary causative factors which can be targeted for early diagnosis and/or for prevention of disease progression.

Keywords: Alzheimer's type dementia, iron, gut dysbiosis, iron dysregulation and dormant microbes hypothesis, inflammation

---

[1]Presence of microbes in the wrong place, i.e., sterile environments such as blood.

INTRODUCTION

Alzheimer's type dementia (AD) is the most prevalent example of dementia, accounting for 75% of all cases (Qui et al., 2009), with an estimated global economic impact of $604 billion per year (Langa, 2015). In 2013 this neurodegenerative disorder was diagnosed in 44.4 million individuals worldwide. This number is expected to increase to 75.6 million by 2030 (Vradenburg, 2015; Pretorius et al., 2016a). The increasing aging population and anticipated increase in prevalence of AD has severe socio-economic implications (Prince et al., 2014). Familial AD can be promoted by mutations of the amyloid precursor protein (APP), presenilin (Bu et al., 2015) and apolipoprotein E (Ayton et al., 2015) genes, however, most AD patients suffer from the sporadic form, and even after decades of research, the etiology and pathogenesis of this disease remains largely unknown (Makin, 2018), and with essentially no existing disease-modifying treatments (Vogt et al., 2017). Despite the differences between familial and sporadic AD, the resultant neuropathology is shared by both (Pritchard et al., 2017).

Vascular dementia (VaD), also known as multi-infarct dementia, is caused by obstructions in the supply of blood to the brain, which over time results in stepwise neurodegeneration (Karantzoulis and Galvin, 2011). The pathology of VaD is characterized by atheromas of primarily cerebral arteries and arterioles. Vascular lesions characteristic of VaD often co-exist with AD, with 25–80% of individuals with dementia showing both AD symptoms and cerebrovascular lesions (Jellinger, 2008), a condition termed mixed dementia (MD). In early AD, critically located small vascular lesions in subcortical regions may promote cognitive decline. This suggests a synergistic relation between disorders (Jellinger and Attems, 2007). The distinction between isolated AD, VaD, and MD, where both pathologies coexist in the same individual, remains a controversial issue and one of the most difficult diagnostic challenges (Zekry et al., 2002; Jellinger and Attems, 2007). Additionally the population-based prevalence of MD in prospective and retrospective autopsy studies, ranges from 2 to 58%, emphasizing the coexistence of AD with multiple cerebrovascular lesions in patients with cognitive impairments. Moreover inflammation and alterations of inflammatory biomarkers are common to both AD and VaD (Schmidt et al., 2002). For these reasons, VaD and the pathogenesis thereof, fall under the AD umbrella of this review.

For the individual, AD shortens life expectancy significantly, with the cognitive deficit often causing institutionalization, physical disability and reduced quality of life (Qui et al., 2009; Pritchard et al., 2017). Hallmark features of AD pathology in the brain often include extracellular plaques composed of amyloid-β (Aβ), intracellular neurofibrillary tangles which are composed of hyperphosphorylated tau, basal forebrain cholinergic insufficiency and extensive neuronal and synaptic loss in the cortex and hippocampus (Law et al., 2001; Vogt et al., 2017). Aβ42 peptides either as monomers, dimers or intermediate amyloids stimulate arrays of inflammatory gene expression characteristic of the innate immune system (Zhao et al., 2015). These Aβ42 peptides are not only highly immunogenic, but they may self-aggregate into structures that interact with the plasma membrane and cause uncontrolled seepage of ions into and/or out of the neurons (Zhao and Lukiw, 2015), disrupting their normal physiological functioning.

Another hallmark of AD is activated neuroglial cells which produce significant amounts of inflammatory molecules. At low levels this may have a protective function but the increased expression in AD could induce neurodegeneration (Kamer et al., 2008). This said, cerebral inflammation caused by the activation of glial cells is generally asymptomatic as this occurs in the normal aging brain. According to Barrientos et al. (2016) prolonged production of pro-inflammatory cytokines as well as increased neuroinflammatory responses are common in the normal aging brain. The primary source of this exaggerated response is sensitized microglia. Other causes of this phenomenon may include neuroendocrine system dysregulation and potentiation of neuroinflammatory responses following an immune challenge, due to persistently elevated glucocorticoid levels in older individuals (Barrientos et al., 2016). Excessive age-related glial priming, present in AD, could also be due to microbial infiltration from disturbed microbiomes across a permeabilized blood brain barrier, providing slow inflammatory damage (Pritchard et al., 2017).

Recent research (Dorey et al., 2014; Filiou et al., 2014; Steardo et al., 2015) also suggests that neuro-inflammation may play a central role in the pathological progression of AD. Several neuro-inflammatory mediators including reactive oxygen species, chemokines, cytokines and activated complement are produced and secreted by microglia and astrocytes in the AD brain (Pretorius et al., 2016a). While neuro-inflammation is a part of the normal aging brain, and is a hallmark of acute injury (Lucas et al., 2006) and also of infection (McColl et al., 2009), in AD excessive systemic inflammation also occurs (Pretorius et al., 2016a), simultaneously exacerbating and perpetuating neuro-inflammation. Previous studies have verified that peripheral inflammatory markers such as interferon-γ, tumor necrosis factor-alpha (TNF-α), interleukin-1β (IL-1β), and IL-6 are related to the advancement of AD (Rubio-Perez and Morillas-Ruiz, 2012; Bu et al., 2015).

Some individuals who develop AD seem to possess genetic susceptibilities that are influenced by co-occurring environmental factors (Pritchard et al., 2017). In this review, we rehearse the Iron Dysregulation and Dormant Microbes (IDDM) hypothesis, and its ability to relate events which trigger and promote the pathogenesis of inflammatory conditions such as AD. The IDDM hypothesis emphasizes two main external triggers, namely (1) stress-induced iron dysregulation, and (2) its ability to reactivate dormant or non-replicating microbes which the host had acquired via previous infections or dysbiotic communities. We believe the primary origin of such microbes comes from a dysbiotic gut (Kell and Pretorius, 2015a). These microbes are capable of sloughing off functionally significant inflammagens such as lipopolysaccharide(s) (LPS) from Gram-negative bacteria and lipoteichoic acid (LTA) from Gram-positive bacteria. The consequences of this include significant coagulopathies, for example the amyloidogenic clotting of blood, which increases cell mortality (Kell and Pretorius, 2018). The contents of this manuscript are summarized in **Figure 1**.

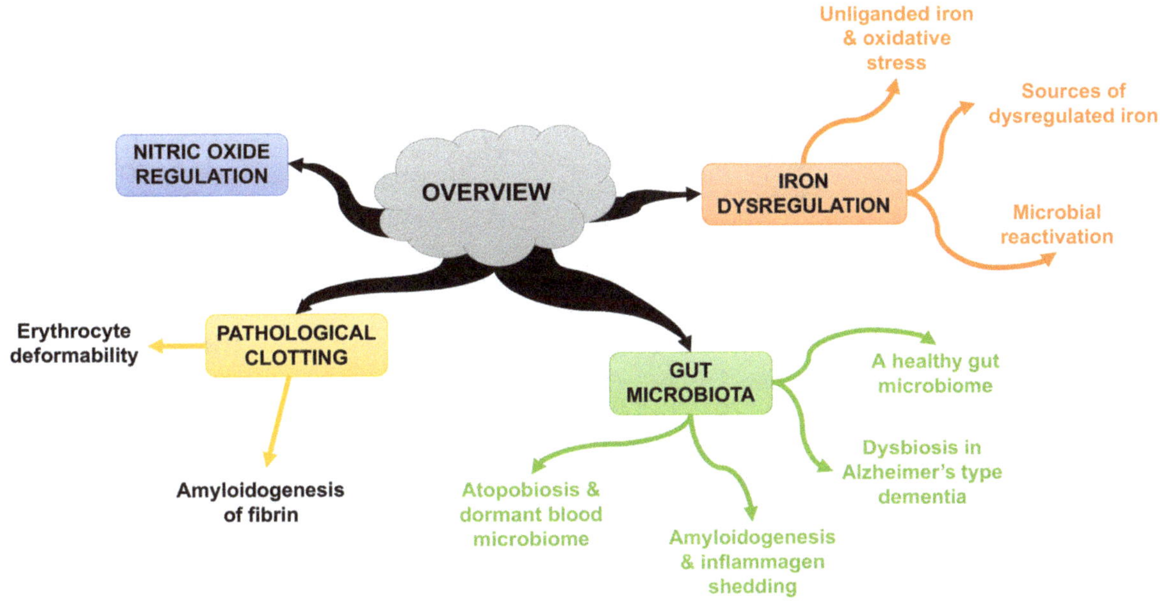

FIGURE 1 | An overview of the contents of this manuscript.

IRON DYSREGULATION

Iron dysregulation is any form of deviation from normal, homeostatic iron metabolism; in particular it includes cerebrospinal fluid ferritin and serum ferritin levels as implicated in Alzheimer's type dementias (Ayton et al., 2015). According to the Alzheimer's Disease Neuroimaging Initiative (ADNI) cohort study, increased ferritin levels, measured in cerebrospinal fluid, were negatively correlated to cognitive performance (Mueller et al., 2005), and these levels predicted conversion of mild cognitive impairment to Alzheimer's disease in 144 individuals over 7 years (Ayton et al., 2015). Furthermore, a strong association between ferritin levels and cerebrospinal fluid apolipoprotein E levels was observed in this study, with the major risk allele, APOE-ε4, inducing 22% higher levels of cerebrospinal fluid ferritin levels when compared to non-ε4 carriers (Ayton et al., 2015). In the same study a modest association between cerebrospinal fluid ferritin and plasma ferritin levels was noted ($p = 0.0002$). Thus, there may be great clinical relevance for the use of systemically elevated serum ferritin (SF) levels as cognitive performance markers (Kell and Pretorius, 2014; Pretorius et al., 2016a).

Causes of Iron Dysregulation

Major sources of iron dysregulation stem from externally induced stressors (Kell and Pretorius, 2018). This form of iron dysregulation can be initiated by several factors that contribute to or cause cell death, such as mechanical damage (Zhang et al., 2013), nutritional stress (Schaffer, 2016), pharmacological stress (Primohamed et al., 2004), and of course oxidative stress (Kerley et al., 2018). Another source of free iron is via heme metabolism, due to the functioning of heme oxygenase-1 (HO-1), which catalyzes the degradation of heme (Pretorius and Kell, 2014). Since upregulation of HO-1 activity occurs in systemic inflammatory disorders in which erythrocytes are lysed, it may also be an important marker of inflammation and iron dysregulation.

Additionally, hepcidin, produced by the liver, is a key regulator of iron metabolism (Michels et al., 2015; Reichert et al., 2017). Decreases in hepcidin levels enhance surface exposure of ferroportin (Ganz and Nemeth, 2012) on enterocytes, macrophages and hepatocytes to increase serum ferritin levels (illustrated by **Figure 2**). Hepcidin expression is induced by inflammatory markers such as LPS, IL-1β, and IL-6, while increases in $1,25(OH)_2D_3$ (calcitriol) levels cause hepcidin levels to decrease (Kell and Pretorius, 2018). According to a report by Bacchetta et al. (2014), decreases in hepcidin levels by $1,25(OH)_2D_3$ are due to suppression of the *HAMP* gene by the vitamin D receptor (VDR). Chromatin immunoprecipitation assays confirmed the binding of VDR to the vitamin D response element within the proximal promotor region of the *HAMP* gene (Bacchetta et al., 2014). While this process is intricate, it appears that alterations in vitamin D metabolism could potentially instigate iron dysregulation.

Intestinal inflammation caused by gut dysbiosis can impact iron homeostasis within the GI tract (Cherayil et al., 2011), however, whether these findings have been extrapolated to serum iron homeostasis has not yet been elucidated. While iron dysregulation within the GI tract and gut dysbiosis potentially exacerbate one another, Constante et al. (2017) concluded that luminal heme originating from gastrointestinal bleeding or dietary components more likely contributes to dysbiosis of the gut microbiota in mice than *vice versa*. However, dietary non-heme iron intake from food has been associated with a 30% increased risk of Parkinson's disease ($p = 0.02$) (Logroscino et al., 2008). In the same study authors also observed that supplemental

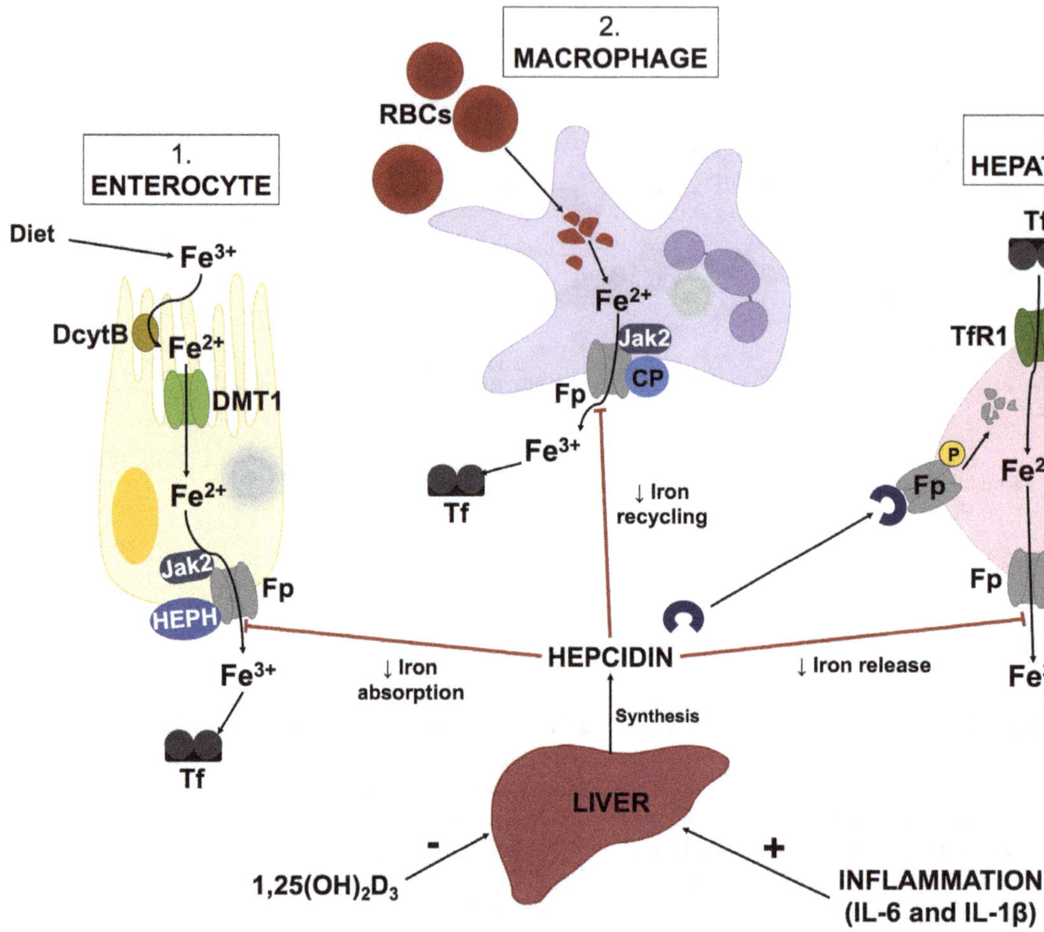

FIGURE 2 | Schematic illustration of the hepcidin-ferroportin axis and its regulation of systemic iron homeostasis. Hepcidin synthesis is regulated at transcriptional level by various stimuli such as inflammatory markers and vitamin D levels. Serum ferritin concentrations are regulated by hepcidin, which causes phosphorylation, internalization and subsequent lysosomal degradation of ferroportitin (Fp), thereby reducing its expression on iron exporting cells. Adapted from Cui et al. (2009) and Mariani et al. (2009) Abbreviations: Fe^{3+}, ferric iron; Fe^{2+}, ferrous cation; DcytB, duodenal cytochrome B; DMT1, divalent metal transporter 1; Jak2, Janus kinase 2; HEPH, hepaestin; Tf, transferritin; RBCs, red blood cells; CP, ceruloplasmin; TfR1, transferritin receptor 1; $1,25(OH)_2D_3$, calcitriol; IL-6, interleukin-6; IL-1β, interleukin-1beta.

iron intake was associated with a borderline increase in Parkinson's disease among men (Logroscino et al., 2008). Nonetheless, the most prominent cause of iron dysregulation in the form of elevated serum ferritin levels is cell death (Kell and Pretorius, 2018).

Unliganded Iron and Oxidative Damage

In AD, iron dysregulation and the benefits of its chelation have been known for decades (Crapper McLachlan et al., 1991), and many reviews point to the role of poorly liganded iron in AD development (Exley, 2006; Castellani et al., 2007, 2012; Kell, 2009, 2010; Sandro and Muckenthaler, 2009; Grunblatt et al., 2011; Weinreb et al., 2011; Peters et al., 2015; Wood, 2015; Belaidi and Bush, 2016). Unliganded iron and the accompanying oxidative damage is causatively related to neuro-inflammation (Bester et al., 2013; Hongkuan et al., 2015). According to Nunomura et al. (2001), neurons with neurofibrillary tangles show a 40–56% decrease in relative 8-hydroxyguanosine (8-OHG) levels when compared to neurons without neurofibrillary tangles in AD patients. 8-OHG is a marker of hydroxyl radical formation (Kell, 2009, 2010), so this finding indicates that oxidative damage is an early event in AD progression, which dissipates with lesion formation (Nunomura et al., 2001). This is further supported by (Moreira et al., 2005) who found one of the earliest pathological events in AD to be an imbalance between free radical scavenging and generation. The relationship between poorly liganded iron and oxidative stress involves iron's catalytic contribution to the Fenton and Haber-Weiss reactions. These reactions are involved in the formation of the highly reactive hydroxyl radical (OH^-), the most biologically detrimental free radical species, specifically with regards to macromolecules such as lipids, proteins and nucleic acids (Moreira et al., 2005; Kell, 2009, 2010; Lipinski and Pretorius, 2013; Pretorius et al., 2016a). Notably, iron chelation can reverse tau protein hyperphosphorylation in mice brains (Guo et al., 2013), thereby reducing the formation of intracellular neurofibrillary tangles.

Microbial Reactivation

Dormancy is extremely common in microbiology, even among non-sporulating bacteria (Kaprelyants et al., 1993; Lewis, 2007; Kell et al., 2015; Kell and Kenny, 2016), for sound evolutionary reasons (Mukamolova et al., 2003). Our major hypothesis involves shared symptoms across numerous chronic inflammatory diseases caused by dormant microbes (Pretorius et al., 2016a). As reviewed in 2016 (Pretorius et al., 2016a), microbial reactivation or resuscitation, which may be autocatalytic (Mukamolova et al., 1998), indicates that these so-called dormant microbes which are non-growing and appear operationally dead (Kell et al., 1998), can recover culturability. Metals, although explicitly involved in production of free radicals and potentially oxidative stress in AD, are also involved in the process of dormant microbe reactivation (Bester et al., 2015; Kell et al., 2015). All microbes (with the possible exception of *Borrelia*) require free available iron to grow. This follows from the *in vivo* limitation of microbial growth in the absence or decreased availability of free iron (Markel et al., 2007; Reid et al., 2009; Chu et al., 2010; Nairz et al., 2010, 2014; Skaar, 2010; Haley and Skaar, 2012; Armitage and Drakesmith, 2014; Subashchandrabose and Mobley, 2015; Damron et al., 2016; Carver, 2018). It is its absence in normal metabolism that causes dormant bacteria to remain in that state. With this in mind, iron dysregulation specifically in the form of high SF levels (Kell and Pretorius, 2014), accelerates AD pathology in two ways (Pretorius et al., 2016a) which suggests the opportunity of its use as a biomarker for early diagnosis and/or a target for slowing down disease progression (Bester et al., 2013).

GUT MICROBIOTA

The human gut microbiome contains approximately 10–100 trillion microbes, outnumbering human genes by 100-fold (Zhu et al., 2010). The gut microbiome forms the largest diffuse organ system in the body, and is more metabolically active than is the liver (Zhao et al., 2015). Through various systemic effects, the well-being and health of the human host is largely impacted by these microbes (Zhao and Lukiw, 2015). However, the human microbiome displays a high degree of variation at inter-individual levels (Costello et al., 2009). For example, even as infants the composition of the gut microbiota is idiosyncratic with significant inter-individual variation being evident from the 1st day after birth (Chong et al., 2018). As a consequence it is has been impossible to define a healthy microbiome (Dave et al., 2012), but, it has become apparent that certain compositions of microbial communities may be able to promote both health and disease (Blum, 2017).

Intriguingly the human gastrointestinal (GI) tract has co-evolved with two major phyla: (1) *Firmicutes* which constitutes 80% and, (2) *Bacteriodetes* which constitutes 20% of all GI tract bacteria (Pritchard et al., 2017; Zhao et al., 2017). There is increasing evidence implicating host–microbiome interactions at all stages of complexity including the central nervous system (Stilling et al., 2014). According to Stilling et al. (2014) gut-microbial products can distress chromatin plasticity, leading to changes in neuronal transcription and host conduct. This is due to the fact that the microbiota is an essential mediator of gene–environment interactions and may themselves be regarded as an epigenetic entity. Current research which supports this view includes reports which have characterized small non-coding RNA secreted from microbial cells in the GI tract (Ghosal et al., 2015; Zhao et al., 2017).

Alterations of the gut microbiota can promote pro-inflammatory cytokine release and increase intestinal permeability, which has also been associated with AD (Pistollato et al., 2016). In particular, changes of gut microbial diversity and density can result in systemic and neuro-inflammation as well as dysfunction of the cerebellum and hippocampus (Pistollato et al., 2016). Considering the multitudes of LPSs and amyloids in the GI tract, it is plausible that the microbiota is involved in the pathogenesis of neurological disorders hallmarked by amyloidogenic features (Tran and Greenwood-Van Meerveld, 2013; Shoemark and Allen, 2015; Zhao and Lukiw, 2015) such as AD.

Dysbiosis

Dysbiosis refers to alteration in the composition of the microbiota and has been implicated in the etiology of various disease states (de Oliveira et al., 2017; Kho and Lal, 2018). Perturbations of the gut microbiota can occur as consequences of antibiotic treatment (especially during infancy), dietary changes, sedentary behavior, food additives, non-steroidal anti-inflammatory and other drugs (Wallace, 2013; Ticinesi et al., 2017; Maier et al., 2018) and various other conditions (Pistollato et al., 2016). Dietary changes, for example, may explain up to 57% of the total structural variation the gut microbiome (Brown et al., 2012). Using a humanized mouse model in which adult human fecal microbiota were transplanted into germ-free mice, Brown et al. (2012) reported a shift in the composition of microbiota after switching the mice from a low-fat, plant polysaccharide-rich diet to a Western diet. While diets rich in refined sugars result in different changes to the microbiota from diets lacking fiber, due to the intricate balance that exists between microbial species, alterations in one species can disrupt the entire microbial community (Brown et al., 2012). Thus, alterations in diet, although modifiable, could potentially be a major hurdle in treatment dysbiosis-related conditions if not adequately addressed. Furthermore, physical activity and its relative intensity can induce or prevent gut dysbiosis by influencing splanchnic blood flow, intestinal permeability and inflammatory cytokine expression (Monda et al., 2017). For example, in mice, even in combination with a high-fat diet, exercise may reduce inflammatory infiltrate into epithelial cells, protecting the integrity of the GI wall (Campbell et al., 2016).

Broad-scale fluctuations in the gut microbiota play significant roles in disease advancement through immune and systemic activation (Vogt et al., 2017). There is considerable evidence for the existence of the gut-brain axis which allows bi-directional communication through various pathways such as neural, endocrine and immune mechanisms (Gareau, 2014; Lyte, 2014; Bienenstock et al., 2015; Köhler et al., 2016; Fung et al., 2017; Sandhu et al., 2017). Within this context, changes in microbial communities could lead to pathophysiological changes in the brain of individuals with AD. Dysbiosis is often associated with increased anxiety and memory impairment due to decreased secretion of neurotrophic factors such as brain-derived neurotrophic factor (Stilling et al., 2014).

Dysbiosis in Alzheimer's Type Dementia

The recognition of dysbiosis and its possible link to neurodegenerative diseases are increasing as our understanding about the gut-brain axis improves (Miklossy and McGeer, 2016). A recent study in which transgenic AD mice were raised under germ-free conditions, indicated that these mice, compared to conventionally-raised AD mice, had less cerebral amyloid deposition (Harach et al., 2017). This indicates that a dysbiotic gut may influence progression of amyloid pathologies.

The gut microbiome diversity of AD patients is notably decreased and compositionally distinct from age- and gender-matched controls (Vogt et al., 2017). In this study Vogt et al. (2017), the authors reported decreases in Firmicutes and *Bifidobacterium* spp. and increased Bacteriodetes in AD patients. *Bifidobacterium* spp. are important in gut health and their beneficial effects are well-documented (Arboleya et al., 2016). For instance, particular *Bifidobacterium* species, such as *B. bifidum, B. cantenulatum, B. breve,* and *B. adolescentis,* have anti-inflammatory properties such as inhibiting LPS-induced IL-8 production and TNFα expression (Khokhlova et al., 2012) Bifidobacteria are also known to reduce intestinal permeability (Underwood et al., 2015). Moreover, *Bifidobacterium* supplementation has shown to decrease intestinal LPS levels and mend the GI-mucosal barrier in mice (Griffiths et al., 2004; Wang et al., 2006). The phylum Bacteriodetes encompasses an abundant and diverse group of Gram-negative bacteria, which have been detected as being increased in patients with Parkinson's disease (Keshavarzian et al., 2015). The shedding of LPS and subsequent induction of inflammation is also associated with the increase in numbers of fraction of these bacteria. Considering these findings, individuals with AD may present with a gut microbial phenotype that has an increased propensity for the translocation of inflammatory bacterial components (Vogt et al., 2017).

Amyloidogenesis

Amyloid by definition is protein that is deposited as an insoluble fibril as a result of successive alterations in the protein folding process, known as amyloidosis. Similarly to prions, there is no change in the primary amino acid sequence of the proteins when they adopt an insoluble amyloid form (Kell and Pretorius, 2018). Interestingly, self-associating amyloidogenic lipoproteins are secreted by most microbial species (Schwartz et al., 2016), and amyloid is one of the main secretory products of the gut microbiome (Zhao et al., 2017). The role of the gut in dissemination of amyloid proteins has been reviewed by Pistollato et al. (2016), in which the authors adopted the unifying prion concept to explain transmission of these prion-like proteins. The cumulative life-long contribution of microbial amyloid to neurodegenerative pathophysiology is little recognized. Progressive production and aggregation of amyloids contributes to the pathogenesis of diseases in which amyloids accumulate, which is often mediated by microglial cells (Zhao et al., 2017). Thus, bacterial amyloids originating from the gut microbiome may enhance inflammatory responses to cerebral accumulation of Aβ and play a role in the pathogenesis of AD (Pistollato et al., 2016).

For example, functional amyloid from *Klebsiella pneumoniae* can depolymerise from its fibrillary state to release oligomers which induce cytotoxicity equal to that caused by pathological Aβ in AD (Shahnawaz and Soto, 2012). The molecular mimicry theory (Ebringer and Rashid, 2009; Proal et al., 2013, 2017) includes microbial curli fibers[2] and Aβ as a protein–protein interaction which could result in cross-seeding, even if these proteins are essentially unalike (Friedland, 2015; Zhao et al., 2015). These extrinsic curli proteins act as pathogen-associated molecular patterns with increased β-pleated sheet structures, and can cross-react with antibodies to Aβ plaques (Miklossy, 2016). It is plausible that extracellular senile plaques, due to their morphological appearance and density, may in fact be constituted of curli-like Aβ compositions. In theory, this gives bacterial phylotypes a more blatant role in AD causality (Pritchard et al., 2017). The influence of gut microbiota on amyloid formation and propagation is more significant throughout aging as both the epithelium of the GI tract and the blood-brain barrier (BBB) increase in permeability to smaller molecules (Tran and Greenwood-Van Meerveld, 2013; Pistollato et al., 2016).

Shedding of Inflammagens

Some of the foremost bacterial species of the GI tract, such as the Gram-negative bacilli *Bacteroides fragilis* and *Escherichia coli,* secrete a multifarious selection of pro-inflammatory neurotoxins which are not only pathogenic but also detrimental to the homeostatic functioning of neurons (Zhao et al., 2017). The shedding of inflammagens such as LPS from gut-microbiota-related dysbiosis causes systemic and neuro-inflammation and promotes gut permeability. Shedding can occur in response to varying physiological and environmental signals with the most extreme example of microbial shedding known as the Jarisch-Herxheimer reaction. This is basically an uninhibited cytokine storm, which is caused by prompt release of inflammagenic material, often following antibiotic treatment of syphilis (Kell and Pretorius, 2018), or other diseases caused by spirochetes. As mentioned earlier, this may promote neuronal dysfunction and apoptosis, impairment of synaptic plasticity and induced vulnerability to cognitive decline (Daulatzai, 2014). Bacterial LPS has also been found in AD hippocampal brain lysates where the mean LPS levels were three-fold higher in the hippocampus of AD patients than in age-matched controls. This was said to increase to 26-fold in advanced AD hippocampal cases (Zhao et al., 2017).

[2] Extracellular bacterial amyloids.

LPSs are sparingly soluble but over a period of time characteristically form large heterogenous aggregates which are exceptionally immunogenic (Zhao et al., 2015). Interestingly the glycosylphosphatidyl-inositol-anchored LPS and microbe-detecting CD41 receptor, which is crucial in the neutralization of invading microbes, is similarly, stimulated by Aβ fibrils (Dowhan, 2014), relating innate-immune signaling with amyloidogenesis in AD. It has also been noted that previous bacterial infections which resulted in the formation of antibodies to amyloids or bacterial inflammagens may predispose central nervous system amyloids to ensuing attack by antibodies, which results in upregulation of neuro-inflammation (Via et al., 2015; Zhao et al., 2015). The inflammagenic potency of LPS is so pronounced that it is frequently used to stimulate *in vivo* AD models (Lee et al., 2008; Catorce and Gevorkian, 2016; Zakaria et al., 2017).

LTA is the cell wall equivalent of LPS in Gram-positive bacteria and is equally capable of inducing an inflammatory response through its interactions with toll-like receptor (TLR) 2 (Kell and Pretorius, 2018). LTA has not been as well studied as LPS with regards to inflammagenesis, however, recent work suggests that LTAs may in fact be more potent than LPSs (Pretorius et al., 2018). The stimulation of inflammatory cytokine production by both LPS and LTA are mediated through TLR binding (reviewed by Kell and Pretorius, 2018). In response to inflammagens, concentrations of acute phase biomarkers and inflammatory cytokines such as TNF-α, IL-1β, IL-6, IL-8, C-reactive protein (CRP), serum amyloid A (SAA), and fibrinogen increase significantly (deRosset and Strutz, 2015; De Buck et al., 2016; Pindjakova et al., 2017).

Additionally, increased BBB permeability typically observed in individuals with AD can be caused by shed bacterial inflammagens. The BBB plays a fundamental role in the initiation and continuance of chronic inflammation during AD (Zenaro et al., 2017). While Aβ accumulation in vasculature results in inflammatory events that increase BBB permeability in AD (Erickson and Banks, 2013), proteolytic enzymes such as carbonic anhydrases, peptidyl deiminases and gingipains, and appendages such as curli fibers, fimbriae and other amyloid-like proteins, which are carried with LPS (Pritchard et al., 2017) and contribute significantly to BBB permeabilization. BBB dysfunction during AD effects Aβ clearance, endothelial cell function, tight junction integrity and may activate glial cells which accelerates migration of leukocytes to the brain (Zenaro et al., 2017). This could stimulate the beginning of chronic neuro-inflammation in AD.

Atopobiosis

Atopobiosis refers to the appearance of some of the gut microbes in the wrong place (Potgieter et al., 2015). The sterility of blood is seemingly a controversial topic. The presence of a "physiological" blood microbiota has been reported by several studies using 16S ribosomal DNA quantitative polymerase chain reactions (Amar et al., 2013; Lelouvier et al., 2016; Martel et al., 2017; Proal and Marshall, 2018). Yet, in these studies the plausible source of these microbes from gut permeability was not investigated. Authors of the same studies have reported that changes in the composition of this blood microbiota can be associated with disease. However, based on immunological and clinical understanding (Ochei and Kolhatkar, 2000) the detection of bacteria in blood is always abnormal (Kinnby and Chavez de Paz, 2016; Andreadou et al., 2017) and thus referred to as atopobiosis (Potgieter et al., 2015). As seen in **Figure 3**, atopobiosis is caused by bacterial translocation in which bacteria move from the GI tract to normally sterile blood and tissues (Potgieter et al., 2015). Once translocation has taken place, these bacteria can cause direct infection and inflammation. The process of bacterial translocation has been reviewed by Potgieter et al. (2015) but can briefly be described by the simultaneous dysfunction of three role players: (1) dendritic cells (2) GI epithelium and, (3) M cells which overlay Peyer's patches. It is a combination of various compromised mucosal defenses that leads to bacterial translocation. When the influx of gut microbes and toxins is particularly abundant, it is often referred to as a "leaky gut" (Maes, 2009; Fasano, 2012; Quigley, 2016; Mu et al., 2017; Kell and Pretorius, 2018) and is due to severely compromised epithelial tight junctions (Fasano, 2012).

Dormant Blood Microbiome

Bacteria that have successfully translocated to the blood have the ability to become dormant and reactivate upon appropriate stimuli, such as iron dysregulation in the form of high SF levels as discussed in section Causes of Iron Dysregulation. In contrast to conventional infections, these bacteria do not multiply but enter dormant states (Kell and Kenny, 2016; Pretorius et al., 2016a; Kell and Pretorius, 2018). This is especially relevant in clinical settings when toxic concentrations of antibiotics promote bacterial persistence or adoption of a dormant state that permits their survival (Kell and Pretorius, 2018). Even though the major source of this dormant blood microbiome has been reviewed here as a dysbiotic and permeabilized GI tract, we also recognize periodontitis, gingivitis, urinary tract infections and even insemination as possible points of microbial infection and subsequent translocation (Kamer et al., 2008; Flores-Mireles et al., 2015; Kenny and Kell, 2017; Pretorius et al., 2017; Pritchard et al., 2017). Current research has drifted toward the correlation between an individual's infectious burden and risk of developing AD, with particular emphasis on herpes simplex virus 1 (HSV1) and human herpesvirus 6 and 7 infections (Honjo et al., 2009; Itzhaki, 2014, 2017; Bu et al., 2015; Itzhaki et al., 2016; Itzhaki and Tabet, 2017; Eimer et al., 2018; Itzhaki and Lathe, 2018; Readhead et al., 2018; Tzeng et al., 2018). Dormant bacteria can survive in leukocytes (Thwaites and Gant, 2011; Liehl et al., 2015) and erythrocytes (Potgieter et al., 2015) to establish the dormant blood microbiome. In Potgieter et al. (2015) transmission electron micrographs of cellular inclusions thought to be L-forms of bacteria inside erythrocytes of individuals diagnosed with AD can be seen (see also Mattman, 2001). **Figure 4** illustrates the association of bacteria with pathological coagulations within the blood of individuals diagnosed with AD. This dormant blood microbiome affects the integrity of the hematological system, promoting pathological coagulation.

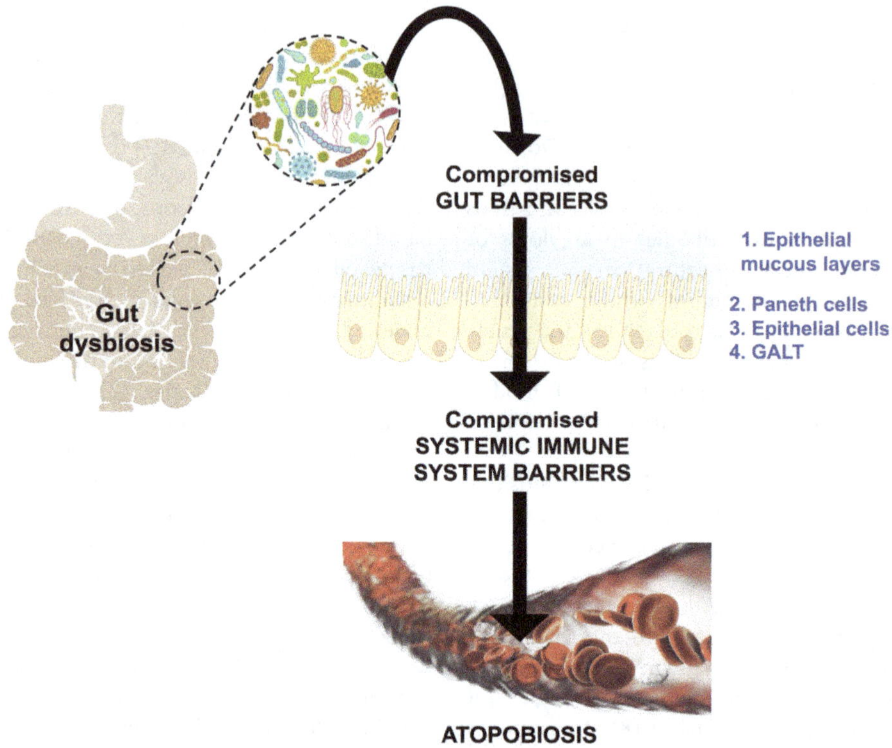

FIGURE 3 | A schematic representation of bacterial translocation from a dysbiotic gastrointestinal tract to normally sterile tissues, such as blood. This occurs due to compromised gut barriers such as the epithelial mucous layer, Paneth cells (which secreted antimicrobial peptides) and epithelial cells and gut associated lymphoid tissue (GALT) as mechanical barriers. Simultaneously, there will be compromised systemic immune system function, which enables microbes to enter into normally sterile tissues via dendritic cells, injured epithelial, M-cells and Peyer's patches. This phenomenon is known as atopobiosis and is implicated in both communicable and non-communicable diseases. Figure adapted from Potgieter et al. (2015).

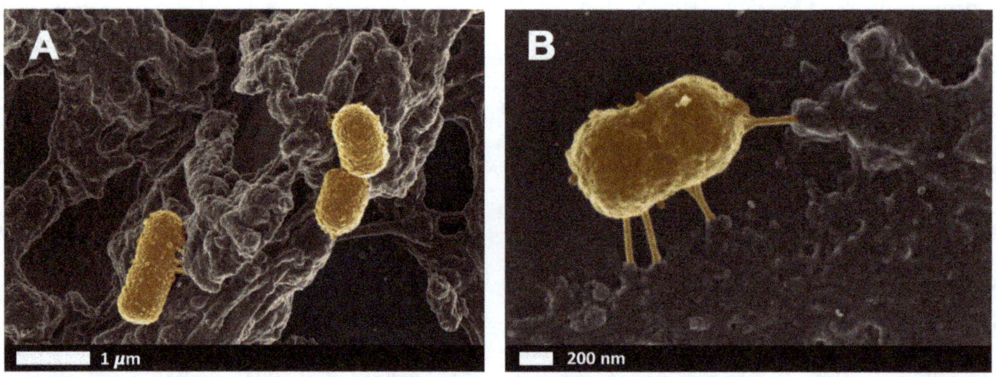

FIGURE 4 | Scanning electron micrographs of bacteria associated with pathological coagulations found within the blood of individuals diagnosed with Alzheimer's disease. Unpublished data from Potgieter et al. (2015). **(A)** low magnification, **(B)** higher magnification.

PATHOLOGICAL COAGULATION

LPS is well known to cause inflammatory cytokine production which can cause hypercoagulation, often referred to as endotoxin-mediated hypercoagulation (Slotta et al., 2008; Kell and Pretorius, 2017). LPS may activate the coagulation pathway via upregulation of tissue factor (TF), which leads to activation of pro-thrombin (Landsem et al., 2015). Two main components of the hematological system namely fibrinogen and erythrocytes and the changes induced during inflammation and AD, will be discussed below.

Fibrinogen

Fibrinogen is the precursor of fibrin and thus plays a major role in thrombosis and hemostasis (Pretorius and Kell, 2014). During inflammation, circulating fibrinogen levels are increased, while fibrinolysis is impaired. Amyloidogenesis of the fibrin fibers occurs, resulting in the formation of dense matted deposits which trap other blood cells and distort their shape. The combination of the increased propensity to form a stiffer fibrin network and reduced fibrinolysis is a feature of numerous inflammatory diseases such as AD (Ahn et al., 2010; Zamolodchikov and Strickland, 2012). **Figure 5** illustrates some of the morphological changes of fibrin fibers due to the addition of LPS.

The presence of excessive (unliganded) iron and the consequential production of hydroxyl radicals is one of the leading causes of altered fibrin cross-linking (Pretorius and Kell, 2014; Kell and Pretorius, 2015b). Dense matted deposits produced in the presence of ferric ions are abnormally resistant to chemical and proteolytic degradation, hypothesized to be due to the existence of intermolecular hydrophobic bonds (Lipinski and Pretorius, 2012). As reviewed, it seems that iron dysregulation may serve as a causative factor for multiple pathologies involved in AD progression. This altered fibrinogen structure, with excessive cross-linking and increased β-pleated sheet structure, has been implicated in the development of neuro-inflammation and memory impairments. Increased fibrinogen levels are a strong indicator of cerebrovascular risk since fibrinogen binds to Aβ which further delays clot degradation (Bester et al., 2013; Pretorius et al., 2016a). In addition, pharmacological inhibition of the fibrinogen–Aβ interaction with Ru-505 altered thrombus structure and paused cognitive decline in mice (Ahn et al., 2014), providing a strong association between pathological clotting and neurodegenerative diseases.

Erythrocytes

The dynamics of erythrocytes represent an important but understudied feature of the cardiovascular system. Central to this is their rheology, viscosity, aggregation and deformability (Baskurt et al., 2011; Pretorius and Kell, 2014). It is thought that alterations in erythrocytes and their rheology can contribute to the pathogenesis of AD by hindering oxygen delivery (Tripathy et al., 2013). Dense matted deposits may also trap erythrocytes, impairing their effective delivery of oxygen to the brain. Proficient oxygen delivery is vital for normal functioning of the brain, underpinned by that fact that 20% of an individual's total oxygen intake is used by the brain. Neurons are particularly susceptible to hypoxic periods, which can cause irreversible neurological consequences (Lipinski and Pretorius, 2013) after only a few minutes. Altered functioning of erythrocytes is also strongly suggested by changes in their size distribution (Ozturk et al., 2013; Weuve et al., 2014; Pilling et al., 2017; Winchester et al., 2018).

As reviewed by Pretorius and Kell (2014), erythrocyte deformability is a complex process which is significantly altered by pathophysiological conditions. Briefly, reduced erythrocyte deformability is an important feature of inflammation in which reactive oxygen species cause degradation of spectrin and band 3, for example, which are important membrane proteins. Since the plasma membrane and the cytoskeleton are responsible for

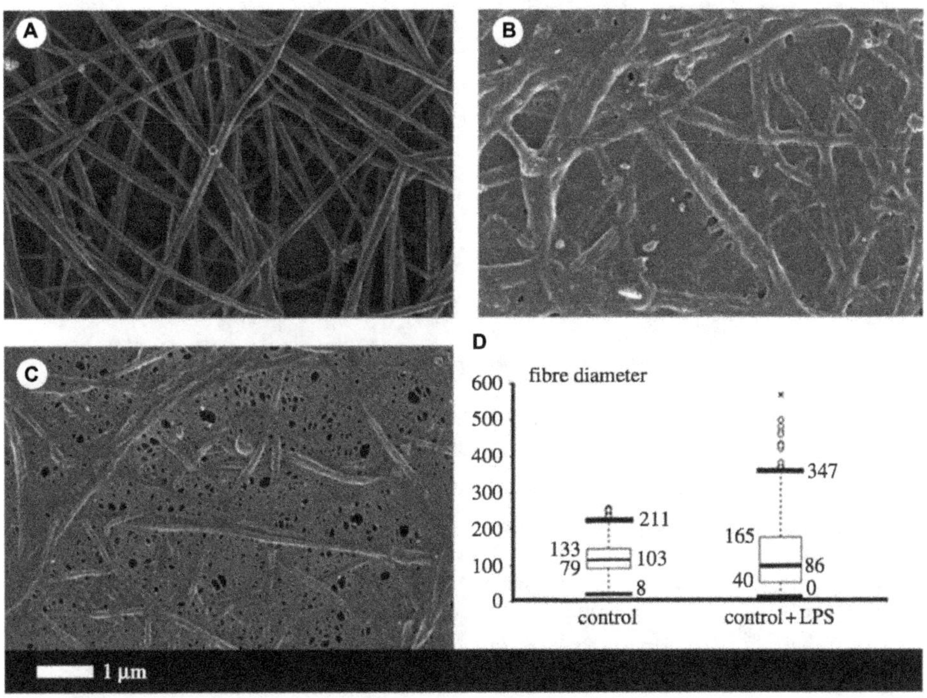

FIGURE 5 | Micrographs from scanning electron microscopy **(A–C)** as well as a box and whisker plot indicating fiber distribution **(D)** taken from Pretorius et al. (2016b) (open access publication). **(A)** Is indicative of healthy fibrin fibers during coagulation (with the addition of thrombin), while **(B,C)** demonstrate the large effect of 0.2 ng/l^{-1} 0111:B4 LPS on fibrin morphology. LPS, lipopolysaccharide. ∗, outlier measurement.

the preservation of erythrocyte shape and stability, modifications of the phospholipid bilayer can affect deformability. In 2010, Mohanty et al. (2010) reported that 15% of erythrocytes in AD were elongated and suggested that a potential link between changes in the erythrocyte proteome could contribute to AD pathology. Deformability and impaired reformability, particularly after erythrocytes have moved through capillaries, reduces their oxygen carrying capacity, potentiating transient states of hypoxia. **Figure 6** illustrates erythrocyte deformability as well as loss of membrane integrity in typical blood samples from individual's diagnosed with AD. It is clear to see how the loss of the typical bi-concave structure of these erythrocytes would impair their physiological functioning.

NITRIC OXIDE REGULATION

The dysregulation of nitric oxide (NO) synthesis is prevalent in many diseased conditions (Cooke and Dzau, 1997; Kolios et al., 2004; Naseem, 2005; Karpuzoglu and Ahmed, 2006; Pacher et al., 2007). Recently, the physiological role of erythrocytes in regulating nitric oxide levels has also been investigated (Saldanha, 2016). Due to the consequences of chronic systemic inflammation and pathological coagulation, such as erythrocyte deformability and lysis, it is plausible that aberrant NO regulation could occur and causatively contribute to AD pathogenesis.

NO is synthesized by three isoforms of nitric oxide synthases. Although NO has vasoactive, immunological and neurophysiological functions, it can be neurotoxic at high concentrations and has been implicated in neurodegenerative diseases (Law et al., 2001). In this regard, erythrocytes have an important role in vascular function. Normally, erythrocytes regulate hemostasis by balancing oxygen delivery and NO scavenging and production. More specifically, hemoglobin (Hb) compartmentalization and encapsulation reduces an erythrocyte's ability to scavenge NO. However, in various diseases hemolysis introduces cell-free Hb into circulation, increasing NO scavenging and inducing hypertension (Helms et al., 2018). A decrease in NO may lead to a reduced ability to learn and

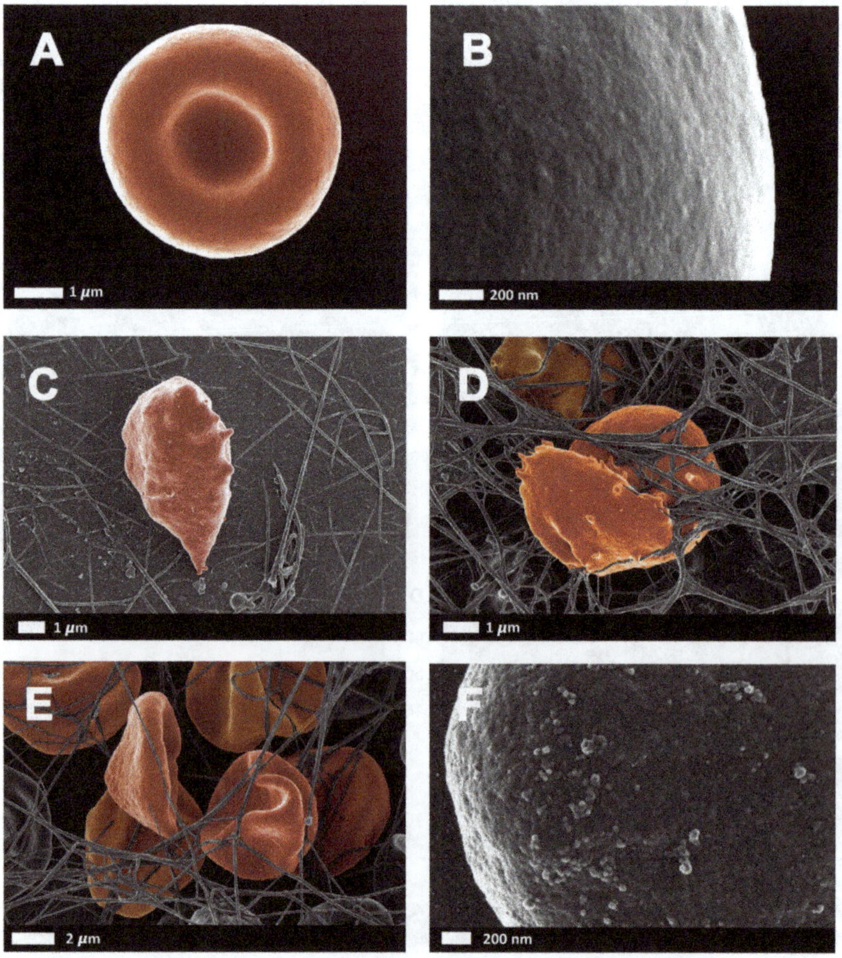

FIGURE 6 | Erythrocytes from healthy individuals **(A–B)** and individuals diagnosed with Alzheimer's type dementia **(C–F)**. **(C)** Serum ferritin: 57 ng.L^{-1} **(D)** Serum ferritin: 256 ng.L^{-1} **(E)** Serum ferritin: 302 ng.L^{-1} **(F)** Serum ferritin: 302 ng.L^{-1} (100,000× machine magnification of erythrocyte membrane). Unpublished data from Bester et al. (2013).

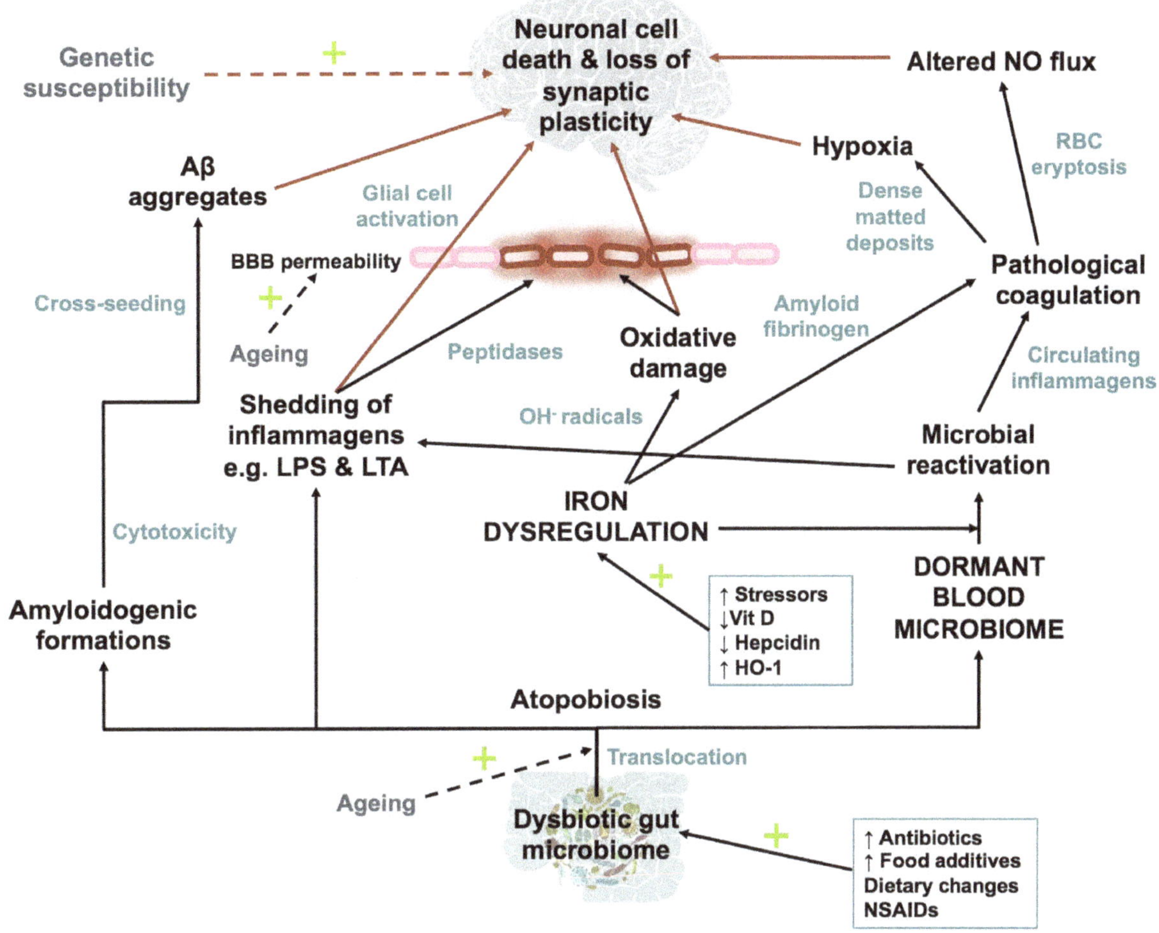

FIGURE 7 | Schematic representation of The Iron Dysregulation and Dormant Microbes hypothesis. With reference to the scheme it is plausible that systemic inflammation caused by stress induced iron dysregulation and subsequent microbial reactivation can lead to increased permeability of the blood brain barrier as well as a neuro-inflammatory environment which promotes neuronal cell death. The red arrows indicate factors which could contribute to synaptic loss and neuronal death. Dashed arrows have not been discussed in detail in this review but are recognized as contributors to the pathogenesis of Alzheimer's-type dementias. Adapted from Kell and Pretorius (2018). Abbreviations: Aβ, amyloid beta; NO, nitric oxide; BBB, blood brain barrier; RBC, red blood cell; OH^-, hydroxyl; LPS, lipopolysaccharide; LTA, lipoteichoic acid; HO-1, heme oxygenase-1 and NSAIDs, non-steroidal anti-inflammatory drugs.

memorize due to impairment of long-term potentiation, since NO is responsible for the synaptic efficiency of pre-synaptic glutamatergic neurons (Panthi et al., 2018). Hypoperfusion of the brain and increased oxidative stress within the vasculature are common phenomena in AD (Edwards and Rickard, 2007) and some researchers have reported abnormalities in NO synthase expression as early symptoms of cognitive impairment and AD (Lüth et al., 2002; Malinski, 2007).

Furthermore, NO can exert its neurotoxic effects through three main mechanisms. Firstly, NO is a free radical which can react with superoxide anions to produce another damaging radical, peroxynitrite (Eliasson et al., 1999). This can produce significant oxidative stress which leads to oxidative damage and eventually neuronal death. Secondly, NO causes nitrosylation in a variety of proteins such as glyceraldehyde-3 phosphate dehydrogenase (GADPH) and protein kinase C (PKC), inhibiting their functioning. Lastly, NO can impair glycolysis and the latter energy manufacturing by potentiating ADP-ribosylation of GADPH (Law et al., 2001) as well as binding aconitase and thereby inhibiting electron transfer in the electron transport chain.

Together, pathological coagulation and altered nitric oxide regulation can enhance the propensity of spontaneous clot formation in cerebral arteries and arterioles. These clots are more resistant to degradation, due to amylodiogenesis of fibrin fibers in the presence of ferric irons, and may thus potentiate transient periods of hypoxia in the brain, promoting the occurrence of MD.

CONCLUSION

While numerous hypotheses for the pathogenesis of AD exist (extensively reviewed by Law et al., 2001; Hardy and Selkoe, 2002; Swerdlow, 2007; Armstrong, 2011;

Dong et al., 2012; Barage and Sonawane, 2015; Selkoe and Hardy, 2016; Area-Gomez and Schon, 2017; Makin, 2018), the IDDM hypothesis (illustrated in **Figure 7**) recognizes that a combination of a dormant blood or tissue microbiome can be re-activated by unliganded iron. This in turn can induce shedding of highly inflammagenic LPS and LTA molecules, from which all known sequlae of AD can be seen to follow.

As reviewed here, dysbiotic bacterial communities from the GI tract or microbes from other sources of infection, translocate into normally sterile tissues and blood to establish a dormant blood microbiome. Characteristic of AD (and many other chronic, inflammatory diseases; Kell, 2009) is iron dysregulation, that amongst many other affects, causes microbial reactivation. Iron dysregulation, specifically in the form of elevated SF levels, which can causatively modulate oxidative damage, the formation of amyloidogenic fibrinogen and the aforementioned microbial reactivation as part of AD pathogenesis. Microbes contribute to amyloidogenic formations, inflammagen shedding, pathological clotting and systemic as well as neuro-inflammation. Various changes to the hematological system ensue, increasing the risk of pathological coagulation and transient hypoxic events in the AD brain. Increasing BBB permeability and glial cell activation initiate the slow inflammatory progression of AD, in combination with loss of synaptic plasticity and neuronal death. While AD is a disease too complex to fit to any particular model, the IDDM hypothesis highlights several causative role players which can be targeted for early diagnosis and/or for prevention of disease progression.

AUTHOR CONTRIBUTIONS

LP wrote the paper. DK co-wrote the paper and edited the paper. EP co-wrote the paper and is the study leader.

FUNDING

Funders include the Biotechnology and Biological Sciences Research Council (Grant No. BB/L025752/1) as well as the National Research Foundation (NRF) of South Africa (91548: Competitive Program) and the Medical Research Council of South Africa (MRC) (Self-Initiated Research Program) for supporting this collaboration.

ACKNOWLEDGMENTS

This is paper 18 in the series "A dormant blood microbiome in chronic, inflammatory disease". We thank the Biotechnology and Biological Sciences Research Council, the National Research Foundation (NRF) of South Africa and the Medical Research Council (MRC) of South Africa, for financially supporting this collaboration.

REFERENCES

Ahn, H. J., Glickman, J. F., Poon, K. L., Zamolodchikov, D., Jno-Charles, O. C., Norris, E. H., et al. (2014). A novel Abeta-fibrinogen interaction inhibitor rescues altered thrombosis and cognitive decline in Alzheimer's disease mice. *J. Exp. Med.* 211, 1049–1062. doi: 10.1084/jem.20131751

Ahn, H. J., Zamolodchikov, D., Cortes-Canteli, M., Norris, E. H., Glickman, J. F., and Strickland, S. (2010). Alzheimer's disease peptide beta-amyloid interacts with fibrinogen and induces its oligomerization. *Proc. Natl. Acad. Sci. U.S.A.* 107, 21812–21817. doi: 10.1073/pnas.1010373107

Amar, J., Lange, C., Payros, G., Garret, C., Chabo, C., Lantieri, O., et al. (2013). Blood microbiota dysbiosis is associated with the onset of cardiovascular events in a large general population: the D.E.S.I.R. study. *PLoS One* 8:e54461. doi: 10.1371/journal.pone.0054461

Andreadou, E., Pantazaki, A. A., Daniilidou, M., and Magba, T. (2017). Rhamnolipids, microbial virulence factors, in Alzheimer's disease. *J. Alzheimers Dis.* 59, 209–222. doi: 10.3233/JAD-161020

Arboleya, S., Watkins, C., Stanton, C., and Ross, R. P. (2016). Gut bifidobacteria populations in human health and aging. *Front. Microbiol.* 7:1204. doi: 10.3389/fmicb.2016.01204

Area-Gomez, E., and Schon, E. A. (2017). On the pathogenesis of Alzheimer's disease: the MAM hypothesis. *FASEB J.* 31, 864–867. doi: 10.1096/fj.201601309

Armitage, A. E., and Drakesmith, H. (2014). The battle for iron. *Science* 346, 1299–1300. doi: 10.1126/science.aaa2468

Armstrong, R. A. (2011). The pathogenesis of Alzheimer's disease: a reevaluation of the "amyloid cascade hypothesis". *Int. J. Alzheimers Dis.* 2011:630865. doi: 10.4061/2011/630865

Ayton, S., Faux, N. G., Bush, A. I., Alzheimer's Disease, and Neuroimaging Initiative. (2015). Ferritin levels in the cerebrospinal fluid predict Alzheimer's disease outcomes and are regulated by APOE. *Nat. Commun.* 6:6760. doi: 10.1038/ncomms7760

Bacchetta, J., Zaritsky, J. J., Sea, J. L., Chun, R. F., Lisse, T. S., Zavala, K., et al. (2014). Suppression of iron-regulatory hepcidin by vitamin D. *J. Am. Soc. Nephrol.* 25, 564–572. doi: 10.1681/ASN.2013040355

Barage, S. H., and Sonawane, K. D. (2015). Amyloid cascade hypothesis: pathogenesis and therapeutic strategies in Alzheimer's disease. *Neuropeptides* 52, 1–18. doi: 10.1016/j.npep.2015.06.008

Barrientos, R. M., Kitt, M. M., Watkins, L. R., and Maier, S. F. (2016). Neuroinflammation in the normal aging hippocampus. *Neuroscience* 309, 84–99. doi: 10.1016/j.neuroscience.2015.03.007

Baskurt, O., Neu, B., and Meiselman, H. J. (2011). *Red Blood Cell Aggregation*, 1st Edn. Boca Raton, FL: CRC Press. doi: 10.1201/b11221

Belaidi, A. A., and Bush, A. I. (2016). Iron neurochemistry in Alzheimer's disease and Parkinson's disease: targets for therapeutics. *J. Neurochem.* 139(Suppl. 1), 179–197. doi: 10.1111/jnc.13425

Bester, J., Buys, A. V., Lipinski, B., Kell, D. B., and Pretorius, E. (2013). High ferritin levels have major effects on the morphology of erythrocytes in Alzheimer's disease. *Front. Aging Neurosci.* 5:88. doi: 10.3389/fnagi.2013.00088

Bester, J., Soma, P., Kell, D. B., and Pretorius, E. (2015). Viscoelastic and ultrastructural characteristics of whole blood and plasma in Alzheimer-type dementia, and the possible role of bacterial lipopolysaccharides (LPS). *Oncotarget* 6, 35285–35303. doi: 10.18632/oncotarget.6074

Bienenstock, J., Kunze, W., and Forsythe, P. (2015). Microbiota and the gut-brain axis. *Nutr. Rev.* 73(Suppl. 1), 28–31. doi: 10.1093/nutrit/nuv019

Blum, H. E. (2017). The human microbiome. *Adv. Med. Sci.* 62, 414–420. doi: 10.1016/j.advms.2017.04.005

Brown, K., DeCoffe, D., Molcan, E., and Gibson, D. L. (2012). Diet-induced dysbiosis of the intestinal microbiota and the effects on immunity and disease. *Nutrients* 4, 1095–1119. doi: 10.3390/nu4081095

Bu, X. L., Yao, X. Q., Jiao, S. S., Zeng, F., Liu, Y. H., Xiang, Y., et al. (2015). A study on the association between infectious burden and Alzheimer's disease. *Eur. J. Neurol.* 22, 1519–1525. doi: 10.1111/ene.12477

Campbell, S. C., Wisniewski, P. J., Noji, M., McGuinness, L. R., Haggblom, M. M., Lightfoot, S. A., et al. (2016). The effect of diet and exercise on intestinal integrity and microbial diversity in mice. *PLoS One* 11:e0150502. doi: 10.1371/journal.pone.0150502

Carver, P. L. (2018). The battle for iron between humans and microbes. *Curr. Med. Chem.* 25, 25–36. doi: 10.2174/0929867324666170720110049

Castellani, R. J., Moreira, P. I., Liu, G., Dobson, J., Perry, G., Smith, M. A., et al. (2007). Iron: the Redox-active center of oxidative stress in Alzheimer disease. *Neurochem. Res.* 32, 1640–1645. doi: 10.1007/s11064-007-9360-7

Castellani, R. J., Moreira, P. I., Perry, G., and Zhu, X. (2012). The role of iron as a mediator of oxidative stress in Alzheimer disease. *Biofactors* 38, 133–138. doi: 10.1002/biof.1010

Catorce, M. N., and Gevorkian, G. (2016). LPS-induced murine neuroinflammation model: main features and suitability for pre-clinical assessment of nutraceuticals. *Curr. Neuropharmacol.* 14, 155–164. doi: 10.2174/1570159X14666151204122017

Cherayil, B. J., Ellenbogen, S., and Shanmugam, N. N. (2011). Iron and intestinal immunity. *Curr. Opin. Gastroenterol.* 27, 523–528. doi: 10.1097/MOG.0b013e32834a4cd1

Chong, C. Y. L., Bloomfield, F. H., and O'Sullivan, J. M. (2018). Factors affecting gastrointestinal microbiome development in neonates. *Nutrients* 10;E274. doi: 10.3390/nu10030274

Chu, B. C., Garcia-Herrero, A., Johanson, T. H., Krewulak, K. D., Lau, C. K., Peacock, R. S., et al. (2010). Siderophore uptake in bacteria and the battle for iron with the host; a bird's eye view. *Biometals* 23, 601–611. doi: 10.1007/s10534-010-9361-x

Constante, M., Fragoso, G., Calvé, A., Samba-Mondonga, M., and Santos, M. M. (2017). Dietary heme induces gut dysbiosis, aggravates colitis, and potentiates the development of adenomas in mice. *Front. Microbiol.* 8:1809. doi: 10.3389/fmicb.2017.01809

Cooke, J. P., and Dzau, V. J. (1997). NITRIC OXIDE SYNTHASE: role in the genesis of vascular disease. *Annu. Rev. Med.* 48, 489–509. doi: 10.1146/annurev.med.48.1.489

Costello, E. K., Lauber, C. L., Hamady, M., Fierer, N., Gordon, J. I., and Knight, R. (2009). Bacterial community variation in human body habitats across space and time. *Science* 326, 1694–1697. doi: 10.1126/science.1177486

Crapper McLachlan, D. R., Dalton, A. J., Kruck, T. P. A., Bell, M. Y., Smith, W. L., Kalow, W., et al. (1991). Intramuscular desferrioxamine in patients with Alzheimer's disease. *Lancet* 337, 1304–1308. doi: 10.1016/0140-6736(91)92978-B

Cui, Y., Wu, Q., and Zhou, Y. (2009). Iron-refractory iron deficiency anemia: new molecular mechanisms. *Kidney Int.* 76, 1137–1141. doi: 10.1038/ki.2009.357

Damron, F. H., Oglesby-Sherrouse, A. G., Wilks, A., and Barbier, M. (2016). Dual-seq transcriptomics reveals the battle for iron during *Pseudomonas aeruginosa* acute murine pneumonia. *Sci. Rep.* 6:39172. doi: 10.1038/srep39172

Daulatzai, M. A. (2014). Role of stress, depression, and aging in cognitive decline and Alzheimer's disease. *Curr. Top. Behav. Neurosci.* 18, 265–296. doi: 10.1007/7854_2014_350

Dave, M., Higgins, P. D., Middha, S., and Rioux, K. P. (2012). The human gut microbiome: current knowledge, challenges, and future directions. *Transl. Res.* 160, 246–257. doi: 10.1016/j.trsl.2012.05.003

De Buck, M., Gouwy, M., Wang, J. M., Van Snick, J., Proost, P., Struyf, S., et al. (2016). The cytokine-serum amyloid A-chemokine network. *Cytokine Growth Factor Rev.* 30, 55–69. doi: 10.1016/j.cytogfr.2015.12.010

de Oliveira, G. L. V., Leite, A. Z., Higuchi, B. S., Gonzaga, M. I., and Mariano, V. S. (2017). Intestinal dysbiosis and probiotic applications in autoimmune diseases. *Immunology* 152, 1–12. doi: 10.1111/imm.12765

deRosset, L., and Strutz, K. L. (2015). Developmental origins of chronic inflammation: a review of the relationship between birth weight and C-reactive protein. *Ann. Epidemiol.* 25, 539–543. doi: 10.1016/j.annepidem.2015.01.003

Dong, S., Duan, Y., Hu, Y., and Zhao, Z. (2012). Advances in the pathogenesis of Alzheimer's disease: a re-evaluation of amyloid cascade hypothesis. *Transl. Neurodegener.* 1:18. doi: 10.1186/2047-9158-1-18

Dorey, E., Chang, N., Liu, Q. Y., Yang, Z., and Zhang, W. (2014). Apolipoprotein E, amyloid-beta, and neuroinflammation in Alzheimer's disease. *Neurosci. Bull.* 30, 317–330. doi: 10.1007/s12264-013-1422-z

Dowhan, W. (2014). Lipids and extracellular materials. *Annu. Rev. Biochem.* 83, 45–49. doi: 10.1146/annurev-biochem-010314-112017

Ebringer, A., and Rashid, T. (2009). Rheumatoid arthritis is caused by Proteus-the molecular mimicry theory and Karl Popper. *Front. Biosci.* 1, 577–586. doi: 10.2741/e56

Edwards, T. M., and Rickard, N. S. (2007). New perspectives on the mechanisms through which nitric oxide may affect learning and memory processes. *Neurosci. Biobehav. Rev.* 31, 413–425. doi: 10.1016/j.neubiorev.2006.11.001

Eimer, W. A., Vijaya Kumar, D. K., Navalpur Shanmugam, N. K., Washicosky, K. J., Rodriguez, A. S., Gyorgy, B., et al. (2018). Alzheimer's disease-associated β-amyloid is rapidly seeded by herpesviridae to protect against brain infection. *Neuron* 99, 56–63.e3. doi: 10.1016/j.neuron.2018.06.030

Eliasson, M. J. L., Haung, Z., Ferrante, R. J., Sasamata, M., Molliver, M. E., and Snyder, S. H. (1999). Neuronal nitric oxide synthase activation and peroxynitrite formation in ischemic stroke linked to neural damage. *J. Neurosci.* 19, 5910–5918. doi: 10.1523/JNEUROSCI.19-14-05910.1999

Erickson, M. A., and Banks, W. A. (2013). Blood-brain barrier dysfunction as a cause and consequence of Alzheimer's disease. *J. Cereb. Blood Flow Metab.* 33, 1500–1513. doi: 10.1038/jcbfm.2013.135

Exley, C. (2006). Aluminium and iron, but neither copper nor zinc, are key to the precipitation of beta-sheets of Abeta42 in senile plaque cores in Alzheimer's disease. *J. Alzheimers Dis.* 10, 173–177. doi: 10.3233/JAD-2006-102-305

Fasano, A. (2012). Leaky gut and autoimmune diseases. *Clin. Rev. Allergy Immunol.* 42, 71–78. doi: 10.1007/s12016-011-8291-x

Filiou, M. D., Arefin, A. S., Moscato, P., and Graeber, M. B. (2014). 'Neuroinflammation' differs categorically from inflammation: transcriptomes of Alzheimer's disease, Parkinson's disease, schizophrenia and inflammatory diseases compared. *Neurogenetics* 15, 201–212. doi: 10.1007/s10048-014-0409-x

Flores-Mireles, A. L., Walker, J. N., Caparon, M., and Hultgren, S. J. (2015). Urinary tract infections: epidemiology, mechanisms of infection and treatment options. *Nat. Rev. Microbiol.* 13, 269–284. doi: 10.1038/nrmicro3432

Friedland, R. P. (2015). Mechanisms of molecular mimicry involving the microbiota in neurodegeneration. *J. Alzheimers Dis.* 45, 349–362. doi: 10.3233/JAD-142841

Fung, T. C., Olson, C. A., and Hsiao, E. Y. (2017). Interactions between the microbiota, immune and nervous systems in health and disease. *Nat. Neurosci.* 20, 145–155. doi: 10.1038/nn.4476

Ganz, T., and Nemeth, E. (2012). Hepcidin and iron homeostasis. *Biochim. Biophys. Acta* 1823, 1434–1443. doi: 10.1016/j.bbamcr.2012.01.014

Gareau, M. G. (2014). Microbiota-gut-brain axis and cognitive function. *Adv. Exp. Med. Biol.* 817, 357–371. doi: 10.1007/978-1-4939-0897-4_16

Ghosal, A., Upadhyaya, B. B., Fritz, J. V., Heintz-Buschart, A., Desai, M. S., Yusuf, D., et al. (2015). The extracellular RNA complement of *Escherichia coli*. *Microbiologyopen* 4, 252–266. doi: 10.1002/mbo3.235

Griffiths, E. A., Duffy, L. C., Schanbacher, F. L., Qiao, H., Dryja, D., Leavens, A., et al. (2004). In vivo effects of bifidobacteria and lactoferrin on gut endotoxin concentration and mucosal immunity in Balb/c mice. *Dig. Dis. Sci.* 49, 579–589. doi: 10.1023/B:DDAS.0000026302.92898.ae

Grunblatt, E., Bartl, J., and Riederer, P. (2011). The link between iron, metabolic syndrome, and Alzheimer's disease. *J. Neural. Transm.* 118, 371–379. doi: 10.1007/s00702-010-0426-3

Guo, C., Wang, P., Zhong, M. L., Wang, T., Huang, X. S., Li, J. Y., et al. (2013). Deferoxamine inhibits iron induced hippocampal tau phosphorylation in the Alzheimer transgenic mouse brain. *Neurochem. Int.* 62, 165–172. doi: 10.1016/j.neuint.2012.12.005

Haley, K. P., and Skaar, E. P. (2012). A battle for iron: host sequestration and *Staphylococcus aureus* acquisition. *Microbes Infect.* 14, 217–227. doi: 10.1016/j.micinf.2011.11.001

Harach, T., Marungruang, N., Duthilleul, N., Cheatham, V., Mc Coy, K. D., Frisoni, G., et al. (2017). Reduction of Abeta amyloid pathology in APPPS1 transgenic mice in the absence of gut microbiota. *Sci. Rep.* 7:1802. doi: 10.1038/srep41802

Hardy, J., and Selkoe, D. J. (2002). The amyloid hypothesis of Alzheimer's disease: progress and problems on the road to therapeutics. *Science* 297, 353–356. doi: 10.1126/science.1072994

Helms, C. C., Gladwin, M. T., and Kim-Shapiro, D. B. (2018). Erythrocytes and vascular function: oxygen and nitric oxide. *Front. Physiol.* 9:125. doi: 10.3389/fphys.2018.00125

Hongkuan, Y., Hongpeng, G., Mingchun, Y., Ziyi, L., Shigeko, T., Daijiro, Y., et al. (2015). Upregulation of mitochondrial ferritin by proinflammatory cytokines: implications for a role in Alzheimer's disease. *J. Alzheimers Dis.* 45, 797–811. doi: 10.3233/JAD-142595

Honjo, K., van Reekum, R., and Verhoeff, N. P. (2009). Alzheimer's disease and infection: do infectious agents contribute to progression of Alzheimer's disease? *Alzheimers Dement.* 5, 348–360. doi: 10.1016/j.jalz.2008.12.001

Itzhaki, R. F. (2014). Herpes simplex virus type 1 and Alzheimer's disease: increasing evidence for a major role of the virus. *Front. Aging Neurosci.* 6:202. doi: 10.3389/fnagi.2014.00202

Itzhaki, R. F. (2017). Herpes simplex virus type 1 and Alzheimer's disease: possible mechanisms and signposts. *FASEB J.* 31, 3216–3226. doi: 10.1096/fj.201700360

Itzhaki, R. F., and Lathe, R. (2018). Herpes viruses and senile dementia: first population evidence for a causal link. *J. Alzheimers Dis.* 64, 363–366. doi: 10.3233/JAD-180266

Itzhaki, R. F., Lathe, R., Balin, B. J., Ball, M. J., Bearer, E. L., Braak, H., et al. (2016). Microbes and Alzheimer's disease. *J. Alzheimers Dis.* 51, 979–984. doi: 10.3233/JAD-160152

Itzhaki, R. F., and Tabet, N. (2017). Herpes simplex encephalitis and Alzheimer's disease: is there a link? *J. Neurol. Sci.* 380, 20–21. doi: 10.1016/j.jns.2017.06.046

Jellinger, K. A. (2008). Morphologic diagnosis of "vascular dementia" - a critical update. *J. Neurol. Sci.* 270, 1–12. doi: 10.1016/j.jns.2008.03.006

Jellinger, K. A., and Attems, J. (2007). Neuropathological evaluation of mixed dementia. *J. Neurol. Sci.* 257, 80–87. doi: 10.1016/j.jns.2007.01.045

Kamer, A. R., Craig, R. G., Dasanayake, A. P., Brys, M., Glodzik-Sobanska, L., and de Leon, M. J. (2008). Inflammation and Alzheimer's disease: possible role of periodontal diseases. *Alzheimers Dement.* 4, 242–250. doi: 10.1016/j.jalz.2007.08.004

Kaprelyants, A. S., Gottschal, J. C., and Kell, D. B. (1993). Dormancy in non-sporulating bacteria. *FEMS Microbiol. Rev.* 104, 271–286. doi: 10.1111/j.1574-6968.1993.tb05871.x

Karantzoulis, S., and Galvin, J. E. (2011). Distinguishing Alzheimer's disease from other major forms of dementia. *Expert Rev. Neurother.* 11, 1579–1591. doi: 10.1586/ern.11.155

Karpuzoglu, E., and Ahmed, S. A. (2006). Estrogen regulation of nitric oxide and inducible nitric oxide synthase (iNOS) in immune cells: implications for immunity, autoimmune diseases, and apoptosis. *Nitric Oxide* 15, 177–186. doi: 10.1016/j.niox.2006.03.009

Kell, D., Potgieter, M., and Pretorius, E. (2015). Individuality, phenotypic differentiation, dormancy and 'persistence' in culturable bacterial systems: commonalities shared by environmental, laboratory, and clinical microbiology. *F1000Res.* 4:179. doi: 10.12688/f1000research.6709.2

Kell, D. B. (2009). Iron behaving badly: inappropriate iron chelation as a major contributor to the aetiology of vascular and other progressive inflammatory and degenerative diseases. *BMC Med. Genomics* 2:2. doi: 10.1186/1755-8794-2-2

Kell, D. B. (2010). Towards a unifying, systems biology understanding of large-scale cellular death and destruction caused by poorly liganded iron: Parkinson's, Huntington's, Alzheimer's, prions, bactericides, chemical toxicology and others as examples. *Arch. Toxicol.* 84, 825–889. doi: 10.1007/s00204-010-0577-x

Kell, D. B., Kaprelyants, A. S., Weichart, D. H., Harwood, C. R., and Barer, M. R. (1998). Viability and activity in readily culturable bacteria- a review and discussion of the practical issues. *Antonie Van Leeuwenhoek* 73, 169–187. doi: 10.1023/A:1000664013047

Kell, D. B., and Kenny, L. C. (2016). A dormant microbial component in the development of preeclampsia. *Front. Med.* 3:60. doi: 10.3389/fmed.2016.00060

Kell, D. B., and Pretorius, E. (2014). Serum ferritin is an important inflammatory disease marker, as it is mainly a leakage product from damaged cells. *Metallomics* 6, 748–773. doi: 10.1039/c3mt00347g

Kell, D. B., and Pretorius, E. (2015a). On the translocation of bacteria and their lipopolysaccharides between blood and peripheral locations in chronic, inflammatory diseases: the central roles of LPS and LPS-induced cell death. *Integr. Biol.* 7, 1339–1377. doi: 10.1039/c5ib00158g

Kell, D. B., and Pretorius, E. (2015b). The simultaneous occurrence of both hypercoagulability and hypofibrinolysis in blood and serum during systemic inflammation, and the roles of iron and fibrin(ogen). *Integr. Biol.* 7, 24–52. doi: 10.1039/c4ib00173g

Kell, D. B., and Pretorius, E. (2017). Proteins behaving badly. Substoichiometric molecular control and amplification of the initiation and nature of amyloid fibril formation: lessons from and for blood clotting. *Prog. Biophys. Mol. Biol.* 123, 16–41. doi: 10.1016/j.pbiomolbio.2016.08.006

Kell, D. B., and Pretorius, E. (2018). No effects without causes: the Iron Dysregulation and Dormant Microbes hypothesis for chronic, inflammatory diseases. *Biol. Rev. Camb. Philos. Soc.* 93, 1518–1557. doi: 10.1111/brv.12407

Kenny, L. C., and Kell, D. B. (2017). Immunological tolerance, pregnancy, and preeclampsia: the roles of semen microbes and the father. *Front. Med.* 4:239. doi: 10.3389/fmed.2017.00239

Kerley, R. N., McCarthy, C., Kell, D. B., and Kenny, L. C. (2018). The potential therapeutic effects of ergothioneine in pre-eclampsia. *Free Radic. Biol. Med.* 117, 145–157. doi: 10.1016/j.freeradbiomed.2017.12.030

Keshavarzian, A., Green, S. J., Engen, P. A., Voigt, R. M., Naqib, A., Forsyth, C. B., et al. (2015). Colonic bacterial composition in Parkinson's disease. *Mov. Disord.* 30, 1351–1360. doi: 10.1002/mds.26307

Kho, Z. Y., and Lal, S. K. (2018). The human gut microbiome - a potential controller of wellness and disease. *Front. Microbiol.* 9:1835. doi: 10.3389/fmicb.2018.01835

Khokhlova, E. V., Smeianov, V. V., Efimov, B. A., Kafarskaia, L. I., Pavlova, S. I., and Shkoporov, A. N. (2012). Anti-inflammatory properties of intestinal Bifidobacterium strains isolated from healthy infants. *Microbiol. Immunol.* 56, 27–39. doi: 10.1111/j.1348-0421.2011.00398.x

Kinnby, B., and Chavez de Paz, L. E. (2016). Plasminogen coating increases initial adhesion of oral bacteria in vitro. *Microb. Pathog.* 100, 10–16. doi: 10.1016/j.micpath.2016.08.002

Köhler, C. A., Maes, M., Slyepchenko, A., Berk, M., Solmi, M., Lanctôt, K. L., et al. (2016). The gut-brain axis, including the microbiome, leaky gut and bacterial translocation: mechanisms and pathophysiological role in Alzheimer's disease. *Curr. Pharm. Des.* 22, 6152–6166. doi: 10.2174/1381612822666160907093807

Kolios, G., Valatas, V., and Ward, S. G. (2004). Nitric oxide in inflammatory bowel disease: a universal messenger in an unsolved puzzle. *Immunology* 113, 427–437. doi: 10.1111/j.1365-2567.2004.01984.x

Landsem, A., Fure, H., Christiansen, D., Nielsen, E. W., Osterud, B., Mollnes, T. E., et al. (2015). The key roles of complement and tissue factor in *Escherichia coli*-induced coagulation in human whole blood. *Clin. Exp. Immunol.* 182, 81–89. doi: 10.1111/cei.12663

Langa, K. M. (2015). Is the risk of Alzheimer's disease and dementia declining? *Alzheimers Res. Ther.* 7:34. doi: 10.1186/s13195-015-0118-1

Law, A., Gauthier, S., and Quirion, R. (2001). Say NO to Alzheimer's disease: the putative links between nitric oxide and dementia of the Alzheimer's type. *Brain Res. Rev.* 35, 73–96. doi: 10.1016/S0165-0173(00)00051-5

Lee, J. W., Lee, Y. K., Yuk, D. Y., Choi, D. Y., Ban, S. B., Oh, K. W., et al. (2008). Neuro-inflammation induced by lipopolysaccharide causes cognitive impairment through enhancement of beta-amyloid generation. *J. Neuroinflammation* 5:37. doi: 10.1186/1742-2094-5-37

Lelouvier, B., Servant, F., Paisse, S., Brunet, A. C., Benyahya, S., Serino, M., et al. (2016). Changes in blood microbiota profiles associated with liver fibrosis in obese patients: a pilot analysis. *Hepatology* 64, 2015–2027. doi: 10.1002/hep.28829

Lewis, K. (2007). Persister cells, dormancy and infectious disease. *Nat. Rev. Microbiol.* 5, 48–56. doi: 10.1038/nrmicro1557

Liehl, P., Zuzarte-Luis, V., and Mota, M. M. (2015). Unveiling the pathogen behind the vacuole. *Nat. Rev. Microbiol.* 13, 589–598. doi: 10.1038/nrmicro3504

Lipinski, B., and Pretorius, E. (2012). Novel pathway of iron-induced blood coagulation: implications for diabetes mellitus and its complications. *Pol. Arch. Med. Wewn.* 122, 115–122. doi: 10.20452/pamw.1201

Lipinski, B., and Pretorius, E. (2013). The role of iron-induced fibrin in the pathogenesis of Alzheimer's disease and the protective role of magnesium. *Front. Hum. Neurosci.* 7:735. doi: 10.3389/fnhum.2013.00735

Logroscino, G., Gao, X., Chen, H., Wing, A., and Ascherio, A. (2008). Dietary iron intake and risk of Parkinson's disease. *Am. J. Epidemiol.* 168, 1381–1388. doi: 10.1093/aje/kwn273

Lucas, S. M., Rothwell, N. J., and Gibson, R. M. (2006). The role of inflammation in CNS injury and disease. *Br. J. Pharmacol.* 147(Suppl. 1), S232–S240. doi: 10.1038/sj.bjp.0706400

Lüth, H., Münch, G., and Arendt, T. (2002). Aberrant expression of NOS isoforms in Alzheimer's disease is structurally related to nitrotyrosine formation. *Brain Res.* 953, 135–143. doi: 10.1016/S0006-8993(02)03280-8

Lyte, M. (2014). Microbial endocrinology and the microbiota-gut-brain axis. *Adv. Exp. Med. Biol.* 817, 3–24. doi: 10.1007/978-1-4939-0897-4_1

Maes, M. (2009). Leaky gut in chronic fatigue syndrome: a review. *Act. Nerv. Super. Rediviva* 51, 21–28.

Maier, L., Pruteanu, M., Kuhn, M., Zeller, G., Telzerow, A., Anderson, E. E., et al. (2018). Extensive impact of non-antibiotic drugs on human gut bacteria. *Nature* 555, 623–628. doi: 10.1038/nature25979

Makin, S. (2018). The amyloid hypothesis on trial. *Nature* 559, S4–S7. doi: 10.1038/d41586-018-05719-4

Malinski, T. (2007). Nitric oxide and nitroxidative stress in Alzheimer's disease. *J. Alzheimers Dis.* 11, 207–218. doi: 10.3233/JAD-2007-11208

Mariani, R., Trombini, P., Pozzi, M., and Piperno, A. (2009). Iron metabolism in thalassemia and sickle cell disease. *Mediterr. J. Hematol. Infect. Dis.* 1:e2009006. doi: 10.4084/MJHID.2009.006

Markel, T. A., Crisostomo, P. R., Wang, M., Herring, C. M., Meldrum, K. K., Lillemoe, K. D., et al. (2007). The struggle for iron: gastrointestinal microbes modulate the host immune response during infection. *J. Leukoc. Biol.* 81, 393–400. doi: 10.1189/jlb.0906579

Martel, J., Wu, C. Y., Huang, P. R., Cheng, W. Y., and Young, J. D. (2017). Pleomorphic bacteria-like structures in human blood represent non-living membrane vesicles and protein particles. *Sci. Rep.* 7:10650. doi: 10.1038/s41598-017-10479-8

Mattman, L. (2001). *Cell Wall Deficient forms: Stealth Pathogens*, 3rd Edn. Boca Raton, FL: CRC Press.

McColl, B. W., Allan, S. M., and Rothwell, N. J. (2009). Systemic infection, inflammation and acute ischemic stroke. *Neuroscience* 158, 1049–1061. doi: 10.1016/j.neuroscience.2008.08.019

Michels, K., Nemeth, E., Ganz, T., and Mehrad, B. (2015). Hepcidin and host defense against infectious diseases. *PLoS Pathog.* 11:e1004998. doi: 10.1371/journal.ppat.1004998

Miklossy, J. (2016). Bacterial amyloid and DNA are important constituents of senile plaques: further evidence of the spirochetal and biofilm nature of senile plaques. *J. Alzheimers Dis.* 53, 1459–1473. doi: 10.3233/JAD-160451

Miklossy, J., and McGeer, P. L. (2016). Common mechanisms involved in Alzheimer's disease and type 2 diabetes: a key role of chronic bacterial infection and inflammation. *Aging* 8, 575–588. doi: 10.18632/aging.100921

Mohanty, J. G., Shukla, H. D., Williamson, J. D., Launer, L. J., Saxena, S., and Rifkind, J. M. (2010). Alterations in the red blood cell membrane proteome in Alzheimer's subjects reflect disease-related changes and provide insight into altered cell morphology. *Proteome Sci.* 8:11. doi: 10.1186/1477-5956-8-11

Monda, V., Villano, I., Messina, A., Valenzano, A., Esposito, T., Moscatelli, F., et al. (2017). Exercise modifies the gut microbiota with positive health effects. *Oxid. Med. Cell. Longev.* 2017:3831972. doi: 10.1155/2017/3831972

Moreira, P. I., Honda, K., Liu, Q., Santos, M. S., Oliveira, C. R., Gjumrakch, A., et al. (2005). Oxidative stress: the old enemy in Alzheimer's disease pathophysiology. *Curr. Alzheimer Res.* 2, 430–438. doi: 10.2174/156720505774330537

Mu, Q., Kirby, J., Reily, C. M., and Luo, X. M. (2017). Leaky gut as a danger signal for autoimmune diseases. *Front. Immunol.* 8:598. doi: 10.3389/fimmu.2017.00598

Mueller, S. G., Weiner, M. W., Thal, L. J., Petersen, R. C., Jack, C., Jagust, W., et al. (2005). The Alzheimer's disease neuroimaging initiative. *Neuroimaging Clin. N. Am.* 15, 869–881. doi: 10.1016/j.nic.2005.09.008

Mukamolova, G. V., Kaprelyants, A. S., Kell, D. B., and Young, M. (2003). Adoption of the transiently non-culturable state - a bacterial survival strategy? *Adv. Microb. Physiol.* 47, 65–129. doi: 10.1016/S0065-2911(03)47002-1

Mukamolova, G. V., Kaprelyants, A. S., Young, D. I., Young, M., and Kell, D. B. (1998). A bacterial cytokine. *Proc. Natl. Acad. Sci. U.S.A.* 95, 8916–8921. doi: 10.1073/pnas.95.15.8916

Nairz, M., Haschka, D., Demetz, E., and Weiss, G. (2014). Iron at the interface of immunity and infection. *Front. Pharmacol.* 5:152. doi: 10.3389/fphar.2014.00152

Nairz, M., Schroll, A., Sonnweber, T., and Weiss, G. (2010). The struggle for iron - a metal at the host-pathogen interface. *Cell Microbiol.* 12, 1691–1702. doi: 10.1111/j.1462-5822.2010.01529.x

Naseem, K. M. (2005). The role of nitric oxide in cardiovascular diseases. *Mol. Aspects Med.* 26, 33–65. doi: 10.1016/j.mam.2004.09.003

Nunomura, A., Perry, G., Aliev, G., Hirai, K., Takeda, A., Balraj, E. K., et al. (2001). Oxidative damage is the earliest event in Alzheimer disease. *J. Neuropathol. Exp. Neurol.* 60, 759–767. doi: 10.1093/jnen/60.8.759

Ochei, J., and Kolhatkar, A. (eds). (2000). "Pus abscess and wound drain," in *Medical Laboratory Science: Theory and Practice*, (New Delhi: Tata McGraw-Hill Publishing Company Limited), 622.

Ozturk, Z. A., Unal, A., Yigiter, R., Yesil, Y., Kuyumcu, M. E., Neyal, M., et al. (2013). Is increased red cell distribution width (RDW) indicating the inflammation in Alzheimer's disease (AD)? *Arch. Gerontol. Geriatr.* 56, 50–54. doi: 10.1016/j.archger.2012.10.002

Pacher, P., Beckman, J. S., and Liaudet, L. (2007). Nitric oxide and peroxynitrite in health and disease. *Physiol. Rev.* 87, 315–424. doi: 10.1152/physrev.00029.2006

Panthi, S., Manandhar, S., and Gautam, K. (2018). Hydrogen sulfide, nitric oxide, and neurodegenerative disorders. *Transl. Neurodegener.* 7:3. doi: 10.1186/s40035-018-0108-x

Peters, D. G., Connor, J. R., and Meadowcroft, M. D. (2015). The relationship between iron dyshomeostasis and amyloidogenesis in Alzheimer's disease: two sides of the same coin. *Neurobiol. Dis.* 81, 49–65. doi: 10.1016/j.nbd.2015.08.007

Pilling, L. C., Atkins, J. L., Duff, M. O., Beaumont, R. N., Jones, S. E., Tyrrell, J., et al. (2017). Red blood cell distribution width: genetic evidence for aging pathways in 116,666 volunteers. *PLoS One* 12:e0185083. doi: 10.1371/journal.pone.0185083

Pindjakova, J., Sartini, C., Lo Re, O., Rappa, F., Coupe, B., Lelouvier, B., et al. (2017). Gut dysbiosis and adaptive immune response in diet-induced obesity vs. Systemic inflammation. *Front. Microbiol.* 8:1157. doi: 10.3389/fmicb.2017.01157

Pistollato, F., Sumalla Cano, S., Elio, I., Masias Vergara, M., Giampieri, F., and Battino, M. (2016). Role of gut microbiota and nutrients in amyloid formation and pathogenesis of Alzheimer disease. *Nutr. Rev.* 74, 624–634. doi: 10.1093/nutrit/nuw023

Potgieter, M., Bester, J., Kell, D. B., and Pretorius, E. (2015). The dormant blood microbiome in chronic, inflammatory diseases. *FEMS Microbiol. Rev.* 39, 567–591. doi: 10.1093/femsre/fuv013

Pretorius, E., Akeredolu, O. O., Soma, P., and Kell, D. B. (2017). Major involvement of bacterial components in rheumatoid arthritis and its accompanying oxidative stress, systemic inflammation and hypercoagulability. *Exp. Biol. Med.* 242, 355–373. doi: 10.1177/1535370216681549

Pretorius, E., Bester, J., and Kell, D. B. (2016a). A bacterial component to Alzheimer's-type dementia seen via a systems biology approach that links iron dysregulation and inflammagen shedding to disease. *J. Alzheimers Dis.* 53, 1237–1256. doi: 10.3233/JAD-160318

Pretorius, E., Mbotwe, S., Bester, J., Robinson, C. J., and Kell, D. B. (2016b). Acute induction of anomalous and amyloidogenic blood clotting by molecular amplification of highly substoichiometric levels of bacterial lipopolysaccharide. *J. R. Soc. Interface* 13:20160539. doi: 10.1098/rsif.2016.0539

Pretorius, E., and Kell, D. B. (2014). Diagnostic morphology: biophysical indicators for iron-driven inflammatory diseases. *Integr. Biol.* 6, 486–510. doi: 10.1039/c4ib00025k

Pretorius, E., Page, M. J., Hendricks, L., Nkosi, N. B., Benson, S. R., and Kell, D. B. (2018). Both lipopolysaccharide and lipoteichoic acids potently induce anomalous fibrin amyloid formation: assessment with novel Amytracker stains. *J. R. Soc. Interface* 15:20170941. doi: 10.1098/rsif.2017.0941

Primohamed, M., James, S., Meakin, S., Green, C., Scott, A. K., Walley, T. J., et al. (2004). Adverse drug reactions as cause of admission to hospital-prospective analysis of 18 820 patients. *BMJ* 329, 15–19. doi: 10.1136/bmj.329.7456.15

Prince, M., Albanese, E., Guerchet, M., and Prina, M. (2014). World Alzheimer report 2014. *Alzheimers Dis. Int.* 2014, 104.

Pritchard, A. B., Crean, S., Olsen, I., and Singhrao, S. K. (2017). Periodontitis, microbiomes and their role in Alzheimer's disease. *Front. Aging Neurosci.* 9:336. doi: 10.3389/fnagi.2017.00336

Proal, A. D., Albert, P. J., and Marshall, T. G. (2013). The human microbiome and autoimmunity. *Curr. Opin. Rheumatol.* 25, 234–240. doi: 10.1097/BOR.0b013e32835cedbf

Proal, A. D., Lindseth, I. A., and Marshall, T. G. (2017). Microbe-microbe and host-microbe interactions drive microbiome dysbiosis and inflammatory processes. *Discov. Med.* 23, 51–60.

Proal, A. D., and Marshall, T. G. (2018). Re-framing the theory of autoimmunity in the era of the microbiome: persistent pathogens, autoantibodies, and molecular mimicry. *Discov. Med.* 140, 299–308.

Qui, C., Kivipelto, M., and von Strauss, E. (2009). Epidemiology of Alzheimer's disease: occurrence, determinants, and strategies toward intervention. *Dialogues Clin. Neurosci.* 11, 111–128.

Quigley, E. M. (2016). Leaky gut - concept or clinical entity? *Curr. Opin. Gastroenterol.* 32, 74–79. doi: 10.1097/MOG.0000000000000243

Readhead, B., Haure-Mirande, J. V., Funk, C. C., Richards, M. A., Shannon, P., Haroutunian, V., et al. (2018). Multiscale analysis of independent Alzheimer's cohorts finds disruption of molecular, genetic, and clinical networks by human Herpesvirus. *Neuron* 99, 64–82.e7. doi: 10.1016/j.neuron.2018.05.023

Reichert, C. O., da Cunha, J., Levy, D., Bydlowski, S. P., and Spada, C. (2017). Hepcidin: homeostasis and diseases related to iron metabolism. *Acta Haematol.* 137, 220–236. doi: 10.1159/000471838

Reid, D. W., Anderson, G. J., and Lamont, I. L. (2009). Role of lung iron in determining the bacterial and host struggle in cystic fibrosis. *Am. J. Physiol. Lung Cell. Mol. Physiol.* 297, L795–L802. doi: 10.1152/ajplung.00132.2009

Rubio-Perez, J. M., and Morillas-Ruiz, J. M. (2012). A review: inflammatory process in Alzheimer's disease, role of cytokines. *ScientificWorldJournal.* 2012:756357. doi: 10.1100/2012/756357

Saldanha, C. (2016). Physiological role of erythrocyte nitric oxide. *Clin. Hemorheol. Microcirc.* 64, 517–520. doi: 10.3233/CH-168028

Sandhu, K. V., Sherwin, E., Schellekens, H., Stanton, C., Dinan, T. G., and Cryan, J. F. (2017). Feeding the microbiota-gut-brain axis: diet, microbiome, and neuropsychiatry. *Transl. Res.* 179, 223–244. doi: 10.1016/j.trsl.2016.10.002

Sandro, A., and Muckenthaler, M. U. (2009). Iron toxicity in diseases of aging: Alzheimer's disease, Parkinson's disease and atherosclerosis. *J. Alzheimers Dis.* 14, 879–895. doi: 10.3233/JAD-2009-1010

Schaffer, J. E. (2016). Lipotoxicity: many roads to cell dysfunction and cell death: introduction to a thematic review series. *J. Lipid Res.* 57, 1327–1328. doi: 10.1194/jlr.E069880

Schmidt, R., Schmidt, H., Curb, J. D., Masaki, K., White, L. R., and Launer, L. J. (2002). Early inflammation and dementia: a 25-year follow-up of the Honolulu-Asia Aging Study. *Ann. Neurol.* 52, 168–174. doi: 10.1002/ana.10265

Schwartz, K., Ganesan, M., Payne, D. E., Solomon, M. J., and Boles, B. R. (2016). Extracellular DNA facilitates the formation of functional amyloids in *Staphylococcus aureus* biofilms. *Mol. Microbiol.* 99, 123–134. doi: 10.1111/mmi.13219

Selkoe, D. J., and Hardy, J. (2016). The amyloid hypothesis of Alzheimer's disease at 25 years. *EMBO Mol. Med.* 8, 595–608. doi: 10.15252/emmm.201606210

Shahnawaz, M., and Soto, C. (2012). Microcin amyloid fibrils A are reservoir of toxic oligomeric species. *J. Biol. Chem.* 287, 11665–11676. doi: 10.1074/jbc.M111.282533

Shoemark, D. K., and Allen, S. J. (2015). The microbiome and disease: reviewing the links between the oral microbiome, aging, and Alzheimer's disease. *J. Alzheimers Dis.* 43, 725–738. doi: 10.3233/JAD-141170

Skaar, E. P. (2010). The battle for iron between bacterial pathogens and their vertebrate hosts. *PLoS Pathog.* 6:e1000949. doi: 10.1371/journal.ppat.1000949

Slotta, J. E., Braun, O. O., Menger, M. D., and Thorlacius, H. (2008). Central role of Rho kinase in lipopolysaccharide-induced platelet capture on venous endothelium. *J. Investig. Med.* 56, 720–725. doi: 10.2310/JIM.0b013e31816c3e81

Steardo, L. Jr., Bronzuoli, M. R., Iacomino, A., Esposito, G., Steardo, L., and Scuderi, C. (2015). Does neuroinflammation turn on the flame in Alzheimer's disease? Focus on astrocytes. *Front. Neurosci.* 9:259. doi: 10.3389/fnins.2015.00259

Stilling, R. M., Dinan, T. G., and Cryan, J. F. (2014). Microbial genes, brain & behaviour - epigenetic regulation of the gut-brain axis. *Genes Brain Behav.* 13, 69–86. doi: 10.1111/gbb.12109

Subashchandrabose, S., and Mobley, H. L. (2015). Back to the metal age: battle for metals at the host-pathogen interface during urinary tract infection. *Metallomics* 7, 935–942. doi: 10.1039/c4mt00329b

Swerdlow, R. H. (2007). Pathogenesis of Alzheimer's disease. *Clin. Interve. Aging* 2, 347–359.

Thwaites, G. E., and Gant, V. (2011). Are bloodstream leukocytes Trojan Horses for the metastasis of *Staphylococcus aureus*? *Nat. Rev. Microbiol.* 9, 215–222. doi: 10.1038/nrmicro2508

Ticinesi, A., Milani, C., Lauretani, F., Nouvenne, A., Mancabelli, L., Lugli, G. A., et al. (2017). Gut microbiota composition is associated with polypharmacy in elderly hospitalized patients. *Sci. Rep.* 7:11102. doi: 10.1038/s41598-017-10734-y

Tran, L., and Greenwood-Van Meerveld, B. (2013). Age-associated remodeling of the intestinal epithelial barrier. *J. Gerontol. A Biol. Sci. Med. Sci.* 68, 1045–1056. doi: 10.1093/gerona/glt106

Tripathy, D., Sanchez, A., Yin, X., Luo, J., Martinez, J., and Grammas, P. (2013). Thrombin, a mediator of cerebrovascular inflammation in AD and hypoxia. *Front. Aging Neurosci.* 5:19. doi: 10.3389/fnagi.2013.00019

Tzeng, N. S., Chung, C. H., Lin, F. H., Chiang, C. P., Yeh, C. B., Lu, R. B., et al. (2018). Anti-herpetic medications and reduced risk of dementia in patients with herpes simplex virus infections-a nationwide, population-based cohort study in Taiwan. *Neurotherapeutics* 15, 417–429. doi: 10.1007/s13311-018-0611-x

Underwood, M. A., German, J. B., Lebrilla, C. B., and Mills, D. A. (2015). *Bifidobacterium longum* subspecies infantis: champion colonizer of the infant gut. *Pediatr. Res.* 77, 229–235. doi: 10.1038/pr.2014.156

Via, A., Uyar, B., Brun, C., and Zanzoni, A. (2015). How pathogens use linear motifs to perturb host cell networks. *Trends Biochem. Sci.* 40, 36–48. doi: 10.1016/j.tibs.2014.11.001

Vogt, N. M., Kerby, R. L., Dill-McFarland, K. A., Harding, S. J., Merluzzi, A. P., Johnson, S. C., et al. (2017). Gut microbiome alterations in Alzheimer's disease. *Sci. Rep.* 7:13537. doi: 10.1038/s41598-017-13601-y

Vradenburg, G. (2015). A pivotal moment in Alzheimer's disease and dementia: how global unity of purpose and action can beat the disease by 2025. *Expert Rev. Neurother.* 15, 73–82. doi: 10.1586/14737175.2015.995638

Wallace, J. L. (2013). Polypharmacy of osteoarthritis: the perfect intestinal storm. *Dig. Dis. Sci.* 58, 3088–3093. doi: 10.1007/s10620-013-2777-8

Wang, Z., Xiao, G., Yao, Y., Guo, S., Lu, K., and Sheng, Z. (2006). The role of bifidobacteria in gut barrier function after thermal injury in rats. *J. Trauma* 61, 650–657. doi: 10.1097/01.ta.0000196574.70614.27

Weinreb, O., Mandel, S., Bar-Am, O., and Amit, T. (2011). Iron-chelating backbone coupled with monoamine oxidase inhibitory moiety as novel pluripotential therapeutic agents for Alzheimer's disease: a tribute to Moussa Youdim. *J. Neural Transm.* 118, 479–492. doi: 10.1007/s00702-011-0597-6

Weuve, J., Mendes de Leon, C. F., Bennett, D. A., Dong, X., and Evans, D. A. (2014). The red cell distribution width and anemia in association with prevalent dementia. *Alzheimer Dis. Assoc. Disord.* 28, 99–105. doi: 10.1097/WAD.0b013e318299673c

Winchester, L. M., Powell, J., Lovestone, S., and Nevado-Holgado, A. J. (2018). Red blood cell indices and anaemia as causative factors for cognitive function deficits and for Alzheimer's disease. *Genome Med.* 10:51. doi: 10.1186/s13073-018-0556-z

Wood, H. (2015). Alzheimer disease: iron–the missing link between ApoE and Alzheimer disease? *Nat. Rev. Neurol.* 11:369. doi: 10.1038/nrneurol.2015.96

Zakaria, R., Yaacob, W. M. W., Othman, Z., Long, I., Ahmad, A. H., and Al-Rahbi, B. (2017). Lipopolysaccharide-induced memory impairment in rats: a model of Alzheimer's disease. *Physiol. Res.* 66, 553–565.

Zamolodchikov, D., and Strickland, S. (2012). Abeta delays fibrin clot lysis by altering fibrin structure and attenuating plasminogen binding to fibrin. *Blood* 119, 3342–3351. doi: 10.1182/blood-2011-11-389668

Zekry, D., Hauw, J., and Gold, G. (2002). Mixed dementia: epidemiology, diagnosis, and treatment. *J. Am. Geriatr. Soc.* 50, 1431–1438. doi: 10.1046/j.1532-5415.2002.50367.x

Zenaro, E., Piacentino, G., and Constantin, G. (2017). The blood-brain barrier in Alzheimer's disease. *Neurobiol. Dis.* 107, 41–56. doi: 10.1016/j.nbd.2016.07.007

Zhang, L., Hu, R., Li, M., Li, F., Meng, H., Zhu, G., et al. (2013). Deferoxamine attenuates iron-induced long-term neurotoxicity in rats with traumatic brain injury. *Neurol. Sci.* 34, 639–645. doi: 10.1007/s10072-012-1090-1

Zhao, Y., Dua, P., and Lukiw, W. J. (2015). Microbial sources of amyloid and relevance to amyloidogenesis and Alzheimer's disease (AD). *J. Alzheimers Dis. Parkinsonism* 5:177.

Zhao, Y., Jaber, V., and Lukiw, W. J. (2017). Secretory products of the human GI tract microbiome and their potential impact on Alzheimer's disease (AD): detection of lipopolysaccharide (LPS) in AD hippocampus. *Front. Cell. Infect. Microbiol.* 7:318. doi: 10.3389/fcimb.2017.00318

Zhao, Y., and Lukiw, W. J. (2015). Microbiome-generated amyloid and potential impact on amyloidogenesis in Alzheimer's disease (AD). *J. Nat. Sci.* 1:e138.

Zhu, B., Wang, X., and Li, L. (2010). Human gut microbiome: the second genome of human body. *Protein Cell* 1, 718–725. doi: 10.1007/s13238-010-0093-z

18

Iron in Neurodegeneration – Cause or Consequence?

Alain Ndayisaba, Christine Kaindlstorfer and Gregor K. Wenning*

Department of Neurology, Medical University of Innsbruck, Innsbruck, Austria

Correspondence:
Gregor K. Wenning
gregor.wenning@i-med.ac.at

Iron dyshomeostasis can cause neuronal damage to iron-sensitive brain regions. Neurodegeneration with brain iron accumulation reflects a group of disorders caused by iron overload in the basal ganglia. High iron levels and iron related pathogenic triggers have also been implicated in sporadic neurodegenerative diseases including Alzheimer's disease (AD), Parkinson's disease (PD), and multiple system atrophy (MSA). Iron-induced dyshomeostasis within vulnerable brain regions is still insufficiently understood. Here, we summarize the modes of action by which iron might act as primary or secondary disease trigger in neurodegenerative disorders. In addition, available treatment options targeting brain iron dysregulation and the use of iron as biomarker in prodromal stages are critically discussed to address the question of cause or consequence.

Keywords: iron, neurodegeneration, neurodegenerative mechanisms, mitochondrial dysfunction, autophagic-lysosomal dysfunction, protein aggregation, neuroinflammation

INTRODUCTION

Iron is involved in an abundant number of cellular processes in the brain including mitochondrial respiration, myelin synthesis, DNA synthesis, oxygen transportation, neurotransmitter synthesis and cellular metabolism (Stankiewicz and Brass, 2009; Ward et al., 2014). In the CNS, iron is present in neurons, oligodendrocytes, astroglia and microglia cells.

Within the cell, iron mediates essential functions due to its capability to participate in reaction of electron transfer thereby switching between two states: ferrous (II) and ferric (III) iron. This mechanism represents a double-edge sword because distinct levels of reactive oxygen species (ROS) are produced during these reactions enabling calcium-mediated basal synaptic transmission and long-term potentiation (Muñoz et al., 2011), but on the other hand may catalyze the so-called Fenton reaction, which generates ROS in high amounts detrimental for cellular function and eventually survival (Halliwell, 2006). Thus, tight regulation of intracellular iron homeostasis is required which is facilitated by sequestration of iron into iron-binding proteins like heme, ferritin, neuromelanin, and iron-sulfur clusters among others (Kruszewski, 2003).

Iron levels in the brain and body increase sharply up to 30 years of age due to a metabolic need during the growth process and remain stable during adulthood (Bolognin et al., 2009; Stankiewicz and Brass, 2009; Apostolakis and Kypraiou, 2017). In the aging brain however, region-specific increase of total iron is observed, probably triggered by inflammation, increased blood-brain barrier (BBB) permeability, redistribution of iron within the brain, and changes in iron homeostasis (Conde and Streit, 2006; Farrall and Wardlaw, 2009; Ward et al., 2014) and shows highest iron levels in the basal ganglia. In addition, iron accumulation varies among brain cell types, as neurons, micro- and astroglia accumulate iron over their lifespan, whereas oligodendroglial iron levels remain stable (Connor et al., 1990). Changes in regional iron distribution have been demonstrated consistently in neurodegenerative diseases via magnetic resonance imaging (MRI) (Duyn, 2010) and at post-mortem examinations (Hare et al., 2012) and since aging represents the number one risk factor for neurodegeneration, there may be a link between age-related iron accumulation and neurodegeneration (Zecca et al., 2001, 2004; Ward et al., 2014).

Alzheimer's disease (AD), Parkinson's disease (PD), multiple system atrophy (MSA), dementia with Lewy bodies, amyotrophic lateral sclerosis, Huntington's disease (HD), frontotemporal dementia, corticobasal degeneration, and progressive supranuclear palsy (PSP) are primarily characterized by the deposition of insoluble protein aggregates which colocalize with iron (Coffey et al., 1989; Berg and Hochstrasser, 2006; Muller and Leavitt, 2014; Wang et al., 2016; Fernández et al., 2017; Lee et al., 2017; Sheelakumari et al., 2017; Kaindlstorfer et al., 2018; Lane et al., 2018; Moreau et al., 2018), suggesting a link between those clinically and pathologically distinct disease entities. This raises the question whether iron dyshomeostasis represents a critical factor in initiating neurodegeneration, whether it contributes to acceleration of widespread pathology as a result of nerve cell death and the consecutive release of intracellular components or whether neurodegeneration and iron accumulation constitute two completely unrelated events appearing in parallel.

In this review we aim to outline the potential links between pathophysiological mechanisms and the role of iron in neurodegeneration.

BRAIN IRON METABOLISM IN HEALTH AND AGING

Both excess and deficiency of iron lead to impaired brain function, thus tight regulation of iron metabolism is critical.

Iron enters the brain either bound to transferrin, thereby crossing the BBB or the blood-cerebrospinal fluid (CSF) barrier (Moos and Morgan, 2000), or possibly unbound, especially in conditions that result in iron overload as transferrin becomes saturated with iron. The exact uptake mechanisms in the latter case are unknown, but it is hypothesized that free serum iron might be reduced by cellular reductants such as ascorbate (Lane and Lawen, 2008; Lane et al., 2010; Lane and Richardson, 2014) to then be imported by divalent metal transporter 1 (DMT1) or ZRT/IRT-like proteins (ZIPs) like ZIP14 or ZIP8 (Jenkitkasemwong et al., 2012). Iron uptake into astroglia is thought to be mediated mainly by non-Tf bound iron (Ashraf et al., 2018), as TfR1 has so far only been reported *in vitro* (Pelizzoni et al., 2013). DMT1, a transporter located in cellular and endosomal membranes, is found in astrocytes and is believed to facilitate transport of non-transferrin bound iron into the cytoplasm (Xu and Ling, 1994). How iron is exported from the endothelial cells is still elusive (Ward et al., 2014). Within the CSF, iron occurs mainly as holo-transferrin (two ferric iron atoms bound to apo-transferrin) that interacts with TfR1. Neurons internalize the Tf-TfR1 complex into endosomes, where iron is separated from transferrin after acidification, converted into its ferrous form via reductase STEAP3 (Ohgami et al., 2005) and transported into the cytoplasm via DMT1 (Moos and Morgan, 2004).

Iron, prone to contribute to oxidative stress, can be (i) stored within ferritin (Zecca et al., 2004), (ii) imported into mitochondria, probably via so-called mitoferrins and TfR2 (Mastroberardino et al., 2009; Horowitz and Greenamyre, 2010), to enable biosynthesis of heme and iron-sulfur clusters and contribute in the respiratory chain reaction, or (iii) be released from the cell via ferroportin 1 (Ward et al., 2014). Intracellular iron homeostasis is tightly modulated by the iron regulatory protein (IRP) and iron-responsive element (IRE) signaling pathways (Pantopoulos, 2004; Zhang D.L. et al., 2014). IRP1 and IRP2 are two RNA-binding proteins that interact with IREs, non-coding sequences of messenger RNA (mRNA) transcripts to alter translation of ferritin, ferroportin and TfR mRNA. Ferritin H and L subunits or ferroportin mRNA transcripts carry IREs within the 5′-untranslated region (UTR), whereas mRNA transcripts for TfR and DMT-1 carry IRE motifs at the 3′-UTR. Cytosolic iron binds to IRPs and induces a conformational change within the molecule that does not allow attachment to IREs. Decreased iron levels on the other hand facilitate IRP–IRE interaction: IRP binding at the 5′-UTR inhibits further mRNA translation of ferritin subunits and ferroportin; at the 3′-UTR, binding protects against endonuclease cleavage (Pantopoulos, 2004; Zhou and Tan, 2017). Ferritin represents the dominant iron storage protein in the CNS, mostly found in glia and also within neurons, whereas neuromelanin (NM) captures large amounts of iron in certain neuronal populations for longer-term storage (Zucca et al., 2017). Recent studies have demonstrated that human poly-(rC)-binding proteins 1–4 (PCBPs 1–4) are implicated in iron transfer to ferritin (Philpott, 2012; Leidgens et al., 2013; Frey et al., 2014; Yanatori et al., 2014), which is a 24 subunit heteropolymer with heavy chains (H-type ferritin) with ferroxidase activity and light chains (L-type ferritin) crucial for subsequent iron storage. H-type ferritin occurs more abundantly in neurons for rapid mobilization and use, whereas in astro- and microglia L-type ferritin predominates for iron storage. In oligodendrocytes, both forms of ferritin are expressed (Ashraf et al., 2018). Neuromelanin (NM), a dark brown pigment, is present in dopaminergic neurons of the substantia nigra, the noradrenergic neurons of locus coeruleus, the ventral tegmental area, the ventral reticular formation and the nucleus of the solitary tract in the medulla oblongata (Zecca et al., 2004; Fedorow et al., 2005), but it has also been detected in the putamen, premotor cortex and cerebellum in lower amounts (Zecca et al., 2008; Engelen et al., 2012). Ferritin degradation by the autophagy-lysosome system (Asano et al., 2011) initiates iron release which can then be reutilized or exported, mainly through ferroportin 1 (Biasiotto et al., 2016). This requires ferroxidases ceruloplasmin and hephaestin to oxidize iron for export (Hentze et al., 2004). In addition, heme-oxygenase 1 represents a stress protein which degrades heme to ferrous iron in order to maintain iron homeostasis (Nitti et al., 2018). Systemic ferroportin levels are regulated by circulating hepcidin, the main iron regulatory hormone in the body - during iron overload and inflammation, hepcidin induces ferroportin internalization and degradation (Wang and Pantopoulos, 2011). The origin of hepcidin within the brain is unknown, It may be locally produced or systemically derived by passing the BBB (Vela, 2018). Conditional ferroportin knock-out mice for example do not show any significant intracellular iron accumulation in the brain, nor do they show behavioral or histological deficits compared to wildtype mice (Matak et al., 2016), suggesting that other cellular iron export mechanisms exist.

Iron accumulates as a function of the aging brain and thereby the levels of labile, potentially harmful iron increase (Ward et al., 2014). Iron accumulating at toxic levels within neurons, as seen in neurodegeneration, may lead to cell death via apoptosis, autophagy, necrosis or ferroptosis, a recently discovered mechanism of iron-mediated cell death distinct from apoptosis (Dixon et al., 2012). In glial cells however, iron accumulation triggers the release of pro-inflammatory cytokines, thereby creating a pro-inflammatory environment (Williams et al., 2012) which promotes neurodegeneration (Xu et al., 2012).

The underlying mechanisms of age and disease related region and cell specific differences in iron levels have not been fully elucidated yet, but the distinct iron richness of the basal ganglia may explain its increased vulnerability to neurodegeneration (Hallgren and Sourander, 1958; Zecca et al., 2004; Xu et al., 2012). In neurons of substantia nigra and locus coeruleus, premotor cortex, putamen, and cerebellum, neuromelanin levels are increased for sequestration of iron, however neuromelanin may itself exhibit toxic functions which are further explained in later sections (Zecca et al., 2004, 2008).

Astro- and microglia exhibit increased iron deposition and ferritin concentrations throughout their lifespan. In contrast, oligodendrocytes that constitute the main iron reservoir in the CNS (Connor et al., 1990; Kaindlstorfer et al., 2018) do not accumulate iron by aging. Iron is essential in the development of oligodendrocytes to allow proper axon myelination, as iron deficiency induces hypomyelination that persists even after the iron imbalance has been corrected (Todorich et al., 2009). The role of iron in oligodendrocytes is further exemplified by Tim-2, a receptor selective for H-ferritin uptake (Todorich et al., 2008). Neuroinflammation in the elderly brain is induced via activated microglia, a lot of which are ferritin-positive (Kaneko et al., 1989). Of those, most exhibit a dystrophic-type morphology, and it has been suggested that iron uptake into the activated microglia cells may represent another source of toxic iron, as seen in neurodegenerative diseases (Rathnasamy et al., 2013; McCarthy et al., 2018; Refolo et al., 2018).

IRON IN NEURODEGENERATIVE DISEASES – A ONE-SIZE-FITS-ALL?

Iron accumulation as a hallmark feature has been confirmed in many neurodegenerative diseases. **Figure 1** depicts dysfunctional pathways colocalizing with iron accumulation in neurodegeneration. Here, we review the contribution of iron to key mechanisms in neurodegeneration and evaluate its impact on pathogenesis.

Iron and Mitochondrial Dysfunction

Mitochondria provide neurons and glia with energy in the form of ATP via oxidative phosphorylation of glucose. Functional disruption of this pathway is likely to contribute to neurodegeneration. In PD, environmental toxins that disrupt mitochondrial complex I function like rotenone induce parkinsonism (Talpade et al., 2000; Dauer and Przedborski, 2003). Also, genetic causes of early-onset PD including PARK2, PINK1, and DJ-1 may interfere with mitochondrial autophagy, thus leading to mitochondrial dysfunction (Batlevi and La Spada, 2011). Moreover, transcriptional dysregulation of coactivator PGC-1α and PPAR transcription factors, including PPAR-δ (Dickey et al., 2016) may play an important role in sporadic AD (Katsouri et al., 2016), PD, and HD. Vulnerability of neural tissue to mitochondrial dysfunction is further demonstrated in single-gene mutations causative of systemic defects in mitochondrial quality control, that can trigger neurodegeneration without having an effect on peripheral tissue (Batlevi and La Spada, 2011). In an iPSC-model of familial PD, accumulation of oxidized dopamine as an effect of mitochondrial oxidative stress has downstream effects on lysosomal function and α-synuclein (α-syn) aggregation (Burbulla et al., 2017). Inversely, lysosomal dysfunction resulting in insufficient mitophagy shows that dysfunction of one system inevitably impairs the other (Plotegher and Duchen, 2017). A large part of intracellular iron is utilized for synthesis of heme and iron-sulfur clusters in mitochondria (Singh et al., 2014). Thus, iron homeostasis is heavily dependent upon proper mitochondrial function.

Neurodegeneration with brain iron accumulation comprises a number of pediatric and adult neurological diseases characterized by parkinsonism and dementia, and excessive iron accumulation in the basal ganglia among other regions (Hogarth, 2015). Distinct genetic causes have been described within this disease spectrum, yet no direct link between neurodegeneration and iron accumulation can be spanned in most forms. Mutations in PANK2, a gene implicated in coenzyme A biosynthesis, lipids synthesis and citric acid cycle (Zhou et al., 2001), results in panthoten kinase-associated neurodegeneration (PKAN). Though this mutation may not affect iron homeostasis directly, subsequent iron accumulation suggests that mitochondrial dysfunction may trigger iron dyshomeostasis. In iPSC-derived neurons from a PKAN patient, early disease stage phenotype is reflected by mitochondrial deficiency but absent iron dysregulation and iron chelation treatment causes further exacerbation of cellular dysfunction through iron deficiency (Arber et al., 2017).

In Friedreich's ataxia, expansions of unstable nucleotide repeats in the FXN gene result in reduced expression of frataxin (Campuzano et al., 1996), a protein thought to act as molecular chaperone in iron-sulfur clusters and heme biosynthesis as well as iron storage site (Alsina et al., 2018). Thus, lack of frataxin leads to mitochondrial iron overload and generation of ROS, which in turn impairs mitochondrial function creating a vicious cycle (Horowitz and Greenamyre, 2010). Decreased levels of frataxin were also observed in HD human and mouse brains, together with an increase of iron uptake protein mitoferrin 2 and mitochondrial iron accumulation (Agrawal et al., 2018). Interestingly, neonatal iron supplementation increases mitochondrial iron accumulation and mitochondrial dysfunction exacerbating neurodegeneration in HD mice. From

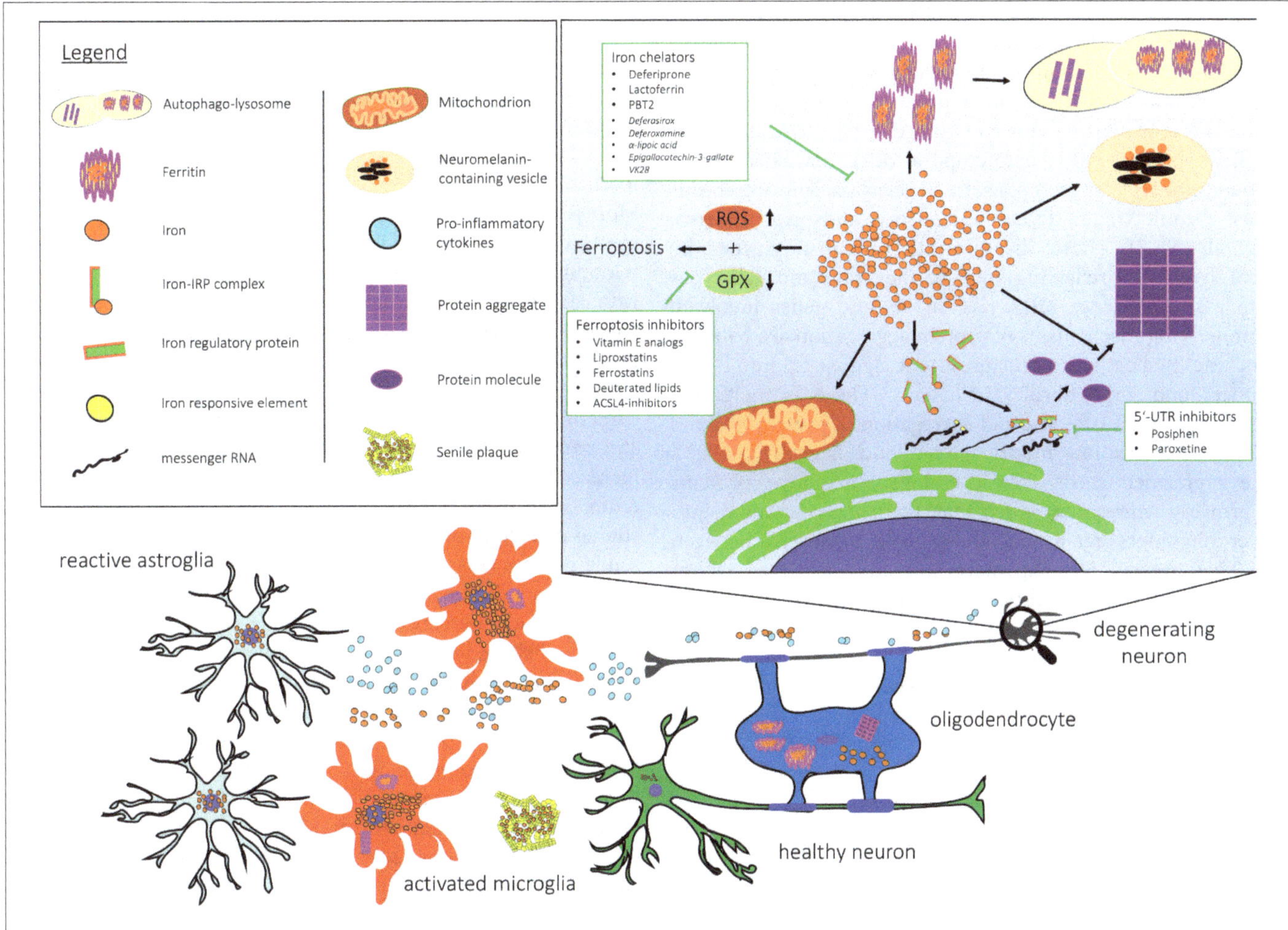

FIGURE 1 | Cellular and subcellular dysregulation linked with brain iron accumulation. 5′-UTR, 5′ untranslated region; ACSL-4, Acyl-CoA Synthetase Long Chain Family Member 4; GPX, gluthathione peroxidase; RNA, ribonucleic acid; ROS, reactive oxygen species.

this dataset it is difficult to conclude whether early-life iron exposure may cause mitochondrial dysfunction as an initiating step of neurodegeneration. It has been discussed that iron fortified infant formula within a critical window of susceptibility to iron overload may contribute to neurodegeneration in later life (Hare et al., 2015). Still, this remains highly speculative without evidence from prospective studies, but might indicate a causal role of iron in mitochondrial dysfunction. In a *Drosophila* model of Friedreich's ataxia, upregulation of mitoferrin associated with frataxin deficiency is observed. Interestingly, targeted downregulation of mitoferrin ameliorates the phenotype while worsening overall life span, indicating that due to its physiological function dysregulation of mitoferrin has detrimental consequences (Navarro et al., 2015). Knockdown of mitoferrin-1 in an Alzheimer model of *Caenorhabditis* elegans reduces paralysis rate and slows progression of AD by decreasing mitochondrial iron accumulation and ROS generation (Huang et al., 2018), showing that mitochondrial iron homeostasis may substantially impact neurodegeneration.

Another aspect favoring a causal role of iron in mitochondrial dysfunction is that damage of mitochondrial DNA due to oxidative stress is detected consistently at an early stage of neurodegeneration, and its vulnerability can be explained by a lack of protective histones (Shokolenko et al., 2009). Dysfunctional mitochondria produce less heme and ISCs, which causes activation of IRPs and further iron accumulation leading to positive feedback loop (Mena et al., 2015). In nigral dopaminergic neurons of human PD and the rotenone mouse model, transferrin accumulates intracellularly and large parts locate in mitochondria, which may be explained by the expression of TfR2 in the mitochondrial membrane of substantia nigra dopaminergic neurons (Mastroberardino et al., 2009). Elevated ROS levels in mitochondria oxidize holo-transferrin, which then tends to release ferrous, redox-reactive iron (Mastroberardino et al., 2009). Treating rats and monkeys with rotenone leads to downregulation of TfR1 in the presence of iron accumulation, whereas TfR2 levels remain elevated (Mastroberardino et al., 2009), supporting previous findings on TfR2 stability during iron overload in hepatic tissue (Fleming et al., 2000; Mifuji et al., 2006). TfR2 stability in conditions of neurodegeneration might thus exacerbate mitochondrial dysfunction, which in turn further affects iron handling.

Iron, Protein Misfolding, and Aggregation

Neurodegenerative diseases are characterized by extra- and/or intracellular accumulation of abnormally folded proteins and selective regional cell death in a progressive and predictable fashion (Fu et al., 2018). This includes AD, PD, MSA, dementia with Lewy bodies, PSP, frontotemporal dementia, corticobasal degeneration, HD, amyotrophic lateral sclerosis, spinocerebellar ataxias, chronic traumatic encephalopathy, and prion diseases (Fu et al., 2018). These disease entities are distinguished by clinical symptoms reflecting areas of the brain and cell types affected, by prevalence rates, risk factors and genes involved. The underlying mechanisms of protein aggregation are believed to include β-sheet-rich structures that aggregate into small oligomers and large fibrillar inclusions. There is increasing evidence that the misfolding and aggregation of proteins follows the seeding-nucleation model (Jarrett and Lansbury, 1993), where preformed seeds recruit endogenous native proteins into growing aggregates, which may then be fragmented into smaller oligomers again that are capable to spread between cells. This concept is being more and more accepted within the neuroscience community. Yet, it does not explain initial mechanisms underlying misfolding of distinct disease-associated proteins in sporadic neurodegeneration. Here, we summarize the current knowledge of interactions between iron and proteins implicated in neurodegenerative diseases.

Iron and α-Synuclein

Central to the pathogenesis of PD is the 17 kDa protein α-synuclein, which accumulates mainly into neuronal cytoplasmic inclusions termed Lewy bodies (Spillantini et al., 1997). Interestingly, α-synuclein can bind both ferrous and ferric iron (Peng et al., 2010), however only latter has been shown to promote aggregation (Levin et al., 2011). Phosphorylated α-synuclein at residue S129 is associated with Lewy bodies, and even though its role in PD pathogenesis has not been fully elucidated yet, it has been shown that phosphorylated synuclein exhibits increased binding affinity toward ferrous iron at the c-terminus (Lu et al., 2011). Iron and free radical generators like dopamine are able to induce aggregation of the wildtype protein in an *in vitro* model, and this effect is exacerbated by the cooccurrence of α-synuclein mutations A53T and A30P, suggesting a detrimental interplay in genetic forms of PD (Ostrerova-Golts et al., 2000). Importantly, α-synuclein possesses and IRE and IRP complexes during iron overload increase its translation resulting in elevated total α-synuclein burden (Friedlich et al., 2007; Zhou and Tan, 2017). On the other hand, it has been reported that α-synuclein exhibits ferrireductase activity that is increased in point mutations (A53T, A30P, or E46K), which may result in altered iron uptake and metabolism in the presence of divalent metal transporter 1 (Davies et al., 2011). In *Saccharomyces cerevisiae* and *Caenorhabditis elegans* models of Parkinson's disease, expression of α-synuclein may phenocopy a high iron condition by inhibiting recycling of iron transporter ortholog of ferroportin or membrane-bound ortholog of ceruloplasmin from endocytic vesicles back to the cell membrane. Iron chelation with desferoxamine partially rescued dopaminergic neurotoxicity in *Caenorhabditis elegans* (Patel et al., 2018).

Taken together, there seems to be an intricate interplay between α-synuclein and iron, both of which promote disease progression in synucleinopathies synergistically.

Iron and Aβ

More than half a decade ago Goodman provided first evidence for iron accumulation in senile plaques of post-mortem AD brains (Goodman, 1953), and more recently, brain imaging of patients with early stage AD demonstrated increased iron concentrations co-localizing with Aβ plaques which may both promote disease development and progression.

Long-term treatment of APP mice with 3,5,5-trimethyhexanoyl ferrocene reveal accelerated plaque formation and more senile morphology, microglial iron inclusions and increased amounts of Aβ (Peters et al., 2018). Although the redox state of iron located in plaques is still elusive, recent studies detected iron oxide magnetite nanoparticles in the core of senile plaques (Plascencia-Villa et al., 2016; Everett et al., 2018). Furthermore, Telling et al. (2017) provide evidence for a direct iron–amyloid interaction within senile plaques. Increased iron levels are believed to enhance Aβ production via downregulation of furin, a proprotein convertase participating in α-secretase-dependent APP processing, which in turn activates β-secretase implicated in Aβ generation (Silvestri and Camaschella, 2008). SH5SY cells exposed to ferric ammonium citrate confirm an increase in β-secretase levels coupled with enhanced $A\beta_{42}$ production, in addition iron treatment promotes accumulation of APP (Banerjee et al., 2014). Interestingly however, in a recent study ferric iron treatment in rat cortical neurons facilitates non-amyloidogenic processing of APP via α-secretase, intracellular localization of sAPPα impaired enzymatic activity of β-secretase, and thus decreases levels of sAPPβ and Aβ (Chen et al., 2018). Boopathi and Kolandaivel (2016) show that ferrous iron induces a structural conformation in Aβ toward a β-sheet structure which tends to form oligomers and fibrils, whereas other groups demonstrate that ferric iron promotes aggregation of both $A\beta_{40}$ and $A\beta_{42}$ as well as cytotoxicity *in vitro* (Tahmasebinia and Emadi, 2017; Galante et al., 2018). $A\beta_{42}$ promotes magnetite nanoparticle formation (Tahirbegi et al., 2016), thus coming full circle and providing evidence for a causative role of iron in AD pathogenesis. The IRP-IRE signaling pathway is also involved in proteostasis of APP (Rogers et al., 2008). Thus, sustained iron overload may result in elevated Aβ-levels, the core constituent of extracellular plaques in AD. Intriguingly, genetic manipulation of iron metabolism substantially influences Aβ toxicity in model organisms. Overexpression of ferritin heavy chain, but also iron chelation, rescue Aβ-mediated toxicity in a Drosophila model expressing Aβ (Rival et al., 2009; Liu et al., 2011).

Iron and Tau

Tauopathies including AD, PSP, corticobasal degeneration, frontotemporal dementia, but also PD and HD, are characterized by neurofibrillary tangles, the core of which consists of paired helical filaments composed of hyperphosphorylated tau. Tau facilitates microtubule stabilization and regulation, regulation of axonal transport (Magnani et al., 2007; Dixit et al., 2008) and likely plays a role in neurotransmission and iron metabolism by the trafficking of APP to the cell surface (Lei et al., 2012).

These functions may be disrupted following hyperphosphorylation of tau, and iron has been shown to mediate this modification depending on its redox state. Whereas Fe (II) forms a reversible interaction through threonine residues, Fe (III) induces an irreversible conformational change, both of which promote aggregation of tau (Ahmadi et al., 2017). Hyperphosphorylation of tau, one of the key steps toward aggregation, may be induced by iron via (CDK25)/P25 complex and GSK-3β (Xie et al., 2012; Guo et al., 2013). In addition, Fe (III) may mediate nitration of tau, which prevents microtubule stabilization and is commonly found in neurofibrillary tangles and senile plaques (Nakamura and Lipton, 2011). Tau accumulation in tangles on the other hand leads to induction of heme-oxygenase 1, an antioxidant that promotes release of the redox-active Fe (II), which releases free radicals to generate oxidative stress (Ward et al., 2014). This in turn promotes tau hyperphosphorylation and aggregation (Lane et al., 2018). Intracellular iron accumulation, a common feature in tauopathies, leads to loss of tau function, which prevents iron export through impaired transport of APP to the cell membrane, where it stabilizes ferroportin (Wong et al., 2014) resulting in a vicious cycle of iron accumulation and tau pathology.

Iron and Autophagic-Lysosomal Dysfunction

Autophagic-lysosomal dysfunction is a hallmark feature of neurodegenerative proteinopathies, either due to mutations directly affecting the autophagy-lysosome machinery, or secondary to aggregation of misfolded proteins. Iron dyshomeostasis may occur as a consequence of inadequate ferritinophagy, a term coined to describe the lysosomal degradation of ferritin molecules mediated via nuclear receptor co-activator 4 (NCOA4) (Mancias et al., 2014; Biasiotto et al., 2016). As both autophagy activation and inhibition have been reported in neurodegeneration, aberrant ferritinophagy may lead to iron dyshomeostasis manifesting as iron deficiency or overload, both of which exert deleterious effects on cell survival. In line with that, quantifications of ferritin levels in substantia nigra of PD brain reveal contradictory findings in the literature (Zecca et al., 2001; Koziorowski et al., 2007; Sian-Hülsmann et al., 2011; Friedman and Galazka-Friedman, 2012; Galazka-Friedman et al., 2012). NCOA4 levels, targeting ferritin heavy chain 1 for ferritin degradation, may be critical for ferritinophagy as factors such as oxidative stress regulate NCOA4 gene transcription (Sharifi et al., 2008). Pharmacological inhibition of autophagy leads to NCOA4 accumulation (Dowdle et al., 2014), probably as a compensatory mechanism. In addition, NCOA4-depletion seems to have a protective effect during oxidative stress (Mancias et al., 2014), possibly contrabalancing transcriptional and translational regulation of ferritin in situations of stress (Torti and Torti, 2002). Another part of the autophagic machinery slowly accumulating iron high amounts of iron, copper and zinc as well as various toxins over the course of several decades constitutes neuromelanin (Zecca et al., 2008). In addition, intracellular dopamine in excess can be metabolized into the more stable NM molecule. However, externalization of neuromelanin organelles and subsequent release of content as seen in PD activates microglia, which may accelerate further cell death and release of neuromelanin-containing vesicles, thereby creating a self-perpetuating cycle (Zhang W. et al., 2013; Zucca et al., 2017). Recent data suggests that neuromelanin-containing vesicles in PD may represent a specialized autolysosomal compartment, where proteins and lipids not otherwise degraded are accumulated in a very slow turnover rhythm (Zucca et al., 2018). Neuromelanin accumulates within vesicles over time, and in PD, and a strong correlation between nigral cell loss and amount of pigmented neuromelanin-immunoreactive neurons could be shown, providing first evidence that neuromelanin-pigmented cells may exhibit increased vulnerability during PD pathogenesis (Zucca et al., 2018). One possible explanation is that at a certain threshold of iron level in PD brains buffering capacities in the form of NM and ferritin are exhausted (Good et al., 1992; Jellinger et al., 1992), and then redox-active iron is freed and may have deleterious consequences and significantly contributes to subsequent pathology (Faucheux et al., 2003).

Iron and Neuroinflammation

Microglia are in a constant cross-talk with neurons and are capable of sensing neuronal dyshomeostasis. Microglial activation is a healthy reaction against disease and injury, accompanied by the release of pro- and anti-inflammatory factors, ROS and recruitment molecules (Colton and Gilbert, 1987; Graeber et al., 1988; Hurley et al., 1999). Chronic neuroinflammation however, a hallmark feature of neurodegenerative diseases, creates a pro-apoptotic environment resulting in neuronal death and thus becomes a driver of neurodegeneration itself (Lull and Block, 2010). AD and PD brains show extensive proliferation of reactive macrophages and activated microglia. In addition to the cocktail of cytokines and ROS released by microglia cells, they also produce high levels of NAPDH oxidase and nitric oxide synthase, two main players of oxidative stress and ROS generation during inflammation (Urrutia et al., 2014).

Interestingly, microglia turn out to be far more efficient in sequestering iron compared to other brain cell types, as levels of ferritin induced by iron exposure in an organotypic slice culture model are highest in microglia and oligodendrocytes, whereas ferritin is rarely detected in astrocytes and, surprisingly, never in neurons (Healy et al., 2016).

Exposing cultured neurons to ferric iron reveals accumulation of iron, however microglia accumulates eightfold more iron than neurons and 4.7-fold more than cultured astrocytes after 24 h (Bishop et al., 2011). Activated microglia in substantia nigra of post-mortem PD brains exhibit enhanced ferritin immunoreactivity (Mirza et al., 2000), yet iron burden does not correlate with ferritin in a linear fashion, as high iron saturation in microglia may be achieved despite low ferritin baseline, as seen in conditions of acute oxidative stress (Mehlhase et al., 2005; Thomsen et al., 2015). In neurodegeneration, iron-containing microglia co-localize with affected areas (Andersen et al., 2014) and there is some intriguing evidence pointing toward a substantial contribution of microglia-associated iron in disease. Ferrous iron in primary midbrain cultures causes progressive dopaminergic neurodegeneration mediated by microglial β-nicotinamide adenine dinucleotide phosphate oxidase 2, a superoxide generator, and inhibition of the enzyme prevents neurotoxicity reflected in decreased levels of superoxide (Zhang W. et al., 2014). Intriguingly however, Wang et al. report that iron accumulation in microglia alone is not sufficient to trigger release of proinflammatory cytokines TNF-α, IL-1β, and IL-6, instead MPP+ is required to trigger enzymatic release, which is then aggravated if iron accumulation is present (Wang et al., 2013). Inflammatory stimuli including TNF-α, IL-β and toll-like receptor-4 agonist lipopolysaccharide (Yang et al., 2002) on the other hand are able to trigger neuronal iron accumulation via alteration of DMT1 and FPN mRNA levels (Urrutia et al., 2013). This is supported by another study showing increased DMT1 and TfR1 and decreased FPN1 protein levels following TNF-α or IL-1β treatment (Wang et al., 2013).

Increased iron uptake in substantia nigra in PD patients has been linked with altered expression of lactoferrin receptor on vulnerable dopaminergic neurons (Faucheux et al., 1995). In addition, lactoferrin has been implicated in AD pathogenesis due to its presence in senile plaques and neurofibrillary tangles in the limbic system (Wang et al., 2015). Lactoferrin is produced only by activated microglia (Fillebeen et al., 2001; An et al., 2009; Wang et al., 2015) and it is suggested that it may have a protective function in neurodegeneration by modulating mitochondrial calcium homeostasis (Fillebeen et al., 1999; Rousseau et al., 2013) rather than sole iron chelation following MPP+ injury (Wang et al., 2015).

Astroglia as part of the BBB are involved in strict separation and regulation of brain iron metabolism from the periphery (Moos et al., 2007; Burkhart et al., 2016). They express coeruloplasmin to facilitate iron uptake and distribution (McCarthy and Kosman, 2015) and hephaestin, indicating ferroxidase activity (Wang et al., 2007). However, astroglia contain relatively small amounts of ferritin and iron (Mirza et al., 2000; Zecca et al., 2004; Bartzokis et al., 2007), yet *in vitro* studies in cultured astrocytes show that cultured astrocytes are surprisingly resistant to ferrous iron compared to neurons and oligodendrocytes, even though intracellular iron burden is comparable (Kress et al., 2002; Oshiro et al., 2008). Possibly this is due to an extensive antioxidative system including metallothioneins (Waller et al., 2018). Astroglia possess heme oxygenase-1, which has been shown to be neuroprotective in different models of PD by impeding oxidative stress (Xu et al., 2016; Yu et al., 2016), it has to be noted however that during the degradation of heme catalyzed by the enzyme, bio-reactive iron is released to participate in Fenton's reaction (Cuadrado and Rojo, 2008). Astroglial increase of iron levels is observed in substantia nigra of PD (Jellinger et al., 1990), which is accompanied by astroglial activation, reflected in part by the up-regulation of lipocalin-2, which, if overexpressed in experimental conditions, initiates nigrostriatal dopaminergic neurodegeneration that is aggravated following iron treatment (Kim et al., 2016). Neurotrophic factors BDNF and GDNF, produced by astroglia besides oligodendrocytes, prevent neuronal iron accumulation by affecting IRPs linked with DMT1 expression (Zhang H.Y. et al., 2014), highlighting the crucial role of astroglial health on iron regulation. In case of iron accumulation, exemplified by a study from Rathore et al. including treatment of rat astrocytes with ferrous iron, increased expression of DMT1, ferroportin and both ferritin subunits are observed. However, co-treatment with TNF-α diminished the increase in H-ferritin, whereas the elevated L-ferritin levels are not altered (Rathore et al., 2012). This raises the question whether microglial activation in form of TNF-α secretion might impair astroglial iron handling and storage. In the 6-OHDA neurotoxin rat model of PD, altered BBB permeability is associated with microglial iron accumulation and increased levels of L-ferritin besides neurodegeneration in substantia nigra (Olmedo-Díaz et al., 2017). Using Mössbauer spectrometry, Friedman et al. (2011) determine decreased levels of L-ferritin in substantia nigra in PD brains in contrast to experimental results.

Iron as cause of neuroinflammation has also been shown in ALS by introducing the G93A mutation of ALS-associated human superoxide dismutase 1 (SOD1) in mice, which results in iron accumulation of ventral motor neurons. Intriguingly, an increase in the enzymatic activity of TNF-α - converting enzyme and subsequent enhanced secretion of soluble TNF-α is observed triggered by iron whereas chelation with deferoxamine mesylate delays disease onset and prolongs overall lifespan (Milanese et al., 2014).

Ferroptosis in Neurodegeneration

Ferroptosis represents a recently discovered form of cell death independent of the caspase pathway and involves iron dysregulation, lipid peroxidation and inflammation as major hallmarks (Dixon, 2017). Central to this phenomenon is the depletion of glutathione, an antioxidant that buffers ROS and binds to labile iron (Hider and Kong, 2011) to prevent Fenton reaction with subsequent ROS production. This imbalance in cellular redox homeostasis causes the accumulation of lipid ROS and thus lipid peroxidation (Gao et al., 2016; Abdalkader et al., 2018). Morphological changes reflecting the consequences include reduced mitochondrial volume (Dixon et al., 2012; Xie et al., 2016), reduced density of mitochondrial membranes (Xie et al., 2016), chromatin condensation (Dixon et al., 2012), cytoplasmic swelling, and eventually rupture of mitochondrial outer membrane (Friedmann Angeli et al., 2014; Xie et al., 2016) and plasma membrane (Dixon et al., 2012). A number of potent inducers of ferroptosis have been identified (Stockwell et al., 2017), among which the small molecule erastin potently induces ferroptosis via inhibition of the xCT cystine/glutamate antiporter, as cystine is essential for glutathione synthesis. Reduced gluthatione is utilized by glutathione peroxidase GPX4 (Yang et al., 2014) to detoxify phospholipid hydroperoxides and hydrogen peroxides (Ursini and Bindoli, 1987). Interestingly, GPX4 knock-out in mice revealed not only iron dysregulation, lipid peroxidation and inflammation, but in addition early signs of an AD phenotype including behavior dysfunction and hippocampal neurodegeneration (Seiler et al., 2008; Hambright et al., 2017). The deleterious effects on neuronal health and survival upon ablation of GPX4 in motor neurons might confer a role of ferroptosis to degenerative motor neuron diseases like amyotrophic lateral sclerosis (Chen et al., 2015).

Key features of ferroptosis including lipid peroxidation and reduced glutathione levels have been detected previously in the substantia nigra in PD (Dexter et al., 1989; Jenner et al., 1992) and colocalize with accumulated iron. According or Jenner et al. these findings may represent early events in the disease (Jenner et al., 1992). In addition, mitochondrial damage, commonly observed in PD as well, may be mediated by the interaction of α-synuclein with mitochondrial membranes, thus aggravating mitochondrial vulnerability and oxidative stress further (Parihar et al., 2008).

Therefore, targeting ferroptosis in neurodegeneration may represent an attractive target for disease modification. Potential candidates include vitamin E analogs, liproxstatins and ferrostatins, deuterated lipids and ACSL4 (Acyl-CoA Synthetase Long Chain Family Member 4) inhibitors (Angeli et al., 2017).

CAN IRON CAUSE NEURODEGENERATION?

Based on the literature reviewed to this point it is certain that iron contributes substantially to neurodegeneration, however so far, no compelling evidence was provided to attribute a causal role to iron, which would imply (1) detection at an early stage if not as first sign, and (2) evidence for disease modification if targeted appropriately. We aim to address both issues based on current knowledge and progress made to this point.

Targeting Iron Dyshomeostasis for Disease Modification in Neurodegeneration

In the past few years numerous targets for treatment of iron dysregulation have been identified including reduction of iron burden but also inhibition of downstream effects. However, the numerous physiological functions of iron and defects resulting from aggressive iron depletion need to be considered. Therefore, the following features of treatment of brain iron dyshomeostasis could be taken into account: ability to pass BBB and consecutive cell membranes; chelation of excess iron with moderate affinity to avoid depletion of transferrin and iron-associated proteins; prevention of side effects due to iron removal in areas lacking iron overload (Boddaert et al., 2007; Hamilton et al., 2017; Loza-Rosas et al., 2017). Here, we will discuss potential candidates based on those selection criteria.

Deferiprone

Deferiprone is an iron chelator currently in use for systemic iron overload conditions like thalassemia major, but its benefit in neurodegenerative conditions lacking systemic iron dysregulation has been shown in a small trial in 9 patients with Friedreich's ataxia, who received deferiprone for 6 months. Treatment results in decreased iron load in dentate nuclei as visualized by MRI, an area implicated in neurodegeneration. Moreover, motor skills and signs of neuropathy are improved especially in the younger patients, and no severe side effects are reported (Boddaert et al., 2007). Deferiprone acts as "conservative iron chelator" by redistributing iron from overloaded areas to areas deprived of iron, thereby keeping overall iron levels stable (Cabantchik et al., 2013). In a 12 months double-blind pilot study (FAIRPARK-I), 40 PD patients were recruited, and treatment with deferiprone reduces substantia nigra hyperechogenicity in MRI and shows clinical improvement determined by the Unified PD Rating Scale (UPDRS) (Devos et al., 2014).

Interestingly however, in another phase II trial on deferiprone 22 early-disease patients (Martin-Bastida et al., 2017) reveal no change in iron content of putamen, striatum nor substantia nigra except for 3 cases. In dentate and caudate nuclei decreased iron load is determined by MRI. In this study, no improvement in motor-UPDRS is observed, even though a trend is achieved in the high dose-tier (30 mg/kg). An ongoing phase III trial, FAIRPARK-II, will reveal further insights into the potential benefits of deferiprone in PD.

Lactoferrin

Lactoferrin (LF) is an iron-binding glycoprotein with 60% amino acid sequence homology to transferrin (Metz-Boutigue et al., 1984). However, LF affinity for iron is 300 times higher than transferrin (Dhennin-Duthille et al., 2000) and it can act by binding two iron, zinc, copper particles or other metals. In AD brain, abnormal LF content was described already a few decades ago (Brown et al., 1985) and in 2010 Wang et al. could show that LF is present in AD model mice, but not healthy wildtype mice (Wang et al., 2010). There is a strong correlation between LF and Aβ, as LF levels increase following generation of Aβ, and with Aβ plaque formation lactoferrin continues to accumulate (van de Looij et al., 2014).

There is evidence of a protective function of lactoferrin as exogenous application results in reduced Aβ deposition and improvement of cognitive decline in AD mice via enhanced non-amyloidogenic processing of APP and α -secretase expression and activity through ERK/1/2-CREB and HIF-1α pathways (Guo et al., 2017). In MPTP mice modeling PD, administration of LF results in reduction of MPTP-induced iron accumulation via suppressed upregulation of DMT1 and TfR. Furthermore, neuroprotection is mediated by an increase in BDNF and HIF-1α with downstream activation of ERK/1/2-CREB pathway (Xu et al., 2018). In addition, LF receptors are found at the BBB, therefore LF may also be utilized as carrier for iron chelators that would otherwise be excluded from CNS. Kamalinia et al. conjugated LF with deferasirox to inject into AD mice, which ameliorates memory function, reduces Aβ levels, and leads to attenuation of apoptosis markers and increase in autophagy (Kamalinia et al., 2013). In a recent pilot study 50 AD patients were treated with lactoferrin for 3 months to find significant improvement in antioxidant and anti-inflammatory markers in serum, and decrease in $A\beta_{42}$, phosphorylated tau, interleukin-6 and caspase-3 as well as improved cognitive function (Mohamed et al., 2019), possibly opening the doors toward new treatments in AD, however further follow-up data are required.

PBT2

Metal chaperone PBT2 is a derivate of clioquinol, an iron, copper and zinc chelator. In a phase II trial for AD clioquinol improved cognition and decreased Aβ plasma levels (Ritchie et al., 2003), however in a transgenic AD mouse model toxicity manifested by myelinopathy was observed (Zhang Y.H. et al., 2013). PBT2 on the other hand improved cognition and decreased intracerebral Aβ levels in preclinical AD models (Adlard et al., 2011, 2014). A phase II trial in 78 AD patients revealed significant reduction in CSF $A\beta_{42}$ and improved cognition by two measures of executive function (Lannfelt et al., 2008; Faux et al., 2010).

IRE (5′UTR) Inhibitors

Another promising target in the self-perpetuating cycle of iron and disease-associated protein accumulation represents the inhibition of the IRE in the 5′-UTR of α-synuclein and APP (Zhou and Tan, 2017). Two compounds have now been tested in clinical trials, these include Posiphen, a phenyl carbamoyl analog of (+)-physostigmine, second-generation 8-hydroxyquinoline analog metal chaperone PBT2, and paroxetine, an antidepressant of the selective serotonin-reuptake inhibitor class.

Posiphen potently inhibits translation of APP and α-synuclein in preclinical models (Shaw et al., 2001; Yu et al., 2013; Teich et al., 2018). In a phase I human trial and a small non-randomized study of five subjects with mild cognitive impairment, administration of posiphen is well tolerated and decreases levels of sAPPα, sAPPβ, total and phosphorylated tau, and inflammatory marker in CSF. In addition, a trend toward lower $A\beta_{42}$ is observed (Maccecchini et al., 2012).

Besides, paroxetine is widely used in the treatment of depression acting through selective inhibition of serotonine reuptake and may represent a suitable candidate for drug repurposing in AD. Preclinical *in vitro* and *in vivo* evidence supports the effects of paroxetine as chemical IRE modulator on APP expression (Payton et al., 2003; Tucker et al., 2006; Bandyopadhyay and Rogers, 2014), and its clinical safety has obviously been proven due to its indication in depression.

Iron as MRI Biomarker for Disease Progression

One of the major drawbacks in therapeutic research of neurodegenerative diseases is a lack of biomarkers for earlier diagnosis, providing a chance for successful disease-modifying treatments. Advances in MRI technology to facilitate more accurate and specific detection of iron may help to determine the biomarker status of iron accumulation at preclinical stages of neurodegeneration. For an extensive review on the use of MRI for brain iron detection we refer to excellent reviews (Schweser et al., 2011; Schipper, 2012).

In premotor PD patients, MRI scans revealed increased echogenicity in substantia nigra, probably indicative of labile iron (Berg et al., 2011). De Marzi et al. (2016) investigated a cohort of patients with idiopathic rapid eye movement sleep behavior disorder (iRBD), a majority of which went on to develop PD. Interestingly, loss of dorsolateral nigral hyperintensity in a T2* map, a sign for low neuromelanin reflecting the loss of dopaminergic neurons (Blazejewska et al., 2013), was determined both in iRBD as well as in PD patients, indicating that loss of dorsolateral nigral hyperintensity may represent a promising biomarker for prodromal PD (De Marzi et al., 2016). In a cohort with carriers of the apolipoprotein ε4 allele at risk for AD and patients with mild cognitive impairment, representing early stage AD, quantitative susceptibility mapping MRI revealed higher Ab plaque load as well as increased iron concentrations colocalizing with Ab plaques both in cortical as well as sub-cortical brain areas (van Bergen et al., 2016). In Huntington's disease however, examination of premanifest gene carriers and early Huntington's disease patients exhibit no differences in iron content in asymptomatic carriers, whereas in early patients a lower R2* parameter value, indicating alterations in iron burden, was observed. In this case, iron measurement by MRI may rather be a marker of disease progression (Di Paola et al., 2014). In genetically and phenotypically distinct disorders like ALS with variable upper and lower motor neuron affection, a reliable biomarker is urgently needed for both early and accurate diagnosis. MRI in ALS patient cohorts shows hypointensity in deep layers of motor cortex, and increased hypointensity correlates with more severe affection of upper motor neurons (Kwan et al., 2012). Direct comparison of MRI signal changes in ALS with histological examination of post-mortem ALS brains revealed that motor cortex hypointensity corresponds to microglial iron accumulation, which may have utility as marker for disease progression (Pallebage-Gamarallage et al., 2018). Taken together, brain iron detection via MRI will be a powerful tool in the future both for early diagnosis and for evaluation of disease progression in neurodegenerative disorders. Detection of biochemical or structural components implicated in the disease process in addition to brain iron have immense potential to elucidate early pathophysiological changes in the otherwise inaccessible brain.

CONCLUSION AND OUTLOOK

Experimental data show that many neurodegenerative diseases represent conditions of multifactorial cellular dysfunction associated with iron dyshomeostasis present already at early disease stages, yet preclinical models may not be able to answer what comes first in sporadic neurodegenerative diseases. Intriguingly however, iron substantially contributes to and drives many aspects of neurodegeneration, plus, genetic modification of iron metabolism resulted in rescue of neurodegeneration in different animal models, indicating a causal role of iron in neurodegenerative disorders. Advances in MRI technology to facilitate more accurate and specific detection of iron hold great promise to implement iron as a biomarker for preclinical stages of neurodegeneration, probably a crucial treatment window for upcoming therapies. Moreover, CSF levels of iron related proteins in sporadic neurodegenerative diseases may aid in early diagnosis in the future, like CSF ferritin in AD (Ayton et al., 2015, 2017). Currently, a number of various promising compounds targeting different aspects of iron dysregulation besides conventional iron chelation are being tested at different clinical and preclinical trial stages. Recently discovered mechanisms like ferroptosis may pose promising targets for disease modification via ferrostatins in the future.

AUTHOR CONTRIBUTIONS

AN wrote the manuscript. CK and GW edited and revised the manuscript.

FUNDING

This study was supported by grant F4414 of the Austrian Science Fund (FWF).

REFERENCES

Abdalkader, M., Lampinen, R., Kanninen, K. M., Malm, T. M., and Liddell, J. R. (2018). Targeting Nrf2 to suppress ferroptosis and mitochondrial dysfunction in neurodegeneration. *Front. Neurosci.* 12:466. doi: 10.3389/fnins.2018.00466

Adlard, P. A., Bica, L., White, A. R., Nurjono, M., Filiz, G., Crouch, P. J., et al. (2011). Metal ionophore treatment restores dendritic spine density and synaptic protein levels in a mouse model of Alzheimer's disease. *PLoS One* 6:e17669. doi: 10.1371/journal.pone.0017669

Adlard, P. A., Sedjahtera, A., Gunawan, L., Bray, L., Hare, D., Lear, J., et al. (2014). A novel approach to rapidly prevent age-related cognitive decline. *Aging Cell* 13, 351–359. doi: 10.1111/acel.12178

Agrawal, S., Fox, J., Thyagarajan, B., and Fox, J. H. (2018). Brain mitochondrial iron accumulates in Huntington's disease, mediates mitochondrial dysfunction, and can be removed pharmacologically. *Free Radic. Biol. Med.* 120, 317–329. doi: 10.1016/j.freeradbiomed.2018.04.002

Ahmadi, S., Ebralidze, I. I., She, Z., and Kraatz, H.-B. (2017). Electrochemical studies of tau protein-iron interactions—Potential implications for Alzheimer's Disease. *Electrochim. Acta* 236, 384–393. doi: 10.1016/j.electacta.2017.03.175

Alsina, D., Purroy, R., Ros, J., and Tamarit, J. (2018). Iron in Friedreich ataxia: a central role in the pathophysiology or an epiphenomenon? *Pharmaceuticals* 11:E89. doi: 10.3390/ph11030089

An, L., Sato, H., Konishi, Y., Walker, D. G., Beach, T. G., Rogers, J., et al. (2009). Expression and localization of lactotransferrin messenger RNA in the cortex of Alzheimer's disease. *Neurosci. Lett.* 452, 277–280. doi: 10.1016/j.neulet.2009.01.071

Andersen, H. H., Johnsen, K. B., and Moos, T. (2014). Iron deposits in the chronically inflamed central nervous system and contributes to neurodegeneration. *Cell. Mol. Life Sci.* 71, 1607–1622. doi: 10.1007/s00018-013-1509-8

Angeli, J. P. F., Shah, R., Pratt, D. A., and Conrad, M. (2017). Ferroptosis inhibition: mechanisms and opportunities. *Trends Pharmacol. Sci.* 38, 489–498. doi: 10.1016/j.tips.2017.02.005

Apostolakis, S., and Kypraiou, A. M. (2017). Iron in neurodegenerative disorders: being in the wrong place at the wrong time? *Rev. Neurosci.* 28, 893–911. doi: 10.1515/revneuro-2017-0020

Arber, C., Angelova, P. R., Wiethoff, S., Tsuchiya, Y., Mazzacuva, F., Preza, E., et al. (2017). iPSC-derived neuronal models of PANK2-associated neurodegeneration reveal mitochondrial dysfunction contributing to early disease. *PLoS One* 12:e0184104. doi: 10.1371/journal.pone.0184104

Asano, T., Komatsu, M., Yamaguchi, Y., Ishikawa-Iwai, F., Mizushima, N., and Iwai, K. (2011). Distinct mechanisms of ferritin delivery to lysosomes in iron-depleted and iron-replete cells. *Mol. Cell. Biol.* 31, 2040–2052. doi: 10.1128/MCB.01437-10

Ashraf, A., Clark, M., and So, P. W. (2018). The aging of iron man. *Front. Aging Neurosci.* 10:65. doi: 10.3389/fnagi.2018.00065

Ayton, S., Faux, N. G., and Bush, A. I. (2017). Association of cerebrospinal fluid ferritin level with preclinical cognitive decline in APOE-ε4 carriers. *JAMA Neurol.* 74, 122–125. doi: 10.1001/jamaneurol.2016.4406

Ayton, S., Faux, N. G., Bush, A. I., and Alzheimer's Disease Neuroimaging Initiative. (2015). Ferritin levels in the cerebrospinal fluid predict Alzheimer's disease outcomes and are regulated by APOE. *Nat. Commun.* 6:6760. doi: 10.1038/ncomms7760

Bandyopadhyay, S., and Rogers, J. T. (2014). Alzheimer's disease therapeutics targeted to the control of amyloid precursor protein translation: maintenance of brain iron homeostasis. *Biochem. Pharmacol.* 88, 486–494. doi: 10.1016/j.bcp.2014.01.032

Banerjee, P., Sahoo, A., Anand, S., Ganguly, A., Righi, G., Bovicelli, P., et al. (2014). Multiple mechanisms of iron-induced amyloid beta-peptide accumulation in SHSY5Y cells: protective action of negletein. *Neuromolecular Med.* 16, 787–798. doi: 10.1007/s12017-014-8328-4

Bartzokis, G., Tishler, T. A., Lu, P. H., Villablanca, P., Altshuler, L. L., Carter, M., et al. (2007). Brain ferritin iron may influence age- and gender-related risks of neurodegeneration. *Neurobiol. Aging* 28, 414–423. doi: 10.1016/j.neurobiolaging.2006.02.005

Batlevi, Y., and La Spada, A. R. (2011). Mitochondrial autophagy in neural function, neurodegenerative disease, neuron cell death, and aging. *Neurobiol. Dis.* 43, 46–51. doi: 10.1016/j.nbd.2010.09.009

Berg, D., and Hochstrasser, H. (2006). Iron metabolism in Parkinsonian syndromes. *Mov. Disord.* 21, 1299–1310. doi: 10.1002/mds.21020

Berg, D., Seppi, K., Behnke, S., Liepelt, I., Schweitzer, K., Stockner, H., et al. (2011). Enlarged substantia nigra hyperechogenicity and risk for Parkinson disease: a 37-month 3-center study of 1847 older persons. *Arch. Neurol.* 68, 932–937. doi: 10.1001/archneurol.2011.141

Biasiotto, G., Di Lorenzo, D., Archetti, S., and Zanella, I. (2016). Iron and neurodegeneration: is ferritinophagy the link? *Mol. Neurobiol.* 53, 5542–5574. doi: 10.1007/s12035-015-9473-y

Bishop, G. M., Dang, T. N., Dringen, R., and Robinson, S. R. (2011). Accumulation of non-transferrin-bound iron by neurons, astrocytes, and microglia. *Neurotox. Res.* 19, 443–451. doi: 10.1007/s12640-010-9195-x

Blazejewska, A. I., Schwarz, S. T., Pitiot, A., Stephenson, M. C., Lowe, J., Bajaj, N., et al. (2013). Visualization of nigrosome 1 and its loss in PD: pathoanatomical correlation and in vivo 7 T MRI. *Neurology* 81, 534–540. doi: 10.1212/WNL.0b013e31829e6fd2

Boddaert, N., Le Quan Sang, K. H., Rötig, A., Leroy-Willig, A., Gallet, S., Brunelle, F., et al. (2007). Selective iron chelation in Friedreich ataxia: biologic and clinical implications. *Blood* 110, 401–408. doi: 10.1182/blood-2006-12-065433

Bolognin, S., Messori, L., and Zatta, P. (2009). Metal ion physiopathology in neurodegenerative disorders. *Neuromolecular Med.* 11, 223–238. doi: 10.1007/s12017-009-8102-1

Boopathi, S., and Kolandaivel, P. (2016). Fe(2+) binding on amyloid β-peptide promotes aggregation. *Proteins* 84, 1257–1274. doi: 10.1002/prot.25075

Brown, R. D., Rickard, K. A., and Kronenberg, H. (1985). Lactoferrin in the myeloproliferative disorders: a search for granulopoietic regulator defects. *Br. J. Haematol.* 59, 617–626. doi: 10.1111/j.1365-2141.1985.tb07356.x

Burbulla, L. F., Song, P., Mazzulli, J. R., Zampese, E., Wong, Y. C., Jeon, S., et al. (2017). Dopamine oxidation mediates mitochondrial and lysosomal dysfunction in Parkinson's disease. *Science* 357, 1255–1261. doi: 10.1126/science.aam9080

Burkhart, A., Skjørringe, T., Johnsen, K. B., Siupka, P., Thomsen, L. B., Nielsen, M. S., et al. (2016). Expression of iron-related proteins at the neurovascular unit supports reduction and reoxidation of iron for transport through the blood-brain barrier. *Mol. Neurobiol.* 53, 7237–7253. doi: 10.1007/s12035-015-9582-7

Cabantchik, Z. I., Munnich, A., Youdim, M. B., and Devos, D. (2013). Regional siderosis: a new challenge for iron chelation therapy. *Front. Pharmacol.* 4:167. doi: 10.3389/fphar.2013.00167

Campuzano, V., Montermini, L., Molt, M. D., Pianese, L., Cossée, M., Cavalcanti, F., et al. (1996). Friedreich's ataxia: autosomal recessive disease caused by an intronic GAA triplet repeat expansion. *Science* 271, 1423–1427. doi: 10.1126/science.271.5254.1423

Chen, L., Hambright, W. S., Na, R., and Ran, Q. (2015). Ablation of the ferroptosis inhibitor glutathione peroxidase 4 in neurons results in rapid motor neuron degeneration and paralysis. *J. Biol. Chem.* 290, 28097–28106. doi: 10.1074/jbc.M115.680090

Chen, Y. T., Chen, W. Y., Huang, X. T., Xu, Y. C., and Zhang, H. Y. (2018). Iron dysregulates APP processing accompanying with sAPPα cellular retention and β-secretase inhibition in rat cortical neurons. *Acta Pharmacol. Sin.* 39, 177–183. doi: 10.1038/aps.2017.113

Coffey, C. E., Alston, S., Heinz, E. R., and Burger, P. C. (1989). Brain iron in progressive supranuclear palsy: clinical, magnetic resonance imaging, and neuropathological findings. *J. Neuropsychiatry Clin. Neurosci.* 1, 400–404. doi: 10.1176/jnp.1.4.400

Colton, C. A., and Gilbert, D. L. (1987). Production of superoxide anions by a CNS macrophage, the microglia. *FEBS Lett.* 223, 284–288. doi: 10.1016/0014-5793(87)80305-8

Conde, J. R., and Streit, W. J. (2006). Microglia in the aging brain. *J. Neuropathol. Exp. Neurol.* 65, 199–203. doi: 10.1097/01.jnen.0000202887.22082.63

Connor, J. R., Menzies, S. L., St Martin, S. M., and Mufson, E. J. (1990). Cellular distribution of transferrin, ferritin, and iron in normal and aged human brains. *J. Neurosci. Res.* 27, 595–611. doi: 10.1002/jnr.490270421

Cuadrado, A., and Rojo, A. I. (2008). Heme oxygenase-1 as a therapeutic target in neurodegenerative diseases and brain infections. *Curr. Pharm. Des.* 14, 429–442. doi: 10.2174/138161208783597407

Dauer, W., and Przedborski, S. (2003). Parkinson's disease: mechanisms and models. *Neuron* 39, 889–909. doi: 10.1016/S0896-6273(03)00568-3

Davies, P., Moualla, D., and Brown, D. R. (2011). Alpha-synuclein is a cellular ferrireductase. *PLoS One* 6:e15814. doi: 10.1371/journal.pone.0015814

De Marzi, R., Seppi, K., Högl, B., Müller, C., Scherfler, C., Stefani, A., et al. (2016). Loss of dorsolateral nigral hyperintensity on 3.0 tesla susceptibility-weighted imaging in idiopathic rapid eye movement sleep behavior disorder. *Ann. Neurol.* 79, 1026–1030. doi: 10.1002/ana.24646

Devos, D., Moreau, C., Devedjian, J. C., Kluza, J., Petrault, M., Laloux, C., et al. (2014). Targeting chelatable iron as a therapeutic modality in Parkinson's disease. *Antioxid. Redox Signal.* 21, 195–210. doi: 10.1089/ars.2013.5593

Dexter, D. T., Wells, F. R., Lees, A. J., Agid, F., Agid, Y., Jenner, P., et al. (1989). Increased nigral iron content and alterations in other metal ions occurring in brain in Parkinson's disease. *J. Neurochem.* 52, 1830–1836. doi: 10.1111/j.1471-4159.1989.tb07264.x

Dhennin-Duthille, I., Masson, M., Damiens, E., Fillebeen, C., Spik, G., and Mazurier, J. (2000). Lactoferrin upregulates the expression of CD4 antigen through the stimulation of the mitogen-activated protein kinase in the human lymphoblastic T Jurkat cell line. *J. Cell. Biochem.* 79, 583–593. doi: 10.1002/1097-4644(20001215)79:4<583::AID-JCB70>3.0.CO;2-9

Di Paola, M., Phillips, O. R., Sanchez-Castaneda, C., Di Pardo, A., Maglione, V., Caltagirone, C., et al. (2014). MRI measures of corpus callosum iron and myelin in early Huntington's disease. *Hum. Brain Mapp.* 35, 3143–3151. doi: 10.1002/hbm.22391

Dickey, A. S., Pineda, V. V., Tsunemi, T., Liu, P. P., Miranda, H. C., Gilmore-Hall, S. K., et al. (2016). PPAR-δ is repressed in Huntington's disease, is required for normal neuronal function and can be targeted therapeutically. *Nat. Med.* 22, 37–45. doi: 10.1038/nm.4003

Dixit, R., Ross, J. L., Goldman, Y. E., and Holzbaur, E. L. (2008). Differential regulation of dynein and kinesin motor proteins by tau. *Science* 319, 1086–1089. doi: 10.1126/science.1152993

Dixon, S. J. (2017). Ferroptosis: bug or feature? *Immunol. Rev.* 277, 150–157. doi: 10.1111/imr.12533

Dixon, S. J., Lemberg, K. M., Lamprecht, M. R., Skouta, R., Zaitsev, E. M., Gleason, C. E., et al. (2012). Ferroptosis: an iron-dependent form of nonapoptotic cell death. *Cell* 149, 1060–1072. doi: 10.1016/j.cell.2012.03.042

Dowdle, W. E., Nyfeler, B., Nagel, J., Elling, R. A., Liu, S., Triantafellow, E., et al. (2014). Selective VPS34 inhibitor blocks autophagy and uncovers a role for NCOA4 in ferritin degradation and iron homeostasis in vivo. *Nat. Cell Biol.* 16, 1069–1079. doi: 10.1038/ncb3053

Duyn, J. H. (2010). Study of brain anatomy with high-field MRI: recent progress. *Magn. Reson. Imaging* 28, 1210–1215. doi: 10.1016/j.mri.2010.02.007

Engelen, M., Vanna, R., Bellei, C., Zucca, F. A., Wakamatsu, K., Monzani, E., et al. (2012). Neuromelanins of human brain have soluble and insoluble components with dolichols attached to the melanic structure. *PLoS One* 7:e48490. doi: 10.1371/journal.pone.0048490

Everett, J., Collingwood, J. F., Tjendana-Tjhin, V., Brooks, J., Lermyte, F., Plascencia-Villa, G., et al. (2018). Nanoscale synchrotron X-ray speciation of iron and calcium compounds in amyloid plaque cores from Alzheimer's disease subjects. *Nanoscale* 10, 11782–11796. doi: 10.1039/c7nr06794a

Farrall, A. J., and Wardlaw, J. M. (2009). Blood-brain barrier: ageing and microvascular disease–systematic review and meta-analysis. *Neurobiol. Aging* 30, 337–352. doi: 10.1016/j.neurobiolaging.2007.07.015

Faucheux, B. A., Herrero, M. T., Villares, J., Levy, R., Javoy-Agid, F., Obeso, J. A., et al. (1995). Autoradiographic localization and density of [125I]ferrotransferrin binding sites in the basal ganglia of control subjects, patients with Parkinson's disease and MPTP-lesioned monkeys. *Brain Res.* 691, 115–124. doi: 10.1016/0006-8993(95)00629-5

Faucheux, B. A., Martin, M. E., Beaumont, C., Hauw, J. J., Agid, Y., and Hirsch, E. C. (2003). Neuromelanin associated redox-active iron is increased in the substantia nigra of patients with Parkinson's disease. *J. Neurochem.* 86, 1142–1148. doi: 10.1046/j.1471-4159.2003.01923.x

Faux, N. G., Ritchie, C. W., Gunn, A., Rembach, A., Tsatsanis, A., Bedo, J., et al. (2010). PBT2 rapidly improves cognition in Alzheimer's disease: additional phase II analyses. *J. Alzheimers Dis.* 20, 509–516. doi: 10.3233/JAD-2010-1390

Fedorow, H., Tribl, F., Halliday, G., Gerlach, M., Riederer, P., and Double, K. L. (2005). Neuromelanin in human dopamine neurons: comparison with peripheral melanins and relevance to Parkinson's disease. *Prog. Neurobiol.* 75, 109–124. doi: 10.1016/j.pneurobio.2005.02.001

Fernández, B., Ferrer, I., Gil, F., and Hilfiker, S. (2017). Biomonitorization of iron accumulation in the substantia nigra from Lewy body disease patients. *Toxicol. Rep.* 4, 188–193. doi: 10.1016/j.toxrep.2017.03.005

Fillebeen, C., Mitchell, V., Dexter, D., Benaissa, M., Beauvillain, J., Spik, G., et al. (1999). Lactoferrin is synthesized by mouse brain tissue and its expression is enhanced after MPTP treatment. *Brain Res. Mol. Brain Res.* 72, 183–194. doi: 10.1016/S0169-328X(99)00221-1

Fillebeen, C., Ruchoux, M. M., Mitchell, V., Vincent, S., Benaïssa, M., and Pierce, A. (2001). Lactoferrin is synthesized by activated microglia in the human substantia nigra and its synthesis by the human microglial CHME cell line is upregulated by tumor necrosis factor alpha or 1-methyl-4-phenylpyridinium treatment. *Brain Res. Mol. Brain Res.* 96, 103–113. doi: 10.1016/S0169-328X(01)00216-9

Fleming, R. E., Migas, M. C., Holden, C. C., Waheed, A., Britton, R. S., Tomatsu, S., et al. (2000). Transferrin receptor 2: continued expression in mouse liver in the face of iron overload and in hereditary hemochromatosis. *Proc. Natl. Acad. Sci. U.S.A.* 97, 2214–2219. doi: 10.1073/pnas.040548097

Frey, A. G., Nandal, A., Park, J. H., Smith, P. M., Yabe, T., Ryu, M. S., et al. (2014). Iron chaperones PCBP1 and PCBP2 mediate the metallation of the dinuclear iron enzyme deoxyhypusine hydroxylase. *Proc. Natl. Acad. Sci. U.S.A.* 111, 8031–8036. doi: 10.1073/pnas.1402732111

Friedlich, A. L., Tanzi, R. E., and Rogers, J. T. (2007). The 5′-untranslated region of Parkinson's disease alpha-synuclein messenger RNA contains a predicted iron responsive element. *Mol. Psychiatry* 12, 222–223. doi: 10.1038/sj.mp.4001937

Friedman, A., Arosio, P., Finazzi, D., Koziorowski, D., and Galazka-Friedman, J. (2011). Ferritin as an important player in neurodegeneration. *Parkinsonism Relat. Disord.* 17, 423–430. doi: 10.1016/j.parkreldis.2011.03.016

Friedman, A., and Galazka-Friedman, J. (2012). The history of the research of iron in Parkinsonian substantia nigra. *J. Neural Transm.* 119, 1507–1510. doi: 10.1007/s00702-012-0894-8

Friedmann Angeli, J. P., Schneider, M., Proneth, B., Tyurina, Y. Y., Tyurin, V. A., Hammond, V. J., et al. (2014). Inactivation of the ferroptosis regulator Gpx4 triggers acute renal failure in mice. *Nat. Cell Biol.* 16, 1180–1191. doi: 10.1038/ncb3064

Fu, H., Hardy, J., and Duff, K. E. (2018). Selective vulnerability in neurodegenerative diseases. *Nat. Neurosci.* 21, 1350–1358. doi: 10.1038/s41593-018-0221-2

Galante, D., Cavallo, E., Perico, A., and D'Arrigo, C. (2018). Effect of ferric citrate on amyloid-beta peptides behavior. *Biopolymers* 109:e23224. doi: 10.1002/bip.23224

Galazka-Friedman, J., Bauminger, E. R., Szlachta, K., and Friedman, A. (2012). The role of iron in neurodegeneration–Mössbauer spectroscopy, electron microscopy, enzyme-linked immunosorbent assay and neuroimaging studies. *J. Phys. Condens. Matter* 24:244106. doi: 10.1088/0953-8984/24/24/244106

Gao, M., Monian, P., Pan, Q., Zhang, W., Xiang, J., and Jiang, X. (2016). Ferroptosis is an autophagic cell death process. *Cell Res.* 26, 1021–1032. doi: 10.1038/cr.2016.95

Good, P. F., Olanow, C. W., and Perl, D. P. (1992). Neuromelanin-containing neurons of the substantia nigra accumulate iron and aluminum in Parkinson's disease: a LAMMA study. *Brain Res.* 593, 343–346. doi: 10.1016/0006-8993(92)91334-B

Goodman, L. (1953). Alzheimer's disease; a clinico-pathologic analysis of twenty-three cases with a theory on pathogenesis. *J. Nerv. Ment. Dis.* 118, 97–130. doi: 10.1097/00005053-195308000-00001

Graeber, M. B., Streit, W. J., and Kreutzberg, G. W. (1988). Axotomy of the rat facial nerve leads to increased CR3 complement receptor expression by activated microglial cells. *J. Neurosci. Res.* 21, 18–24. doi: 10.1002/jnr.490210104

Guo, C., Wang, P., Zhong, M. L., Wang, T., Huang, X. S., Li, J. Y., et al. (2013). Deferoxamine inhibits iron induced hippocampal tau phosphorylation in the Alzheimer transgenic mouse brain. *Neurochem. Int.* 62, 165–172. doi: 10.1016/j.neuint.2012.12.005

Guo, C., Yang, Z. H., Zhang, S., Chai, R., Xue, H., Zhang, Y. H., et al. (2017). Intranasal lactoferrin enhances α-secretase-dependent amyloid precursor protein processing via the ERK1/2-CREB and HIF-1α pathways in an Alzheimer's disease mouse model. *Neuropsychopharmacology* 42, 2504–2515. doi: 10.1038/npp.2017.8

Hallgren, B., and Sourander, P. (1958). The effect of age on the non-haemin iron in the human brain. *J. Neurochem.* 3, 41–51. doi: 10.1111/j.1471-4159.1958.tb12607.x

Halliwell, B. (2006). Oxidative stress and neurodegeneration: where are we now? *J. Neurochem.* 97, 1634–1658. doi: 10.1111/j.1471-4159.2006.03907.x

Hambright, W. S., Fonseca, R. S., Chen, L., Na, R., and Ran, Q. (2017). Ablation of ferroptosis regulator glutathione peroxidase 4 in forebrain neurons promotes cognitive impairment and neurodegeneration. *Redox Biol.* 12, 8–17. doi: 10.1016/j.redox.2017.01.021

Hamilton, J. L., Ul-Haq, M. I., Creagh, A. L., Haynes, C. A., and Kizhakkedathu, J. N. (2017). Iron binding and iron removal efficiency of desferrioxamine based polymeric iron chelators: influence of molecular size and chelator density. *Macromol. Biosci.* 17:1600244. doi: 10.1002/mabi.201600244

Hare, D. J., Arora, M., Jenkins, N. L., Finkelstein, D. I., Doble, P. A., and Bush, A. I. (2015). Is early-life iron exposure critical in neurodegeneration? *Nat. Rev. Neurol.* 11, 536–544. doi: 10.1038/nrneurol.2015.100

Hare, D. J., Gerlach, M., and Riederer, P. (2012). Considerations for measuring iron in post-mortem tissue of Parkinson's disease patients. *J. Neural Transm.* 119, 1515–1521. doi: 10.1007/s00702-012-0898-4

Healy, S., McMahon, J., Owens, P., and FitzGerald, U. (2016). Significant glial alterations in response to iron loading in a novel organotypic hippocampal slice culture model. *Sci. Rep.* 6:36410. doi: 10.1038/srep36410

Hentze, M. W., Muckenthaler, M. U., and Andrews, N. C. (2004). Balancing acts: molecular control of mammalian iron metabolism. *Cell* 117, 285–297. doi: 10.1016/S0092-8674(04)00343-5

Hider, R. C., and Kong, X. L. (2011). Glutathione: a key component of the cytoplasmic labile iron pool. *Biometals* 24, 1179–1187. doi: 10.1007/s10534-011-9476-8

Hogarth, P. (2015). Neurodegeneration with brain iron accumulation: diagnosis and management. *J. Mov. Disord.* 8, 1–13. doi: 10.14802/jmd.14034

Horowitz, M. P., and Greenamyre, J. T. (2010). Mitochondrial iron metabolism and its role in neurodegeneration. *J. Alzheimers Dis.* 20(Suppl. 2), S551–S568. doi: 10.3233/JAD-2010-100354

Huang, J., Chen, S., Hu, L., Niu, H., Sun, Q., Li, W., et al. (2018). Mitoferrin-1 is involved in the progression of Alzheimer's disease through targeting mitochondrial iron metabolism in a *Caenorhabditis elegans* model of Alzheimer's disease. *Neuroscience* 385, 90–101. doi: 10.1016/j.neuroscience.2018.06.011

Hurley, S. D., Walter, S. A., Semple-Rowland, S. L., and Streit, W. J. (1999). Cytokine transcripts expressed by microglia in vitro are not expressed by ameboid microglia of the developing rat central nervous system. *Glia* 25, 304–309. doi: 10.1002/(SICI)1098-1136(19990201)25:3<304::AID-GLIA10>3.0.CO;2-W

Jarrett, J. T., and Lansbury, P. T. (1993). Seeding "one-dimensional crystallization" of amyloid: a pathogenic mechanism in Alzheimer's disease and scrapie? *Cell* 73, 1055–1058. doi: 10.1016/0092-8674(93)90635-4

Jellinger, K., Kienzl, E., Rumpelmair, G., Riederer, P., Stachelberger, H., Ben-Shachar, D., et al. (1992). Iron-melanin complex in substantia nigra of Parkinsonian brains: an x-ray microanalysis. *J. Neurochem.* 59, 1168–1171. doi: 10.1111/j.1471-4159.1992.tb08362.x

Jellinger, K., Paulus, W., Grundke-Iqbal, I., Riederer, P., and Youdim, M. B. (1990). Brain iron and ferritin in Parkinson's and Alzheimer's diseases. *J. Neural Transm. Park. Dis. Dement. Sect.* 2, 327–340. doi: 10.1007/BF02252926

Jenkitkasemwong, S., Wang, C. Y., Mackenzie, B., and Knutson, M. D. (2012). Physiologic implications of metal-ion transport by ZIP14 and ZIP8. *Biometals* 25, 643–655. doi: 10.1007/s10534-012-9526-x

Jenner, P., Schapira, A. H., and Marsden, C. D. (1992). New insights into the cause of Parkinson's disease. *Neurology* 42, 2241–2250. doi: 10.1212/WNL.42.12.2241

Kaindlstorfer, C., Jellinger, K. A., Eschlböck, S., Stefanova, N., Weiss, G., and Wenning, G. K. (2018). The relevance of iron in the pathogenesis of multiple system atrophy: a viewpoint. *J. Alzheimers Dis.* 61, 1253–1273. doi: 10.3233/JAD-170601

Kamalinia, G., Khodagholi, F., Atyabi, F., Amini, M., Shaerzadeh, F., Sharifzadeh, M., et al. (2013). Enhanced brain delivery of deferasirox-lactoferrin conjugates for iron chelation therapy in neurodegenerative disorders: in vitro and in vivo studies. *Mol. Pharm.* 10, 4418–4431. doi: 10.1021/mp4002014

Kaneko, Y., Kitamoto, T., Tateishi, J., and Yamaguchi, K. (1989). Ferritin immunohistochemistry as a marker for microglia. *Acta Neuropathol.* 79, 129–136. doi: 10.1007/BF00294369

Katsouri, L., Lim, Y. M., Blondrath, K., Eleftheriadou, I., Lombardero, L., Birch, A. M., et al. (2016). PPARγ-coactivator-1α gene transfer reduces neuronal loss and amyloid-β generation by reducing β-secretase in an Alzheimer's disease model. *Proc. Natl. Acad. Sci. U.S.A.* 113, 12292–12297. doi: 10.1073/pnas.1606171113

Kim, B. W., Jeong, K. H., Kim, J. H., Jin, M., Lee, M. G., Choi, D. K., et al. (2016). Pathogenic upregulation of glial lipocalin-2 in the Parkinsonian dopaminergic system. *J. Neurosci.* 36, 5608–5622. doi: 10.1523/JNEUROSCI.4261-15.2016

Koziorowski, D., Friedman, A., Arosio, P., Santambrogio, P., and Dziewulska, D. (2007). ELISA reveals a difference in the structure of substantia nigra ferritin in Parkinson's disease and incidental Lewy body compared to control. *Parkinsonism Relat. Disord.* 13, 214–218. doi: 10.1016/j.parkreldis.2006.10.002

Kress, G. J., Dineley, K. E., and Reynolds, I. J. (2002). The relationship between intracellular free iron and cell injury in cultured neurons, astrocytes, and oligodendrocytes. *J. Neurosci.* 22, 5848–5855. doi: 10.1523/JNEUROSCI.22-14-05848.2002

Kruszewski, M. (2003). Labile iron pool: the main determinant of cellular response to oxidative stress. *Mutat. Res.* 531, 81–92. doi: 10.1016/j.mrfmmm.2003.08.004

Kwan, J. Y., Jeong, S. Y., Van Gelderen, P., Deng, H. X., Quezado, M. M., Danielian, L. E., et al. (2012). Iron accumulation in deep cortical layers accounts for MRI signal abnormalities in ALS: correlating 7 tesla MRI and pathology. *PLoS One* 7:e35241. doi: 10.1371/journal.pone.0035241

Lane, D. J., and Lawen, A. (2008). Non-transferrin iron reduction and uptake are regulated by transmembrane ascorbate cycling in K562 cells. *J. Biol. Chem.* 283, 12701–12708. doi: 10.1074/jbc.M800713200

Lane, D. J., and Richardson, D. R. (2014). The active role of vitamin C in mammalian iron metabolism: much more than just enhanced iron absorption! *Free Radic. Biol. Med.* 75, 69–83. doi: 10.1016/j.freeradbiomed.2014.07.007

Lane, D. J., Robinson, S. R., Czerwinska, H., Bishop, G. M., and Lawen, A. (2010). Two routes of iron accumulation in astrocytes: ascorbate-dependent ferrous iron uptake via the divalent metal transporter (DMT1) plus an independent route for ferric iron. *Biochem. J.* 432, 123–132. doi: 10.1042/BJ20101317

Lane, D. J. R., Ayton, S., and Bush, A. I. (2018). Iron and Alzheimer's disease: an update on emerging mechanisms. *J. Alzheimers Dis.* 64, S379–S395. doi: 10.3233/JAD-179944

Lannfelt, L., Blennow, K., Zetterberg, H., Batsman, S., Ames, D., Harrison, J., et al. (2008). Safety, efficacy, and biomarker findings of PBT2 in targeting Abeta as a modifying therapy for Alzheimer's disease: a phase IIa, double-blind, randomised, placebo-controlled trial. *Lancet Neurol.* 7, 779–786. doi: 10.1016/S1474-4422(08)70167-4

Lee, S. H., Lyoo, C. H., Ahn, S. J., Rinne, J. O., and Lee, M. S. (2017). Brain regional iron contents in progressive supranuclear palsy. *Parkinsonism Relat. Disord.* 45, 28–32. doi: 10.1016/j.parkreldis.2017.09.020

Lei, P., Ayton, S., Finkelstein, D. I., Spoerri, L., Ciccotosto, G. D., Wright, D. K., et al. (2012). Tau deficiency induces parkinsonism with dementia by impairing APP-mediated iron export. *Nat. Med.* 18, 291–295. doi: 10.1038/nm.2613

Leidgens, S., Bullough, K. Z., Shi, H., Li, F., Shakoury-Elizeh, M., Yabe, T., et al. (2013). Each member of the poly-r(C)-binding protein 1 (PCBP) family exhibits iron chaperone activity toward ferritin. *J. Biol. Chem.* 288, 17791–17802. doi: 10.1074/jbc.M113.460253

Levin, J., Högen, T., Hillmer, A. S., Bader, B., Schmidt, F., Kamp, F., et al. (2011). Generation of ferric iron links oxidative stress to α-synuclein oligomer formation. *J. Parkinsons Dis.* 1, 205–216. doi: 10.3233/JPD-2011-11040

Liu, B., Moloney, A., Meehan, S., Morris, K., Thomas, S. E., Serpell, L. C., et al. (2011). Iron promotes the toxicity of amyloid beta peptide by impeding its ordered aggregation. *J. Biol. Chem.* 286, 4248–4256. doi: 10.1074/jbc.M110.158980

Loza-Rosas, S. A., Vázquez-Salgado, A. M., Rivero, K. I., Negrón, L. J., Delgado, Y., Benjam, J. A., et al. (2017). Expanding the therapeutic potential of the iron chelator deferasirox in the development of aqueous stable Ti(IV) anticancer complexes. *Inorg. Chem.* 56, 7788–7802. doi: 10.1021/acs.inorgchem.7b00542

Lu, Y., Prudent, M., Fauvet, B., Lashuel, H. A., and Girault, H. H. (2011). Phosphorylation of α-synuclein at Y125 and S129 alters its metal binding properties: implications for understanding the role of α-synuclein in the pathogenesis of Parkinson's disease and related disorders. *ACS Chem. Neurosci.* 2, 667–675. doi: 10.1021/cn200074d

Lull, M. E., and Block, M. L. (2010). Microglial activation and chronic neurodegeneration. *Neurotherapeutics* 7, 354–365. doi: 10.1016/j.nurt.2010.05.014

Maccecchini, M. L., Chang, M. Y., Pan, C., John, V., Zetterberg, H., and Greig, N. H. (2012). Posiphen as a candidate drug to lower CSF amyloid precursor protein, amyloid-β peptide and τ levels: target engagement, tolerability and pharmacokinetics in humans. *J. Neurol. Neurosurg. Psychiatry* 83, 894–902. doi: 10.1136/jnnp-2012-302589

Magnani, E., Fan, J., Gasparini, L., Golding, M., Williams, M., Schiavo, G., et al. (2007). Interaction of tau protein with the dynactin complex. *EMBO J.* 26, 4546–4554. doi: 10.1038/sj.emboj.7601878

Mancias, J. D., Wang, X., Gygi, S. P., Harper, J. W., and Kimmelman, A. C. (2014). Quantitative proteomics identifies NCOA4 as the cargo receptor mediating ferritinophagy. *Nature* 509, 105–109. doi: 10.1038/nature13148

Martin-Bastida, A., Ward, R. J., Newbould, R., Piccini, P., Sharp, D., Kabba, C., et al. (2017). Brain iron chelation by deferiprone in a phase 2 randomised double-blinded placebo controlled clinical trial in Parkinson's disease. *Sci. Rep.* 7:1398. doi: 10.1038/s41598-017-01402-2

Mastroberardino, P. G., Hoffman, E. K., Horowitz, M. P., Betarbet, R., Taylor, G., Cheng, D., et al. (2009). A novel transferrin/TfR2-mediated mitochondrial iron transport system is disrupted in Parkinson's disease. *Neurobiol. Dis.* 34, 417–431. doi: 10.1016/j.nbd.2009.02.009

Matak, P., Matak, A., Moustafa, S., Aryal, D. K., Benner, E. J., Wetsel, W., et al. (2016). Disrupted iron homeostasis causes dopaminergic neurodegeneration in mice. *Proc. Natl. Acad. Sci. U.S.A.* 113, 3428–3435. doi: 10.1073/pnas.1519473113

McCarthy, R. C., and Kosman, D. J. (2015). Mechanisms and regulation of iron trafficking across the capillary endothelial cells of the blood-brain barrier. *Front. Mol. Neurosci.* 8:31. doi: 10.3389/fnmol.2015.00031

McCarthy, R. C., Sosa, J. C., Gardeck, A. M., Baez, A. S., Lee, C. H., and Wessling-Resnick, M. (2018). Inflammation-induced iron transport and metabolism by brain microglia. *J. Biol. Chem.* 293, 7853–7863. doi: 10.1074/jbc.RA118.001949

Mehlhase, J., Sandig, G., Pantopoulos, K., and Grune, T. (2005). Oxidation-induced ferritin turnover in microglial cells: role of proteasome. *Free Radic. Biol. Med.* 38, 276–285. doi: 10.1016/j.freeradbiomed.2004.10.025

Mena, N. P., Urrutia, P. J., Lourido, F., Carrasco, C. M., and Núñez, M. T. (2015). Mitochondrial iron homeostasis and its dysfunctions in neurodegenerative disorders. *Mitochondrion* 21, 92–105. doi: 10.1016/j.mito.2015.02.001

Metz-Boutigue, M. H., Jollès, J., Mazurier, J., Schoentgen, F., Legrand, D., Spik, G., et al. (1984). Human lactotransferrin: amino acid sequence and structural comparisons with other transferrins. *Eur. J. Biochem.* 145, 659–676. doi: 10.1111/j.1432-1033.1984.tb08607.x

Mifuji, R., Kobayashi, Y., Ma, N., Qiang, Q. L., Urawa, N., Horiike, S., et al. (2006). Role of transferrin receptor 2 in hepatic accumulation of iron in patients with chronic hepatitis C. *J. Gastroenterol. Hepatol.* 21(1 Pt 1), 144–151. doi: 10.1111/j.1440-1746.2005.04151.x

Milanese, M., Giribaldi, F., Melone, M., Bonifacino, T., Musante, I., Carminati, E., et al. (2014). Knocking down metabotropic glutamate receptor 1 improves survival and disease progression in the SOD1(G93A) mouse model of amyotrophic lateral sclerosis. *Neurobiol. Dis.* 64, 48–59. doi: 10.1016/j.nbd.2013.11.006

Mirza, B., Hadberg, H., Thomsen, P., and Moos, T. (2000). The absence of reactive astrocytosis is indicative of a unique inflammatory process in Parkinson's disease. *Neuroscience* 95, 425–432. doi: 10.1016/S0306-4522(99)00455-8

Mohamed, W. A., Salama, R. M., and Schaalan, M. F. (2019). A pilot study on the effect of lactoferrin on Alzheimer's disease pathological sequelae: impact of the p-Akt/PTEN pathway. *Biomed. Pharmacother.* 111, 714–723. doi: 10.1016/j.biopha.2018.12.118

Moos, T., and Morgan, E. H. (2000). Transferrin and transferrin receptor function in brain barrier systems. *Cell. Mol. Neurobiol.* 20, 77–95. doi: 10.1023/A:1006948027674

Moos, T., and Morgan, E. H. (2004). The significance of the mutated divalent metal transporter (DMT1) on iron transport into the Belgrade rat brain. *J. Neurochem.* 88, 233–245. doi: 10.1046/j.1471-4159.2003.02142.x

Moos, T., Rosengren Nielsen, T., Skjørringe, T., and Morgan, E. H. (2007). Iron trafficking inside the brain. *J. Neurochem.* 103, 1730–1740. doi: 10.1111/j.1471-4159.2007.04976.x

Moreau, C., Danel, V., Devedjian, J. C., Grolez, G., Timmerman, K., Laloux, C., et al. (2018). Could conservative iron chelation lead to neuroprotection in amyotrophic lateral sclerosis? *Antioxid. Redox Signal.* 29, 742–748. doi: 10.1089/ars.2017.7493

Muller, M., and Leavitt, B. R. (2014). Iron dysregulation in Huntington's disease. *J. Neurochem.* 130, 328–350. doi: 10.1111/jnc.12739

Muñoz, P., Humeres, A., Elgueta, C., Kirkwood, A., Hidalgo, C., and Núñez, M. T. (2011). Iron mediates N-methyl-D-aspartate receptor-dependent stimulation of calcium-induced pathways and hippocampal synaptic plasticity. *J. Biol. Chem.* 286, 13382–13392. doi: 10.1074/jbc.M110.213785

Nakamura, T., and Lipton, S. A. (2011). Redox modulation by S-nitrosylation contributes to protein misfolding, mitochondrial dynamics, and neuronal synaptic damage in neurodegenerative diseases. *Cell Death Differ.* 18, 1478–1486. doi: 10.1038/cdd.2011.65

Navarro, J. A., Botella, J. A., Metzendorf, C., Lind, M. I., and Schneuwly, S. (2015). Mitoferrin modulates iron toxicity in a *Drosophila* model of Friedreich's ataxia. *Free Radic. Biol. Med.* 85, 71–82. doi: 10.1016/j.freeradbiomed.2015.03.014

Nitti, M., Piras, S., Brondolo, L., Marinari, U. M., Pronzato, M. A., and Furfaro, A. L. (2018). Heme oxygenase 1 in the nervous system: does it favor neuronal cell survival or induce neurodegeneration? *Int. J. Mol. Sci.* 19:E2260. doi: 10.3390/ijms19082260

Ohgami, R. S., Campagna, D. R., Greer, E. L., Antiochos, B., McDonald, A., Chen, J., et al. (2005). Identification of a ferrireductase required for efficient transferrin-dependent iron uptake in erythroid cells. *Nat. Genet.* 37, 1264–1269. doi: 10.1038/ng1658

Olmedo-Díaz, S., Estévez-Silva, H., Orädd, G., Af Bjerkén, S., Marcellino, D., and Virel, A. (2017). An altered blood-brain barrier contributes to brain iron accumulation and neuroinflammation in the 6-OHDA rat model of Parkinson's disease. *Neuroscience* 362, 141–151. doi: 10.1016/j.neuroscience.2017.08.023

Oshiro, S., Kawamura, K., Zhang, C., Sone, T., Morioka, M. S., Kobayashi, S., et al. (2008). Microglia and astroglia prevent oxidative stress-induced neuronal cell death: implications for aceruloplasminemia. *Biochim. Biophys. Acta* 1782, 109–117. doi: 10.1016/j.bbadis.2007.12.002

Ostrerova-Golts, N., Petrucelli, L., Hardy, J., Lee, J. M., Farer, M., and Wolozin, B. (2000). The A53T alpha-synuclein mutation increases iron-dependent aggregation and toxicity. *J. Neurosci.* 20, 6048–6054. doi: 10.1523/JNEUROSCI.20-16-06048.2000

Pallebage-Gamarallage, M., Foxley, S., Menke, R. A. L., Huszar, I. N., Jenkinson, M., Tendler, B. C., et al. (2018). Dissecting the pathobiology of altered MRI signal in amyotrophic lateral sclerosis: a post mortem whole brain sampling strategy for the integration of ultra-high-field MRI and quantitative neuropathology. *BMC Neurosci.* 19:11. doi: 10.1186/s12868-018-0416-1

Pantopoulos, K. (2004). Iron metabolism and the IRE/IRP regulatory system: an update. *Ann. N. Y. Acad. Sci.* 1012, 1–13. doi: 10.1196/annals.1306.001

Parihar, M. S., Kunz, E. A., and Brewer, G. J. (2008). Age-related decreases in NAD(P)H and glutathione cause redox declines before ATP loss during glutamate treatment of hippocampal neurons. *J. Neurosci. Res.* 86, 2339–2352. doi: 10.1002/jnr.21679

Patel, D., Xu, C., Nagarajan, S., Liu, Z., Hemphill, W. O., Shi, R., et al. (2018). Alpha-synuclein inhibits Snx3-retromer-mediated retrograde recycling of iron transporters in *S. cerevisiae* and *C. elegans* models of Parkinson's disease. *Hum. Mol. Genet.* 27, 1514–1532. doi: 10.1093/hmg/ddy059

Payton, S., Cahill, C. M., Randall, J. D., Gullans, S. R., and Rogers, J. T. (2003). Drug discovery targeted to the Alzheimer's APP mRNA 5′-untranslated region: the action of paroxetine and dimercaptopropanol. *J. Mol. Neurosci.* 20, 267–275. doi: 10.1385/JMN:20:3:267

Pelizzoni, I., Zacchetti, D., Campanella, A., Grohovaz, F., and Codazzi, F. (2013). Iron uptake in quiescent and inflammation-activated astrocytes: a potentially neuroprotective control of iron burden. *Biochim. Biophys. Acta* 1832, 1326–1333. doi: 10.1016/j.bbadis.2013.04.007

Peng, Y., Wang, C., Xu, H. H., Liu, Y. N., and Zhou, F. (2010). Binding of alpha-synuclein with Fe(III) and with Fe(II) and biological implications of the resultant complexes. *J. Inorg. Biochem.* 104, 365–370. doi: 10.1016/j.jinorgbio.2009.11.005

Peters, D. G., Pollack, A. N., Cheng, K. C., Sun, D., Saido, T., Haaf, M. P., et al. (2018). Dietary lipophilic iron alters amyloidogenesis and microglial morphology in Alzheimer's disease knock-in APP mice. *Metallomics* 10, 426–443. doi: 10.1039/c8mt00004b

Philpott, C. C. (2012). Coming into view: eukaryotic iron chaperones and intracellular iron delivery. *J. Biol. Chem.* 287, 13518–13523. doi: 10.1074/jbc.R111.326876

Plascencia-Villa, G., Ponce, A., Collingwood, J. F., Arellano-Jiménez, M. J., Zhu, X., Rogers, J. T., et al. (2016). High-resolution analytical imaging and electron holography of magnetite particles in amyloid cores of Alzheimer's disease. *Sci. Rep.* 6:24873. doi: 10.1038/srep24873

Plotegher, N., and Duchen, M. R. (2017). Crosstalk between lysosomes and mitochondria in Parkinson's disease. *Front. Cell. Dev. Biol.* 5:110. doi: 10.3389/fcell.2017.00110

Rathnasamy, G., Ling, E. A., and Kaur, C. (2013). Consequences of iron accumulation in microglia and its implications in neuropathological conditions. *CNS Neurol. Disord. Drug Targets* 12, 785–798. doi: 10.2174/18715273113126660169

Rathore, K. I., Redensek, A., and David, S. (2012). Iron homeostasis in astrocytes and microglia is differentially regulated by TNF-α and TGF-β1. *Glia* 60, 738–750. doi: 10.1002/glia.22303

Refolo, V., Bez, F., Polissidis, A., Kuzdas-Wood, D., Sturm, E., Kamaratou, M., et al. (2018). Progressive striatonigral degeneration in a transgenic mouse model of multiple system atrophy: translational implications for interventional therapies. *Acta Neuropathol. Commun.* 6:2. doi: 10.1186/s40478-017-0504-y

Ritchie, C. W., Bush, A. I., Mackinnon, A., Macfarlane, S., Mastwyk, M., MacGregor, L., et al. (2003). Metal-protein attenuation with iodochlorhydroxyquin (clioquinol) targeting Abeta amyloid deposition and toxicity in Alzheimer disease: a pilot phase 2 clinical trial. *Arch. Neurol.* 60, 1685–1691. doi: 10.1001/archneur.60.12.1685

Rival, T., Page, R. M., Chandraratna, D. S., Sendall, T. J., Ryder, E., Liu, B., et al. (2009). Fenton chemistry and oxidative stress mediate the toxicity of the beta-amyloid peptide in a *Drosophila* model of Alzheimer's disease. *Eur. J. Neurosci.* 29, 1335–1347. doi: 10.1111/j.1460-9568.2009.06701.x

Rogers, J. T., Bush, A. I., Cho, H. H., Smith, D. H., Thomson, A. M., Friedlich, A. L., et al. (2008). Iron and the translation of the amyloid precursor protein (APP) and ferritin mRNAs: riboregulation against neural oxidative damage in Alzheimer's disease. *Biochem. Soc. Trans.* 36(Pt 6), 1282–1287. doi: 10.1042/BST0361282

Rousseau, E., Michel, P. P., and Hirsch, E. C. (2013). The iron-binding protein lactoferrin protects vulnerable dopamine neurons from degeneration by preserving mitochondrial calcium homeostasis. *Mol. Pharmacol.* 84, 888–898. doi: 10.1124/mol.113.087965

Schipper, H. M. (2012). Neurodegeneration with brain iron accumulation - clinical syndromes and neuroimaging. *Biochim. Biophys. Acta* 1822, 350–360. doi: 10.1016/j.bbadis.2011.06.016

Schweser, F., Deistung, A., Lehr, B. W., and Reichenbach, J. R. (2011). Quantitative imaging of intrinsic magnetic tissue properties using MRI signal phase: an approach to in vivo brain iron metabolism? *Neuroimage* 54, 2789–2807. doi: 10.1016/j.neuroimage.2010.10.070

Seiler, A., Schneider, M., Förster, H., Roth, S., Wirth, E. K., Culmsee, C., et al. (2008). Glutathione peroxidase 4 senses and translates oxidative stress into 12/15-lipoxygenase dependent- and AIF-mediated cell death. *Cell Metab.* 8, 237–248. doi: 10.1016/j.cmet.2008.07.005

Sharifi, N., Hurt, E. M., Thomas, S. B., and Farrar, W. L. (2008). Effects of manganese superoxide dismutase silencing on androgen receptor function and gene regulation: implications for castration-resistant prostate cancer. *Clin. Cancer Res.* 14, 6073–6080. doi: 10.1158/1078-0432.CCR-08-0591

Shaw, K. T., Utsuki, T., Rogers, J., Yu, Q. S., Sambamurti, K., Brossi, A., et al. (2001). Phenserine regulates translation of beta -amyloid precursor protein mRNA by a putative interleukin-1 responsive element, a target for drug development. *Proc. Natl. Acad. Sci. U.S.A.* 98, 7605–7610. doi: 10.1073/pnas.131152998

Sheelakumari, R., Kesavadas, C., Varghese, T., Sreedharan, R. M., Thomas, B., Verghese, J., et al. (2017). Assessment of iron deposition in the brain in frontotemporal dementia and its correlation with behavioral traits. *AJNR Am. J. Neuroradiol.* 38, 1953–1958. doi: 10.3174/ajnr.A5339

Shokolenko, I., Venediktova, N., Bochkareva, A., Wilson, G. L., and Alexeyev, M. F. (2009). Oxidative stress induces degradation of mitochondrial DNA. *Nucleic Acids Res.* 37, 2539–2548. doi: 10.1093/nar/gkp100

Sian-Hülsmann, J., Mandel, S., Youdim, M. B., and Riederer, P. (2011). The relevance of iron in the pathogenesis of Parkinson's disease. *J. Neurochem.* 118, 939–957. doi: 10.1111/j.1471-4159.2010.07132.x

Silvestri, L., and Camaschella, C. (2008). A potential pathogenetic role of iron in Alzheimer's disease. *J. Cell. Mol. Med.* 12, 1548–1550. doi: 10.1111/j.1582-4934.2008.00356.x

Singh, N., Haldar, S., Tripathi, A. K., Horback, K., Wong, J., Sharma, D., et al. (2014). Brain iron homeostasis: from molecular mechanisms to clinical significance and therapeutic opportunities. *Antioxid. Redox Signal.* 20, 1324–1363. doi: 10.1089/ars.2012.4931

Spillantini, M. G., Schmidt, M. L., Lee, V. M., Trojanowski, J. Q., Jakes, R., and Goedert, M. (1997). Alpha-synuclein in Lewy bodies. *Nature* 388, 839–840. doi: 10.1038/42166

Stankiewicz, J. M., and Brass, S. D. (2009). Role of iron in neurotoxicity: a cause for concern in the elderly? *Curr. Opin. Clin. Nutr. Metab. Care* 12, 22–29. doi: 10.1097/MCO.0b013e32831ba07c

Stockwell, B. R., Friedmann Angeli, J. P., Bayir, H., Bush, A. I., Conrad, M., Dixon, S. J., et al. (2017). Ferroptosis: a regulated cell death nexus linking metabolism, redox biology, and disease. *Cell* 171, 273–285. doi: 10.1016/j.cell.2017.09.021

Tahirbegi, I. B., Pardo, W. A., Alvira, M., Mir, M., and Samitier, J. (2016). Amyloid Aβ 42, a promoter of magnetite nanoparticle formation in Alzheimer's disease. *Nanotechnology* 27:465102. doi: 10.1088/0957-4484/27/46/465102

Tahmasebinia, F., and Emadi, S. (2017). Effect of metal chelators on the aggregation of beta-amyloid peptides in the presence of copper and iron. *Biometals* 30, 285–293. doi: 10.1007/s10534-017-0005-2

Talpade, D. J., Greene, J. G., Higgins, D. S., and Greenamyre, J. T. (2000). In vivo labeling of mitochondrial complex I (NADH:ubiquinone oxidoreductase) in rat brain using [(3)H]dihydrorotenone. *J. Neurochem.* 75, 2611–2621. doi: 10.1046/j.1471-4159.2000.0752611.x

Teich, A. F., Sharma, E., Barnwell, E., Zhang, H., Staniszewski, A., Utsuki, T., et al. (2018). Translational inhibition of APP by Posiphen: efficacy, pharmacodynamics, and pharmacokinetics in the APP/PS1 mouse. *Alzheimers Dement.* 4, 37–45. doi: 10.1016/j.trci.2017.12.001

Telling, N. D., Everett, J., Collingwood, J. F., Dobson, J., van der Laan, G., Gallagher, J. J., et al. (2017). Iron biochemistry is correlated with amyloid plaque morphology in an established mouse model of Alzheimer's disease. *Cell Chem. Biol.* 24, 1205–1215.e3. doi: 10.1016/j.chembiol.2017.07.014

Thomsen, M. S., Andersen, M. V., Christoffersen, P. R., Jensen, M. D., Lichota, J., and Moos, T. (2015). Neurodegeneration with inflammation is accompanied by accumulation of iron and ferritin in microglia and neurons. *Neurobiol. Dis.* 81, 108–118. doi: 10.1016/j.nbd.2015.03.013

Todorich, B., Pasquini, J. M., Garcia, C. I., Paez, P. M., and Connor, J. R. (2009). Oligodendrocytes and myelination: the role of iron. *Glia* 57, 467–478. doi: 10.1002/glia.20784

Todorich, B., Zhang, X., Slagle-Webb, B., Seaman, W. E., and Connor, J. R. (2008). Tim-2 is the receptor for H-ferritin on oligodendrocytes. *J. Neurochem.* 107, 1495–1505. doi: 10.1111/j.1471-4159.2008.05678.x

Torti, F. M., and Torti, S. V. (2002). Regulation of ferritin genes and protein. *Blood* 99, 3505–3516. doi: 10.1182/blood.V99.10.3505

Tucker, S., Ahl, M., Cho, H. H., Bandyopadhyay, S., Cuny, G. D., Bush, A. I., et al. (2006). RNA therapeutics directed to the non coding regions of APP mRNA, in vivo anti-amyloid efficacy of paroxetine, erythromycin, and N-acetyl cysteine. *Curr. Alzheimer Res.* 3, 221–227. doi: 10.2174/156720506777632835

Urrutia, P., Aguirre, P., Esparza, A., Tapia, V., Mena, N. P., Arredondo, M., et al. (2013). Inflammation alters the expression of DMT1, FPN1 and hepcidin, and it causes iron accumulation in central nervous system cells. *J. Neurochem.* 126, 541–549. doi: 10.1111/jnc.12244

Urrutia, P. J., Mena, N. P., and Núñez, M. T. (2014). The interplay between iron accumulation, mitochondrial dysfunction, and inflammation during the execution step of neurodegenerative disorders. *Front. Pharmacol.* 5:38. doi: 10.3389/fphar.2014.00038

Ursini, F., and Bindoli, A. (1987). The role of selenium peroxidases in the protection against oxidative damage of membranes. *Chem. Phys. Lipids* 44, 255–276. doi: 10.1016/0009-3084(87)90053-3

van Bergen, J. M., Li, X., Hua, J., Schreiner, S. J., Steininger, S. C., Quevenco, F. C., et al. (2016). Colocalization of cerebral iron with amyloid beta in mild cognitive impairment. *Sci. Rep.* 6:35514. doi: 10.1038/srep35514 van de Looij, Y., Ginet, V., Chatagner, A., Toulotte, A., Somm, E., Hüppi, P. S., et al. (2014). Lactoferrin during lactation protects the immature hypoxic-ischemic rat brain. *Ann. Clin. Transl. Neurol.* 1, 955–967. doi: 10.1002/acn3.138

Vela, D. (2018). The dual role of hepcidin in brain iron load and inflammation. *Front. Neurosci.* 12:740. doi: 10.3389/fnins.2018.00740

Waller, R., Murphy, M., Garwood, C. J., Jennings, L., Heath, P. R., Chambers, A., et al. (2018). Metallothionein-I/II expression associates with the astrocyte DNA damage response and not Alzheimer-type pathology in the aging brain. *Glia* 66, 2316–2323. doi: 10.1002/glia.23465

Wang, J., Bi, M., Liu, H., Song, N., and Xie, J. (2015). The protective effect of lactoferrin on ventral mesencephalon neurons against MPP + is not connected with its iron binding ability. *Sci. Rep.* 5:10729. doi: 10.1038/srep10729

Wang, J., Jiang, H., and Xie, J. X. (2007). Ferroportin1 and hephaestin are involved in the nigral iron accumulation of 6-OHDA-lesioned rats. *Eur. J. Neurosci.* 25, 2766–2772. doi: 10.1111/j.1460-9568.2007.05515.x

Wang, J., and Pantopoulos, K. (2011). Regulation of cellular iron metabolism. *Biochem. J.* 434, 365–381. doi: 10.1042/BJ20101825

Wang, J., Song, N., Jiang, H., and Xie, J. (2013). Pro-inflammatory cytokines modulate iron regulatory protein 1 expression and iron transportation through reactive oxygen/nitrogen species production in ventral mesencephalic neurons. *Biochim. Biophys. Acta* 1832, 618–625. doi: 10.1016/j.bbadis.2013.01.021

Wang, J. Y., Zhuang, Q. Q., Zhu, L. B., Zhu, H., Li, T., Li, R., et al. (2016). Meta-analysis of brain iron levels of Parkinson's disease patients determined by postmortem and MRI measurements. *Sci. Rep.* 6:36669. doi: 10.1038/srep36669

Wang, L., Sato, H., Zhao, S., and Tooyama, I. (2010). Deposition of lactoferrin in fibrillar-type senile plaques in the brains of transgenic mouse models of Alzheimer's disease. *Neurosci. Lett.* 481, 164–167. doi: 10.1016/j.neulet.2010.06.079

Ward, R. J., Zucca, F. A., Duyn, J. H., Crichton, R. R., and Zecca, L. (2014). The role of iron in brain ageing and neurodegenerative disorders. *Lancet Neurol.* 13, 1045–1060. doi: 10.1016/S1474-4422(14)70117-6

Williams, R., Buchheit, C. L., Berman, N. E., and LeVine, S. M. (2012). Pathogenic implications of iron accumulation in multiple sclerosis. *J. Neurochem.* 120, 7–25. doi: 10.1111/j.1471-4159.2011.07536.x

Wong, B. X., Tsatsanis, A., Lim, L. Q., Adlard, P. A., Bush, A. I., and Duce, J. A. (2014). β-Amyloid precursor protein does not possess ferroxidase activity but does stabilize the cell surface ferrous iron exporter ferroportin. *PLoS One* 9:e114174. doi: 10.1371/journal.pone.0114174

Xie, L., Zheng, W., Xin, N., Xie, J. W., Wang, T., and Wang, Z. Y. (2012). Ebselen inhibits iron-induced tau phosphorylation by attenuating DMT1 up-regulation and cellular iron uptake. *Neurochem. Int.* 61, 334–340. doi: 10.1016/j.neuint.2012.05.016

Xie, Y., Hou, W., Song, X., Yu, Y., Huang, J., Sun, X., et al. (2016). Ferroptosis: process and function. *Cell Death Differ.* 23, 369–379. doi: 10.1038/cdd.2015.158

Xu, J., Jia, Z., Knutson, M. D., and Leeuwenburgh, C. (2012). Impaired iron status in aging research. *Int. J. Mol. Sci.* 13, 2368–2386. doi: 10.3390/ijms13022368

Xu, J., and Ling, E. A. (1994). Studies of the ultrastructure and permeability of the blood-brain barrier in the developing corpus callosum in postnatal rat brain using electron dense tracers. *J. Anat.* 184(Pt 2), 227–237.

Xu, S. F., Zhang, Y. H., Wang, S., Pang, Z. Q., Fan, Y. G., Li, J. Y., et al. (2018). Lactoferrin ameliorates dopaminergic neurodegeneration and motor deficits in MPTP-treated mice. *Redox Biol.* 21:101090. doi: 10.1016/j.redox.2018.101090

Xu, X., Song, N., Wang, R., Jiang, H., and Xie, J. (2016). Preferential heme oxygenase-1 activation in striatal astrocytes antagonizes dopaminergic neuron degeneration in MPTP-intoxicated mice. *Mol. Neurobiol.* 53, 5056–5065. doi: 10.1007/s12035-015-9437-2

Yanatori, I., Yasui, Y., Tabuchi, M., and Kishi, F. (2014). Chaperone protein involved in transmembrane transport of iron. *Biochem. J.* 462, 25–37. doi: 10.1042/BJ20140225

Yang, F., Liu, X. B., Quinones, M., Melby, P. C., Ghio, A., and Haile, D. J. (2002). Regulation of reticuloendothelial iron transporter MTP1 (Slc11a3) by inflammation. *J. Biol. Chem.* 277, 39786–39791. doi: 10.1074/jbc.M201485200

Yang, W. S., SriRamaratnam, R., Welsch, M. E., Shimada, K., Skouta, R., Viswanathan, V. S., et al. (2014). Regulation of ferroptotic cancer cell death by GPX4. *Cell* 156, 317–331. doi: 10.1016/j.cell.2013.12.010

Yu, Q. S., Reale, M., Kamal, M. A., Holloway, H. W., Luo, W., Sambamurti, K., et al. (2013). Synthesis of the Alzheimer drug Posiphen into its primary metabolic products (+)-N1-norPosiphen, (+)-N8-norPosiphen and (+)-N1, N8-bisnorPosiphen, their inhibition of amyloid precursor protein, α-Synuclein synthesis, interleukin-1β release, and cholinergic action. *Antiinflamm. Antiallergy Agents Med. Chem.* 12, 117–128. doi: 10.2174/1871523011312020003

Yu, X., Song, N., Guo, X., Jiang, H., Zhang, H., and Xie, J. (2016). Differences in vulnerability of neurons and astrocytes to heme oxygenase-1 modulation: implications for mitochondrial ferritin. *Sci. Rep.* 6:24200. doi: 10.1038/srep24200

Zecca, L., Bellei, C., Costi, P., Albertini, A., Monzani, E., Casella, L., et al. (2008). New melanic pigments in the human brain that accumulate in aging and block environmental toxic metals. *Proc. Natl. Acad. Sci. U.S.A.* 105, 17567–17572. doi: 10.1073/pnas.0808768105

Zecca, L., Gallorini, M., Schünemann, V., Trautwein, A. X., Gerlach, M., Riederer, P., et al. (2001). Iron, neuromelanin and ferritin content in the substantia nigra of normal subjects at different ages: consequences for iron storage and neurodegenerative processes. *J. Neurochem.* 76, 1766–1773. doi: 10.1046/j.1471-4159.2001.00186.x

Zecca, L., Stroppolo, A., Gatti, A., Tampellini, D., Toscani, M., Gallorini, M., et al. (2004). The role of iron and copper molecules in the neuronal vulnerability of locus coeruleus and substantia nigra during aging. *Proc. Natl. Acad. Sci. U.S.A.* 101, 9843–9848. doi: 10.1073/pnas.0403495101

Zhang, D. L., Ghosh, M. C., and Rouault, T. A. (2014). The physiological functions of iron regulatory proteins in iron homeostasis - an update. *Front. Pharmacol.* 5:124. doi: 10.3389/fphar.2014.00124

Zhang, H. Y., Song, N., Jiang, H., Bi, M. X., and Xie, J. X. (2014). Brain-derived neurotrophic factor and glial cell line-derived neurotrophic factor inhibit ferrous iron influx via divalent metal transporter 1 and iron regulatory protein 1 regulation in ventral mesencephalic neurons. *Biochim. Biophys. Acta* 1843, 2967–2975. doi: 10.1016/j.bbamcr.2014.09.010

Zhang, W., Yan, Z. F., Gao, J. H., Sun, L., Huang, X. Y., Liu, Z., et al. (2014). Role and mechanism of microglial activation in iron-induced selective and progressive dopaminergic neurodegeneration. *Mol. Neurobiol.* 49, 1153–1165. doi: 10.1007/s12035-013-8586-4

Zhang, W., Zecca, L., Wilson, B., Ren, H. W., Wang, Y. J., Wang, X. M., et al. (2013). Human neuromelanin: an endogenous microglial activator for dopaminergic neuron death. *Front. Biosci.* 5, 1–11. doi: 10.2741/E591

Zhang, Y. H., Raymick, J., Sarkar, S., Lahiri, D. K., Ray, B., Holtzman, D., et al. (2013). Efficacy and toxicity of clioquinol treatment and A-beta 42 inoculation in the APP/PSI mouse model of Alzheimer's disease. *Curr. Alzheimer Res.* 10, 494–506. doi: 10.2174/1567205011310050005

Zhou, B., Westaway, S. K., Levinson, B., Johnson, M. A., Gitschier, J., and Hayflick, S. J. (2001). A novel pantothenate kinase gene (PANK2) is defective in Hallervorden-Spatz syndrome. *Nat. Genet.* 28, 345–349. doi: 10.1038/ng572

Zhou, Z. D., and Tan, E. K. (2017). Iron regulatory protein (IRP)-iron responsive element (IRE) signaling pathway in human neurodegenerative diseases. *Mol. Neurodegener.* 12:75. doi: 10.1186/s13024-017-0218-4

Zucca, F. A., Segura-Aguilar, J., Ferrari, E., Muñoz, P., Paris, I., Sulzer, D., et al. (2017). Interactions of iron, dopamine and neuromelanin pathways in brain aging and Parkinson's disease. *Prog. Neurobiol.* 155, 96–119. doi: 10.1016/j.pneurobio.2015.09.012

Zucca, F. A., Vanna, R., Cupaioli, F. A., Bellei, C., De Palma, A., Di Silvestre, D., et al. (2018). Neuromelanin organelles are specialized autolysosomes that accumulate undegraded proteins and lipids in aging human brain and are likely involved in Parkinson's disease. *NPJ Parkinsons Dis.* 4:17. doi: 10.1038/s41531-018-0050-8

Permissions

All chapters in this book were first published by Frontiers; hereby published with permission under the Creative Commons Attribution License or equivalent. Every chapter published in this book has been scrutinized by our experts. Their significance has been extensively debated. The topics covered herein carry significant findings which will fuel the growth of the discipline. They may even be implemented as practical applications or may be referred to as a beginning point for another development.

The contributors of this book come from diverse backgrounds, making this book a truly international effort. This book will bring forth new frontiers with its revolutionizing research information and detailed analysis of the nascent developments around the world.

We would like to thank all the contributing authors for lending their expertise to make the book truly unique. They have played a crucial role in the development of this book. Without their invaluable contributions this book wouldn't have been possible. They have made vital efforts to compile up to date information on the varied aspects of this subject to make this book a valuable addition to the collection of many professionals and students.

This book was conceptualized with the vision of imparting up-to-date information and advanced data in this field. To ensure the same, a matchless editorial board was set up. Every individual on the board went through rigorous rounds of assessment to prove their worth. After which they invested a large part of their time researching and compiling the most relevant data for our readers.

The editorial board has been involved in producing this book since its inception. They have spent rigorous hours researching and exploring the diverse topics which have resulted in the successful publishing of this book. They have passed on their knowledge of decades through this book. To expedite this challenging task, the publisher supported the team at every step. A small team of assistant editors was also appointed to further simplify the editing procedure and attain best results for the readers.

Apart from the editorial board, the designing team has also invested a significant amount of their time in understanding the subject and creating the most relevant covers. They scrutinized every image to scout for the most suitable representation of the subject and create an appropriate cover for the book.

The publishing team has been an ardent support to the editorial, designing and production team. Their endless efforts to recruit the best for this project, has resulted in the accomplishment of this book. They are a veteran in the field of academics and their pool of knowledge is as vast as their experience in printing. Their expertise and guidance has proved useful at every step. Their uncompromising quality standards have made this book an exceptional effort. Their encouragement from time to time has been an inspiration for everyone.

The publisher and the editorial board hope that this book will prove to be a valuable piece of knowledge for researchers, students, practitioners and scholars across the globe.

List of Contributors

Yingying Sun, A. Ninh Pham and T. David Waite
Water Research Centre, School of Civil and Environmental Engineering, The University of New South Wales, Sydney, NSW, Australia

Dominic J. Hare
Atomic Pathology Laboratory, Melbourne Dementia Research Centre at the Florey Institute of Neuroscience and Mental Health and The University of Melbourne, Parkville, VIC, Australia
Department of Clinical Pathology, The University of Melbourne, Parkville, VIC, Australia

Maria Daglas and Paul A. Adlard
The Florey Institute of Neuroscience and Mental Health, The University of Melbourne, Parkville, VIC, Australia

Ilaria Simonelli and Patrizio Pasqualetti
Service of Medical Statistics and Information Technology, Fatebenefratelli Foundation for Health Research and Education, AFaR Division, Rome, Italy

Mariacristina Siotto
IRCCS Fondazione Don Carlo Gnocchi, Milan, Italy

Maria Maddalena Filippi and Mariacarla Ventriglia
Fatebenefratelli Foundation for Health Research and Education, AFaR Division, Rome, Italy

Doriana Landi
Multiple Sclerosis Clinical and Research Unit, Department of Systems Medicine, Tor Vergata University, Rome, Italy

Anna Ghazaryan
Fatebenefratelli Foundation for Health Research and Education, AFaR Division, Rome, Italy
Neurology Unit, Campus Bio-Medico University of Rome, Rome, Italy

Stefano Vollaro and Fabrizio Vernieri
Neurology Unit, Campus Bio-Medico University of Rome, Rome, Italy

Mauro Ciro Antonio Rongioletti
Department of Laboratory Medicine, Research and Development Division, "San Giovanni Calibita", Fatebenefratelli Hospital, Rome, Italy

Rosanna Squitti
IRCCS Istituto Centro San Giovanni di Dio Fatebenefratelli, Brescia, Italy

José Vicente Llorens and Pablo Calap-Quintana
Department of Genetics, Faculty of Biological Sciences, University of Valencia, Valencia, Spain
Unit for Psychiatry and Neurodegenerative Diseases, Biomedical Research Institute INCLIVA, Valencia, Spain

Sirena Soriano
Department of Molecular and Human Genetics, Baylor College of Medicine, Houston, TX, United States
Jan and Dan Duncan Neurological Research Institute, Texas Children's Hospital, Houston, TX, United States

Pilar Gonzalez-Cabo
Department of Physiology, Faculty of Medicine and Dentistry, University of Valencia, Valencia, Spain
Center of Biomedical Network Research on Raren Diseases CIBERER, Valencia, Spain
Associated Unit for Rare Diseases INCLIVA-CIPF, Biomedical Research Institute INCLIVA, Valencia, Spain

María Dolores Moltó
Department of Genetics, Faculty of Biological Sciences, University of Valencia, Valencia, Spain
Unit for Psychiatry and Neurodegenerative Diseases, Biomedical Research Institute INCLIVA, Valencia, Spain
Center of Biomedical Network Research on Mental Health CIBERSAM, Valencia, Spain

Karina Joppe, Anna-Elisa Roser and Fabian Maass
Department of Neurology, University Medical Center Göttingen, Göttingen, Germany

Paul Lingor
Department of Neurology, University Medical Center-Göttingen, Göttingen, Germany
Center for Biostructural Imaging of Neurodegeneration,Göttingen, Germany
German Center for Neurodegenerative Diseases, Göttingen, Germany
Rechts der Isar Hospital, Technical University of Munich, Munich, Germany

Marco Tulio Núñez
Iron and Neuroregeneration Laboratory, Department of Biology, Faculty of Sciences, Universidad de Chile, Santiago, Chile

Cecilia Hidalgo
Calcium Signaling Laboratory, Biomedical Research Institute, CEMC, Physiology and Biophysics Program, Institute of Biomedical Sciences, Faculty of Medicine, Universidad de Chile, Santiago, Chile
Department of Neuroscience, Faculty of Medicine, Universidad de Chile, Santiago, Chile

Driton Vela
Department of Physiology, Faculty of Medicine, University of Pristina, Pristina, Kosovo

Camille Petillon
Laboratoire de Biochimie, CHRU de Tours, Tours, France

Rudolf Hergesheimer
INSERM, U1253, Université de Tours, Tours, France

Hervé Puy and Zoubida Karim
Centre de Recherches sur l'Inflammation, Equipe "Hème, Fer et Maladies Inflammatoires", UMR 1149/ ERL CNRS 8252, Université Paris Diderot Paris 7, UFR de Médecine Site Bichat, Paris, France

Philippe Corcia
INSERM, U1253, Université de Tours, Tours, France
Centre SLA, Service de Neurologie, CHRU de Tours, Tours, France

Patrick Vourc'h, Christian Andres and Hélène Blasco
Laboratoire de Biochimie, CHRU de Tours, Tours, France
INSERM, U1253, Université de Tours, Tours, France

Deborah Chiabrando, Veronica Fiorito, Sara Petrillo and Emanuela Tolosano
Molecular Biotechnology Center, Department of Molecular Biotechnology and Health Sciences, University of Torino, Turin, Italy

Sinead Healy, Jill McMahon and Una FitzGerald
Galway Neuroscience Centre, School of Natural Sciences, National University of Ireland Galway, Galway, Ireland

Qian Jiao, Xixun Du, Jie Wei, Yong Li and Hong Jiang
Department of Physiology, Shandong Provincial Key Laboratory of Pathogenesis and Prevention of Neurological Disorders and State Key Disciplines: Physiology, School of Basic Medicine, Qingdao University, Qingdao, China

Lirong Jin, Changpeng Wang, Zhen Huang, Xiaoqin Cheng, Guoqiang Fei and Chunjiu Zhong
Department of Neurology, Zhongshan Hospital, Fudan University, Shanghai, China

Jian Wang, Kai Liu and Mengsu Zeng
Department of Radiology, Zhongshan Hospital, Fudan University, Shanghai, China
Shanghai Medical Imaging Institute, Shanghai, China

Danlan Lian
Department of Radiology, Xiamen Branch, Zhongshan Hospital, Fudan University, Xiamen, China

Ying Zhou and Yuanfang Li
Department of Neurology, Xiamen Branch, Zhongshan Hospital, Fudan University, Xiamen, China

Yong Zhang
MR Research, GE Healthcare, Shanghai, China

Minzhi Lv
Department of Biostatistics, Zhongshan Hospital, Fudan University, Shanghai, China

Núria DeGregorio-Rocasolano and Teresa Gasull
Cellular and Molecular Neurobiology Research Group, Department of Neurosciences, Germans Trias i Pujol Research Institute (IGTP), Badalona, Spain

Octavi Martí-Sistac
Cellular and Molecular Neurobiology Research Group, Department of Neurosciences, Germans Trias i Pujol Research Institute (IGTP), Badalona, Spain
Department of Cellular Biology, Physiology and Immunology, Universitat Autònoma de Barcelona, Bellaterra, Spain

Fari Ryan, Juan G. Zarruk, Lena Lößlein and Samuel David
Centre for Research in Neuroscience, The Research Institute of the McGill University Health Centre, Montreal, QC, Canada

Jae-Hyeok Lee
Department of Neurology, Research Institute for Convergence of Biomedical Science and Technology, Pusan National University Yangsan Hospital, Pusan National University School of Medicine, Yangsan, South Korea

Myung-Sik Lee
Department of Neurology, Gangnam Severance Hospital, Yonsei University College of Medicine, Seoul, South Korea

Jun-Lin Liu, Yong-Gang Fan and Chuang Guo
College of Life and Health Sciences, Northeastern University, Shenyang, China

Zheng-Sheng Yang
Department of Dermatology, First Hospital of Qinhuangdao, Qinhuangdao, China

Zhan-You Wang
College of Life and Health Sciences, Northeastern University, Shenyang, China Key Laboratory of Medical Cell Biology of Ministry of Education, Institute of Health Sciences, China Medical University, Shenyang, China

Lesha Pretorius and Etheresia Pretorius
Department of Physiological Sciences, Stellenbosch University, Stellenbosch, South Africa School of Chemistry, The University of Manchester, Manchester, United Kingdom

Douglas B. Kell
School of Chemistry, The University of Manchester, Manchester, United Kingdom The Manchester Institute of Biotechnology, The University of Manchester, Manchester, United Kingdom

Alain Ndayisaba, Christine Kaindlstorfer and Gregor K. Wenning
Department of Neurology, Medical University of Innsbruck, Innsbruck, Austria

Index

www.ingramcontent.com/pod-product-compliance
Lightning Source LLC
LaVergne TN
LVHW082151200926
848484LV00008B/2138